AUDITORY-VERBAL THERAPY

Science, Research, and Practice

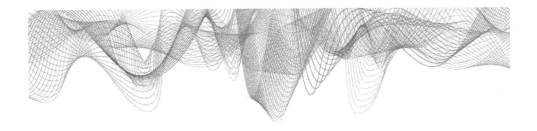

AUDITORY-VERBAL THERAPY

Science, Research, and Practice

Warren Estabrooks,
MEd, Dip Ed Deaf, LSLS Cert. AVT

Helen McCaffrey Morrison,
PhD, CCC/A (Retired), LSLS Cert. AVT

Karen MacIver-Lux,
MA, Aud(C), Reg CASLPO, LSLS Cert. AVT

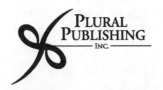

PLURAL
PUBLISHING
INC.

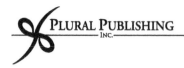

5521 Ruffin Road
San Diego, CA 92123

e-mail: information@pluralpublishing.com
Website: https://www.pluralpublishing.com

Typeset in 10½/13 ITC Garamond by Achorn International
Printed in the United States of America by Integrated Books International

24 23 22 21   2 3 4 5

For permission to use material from this text, contact us by
Telephone: (866) 758-7251
Fax: (888) 758-7255
e-mail: permissions@pluralpublishing.com

Every attempt has been made to contact the copyright holders for material originally printed in another source. If any have been inadvertently overlooked, the publisher will gladly make the necessary arrangements at the first opportunity.

Library of Congress Cataloging-in-Publication Data:
Names: Estabrooks, Warren, editor. | Morrison, Helen McCaffrey, editor. | MacIver-Lux, Karen, editor.
Title: Auditory-verbal therapy : science, research, and practice / [edited by] Warren Estabrooks, Helen McCaffrey Morrison, Karen MacIver-Lux.
Description: San Diego, CA : Plural, [2020] | Includes bibliographical references and index.
Identifiers: LCCN 2020001920 | ISBN 9781635501742 (hardcover) | ISBN 9781635501858 (ebook)
Subjects: MESH: Hearing Loss—rehabilitation | Child | Auditory Perception | Language Therapy—methods | Speech Therapy—methods | Evidence-Based Practice—methods | Infant
Classification: LCC RF290 | NLM WV 271 | DDC 617.8—dc23
LC record available at https://lccn.loc.gov/2020001920

CONTENTS

Part I. Auditory-Verbal Therapy: Foundations and Fundamentals

Part II. Audiology, Hearing Technologies, Speech Acoustics, and Auditory-Verbal Therapy

PREFACE

As one of the editors of *Auditory-Verbal Therapy for Young Children with Hearing Loss and Their Families, and the Practitioners Who Guide Them* (Plural Publishing, 2016), I was fortunate to be part of a global writing team that brought the most current knowledge about Auditory-Verbal Therapy (AVT) to practitioners and parents around the world. In subsequent years, much has changed. The world of science and research and the evolving practice trends in AVT continue to transform the dreams of parents of children who are deaf or hard of hearing into reality, wherever AVT is found. In lieu of a second edition, the concept of a new book about AVT was proposed primarily for the professional community that continually contributes to the worldwide interest in AVT, but also for those anywhere wanting to know more about the exciting progress that drives this evidence-based and evidence-informed intervention for young children who are deaf or hard of hearing and their families.

In a survey of the Listening and Spoken Language Specialist, Certified Auditory-Verbal Therapist (LSLS Cert. AVT) global community, members were asked what they wanted in this new publication. The editors listened, and subsequently for more than two years, *Auditory-Verbal Therapy: Science, Research, and Practice* was planned, developed, and reviewed to offer the reader a blend of some updates on the book of 2016, along with many additional chapters considered highly relevant.

The inspirational work of the pioneers of AVT is woven like a tapestry throughout the pages of this book in which an international cohort of subject matter experts shares the prevailing science, research, and practice of many interrelated disciplines with Auditory-Verbal practitioners, aspiring Auditory-Verbal practitioners, teachers, special educators, audiologists, speech-language pathologists, psychologists, physicians, surgeons, administrators, students, and parents.

In AVT, parents are respected as the child's first and primary models, most enduring teachers, and most significant agents of change. The partnerships and alliances developed and nurtured by parents throughout their Auditory-Verbal journeys are built on a foundation of shared knowledge, kindness, compassion, respect, gratitude, trust, and mutual commitment. Through professional coaching and guidance, parents who choose AVT become engaged with the practitioners in ways that help them realize the outcomes they greatly desire. *Auditory-Verbal Therapy: Science, Research, and Practice* demonstrates how these partnerships help to integrate listening, spoken language, and cognitive and social development into the daily lives of their children.

The authors here advocate that all children who are deaf or hard of hearing deserve the opportunity to acquire spoken language if that is the desired outcome of their parents. For this to happen, a purposeful plan needs to be developed, implemented, adjusted, readjusted, and evaluated throughout the family's lifelong journey.

In 2018, the World Health Organization (WHO) estimated the number of people with hearing loss "to be 466 million persons (6.1% of the world's population), and that 34 million (7%) of these were children (aged 1 to 15 years)." Alarmingly, 60% of children under 15 years of age have hearing loss due to preventable causes; this figure is higher in developing countries (75%) compared with more developed countries (49%). Despite the fact that most children who are deaf or hard of hearing can benefit from hearing technology and early intervention services, global availability of these remains scarce and inequitable. Production of hearing devices meets less than 10% of the global need, and less than 3% of the need in developing countries; intervention and schooling for children who are deaf or hard of hearing in the latter is sadly lacking. WHO estimates that unaddressed hearing loss poses an annual global cost of US$750 billion and predicts that unless action is taken, the projected number of people who are deaf or hard of hearing will grow to 630 million (44.1 million children) by 2030 and may be over 900 million (63 million children) by 2050. The mission of this book is to embrace the future with today's *science, research, and practice,* by encouraging local, national, and global partnerships to bring the outcomes of listening and spoken language to children who are deaf or hard of hearing as effectively and efficiently as possible, wherever they live. The vision is that all barriers to equitable services for young children who are deaf or hard of hearing and their families will disappear. We are all in this together and we have much to do.

"Auditory-Verbal Therapy (AVT) continues to develop along with advances in newborn hearing screening, innovative hearing technologies, creative systems of family-centered intervention, the enhancement of professional preparation for the highly valued Listening and Spoken Language Certified Auditory-Verbal Therapist (LSLS Cert. AVT®) credential, continuous professional improvement, and the prevalence of evidence-based and evidence informed practices. Auditory-Verbal Therapy is accepted and promoted in many parts of the world by researchers, scientists, and practitioners and by parents of children with hearing loss, all who have the same desired outcomes: efficient listening skills; intelligible spoken language; age-appropriate conversational competence equivalent to peers with typical hearing; achievement of promising levels of academic performance; an extensive range of careers and employment opportunities; and greater social and personal interactions within their communities and their cultures." (Estabrooks, 2016)

On behalf of everyone involved in *Auditory-Verbal Therapy: Science, Research, and Practice,* I invite you to gain new knowledge and insights; consolidate what you already know; feel encouraged, appreciated, inspired, and hopeful; and experience a sense of wonder as we all move forward in this new decade—the most exciting time ever for children who are deaf or hard of hearing and their families, for Auditory-Verbal practitioners and those who aspire to be, and for the practice of Auditory-Verbal Therapy.

Warren Estabrooks
Victoria, British Columbia
Canada
Summer, 2020

ACKNOWLEDGMENTS

Our families, our friends, and our circles of support, whose patience, guidance, kindness, and understanding helped us to bring this labor of love to life:

Atkins, Dale	Lux, Martin
Côté, Pierre-Roch	MacIver, Don and Sheila
Estabrooks, Fannie Mae	McCaffrey, Amy
Lux, Emily	Morrison, Michael

Our respected cohort of authors from around the world, for their inspired and dedicated work on this project:

Ashton, Louise	Lenihan, Susan
Childress, Tina	Lim, Stacey
Clark, Frances	McConkey Robbins, Amy
Dickson, Cheryl	McCreery, Ryan
Doucet, Suzanne	Naegle, Olivia
DuBois, Glynnis	Neumann, Sara
Edwards, Carolyne	Norman, Carrie
Eriks-Brophy, Alice	Quayle, Rosie
Fitzpatrick, Elizabeth	Ritter, Kathryn
Flexer, Carol	Robertson, Lyn
Ganek, Hillary	Rosenweig, Elizabeth
Goldblatt, Ellie	Rushbrooke, Emma
Grover, Anita	Sindrey, Dave
Hayward, Denyse	Smith, Joanna
Hogan, Sarah	Smolen, Elaine
Houston, K. Todd	Tannenbaum, Sally
Katz, Lisa	Voss, Jenna
Kenely, Noel	Waite, Monique

Walker, Elizabeth

Warren, Sarah

Wolfe, Jace

Wray, Denise

Zombek, Lindsay

The entire team at Plural Publishing for their encouragement, constant availability, and support

Kelvin Ko for his professional graphic design of the cover

Donya Stubbs for her guidance and work on the survey

Wilder Mayhall Roberts for her helpful peer review

EDITORS

Warren Estabrooks, MEd., Dip Ed Deaf, LSLS Cert. AVT, is President and CEO of **WE Listen International Professional Consulting** in Victoria, British Columbia, Canada. He and his team provide professional education, training, and development in Auditory-Verbal Therapy for practitioners who work with children who are deaf or hard of hearing and their families around the world. For many years, he was Director of the Auditory Learning Centre of the Learning to Listen Foundation at North York General Hospital in Toronto. He was also a Founding Director of Auditory-Verbal International and a Founding Director of the AG Bell Academy for Listening and Spoken Language. He is the Honored Patron of the Warren Estabrooks Centre in Sri Lanka. He is a Canadian of Distinction, recipient of numerous professional and humanitarian awards, and has made significant contributions to the literature.

Helen McCaffrey Morrison, PhD, CCC/A (Retired), LSLS Cert. AVT, is an educator, audiologist, and Auditory-Verbal Therapist. As an Associate Professor at Texas Christian University she taught future educators and speech-language pathologists and published research in both early speech development and Auditory-Verbal practice patterns. Following retirement, she founded **Listening-Speaking-Learning**, mentoring professionals and teaching global online courses. Helen served in the AG Bell Academy as a member of the Certification Committee and the Mentoring Committee. She is a co-author of the Mentor's Guide to Auditory-Verbal Competencies and she received the Health Care Hero Award, Research and Academic Division from the Dallas Business Journal.

Karen MacIver-Lux, MA, Aud(C), Reg CASLPO, LSLS Cert. AVT, is President and CEO of **SoundIntuition**, a Canadian company that provides online training, conferences, and consulting for professionals who work with children and adults who are deaf or hard of hearing and their families. She is also Director of **MacIver-Lux Auditory Learning Services** where she provides a variety of auditory learning services. Formerly, she was Coordinator of Clinical Services at the Learning to Listen Foundation, of which she is a graduate. Karen served as director of the Board of Auditory-Verbal International Inc. and was honored by *Maclean's* magazine as one of the top 100 Canadians.

CONTRIBUTORS

Louise Ashton (nee Honck), MA, MRCSLT, PG Dip AVT, LSLS Cert. AVT, is a Senior Auditory Verbal Practitioner at Auditory Verbal UK in England. She leads Auditory Verbal UK's training programs accredited by the AG Bell Academy for Listening and Spoken Language. Louise provides internal and external clinical supervision and mentoring, uses telepractice as intervention for families that live too far to travel, and presents nationally and internationally. Her particular interests include working with babies and purposeful play.

Tina Childress, AuD, CCC-A, is an educational audiologist in the mainstream and residential school settings. She is also an award-winning presenter, adjunct lecturer and mentor for children and adults, and is active on various local, state, and national Boards and Committees as well as social media. As a late-deafened adult with bilateral cochlear implants, her areas of expertise include (hearing) assistive technology, accessibility (especially in the performing arts), apps, and psychosocial adjustment to hearing loss.

Frances Clark, Cert. MRCSLT, PG Cert. SI, LSLS Cert. AVT, is a Senior Auditory-Verbal Therapist and Clinical Lead at Auditory Verbal UK in London. Frances trained as a Speech Pathologist and Audiologist in South Africa. She is a therapist, mentor, trainer, and presenter. She is a member of the AG Bell global matters committee that promotes access to listen and spoken language across the world. She has a particular interest in Sensory Integration, Theory of Mind, cognition, and professional coaching.

Cheryl L. Dickson, MEd, LSLS Cert. AVT, is an international leader in Auditory-Verbal practice. She is a past President of the AG Bell Academy for Listening and Spoken Language and was chairperson of the AG Bell Mentoring Task Force. She has mentored a number of professionals around the world in preparation for LSLS certification. Cheryl has a number of publications to her credit, some of which can be found on the website of *Cochlear*.

Suzanne P. Doucet, MEd, LSLS Cert. AVT, received her master's degree in Education of children who are deaf or hard of hearing from the Université de Moncton in 1981. She has worked as an itinerant teacher with francophone families in New Brunswick, Canada, for over 30 years. She has co-authored two books and participated in various research projects in the field of education of children who are deaf or hard of hearing. Suzanne is now working as a consultant in auditory-verbal practice.

Glynnis DuBois, RN, BScN, BA, MHSc, Dip AV Studies, SLP Reg CASLPO, is a PhD student at the University of Toronto. She is a clinician in the community and in hospital settings, and is a dance instructor. Glynnis obtained undergraduate degrees in Nursing and Psychology and a Clinical Master's degree in Health Sciences and a postgraduate diploma in Auditory-Verbal Studies. Her research is investigating strategies to support school-readiness skills in preschool children who are deaf or hard of hearing.

Carolyne Edwards, MCISc, MBA, Director, Auditory Management Services, established the first private practice specializing in educational audiology in Canada. She has written numerous publications in the area of educational audiology and counseling. Carolyne has post-graduate training in Gestalt psychotherapy from the Gestalt Institute of Toronto, where she is currently Executive Director and Senior Faculty. She was awarded the Canadian Academy of Audiology's Paul Kuttner Pioneer Award for her contributions to the field of educational audiology.

Alice Eriks-Brophy, BA, BEd, MSc(A), MSc, PhD, professor emerita of speech-language pathology, taught courses in aural rehabilitation and speech sound disorders at the University of Toronto from 2002 to 2018. Her research investigated culturally appropriate service provision for minority children and the influence of family involvement on AVT outcomes. Alice had also been an itinerant teacher at the Montreal Oral School for the Deaf and a classroom teacher, consultant, and researcher working with Indigenous communities in Canada.

Elizabeth M. Fitzpatrick, PhD, LSLS Cert. AVT, is a professor in the Audiology and Speech-Language Pathology Program at the University of Ottawa,

and Senior Scientist at the Children's Hospital of Eastern Ontario Research Institute. Prior to academia, she worked clinically for 20 years as an audiologist and auditory-verbal practitioner. Her research and publications are focused on the epidemiology of pediatric hearing loss, as well as interventions and outcomes in children and adults with hearing loss.

Carol Flexer, PhD, FAAA, CCC-A, LSLS Cert. AVT, received her doctorate in Audiology from Kent State University in 1982. She is a Distinguished Professor Emeritus of Audiology, The University of Akron. An international lecturer in pediatric and educational audiology and author of more than 155 publications including 16 books, Dr. Flexer is a past president of the Educational Audiology Association, the American Academy of Audiology, and the AG Bell Academy for Listening and Spoken Language.

Hillary Ganek, PhD, CCC-SLP, LSLS Cert. AVT, received her doctorate in Rehabilitation Sciences from the University of Toronto. She is a research fellow in the Cochlear Implant Lab at the Hospital for Sick Children in Toronto, Ontario, Canada. Hillary has had the unique experience of studying, teaching, and providing auditory-verbal services in five countries across four continents. Her current research uses daylong audio recordings to investigate the influence of language socialization practices in childhood intervention.

Ellie Goldblatt, MA, PGCE, read history at the University of St. Andrews. She worked as a secondary school teacher, qualifying through the Teach First programme, before joining the UK Civil Service. During this time, she undertook a government secondment at Auditory Verbal UK, developing a cost-benefit analysis of their Auditory-Verbal programme. In 2019, she qualified from the Tavistock and Portman NHS Foundation Trust as a psychodynamic psychotherapist, working with children, young people, and families.

Anita Grover, BA (Economics and Politics), FIDM, FRSA, is the CEO of the charity Auditory-Verbal UK. She leads a dedicated team of LSLS Cert AVTs and staff who are supporting families across the UK and delivering training in Auditory-Verbal practice around the world. She has 20 years' experience working with a succession of UK Government Ministers, business leaders, and not-for-profit organizations leading communications activity on a wide range of economic and social issues.

Denyse V. Hayward, PhD, received her doctorate in Speech-Language Pathology from the University of Alberta in 2003. She is an Associate Professor (Special Education) in the Department of Educational Psychology at the University of Alberta. She is a co-author of the *Test of Early Language and Literacy (TELL)* and the *Sound Access Parent Outcomes Instrument (SAPOI)*. She also co-authored an alphabet book for beginning and struggling readers based on emergent literacy research evidence, *Alphabet Stage*.

Sarah Hogan, DPhil, Clinical Scientist (Audiology), LSLS Cert. AVT, received her doctorate in Auditory Neuroscience from the University of Oxford in 1999 and is an Auditory-Verbal practitioner at Auditory-Verbal UK. She has worked

across a range of settings: as an audiologist in the UK's National Health Service working with adults and children; as a Lecturer in Audiology at Bachelor and Master of Science level; with University Research groups; and within the third sector.

K. Todd Houston, PhD, CCC-SLP, LSLS Cert. AVT, is a Professor of Speech-Language Pathology in the School of Speech-Language Pathology and Audiology at the University of Akron. He also serves as a speech-language pathologist and Listening & Spoken Language Specialist (LSLS) Certified Auditory-Verbal Therapist (Cert. AVT) for the Cochlear Implant Program at Akron Children's Hospital. Dr. Houston also is a co-founder of the 3C Digital Media Network and host of the podcast, *The Listening Brain*.

Lisa Katz, MHSc, SLP(C), Reg CASLPO, LSLS Cert. AVT, is a speech-language pathologist and auditory-verbal therapist in private practice in Toronto, Canada. Previously she worked for the Toronto Infant Hearing Program, as Coordinator of Professional Education at the Learning to Listen Foundation, as a therapist at the CI Program, Hospital for Sick Children, and Consultant to WE Listen International. Lisa has trained professionals globally, presented at many international conferences, and made numerous contributions to the literature.

Noel Kenely, MA, BSc (Hons), MRCSLT, LSLS Cert. AVT, graduated as a speech and language pathologist from the University of Malta in 2004. He has worked with babies and children who are deaf or hard of hearing for 15 years both in Malta and in the United Kingdom where he now resides. He works at Auditory Verbal UK as a therapist and trains professionals in Auditory Verbal therapy. He regularly presents at international conferences on hearing loss and early intervention.

Susan Lenihan, PhD, CED, Professor of Deaf Education at Fontbonne University, prepares teachers, speech-language pathologists, and early interventionists to serve children who are deaf or hard of hearing and their families. She is the editor of the eBook *Preparing to Teach, Committing to Learn*, and she frequently presents on family-centered intervention, professional preparation, and resilience. She serves on the Board of Directors of the AG Bell Association. In 2016, she received the Antonia Brancia Maxon Award for EHDI Excellence.

Stacey R. Lim, AuD, PhD, CCC-A, is an Assistant Professor of Audiology at Central Michigan University, where she teaches graduate-level audiology courses and supervises in the Audiology clinic. Her research and clinical areas of expertise are cochlear implants, pediatric and educational audiology, and aural rehabilitation of children and adults. She was born with a bilateral, profound, sensorineural hearing loss and currently wears a cochlear implant and hearing aid. She and her family attended Auditory-Verbal Therapy.

Amy McConkey Robbins, CCC-SLP, LSLS Cert. AVT, is a private-practice speech-language pathologist. She has authored over 100 publications, including widely used assessment procedures for children who are deaf or hard of hearing. She teaches internationally on spoken language, musical development,

and preventing burnout in serving professions. Her language/music curriculum, *TuneUps*, coauthored with Chris Barton, was voted Most Valuable Product at TherapyTimes.com. Named a Distinguished Alumna of Purdue University, she received the Richard Miyamoto Listening and Spoken Language Service Award.

Ryan W. McCreery, PhD, is the Director of Research at Boys Town National Research Hospital in Omaha, Nebraska. Ryan is also the Director of the Audibility, Perception, and Cognition Laboratory where his team studies perceptual development in children who are deaf or hard of hearing. Ryan received the Early Career Contributions to Research Award from the American Speech-Language-Hearing Association in 2013 and was a co-investigator on the Outcomes of Children with Hearing Loss study.

Olivia G. Naegle, BS, is a third-year Doctor of Audiology student at the University of Memphis School of Communication Sciences and Disorders. Her clinical and research interests include evidence-based practice, and cochlear implants and bone-anchored hearing systems, particularly in the pediatric population. Upon completion of the clinical doctorate program, she plans to pursue a PhD with the intention of focusing on the improvement of clinical practices and outcomes as related to implantable hearing devices.

Sara Neumann, AuD, is a pediatric and cochlear implant audiologist and the Audiology Research Manager and Deaf Education Consultant at Hearts for Hearing in Oklahoma City, Oklahoma. She has co-authored several articles and textbook chapters on pediatric amplification and cochlear implants. Previously, she was an educator of the deaf and hard of hearing for 6 years. Sara has a Bachelor of Science Degree in Deaf Education from Northern Illinois University and a Doctorate of Audiology from Illinois State University.

Carrie Norman, MS, CCC-SLP, LSLS Cert. AVEd, received her Master of Science in Communication Disorders with a Pediatric Aural Habilitation specialization from the University of Texas at Dallas in 2001. She is the President of Collaborative Communications, a private consulting firm dedicated to helping bridge the gap between clinical and educational services for students and families impacted by hearing differences. Her experience spans infancy through high school in both clinical and educational settings.

Rosie Quayle, Cert. MRCSLT, PG Dip AVT, LSLS Cert. AVT, Churchill Fellow, is Clinical Lead Auditory-Verbal Practitioner at Auditory Verbal UK in England, where she oversees the quality of therapy across the clinical team. Rosie contributes to the literature, and presents nationally and internationally. She has developed courses for practitioners seeking Auditory-Verbal certification in the United Kingdom and Europe. Rosie's particular interest is in helping parents with differing learning styles enhance their child's listening and spoken language through play.

Kathryn Ritter, PhD, CED, LSLS Cert. AVT, is currently an Adjunct Associate Professor in the Department of Communication Sciences and Disorders at the University of Alberta. She has 40 years of clinical experience at Glenrose Rehabilitation Hospital, and is a frequent presenter at local, national, and international conferences and workshops. She has published in the areas of Auditory-Verbal practice, mainstreaming children who are deaf or hard of hearing, family support, and instrument development focusing on children with complex needs.

Lyn Robertson, PhD, Emerita Professor of Education, Denison University, Granville, Ohio, received her PhD in Reading from The Ohio State University. She has authored *Literacy Learning for Children Who Are Deaf or Hard of Hearing* (Alexander Graham Bell, 2000), and *Literacy and Deafness* (Plural Publishing, 2009; 2014, 2nd ed.), as well as articles about listening, language, and reading. Lyn has served as board president of the Alexander Graham Bell Association Academy for Listening and Spoken Language.

Elizabeth Rosenzweig, MS, CCC-SLP, LSLS Cert. AVT, is an Auditory-Verbal Therapist in private practice. She serves families around the world via teletherapy and mentors aspiring LSLS professionals. Elizabeth is a member of the National Leadership Consortium in Sensory Disabilities and a PhD candidate at Teachers College, Columbia University. Her research interests include parent coaching and counseling, parent-child interaction, trauma-informed practice, and personnel preparation. She writes on all things about hearing loss.

Emma Rushbrooke, MPhil (Audiology), BA, Dip Aud, LSLS Cert. AVT, RNC, is Clinical Director at Hear and Say in Australia. She has over 20 years' experience working with children who are deaf or hard of hearing. Her Master of Philosophy (University of Queensland) involved researching the validity of remote mapping in children. Emma is the co-editor of the book *Teleprac-tice in Audiology*. She is currently Chair of the AG Bell Academy Board (2019), and her research interests include tele-health, unilateral hearing loss, and implantable technologies.

David Sindrey, MClSc, LSLS Cert. AVT, is an AV practitioner and the author/illustrator of many activities designed for promoting listening and spoken language. His online resources include *The Listening Room* at Advanced Bionics, *Listening Tree*, and *Actividades de Au-dición* for Phonak PIP in Spain. His materials have been translated into six different languages. Mr. Sindrey is now completing a combined Masters of Audiology degree and a PhD in Hearing Science at the University of Western Ontario, Canada.

Joanna Smith, MS, CCC-SLP, LSLS Cert. AVT, is a co-founder and CEO/Executive Director at Hearts for Hearing in Oklahoma City, OK. Prior to the founding of Hearts for Hearing, Joanna served as Program Director of the Hearing Enrichment Language Program and as an Adjunct Assistant Professor at the University of Oklahoma and the University of Central Oklahoma. She frequently presents on the benefits of collaboration when providing care for families impacted by hearing loss.

Elaine Smolen, MAT, LSLS Cert. AVEd, is a PhD candidate and National Leadership Consortium in Sensory Disabilities scholar at Teachers College, Columbia

University. An adjunct faculty member at Teachers College and The College of New Jersey, she also provides consulting and professional mentoring services in the New York area. She has extensive experience in deaf education, having served young children who are deaf or hard of hearing and their families as a head classroom teacher and an itinerant educator.

Sally Tannenbaum, MEd, LSLS Cert. AVT, is an Engagement Manager with MED-EL. Sally is the past Director of the Pediatric Hearing Loss Clinic at the University of Chicago Medicine. She received the Helen Beebe Award for Outstanding Auditory-Verbal Clinician, was a board member on the American Cochlear Implant Alliance, and was a founding director of Auditory-Verbal International. Sally feels blessed to have worked with children who are deaf or hard of hearing and their families for over 35 years.

Jenna Voss, PhD, CED, LSLS Cert. AVEd, is an Assistant Professor and Director of Deaf Education at Fontbonne University. Voss researches and presents on health and educational disparities among children and families experiencing adversity and family-centered early intervention practice. She serves on the Board of Directors of the AG Bell Academy for Listening and Spoken Language. Voss is the co-author of two texts: *Small Talk* and *Case Studies in Deaf Education: Inquiry, Application, and Resources*.

Monique Waite, PhD, BSpath (Hons), completed her PhD in speech-language pathology at the University of Queensland in 2010. A pioneer of research into the application of telepractice in pediatric speech-language pathology, she is currently a Postdoctoral Research Fellow at the University of Queensland, in a position funded by the HEARing Cooperative Research Centre. This position involves leading research in the use of telepractice to improve access and outcomes of children who are deaf or hard of hearing and their families.

Elizabeth A. Walker, PhD, CCC-SLP(A), is an assistant professor at the University of Iowa, where she is the director of the Pediatric Audiology Laboratory. Her NIH-funded research examines the factors that influence individual differences in children who are deaf or hard of hearing. She has published numerous peer-reviewed articles and book chapters and given national and international talks on listening and language outcomes in children who use hearing aids or cochlear implants.

Sarah E. Warren, AuD, PhD, is an Assistant Professor of Audiology in the University of Memphis School of Communication Sciences and Disorders where she is director of the Cochlear Implant Research Lab and Manager of the newly established Midsouth Cochlear Implant Program. Her research areas include clinical outcomes in children and adults with cochlear implants. She also presents and publishes on the topics of aural rehabilitation, interprofessional practice, social determinants of health, and public health.

Jace Wolfe, PhD, is Director of Audiology and Research at Hearts for Hearing in

Oklahoma, and Adjunct Assistant Professor at the University of Oklahoma Health Sciences Center and Salus University. He also teaches in numerous AuD programs. Author/editor of *Cochlear Implants: Audiologic Management and Considerations for Implantable Hearing Devices* and *Programming Cochlear Implants, Second Edition,* Jace has written numerous chapters and peer-reviewed articles, and the *Tot Ten*, a column on pediatric hearing health care and research.

Denise Wray, PhD, CCC-SLP, LSLS Cert. AVT, is a Professor Emerita at the University of Akron where she supervises in the Auditory-Verbal Clinic as well as an ENT Center at Akron Children's Medical Center. Research interests include literacy development in children who are deaf or hard of hearing who are learning to listen and speak using technology. She co-authored over 30 articles and co-directed two grants that developed a specialty in hearing loss for graduate SLP students at UA.

Lindsay Zombek, MS, CCC-SLP, LSLS Cert. AVT, is the Team Lead and a Clinical Specialist in Speech-Language Pathology at University Hospitals Cleveland Medical Center in Cleveland, Ohio. She specializes in aural (re)habilitation services for children and adults who are deaf or hard of hearing and their families with the Cochlear Implant Team. She both presents nationally and writes in various formats on topics related to best practices, brain development, cognition, adult aural rehabilitation, and hearing loss related challenges.

ABOUT THE COVER

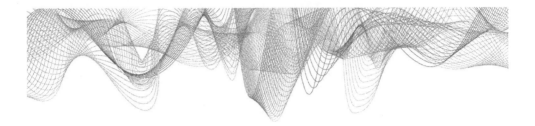

Interwoven soundwaves create a visual imagery of the ups and downs, and highs and lows of being deaf or hard of hearing—from diagnosis to learning to listen and talk, to the fulfillment of personal dreams. Auditory-Verbal Therapy, a journey of lifelong learning, is represented by the warm colors of red, orange, and yellow: AVT's vibrations of energy, happiness, joy, and love. This colorful image defines the strong relationship created by parents, children who are deaf or hard of hearing, and practitioners as they work together to achieve their expected outcomes through Auditory-Verbal Therapy.

Kelvin Ko
Creative Designer
Hong Kong
http://www.kkosc.com

To the pioneers of Auditory-Verbal Therapy

To Auditory-Verbal practitioners and aspiring Auditory-Verbal practitioners everywhere

To the families of children who are deaf or hard of hearing who invite us along on their journeys

In memory of Alice Eriks-Brophy

This book is in honor of Pierre-Roch Côté, my greatest blessing in life. Over many years, his example of service, respect, kindness, and love during many publications, including this one, kept me focused as a messenger of harmony among the professions.

Warren Estabrooks

Part I

AUDITORY-VERBAL THERAPY: FOUNDATIONS AND FUNDAMENTALS

1

AUDITORY-VERBAL THERAPY: AN OVERVIEW

Warren Estabrooks, Helen McCaffrey Morrison, and Karen MacIver-Lux

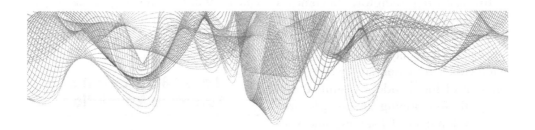

Over the last decade, Auditory-Verbal Therapy (AVT) has advanced in tandem with the rapid development and use of hearing technologies, prolific scientific research, and increased artful early intervention practices, to make the exciting outcomes of listening and spoken conversations for children who are deaf or hard of hearing a greater reality than ever before. In addition, the passion of practitioners around the world to acquire the Listening and Spoken Language—Certified Auditory-Verbal Therapist credential (LSLS Cert. AVT) continues to accelerate an evolution in the professional practice patterns and global knowledge of AVT. In agreement with the October 2019 position statement of the Joint Committee on Infant Hearing (JCIH), this book uses the term *children who are deaf or hard of hearing* because this term "(a) is acceptable to a range of stakeholders, and (b) clearly conveys the intended meaning to the entire community" (JCIH, 2019). This term "includes children who are deaf or hard of hearing whose hearing losses may be congenital or acquired, unilateral or bilateral, of any degree from minimal to profound, and of any type, including conductive, sensory (sensorineural), auditory neuropathy, and mixed hearing condition, whether permanent, transient, or intermittent. This spectrum includes those individuals who identify themselves as being a part of either, or both, the Deaf or hard-of-hearing communities" (JCIH, 2019).

AVT, an evidence-based and evidence-informed early intervention approach for infants, toddlers, and young children who are deaf or hard of hearing and their families, respects *parents as the primary agents of change and primary case managers* in the lives of their children. In AVT the Auditory-Verbal practitioner (the practitioner) and the parents apply specific creative evidence-based strategies in order to promote the optimal and efficient acquisition of spoken language developed primarily through *listening* (Estabrooks, MacIver-Lux, & Rhoades, 2016). *Listening*, therefore, becomes a major force in nurturing the child's personal, social, and academic life. AVT is a holistic intervention in which social interactions are essential for the development of independent cognitive and linguistic functioning and emphasizes the development of listening and spoken language through natural play, singing, games and daily routines, and all the excitement of daily family life. Consequently, AVT can take place anywhere and anytime.

Driven by 10 principles of practice, the mission of AVT is that practitioners will coach and guide parents in ways that help their child who is deaf or hard of hearing to acquire the best hearing access, the most functional auditory skills, and the most intelligible spoken communication that will open the doors to literacy, academic prowess, interpersonal relationships, and the unlimited and independently made choices offered over a lifetime.

The principles of AVT, inspired by the pioneers of the Auditory-Verbal movement, evolved from an illustrious history and continue to guide today's Auditory-Verbal practitioners around the world.

THE HISTORY OF AUDITORY-VERBAL THERAPY

The history of AVT consists of several stories. It's the story of how the AVT principles came to be. It's the story of how AVT got its name. It's the story of the integration of science, technology, medicine, and child development. It's the story of collaboration across professional disciplines. And it's the story of coaching and mentoring, as each generation of practitioners reaches out to the next.

Late 1800s and the Scientific Revolution

The 1800s saw the birth of science as an academic discipline, with numerous discoveries and inventions. Several of these set the stage for the development of AVT. Hermann von Helmholtz (1821–1894) established the science of psychophysics, or the study of the relationship between the measurement of a physical stimulus (e.g., intensity or frequency) and the measurement of perception of that stimulus (e.g., loudness or pitch). Alexander Graham Bell (1847–1922), a polymath with many scientific interests, studied Helmholtz' work in an effort to create a hearing aid for his wife, which led to the invention of the telephone in 1876. Dr. Bell's use of induction coils to transmit sound led to the creation of the first audiometer, by D. E. Hughes in 1879 (Staab, 2017), and a means to demonstrate scientifically that people who are deaf or hard of hearing were able to perceive sound.

Early Twentieth Century—Shifting the Paradigm

In the early twentieth century the scientific discoveries and inventions from the nineteenth century were applied to the diagnosis of hearing loss in children and the subsequent intervention, leading to the discovery that "deaf" children were able to respond to sound and learn from the auditory signal. This shifted the paradigm for work with children who are deaf or hard of hearing. Audition was no longer a sense to be ignored in favor of training visual learning. Audition became the focus.

Victor Urbantschitsch (1847–1921) was the first to explore the efficacy of helping children learn through listening. He entered medical practice at the University of Vienna as an otologist. He observed that children who are deaf or hard of hearing responded to his voice when he spoke directly into their ears, described by him as having *residual hearing* despite having been considered "deaf." Dr. Urbantschitsch went on to devise an approach to training residual hearing, using a systematic method and recording the outcomes. He published his findings in a monograph on *auditory training* (1895, translated by Silverman, 1982) that touched upon a wide range of topics: etiologies of hearing loss, peripheral and central deafness, binaural hearing, the emotional impact of hearing loss, the impact of hearing loss on speech and language, transfer of learning outside the training setting and training personnel. The many topics in Urbantschitsch's monograph set a precedent for the knowledge domains expected to be mastered by today's practicing Auditory-Verbal therapists as well as the topics in this book. Victor Urbantschitsch is considered the father of audiology.

Urbantschitsch's students Max Goldstein (1870–1941) and Emil Froeschels (1884–1972) were particularly inspired by his mentoring and went on to further the development of AVT. Goldstein, an American from St. Louis, studied with Urbantschitsch following his completion of medical school. When Goldstein returned to St. Louis, he applied his *acoustic method* in therapy sessions as part of his medical practice and published his protocols and outcomes (Goldstein, 1939). He advocated for the use of electronic hearing aids for children at a time when there was concern these would be harmful. His approach to therapy emphasized listening rather than the training of lip reading. In addition, Goldstein founded the Central Institute for the Deaf in St. Louis and the medical journal *The Laryngoscope*, which is still in publication.

Dr. Emil Froeschels was Viennese. He developed a practice working with individuals with a variety of speech disorders and was influential in the development of the profession of speech-language pathology. In 1924 he founded the still-existent International Association of Logopedics and Phoniatrics, which supports research and therapy with individuals with speech and voice disorders. Froeschels emigrated to the United States in 1939 when Germany annexed Vienna, first working with Goldstein in St. Louis and then moving to New York. He established a long working relationship with Helen Beebe (see below), a "founding mother" of AVT (Duncan & Rhoades, 2017).

Meanwhile, in the United Kingdom, methods for teaching children with hearing loss were also shifting. The Ewings, Lady Irene (1883–1959) and Sir Alexander (1896–1980), were educators who introduced early identification, parent training in the home, and child-centered teaching of children with hearing loss (described by Lady Ewing as *follow the child's interest*) (Ewing & Ewing, 1947). These fundamental aspects of AVT were considered quite revolutionary (Dawes, 2014). The Ewings also imported the first widely used US clinical audiometer, the Western Electric 2A (Staab, 2017), enabling Sir Alexander to measure thresholds at different frequencies and demonstrate that most "deaf" children had residual hearing. The Ewings and their group developed large table-based hearing aids that parents could take home on loan for use with their children, and developed a teacher-training program that emphasized their parent- and child-centered approach.

Edith Whetnall (1910–1965), an English otologist and educator, extended the work of the Ewings to include an emphasis on infant identification and intervention (Whetnall & Fry, 1954). She stressed that auditory learning developed auditory regions in the cortex (Pollack, 1970) and coined a phrase that is still used in AVT, "listening within earshot." She followed four principles in her work: (1) learning to listen is fundamental to learning spoken language, (2) what is not used early may not be available later, (3) language is best learned in the give and take of communication, and (4) parents and other family members are the principal vehicles of learning to hear and

talk (Hirsh, 1980). Whetnall called her method the *auditory approach* (Whetnall & Fry, 1954).

1950-1980: Pioneers of AVT

AVT as we practice it today coalesced from 1950 to 1980. There were four common elements in the work of practitioners during this time: (1) early identification and optimal acoustic access to sound with hearing technology, (2) learning spoken language through listening, (3) regarding parents as a child's primary teachers and active participants in sessions, and (4) child enrollment in regular education settings from early childhood onward (Pollack & Ernst, 1973). Our pioneers broadened the geographic extent of auditory work far beyond Europe to include locations across North America by establishing centers in Pennsylvania, Colorado, and California in the United States, and Montreal in Canada. Among these pioneers were four individuals who are considered to be the founders of modern AVT—Daniel Ling, Ciwa Griffiths, Helen Beebe, and Doreen Pollack.

Daniel Ling (1926–2003), an audiologist and educator of children with hearing loss from the United Kingdom, trained under the Ewings and spent time observing Dr. Whetnall. Dr. Ling set up an infant hearing program and parent-infant training program and for the first time outside London taught children within a regular education setting (Ling, 1993). Ling was invited to Canada in 1963 to be Principal of the Montreal Oral School, where he introduced auditory-based teaching strategies and developed a program for integrating students into regular education classes. Ling and his wife, Agnes Ling Phillips, established a parent-infant program at McGill University in Montreal and followed with the creation of a graduate program in *aural habilitation* for educators and speech-language pathologists. Ling was the author of numerous research publications and the seminal works *Speech and the Hearing-Impaired Child: Theory and Practice* (1976, 2002) and *Aural Habilitation* (Ling & Ling, 1978).

Ciwa Griffiths (1911–2003), an American, started her career as an educator in regular classrooms (Griffiths, 1991). When a student with hearing loss joined her preschool class, she became interested in learning about ways to best teach her student. During that period of professional development, Dr. Griffiths traveled to the United Kingdom to observe Edith Whetnall and learned about the potential for listening by children with hearing loss. When Griffiths returned home, she established the HEAR Center in Pasadena, California. Like Whetnall, Griffiths called her work the *auditory approach* (Griffiths, 1964).

Helen Beebe (1909–1989), also from the United States, first trained as an educator and later as a speech-language pathologist. During the course of her work in schools for the deaf, Beebe met Emil Froeschels and learned about auditory work. Subsequently, Froeschels became her mentor and colleague for 25 years. She established the Helen Beebe Speech and Hearing Center in Easton, Pennsylvania, and referred to her work as the *unisensory approach*, which highlighted auditory learning as opposed to traditional oral methods (Beebe, 1953).

Doreen Pollack (1920–2005) trained as a speech-language pathologist in London, United Kingdom. She became interested in working with children with hearing loss when her nephew was diagnosed with a severe hearing loss at age 2. Creating a methodology that was influenced by Dr. Goldstein's work (Pollack, 1993), Pollack and her husband moved after World War II to New York City, where she worked at the Columbia Presbyterian Hospital in a new program testing children's hearing and fitting hearing aids and started a parent-child therapy program.

During this time Dr. Hendrik Huizing (1903–1972), an audiologist from the Netherlands, observed Pollack's work while conducting hearing research at Columbia Presbyterian. Huizing was so impressed by the impact that learning through listening made on children's outcomes that, when he returned to the Netherlands, he focused his work on the diagnosis and habilitation of children with hearing loss using Pollack's approach. He called his work *acoupedics*. Huizing is considered one of the first pediatric audiologists and was one of the founders of the International Society of Audiology (Huizing, 2013).

Pollack and her husband moved to Denver, where she began work at the University of Denver, engaged in early identification, fitting hearing aids, and guiding and coaching parents to help their children learn through listening. Pollack adopted Huizing's term, *acoupedics*, to refer to her own methods (Pollack, 1964). In the early 1960s, she started an *acoupedics* program at Denver's Porter Memorial, where she remained until her retirement in 1981 (Turnbull, 2005).

By the 1970s Auditory-Verbal practitioners were increasing in number. A growing body of literature spread the word about this methodology and its outcomes. Mrs. Pollack published her seminal work, *Educational Audiology for the Limited Hearing Infant* (Pollack, 1970). This work laid out seven principles of the *acoupedic approach*: early detection, early fitting with hearing aids, a unisensory approach to training, speech development through the auditory feedback mechanism, the development of language following *typical* patterns, parents as a child's first model, and retention of a typical environment (i.e., regular classroom enrollment). All seven principles were to be in place for a program to be considered *acoupedic*. Pollack copyrighted the term "acoupedics" (Goldberg & Flexer, 2012), establishing an early example of treatment fidelity and standardization of the field. Anyone practicing the acoupedic approach could do so only with her approval. Two subsequent editions of Pollack's book were published (Pollack, 1985; Pollack, Goldberg, & Caleffe-Schenck, 1997).

Practitioners and researchers started coming together to create a community to share experiences and outcomes. In 1973, the A. G. Bell Association for the Deaf hosted a conference on the auditory approach and subsequently published a monograph of the proceedings, *The Auditory Approach* (Griffiths et al., 1973). Later in 1974 and 1979, Ciwa Griffiths organized two international conferences at the HEAR center in Pasadena and brought together speakers from Canada, Denmark, Egypt, Germany, Japan, Mexico, and the United States (Griffiths, 1979).

Professionals and families from around the globe visited the centers created by Griffiths, Beebe, and Pollack to learn more about their methods. The Beebe Center established the Larry Jarret House to house families who traveled to Easton in order to attend weeklong training programs (Goldberg & Talbot, 1993). Pollack conducted summer workshops in Denver for professionals and parents and was awarded a federal training grant in 1978, to train four professionals at a time for 8 months in the *acoupedic approach* (Turnbull, 2005). The Listen Foundation continued this program well past Pollack's retirement through the 1980s, directed by Nancy Caleffe-Schenck (Caleffe-Schenck, 1992).

In 1978, George Fellendorf, former executive director of the Alexander Graham Bell Association for the Deaf and a parent who had worked with Beebe, convened a coalition chaired by Pollack that included Beebe, Ling, and other practitioners of auditory work. The group formed the International Committee on Auditory-Verbal Communication (ICAVC) (Goldberg & Flexer, 2012) and adopted the principles of acoupedic practice (Pollack, 1993). A long discussion ensued to determine the name to give to the work practiced by coalition members (Pollack, 1993). At the time, several terms were in use: auditory training, the acoustic method, the auditory approach, aural habilitation, the unisensory approach, and acoupedics. Dr. Ling suggested a name that was agreed upon by the coalition: the *Auditory-Verbal* approach (Pollack, 1993).

1980–2000: Becoming a Profession

The last two decades of the twentieth century witnessed rapid growth of AVT as a distinct and codified option for families of children with hearing loss. In 1981, the Alexander Graham Bell Association for the Deaf invited ICAVC to join the Association as a special committee (Goldberg, 1993). ICAVC remained with A. G. Bell until 1986 when it was disbanded by ICAVC leadership and, in 1987, re-formed as Auditory-Verbal International (AVI), an autonomous, nonprofit organization. Like ICAVC, AVI adopted Pollack's principles of acoupedic practice as the *Auditory-Verbal Principles*. The ultimate goal of AVI was to promote hearing as the primary route for the acquisition of spoken language skills (Goldberg, 1993).

Several papers were published during this period that further codified AVT. In 1989 AVI approved the Suggested Protocol for Audiological and Hearing Aid Evaluation (Marlowe, 1993), a work that formed the basis for the current Alexander Graham Bell Association's Recommended Protocol for Audiological Assessment, Hearing Aid and Cochlear Implant Evaluation, and Follow-up (A. G. Bell, 2019). In 1990, the Board of Directors of AVI voted to add professional standards and certification of Auditory-Verbal therapists as primary goals (Lake, 2001). A position paper published in 1988 by the Denver-based Auditory-Verbal Network, *A Parent's Guide to Auditory-Verbal Therapy*, was foundational for AVI's work toward developing standards and a path to certification. *A Parent's Guide* described essential aspects and quality indicators of Auditory-Verbal practice: definition of an Auditory-Verbal practitioner, definition of an Auditory-Verbal treatment plan (AVT care plan), and questions parents could ask to ascertain whether the practitioner followed the Auditory-Verbal Principles (Auditory-Verbal Network, 1988). In 1993, *The Volta Review* published a monograph devoted entirely to AVT (Goldberg, 1993).

In 1991 AVI embarked on establishing a certification in AVT. The organization engaged a psychometric company to establish a certification program that included a survey of parents and practitioners regarding the knowledge and skills needed for competent provision of AVT and to create a certification exam. The certification protocol was a precursor to today, with an application process, statement of practice, and letters of recommendation.

In 1994 AVI published the Auditory-Verbal Scope of Practice (AVI, 1994). This paper defined the Auditory-Verbal therapist and the scope of practice of AVT for AVI Certified Auditory-Verbal Therapists (Cert. AVT). The Auditory-Verbal therapist definition listed 10 activities that an Auditory-Verbal therapist must be qualified to carry out. With some adaptations, these 10 activities became the Auditory-Verbal Principles of today. The Scope of Practice described the training and knowledge required for therapists who were certified by AVI. These encompassed eight domains that are similar to the knowledge domains required for current certification for Auditory-Verbal therapists.

The first examination for Auditory-Verbal certification was conducted in 1994 in two sessions. The first session, in Toronto, Ontario, Canada, involved 8 Auditory-Verbal therapists who were involved in creating the exam. The second session took place a few months later in Rochester, New York. A total of 47 individuals from the United States, Canada, and Australia became the first group of Certified Auditory-Verbal Therapists (Cert. AVTs).

In 2003 AVI published the *AVI Standardized Curriculum* for use in training and mentoring professionals in the

Auditory-Verbal approach (AVI, 2003), providing an outline of knowledge domains that an Auditory-Verbal therapist must be able to apply. For 10 years, AVI promoted listening as a way of life and became the certifying body of Auditory-Verbal therapists, until its dissolution in 2004, when the A. G. Bell Academy for Listening and Spoken Language was created solely for the purpose of certification.

In summary, the history of AVT is a history of the synthesis of science, sensory psychology, linguistics, child development, and family support to create a new paradigm that integrates listening into a child's personality (Pollack, 1970). This "new paradigm" is now over 100 years old. Auditory-Verbal certification has been in place for over 25 years, and the practitioners of today owe much to the past and, in particular, to the pioneers. A new generation continues to lead the way forward, as its passionate members shape the future of AVT as a highly regarded, evidence-based, and evidence- informed intervention for children who are deaf or hard of hearing and their families.

THE PRACTICE OF AVT

Auditory-Verbal therapists (practitioners) are obliged to adhere to the Principles of Listening and Spoken Language Specialist (LSLS) Auditory-Verbal Therapy (A. G. Bell Academy, 2017) (see boxed text) when they are practicing AVT. The Principles foster best practices for guiding and coaching families to help their children who are deaf or hard of hearing to reach their highest potential in multiple developmental domains: listening, spoken language, lit-eracy, cognition, and communication in both academic and social settings.

DISCUSSION OF THE PRINCIPLES OF LISTENING AND SPOKEN LANGUAGE— CERTIFIED AUDITORY-VERBAL THERAPY

1. Promote early diagnosis of hearing loss in newborns, infants, toddlers, and young children, followed by immediate audiologic management and AVT.

Auditory-Verbal practitioners advocate early diagnosis of hearing loss, followed by consistent use of appropriately selected and programmed hearing technology, and regularly scheduled AVT sessions in order to optimize the child's overall developmental and life opportunities. Research indicates that early diagnosis of hearing loss, early fitting of appropriate hearing technology, and immediate implementation of family-centered intervention positively influence outcomes in the development of: functional auditory skills and understanding and production of spoken language (Cowan, Edwards, & Ching, 2018); social-emotional wellness (Warner- Czyz, Loy, Pourchot, White, & Cokely, 2018); lit-eracy and educational outcomes (Geers et al., 2017; Goldblat & Pinto, 2017; Robertson, 2014). Children who are identified with hearing loss by 3 months of age and enrolled in family-centered intervention programs by 6 months of age can achieve close to (Ching et al., 2017) or similar language development as children with typical hearing (Fulcher, Purcell, Baker, & Munro, 2012).

Principles of Listening and Spoken Language—Auditory-Verbal Therapy

1. Promote early diagnosis of hearing impairment in newborns, infants, toddlers, and children, followed by immediate audiologic management and Auditory-Verbal therapy.
2. Recommend immediate assessment and use of appropriate, state-of-the-art hearing technology to obtain maximum benefits of auditory stimulation.
3. Guide and coach parents* to help their child use hearing as the primary sensory modality in developing spoken language.
4. Guide and coach parents to become the primary facilitators of their child's listening and spoken language development through active consistent participation in individualized Auditory-Verbal therapy.
5. Create environments that support listening for the acquisition of spoken language throughout the child's daily activities.
6. Guide and coach parents to help their child integrate listening and spoken language into all aspects of the child's life.
7. Guide and coach parents to use natural developmental patterns of audition, speech, language, cognition, and communication.
8. Guide and coach parents to help their child self-monitor spoken language through listening.
9. Administer ongoing formal and informal diagnostic assessments to develop individualized Auditory-Verbal treatment plans, to monitor progress, and to evaluate the effectiveness of the plans for the child and family.
10. Promote education in regular classrooms with typical hearing peers and with appropriate support services from early childhood onwards.

Parents refers to all caregivers in the child's life.
A. G. Bell Academy, 2017, adapted from Pollack (1997), printed by permission.

The Joint Committee on Infant Hearing (JCIH) recommends that all infants be screened at no later than 1 month of age and that those who do not pass the screening have a comprehensive audiological evaluation at no later than 3 months of age (JCIH, 2007). It is also recommended that those infants with confirmed hearing loss begin appropriate intervention (such as AVT) at no later than 6 months of age from health care and education professionals with expertise in hearing loss and deafness in infants and young children. These rec-ommendations fit well with Principle #1 of the LSLS. Cert. AVT.

Children with severe to profound hearing loss who have early and consistent access to cochlear implants prior to 1 year of age have fewer receptive and expressive language deficits than those who have been implanted after the age of 1 year. Language outcomes for those implanted after the age of 1 decline as the age of implantation increases (Ruben, 2018). When auditory neural connections are developed in early infancy with the use of hearing technology, children who are deaf or hard of hearing also achieve better reading skills, educational outcomes, and social-emotional growth over time (Langereis & Vermeulen, 2015; Yoshinago-Itano, 2003; Yoshinago-Itano, Sedy, Wiggin, & Chung, 2017). Indeed, children who receive AVT demonstrate not only similar academic outcomes but similar abilities to interact in all social roles just like their age-matched peers who have typical hearing (Constantinescu-Sharpe et al., 2017).

Geers, Nicholas, Tobey, and Davidson (2016) demonstrated that children who are implanted between 6 and 12 months of age and receive AVT achieve significantly higher scores on all measures of language development as opposed to those implanted between 12 and 18 months. Those advantages were maintained from ages 4.2 to 10.5 years. These researchers also cited evidence from a controlled prospective nationwide (USA) study of children with cochlear implant that those who were using an American Sign Language (ASL) approach statistically demonstrated a disadvantage in spoken language and in reading. In a systematic review, Kaipa and Danser (2016) looked at 14 studies that assessed AVT with implanted children and found that AVT provided significant benefits in three domains: receptive and expressive language, speech perception, and mainstreaming.

Practitioners typically offer weekly AVT sessions, although there are some who do provide them more often and some less often, depending on a number of factors. The frequency and duration of typical AVT sessions have been used as a model for guidelines set forth in a position paper of the American Cochlear Implant Alliance (ACIA), entitled "Pediatric Habilitation Following Co-chlear Implantation" (ACIA, 2015) (Appendix 1). The ACIA position paper cites evidence from the research literature that demonstrates the positive outcomes of AVT as the rationale for the recommendation of one or two 1-hour habilitation sessions per week (Dettman, Wall, Constantinescu, & Dowell, 2013; Dornan et al., 2010; Rhoades, 2001).

2. Recommend immediate assessment and use of appropriate, state-of-the-art hearing technology to obtain maximum benefits of auditory stimulation.

Once hearing loss is identified, immediate assessment and consistent use of appropriately programmed hearing technology is essential so that spoken language is easy to hear, easy to listen to, easy to learn and easy to use. If access to hearing technology is delayed, particularly during developmentally sensitive periods, cortical reorganization will occur (Sharma et al., 2016) and spoken language development will be at risk for delay. Early fitting and consistent use of appropriately selected hearing technology during all of the child's waking hours provide the auditory stimulation necessary to facilitate the development of neural connections in the brain; and these neural connections provide the foundations for spoken language, reading, and academics (Cole & Flexer, 2011). When hearing technology provides adequate audibility to conversational speech across the speech spectrum, listening and spoken language outcomes are better than those with hearing technology that does not provide such access (Tomblin et al., 2014; Walker, Redfern, & Oleson, 2019). Children who demonstrate consistent use of amplification during all waking hours achieved significantly higher scores in vocabulary, grammar, and phonological awareness (Ching, Dillon, Leigh, & Cupples, 2017; Walker et al., 2015). Similarly, consistent access to electrical stimulated information provided by a cochlear implant promotes positive spoken communication outcomes (Li et al., 2014; Wiseman & Warner-Czyz, 2018). Consequently, audiologists, Auditory-Verbal practitioners, and parents form a formidable alliance and continuously assess the effectiveness and appropriateness of all hearing technologies to ensure that the child has consistent and full auditory access to all sounds of speech, all spoken language learning opportunities, and all the other exciting sounds of life.

3. Guide and coach parents to help their child use hearing as the primary sensory modality in developing listening and spoken language.

Currently there is significant evidence to support the validity and value of using hearing (as provided by appropriately selected and programmed hearing technology) as the primary sensory modality for the development of listening and spoken language skills in children who are deaf or hard of hearing. The most compelling evidence is the multisite study conducted by Geers, Mitchell, Warner-Czyz, Wang, and Eisenberg (2017), who demonstrated that children who had been engaged in auditory-based intervention approaches, such as AVT, achieved better speech recognition skills over the first 3 years post-activation of their cochlear implant(s) and exhib-

ited a statistically significant advantage in spoken language and reading near the end of the elementary grades, compared with children who primarily used visual modes of communication such as American Sign Language (ASL). Geers and colleagues also found that over 70% of children exposed to spoken language primarily through listening achieved age-appropriate spoken language compared with only 39% of those exposed to visual modes of communication for 3 or more years. Finally, better early speech perception abilities of the former group were better (mean = 70%) compared with those who did not have early access to hearing (mean = 51%).

In summary, competency in spoken language, social-emotional development, and literacy skills is highly dependent on the level of access the brain has to auditory information and the subsequent development of listening skills. As parents take advantage of opportunities to help their child develop confidence in listening and, later, in becoming independent managers of their hearing technology, children learn to navigate difficult listening environments and to repair communication breakdowns due to mishearing.

4. Guide and coach parents to become the primary facilitators of their child's listening and spoken language development through active consistent participation in individualized Auditory-Verbal Therapy.

Practitioners in AVT recognize that parents are their child's first and most enduring teachers and the *primary agents of change* in their child's listening and spoken language development

(Estabrooks, MacIver-Lux, & Rhoades, 2016; Kaiser & Hancock, 2003). Therefore, AVT is *individually tailored to the specific needs of the child and family*. It is not a prescription of exercises nor is it conducted as group intervention. The higher the level of family participation and engagement in any intervention program, the stronger the child's language and social growth will be (Moeller et al., 2013; Suskind, 2016; Suskind & Leffel, 2013), thus all AVT sessions are conducted jointly with the parents to promote optimal outcomes in audition, speech, language, cognition, and communication.

The practitioner engages in activities with the child and he/she demonstrates strategies that will facilitate the child's development in audition, speech, language, cognition, and communication. Parents then practice the demonstrated strategies with guidance from the practitioner and then on their own with the child. When parents are actively engaged as participants in the AVT session, they learn how to augment their child's listening and language development, how to enhance their responsiveness to all the child's communication attempts, and how to evaluate progress.

The quantity and quality of spoken language parents use can have a profound impact on the child's linguistic development, educational attainment, and cognitive outcomes (Suskind, 2016). Therefore, parents are taught to use spoken language that will support and facilitate their child's receptive and expressive language growth. Practitioners also help parents learn to identify or create meaningful listening and spoken language learning opportunities within the child's daily environment that will facilitate lis-

tening, spoken language, and cognitive growth. Ultimately, it is the parents who are the primary clients in every AVT session. Thus, parent coaching and the guidance skills of the practitioner in AVT are paramount (Fuller & Kaiser, 2019; Graham, Rodger, & Ziviani, 2013; Kaiser & Hancock, 2003; Kaiser & Roberts, 2013) to helping parents to become effective facilitators of their child's listening and spoken communication development.

5. Guide and coach parents to create environments that support listening for the acquisition of spoken language throughout the child's daily activities.

The daily environment of most typical young children is noisy and presents many listening challenges for all children. Full maturation of the structures of the central auditory nervous system (CANS) that enable the child to accurately perceive auditory signals that are degraded and/or presented in non-ideal listening environments is not achieved until children reach late adolescence (Bellis, 2011). Therefore, immature auditory processing skills, along with poor acoustics in the home, nursery school, and/or early childhood classroom, cause children to have difficulty attending to the voices of their peers and caregivers. Children who are deaf or hard of hearing, however, are at an even greater disadvantage. They need to expend even more energy and cognitive resources to understand spoken language than their hearing peers, especially if they have vocabulary and working memory weaknesses (McCreery, Walker, Spratford, Lewis, & Brennan, 2019). An immature CANS impacted by hearing loss and auditory deprivation combined with the child's noisy listening environment increases the likelihood that spoken language will be missed or misheard, resulting in missed spoken language learning opportunities. Children who are deaf or hard of hearing, therefore, during the early stages of listening and spoken language development require spoken language input that's easy to hear and learn. Practitioners demonstrate how the listening environment can be manipulated to make spoken language easier to hear, and subsequently higher level auditory processing skills develop so the child learns to understand degraded speech (due to distance, accented speech, poor-quality recordings, etc.) or speech in the presence of non-ideal listening conditions (car, classroom, restaurant, etc.). Practitioners also coach parents to comfortably use assistance hearing technologies, such as remote microphone hearing assistive technology (RM-HAT) coupled to the child's hearing aids and/or cochlear implants, that help provide optimal audibility to spoken language in the child's daily environments.

6. Guide and coach parents to help their child integrate listening and spoken language into all aspects of the child's life.

A key predictor of a child's linguistic, social-emotional, literacy, and academic competencies is the parents' ability to provide an environment that's rich in meaningful and complex spoken language experiences (Leffel & Suskind, 2013; Roberts et al., 2019; Suskind, 2016; Walker, Redfern, & Oleson, 2019). Additionally, 90% of children's vocabulary

is learned through *overhearing* (Akhtar, Jipson, & Callanan, 2001). If the child does not have consistent bilateral auditory access to spoken language, however, linguistic, social-emotional, literacy, and academic outcomes will be compromised. As a multidimensional approach, AVT focuses on the child's development of listening, talking, and thinking, which then encourages the natural emergence of spoken conversations. Thus, parents in AVT quickly learn to prioritize auditory access and auditory skills development. Doreen Pollack, one of the pioneers of the Auditory-Verbal movement, put it this way, "listening must become an integral part of the child's life" (Pollack, 1970, 1985).

Children's development of conversation and social skills are supported best when they are engaged in meaningful, sustained, and rich language experiences and when the parents are responsive to their children's listening, spoken language, cognitive (Moeller et al., 2013), emotional, and social needs (Mashburn et al., 2008). The practitioner, then, needs to have more than just limited knowledge of the family's daily routines. Therefore, an AVT Care Plan is developed *in partnership with the* parents so they can take advantage of every opportunity for listening and spoken language development. In AVT, practitioners help parents to view their child who is deaf or hard of hearing as a child who *hears with hearing technology and actively listens to learn spoken language.* Parents then learn to transform their child's daily experiences into meaningful spoken language learning opportunities as they come to view their child as *a child who hears and actively listens.* Subsequently, the child learns to value hearing and listening and to view himself/herself the way the parents do. Hence, listening does become part of the child's persona.

7. Guide and coach parents to use natural developmental patterns of audition, speech, language, cognition, and communication.

The planning, delivery, and evaluation of individualized AVT Care Plans are consistent with the developmental stages of children with typical hearing and standard procedures of practitioners. During AVT sessions, the practitioner and parent jointly observe and evaluate the child's current skills and identify those the child has yet to attain but could learn with an adult's help, defined as finding the child's "zone of proximal development" (Vygotsky & Cole, 1981). This process enables the practitioner and parent to select appropriate short-term objectives and long-term goals.

During AVT sessions, the practitioner demonstrates many strategies and, in partnership with the parents, discusses how these can be used most effectively and efficiently in daily routines and activities, in games, in singing, and in book sharing. With consistent active engagement and practice in AVT sessions, parents acquire the confidence to implement strategies that ultimately help their child attain specific short-term and ultimately long-term objectives, based on the natural patterns of development of children with typical hearing. The child's developmental outcomes then dictate new short-term objectives in listening, spoken language, cognition, and communication. Ultimately, the practitioner coaches the parents in ways that will close the listening and spoken language gap between the child's hearing age and chronological age as quickly as possible by developing and cementing neural connections through the provision of linguistically rich auditory information.

8. Guide and coach parents to help their child self-monitor spoken language through listening.

Children typically produce speech and spoken language with the help of *auditory feedback*, the process of listening to others, listening to their own speech production, and making adjustments to their speech and/or language so that it sounds as close as possible to what was modeled or heard. Auditory feedback of one's own speech and spoken language is of great importance for the attainment of auditory goals and the acquisition of fluent spoken language (Liang, Xiao, Feng, & Yan, 2014; Scheerer & Jones, 2018). An effective auditory feedback loop prepares the child for independent verbal communication with minimal need for clarification or interpretation.

During the early stages of development, practitioners encourage parents to imitate their child's vocalizations and spoken language models. These imitations set the stage for the vocal turn taking that takes place in conversations. As the child learns to listen with his or her hearing technology, spoken language and communication skills begin to emerge, then expand, and then become finely tuned. Subsequently, as children acquire more sophisticated listening and linguistic competence, they use listening to self-monitor their own speech and language and self-correct whenever necessary. The ability to self-monitor speech production and spoken language is a lifelong skill that is valuable for facilitating clear communication with others, managing and repairing communication breakdowns, learning new languages, and integrating into their communities of choice.

9. Administer ongoing formal and informal diagnostic assessments to develop individualized Auditory-Verbal treatment plans, to monitor progress, and to evaluate the effectiveness of the plans for the child and family.

Intervention or "treatment" plans are used throughout the medical community and in the social sciences whenever direct services are rendered to an individual. The AVT Care Plan for a young child with hearing loss and his/her family is viewed in a broad context—one that includes the whole family. Consequently, AVT sessions focus on multiple issues that may not be apparent to a casual observer (Ernst, 2012).

AVT is *diagnostic*. Practitioners engage in evidence-based/evidence-informed practice by continuous assessment of the child's and the family's progress, and they identify roadblocks to progress precipitated by challenges additional to hearing loss, changes in hearing technology or hearing status, or by family support requirements. Duncan and Rhoades (2017) indicated that AVT seeks "to explain or establish the functional levels of the development on the child with hearing loss" and that "AVT is considered diagnostic because it has processes of ongoing examination of an individual child's overall progress."

In knowing the outcomes of these diagnostic AVT sessions, the practitioner is able to select the most appropriate short-term and long-term objectives that go far beyond "the perception of acoustic elements to all aspects of spoken language (semantic, pragmatic, and syntactic) and to every area of personal and social development" (Ling, 1989).

The family and the practitioner work together with the child's audiologist, early childhood, preschool, and kindergarten personnel, and additional practitioners to meet the child's individual needs. Ongoing, efficient communication among members enhances opportunities for the child's maximum development.

Parents and practitioners help to create auditory neural architecture in the child's brain by scaffolding the higher-level linguistic skills of reading and writing. Every AVT session helps to monitor the increase of the architecture and build a strong infrastructure. The child's auditory functioning and use of communication in meaningful contexts are recorded to assist the practitioner and parents in finding the *child's zone of proximal development* and subsequently in the planning and delivery of the next steps. In addition to observing, the practitioner administers a battery of tests standardized on children with typical hearing. In conjunction with audiological assessments, these tests help to assess articulation, receptive and expressive vocabulary, receptive and expressive language, and cognitive, pre-literacy, and auditory skills so that rate of progress is monitored. Such objective assessments and measures assist the child's team in determining that AVT is adequately serving the family. When AVT is not appropriate, the practitioner refers the family to another approach and helps to create a transition plan to make the transition as smooth as possible.

10. Promote education in regular schools with peers who have typical hearing and with appropriate services from early childhood onward.

Practitioners guide parents in helping their child to attain the requisite school entry skills in communicative competence, social cognition, and pre-literacy and encourage inclusion in regular educational settings (daycare, preschool, and school). When parents exhibit confidence in helping their child engage in group activities at home and in the community (e.g., baby/parent play groups, playdates, daycare settings) to facilitate social development, optimal social inclusion in school settings is more likely to occur (Constantinescu-Sharpe et al., 2017; Percy-Smith et al., 2008). The social and environmental supports provided by parents, family members, early childhood teachers, and others enhance and expand the child's overall listening, communication, and social competence (National Research Council, 2000) and prepare the child for academic success. Goldblat and Pinto (2017) found positive correlations between academic success and AVT—children who "graduated" from AVT outperformed adolescents and young people who are deaf or hard of hearing who were not in an AVT program.

Inclusion in school typically requires the support services of a hearing resource teacher, educational audiologist, speech-language pathologist, and other school personnel, who work as a collaborative team to create a *safety net* in promoting full brain access to edu-

cational opportunities and to help in fostering and facilitating self-advocacy skills and self-actualization.

LSLS CERT. AVT (LISTENING AND SPOKEN LANGUAGE SPECIALIST: CERTIFIED AUDITORY-VERBAL THERAPIST)

Practitioners who hold the LSLS credential are qualified educators of children who are deaf or hard of hearing, audiologists and/or speech-language pathologists who have chosen to pursue a career supporting the principles of Auditory-Verbal Therapy. They complete a process of certification governed by the *Alexander Graham Bell Academy for Listening and Spoken Language* (A. G. Bell Academy, 2017). Among the various certification requirements, applicants for certification participate in intensive specialized training and mentoring and must pass an examination to obtain the certification known as *Listening and Spoken Language Specialist Certified Auditory-Verbal Therapist (Cert. AVT®)*. LSLS Cert. AVTs are bound by ethical principles and practices under a professional code of ethics and are required to obtain continuing professional education to maintain the certification.

Comprehensive AVT relies on accurate information about the child's hearing loss; auditory, speech, and language skills; learning abilities; social-emotional and cognitive growth; and personal and mental health development. All this information needs to be known by all team members, and especially by the parents. These areas are included in the nine domains of LSLS knowledge required of LSLS Cert. AVTs by the Academy. Current knowledge about hearing loss, hearing technology, and related health and educational issues makes collaboration and partnerships essential (Potter, 2015) and vitally important in AVT. The practitioner works to foster and maintain interprofessional relationships that help families to achieve the positive outcomes they want, as efficiently as possible (Engum & Jeffries, 2012). Certified Auditory-Verbal therapists are often members of one or more multidisciplinary educational/ medical teams that include a variety of doctors, audiologists, speech-language pathologists, teachers, physical therapists, occupational therapists, et al.

As a 501(c)(6) nonprofit organization in the US with the mission of "advancing listening and talking through standards of excellence and international certification of professionals," the Alexander Graham Bell Academy for Listening and Spoken Language offers two certifications: Listening and Spoken Language Specialist Certified Auditory-Verbal Therapist (LSLS Cert. AVT) and Listening and Spoken Language Specialist Certified Auditory-Verbal Educator (LSLS Cert. AVEd). These two professions have commonalities and differences that are reflected in the Principles of Practice specified for each designation.

THE STATE OF AUDITORY-VERBAL THERAPY

While preparing this book, the editors surveyed the global LSLS Cert. AVT community in order to identify current and future practice trends. A market re-search analyst assisted in the construction of the 17-question online survey and data compilation. An invitation and hyperlink to the online survey were distributed to LSLS Cert. AVTs via social media.

A total of 137 LSLS Cert. AVTs responded, representing 24.6% of the practicing 556 LSLS Cert. AVTs at the time of distribution. Respondents were from 16 countries (India, China, Malaysia, Australia, Canada, Argentina, Mexico, Chile, Paraguay, the United Kingdom, Denmark, Germany, Portugal, France, South Africa, and the United States) and across 6 continents, as illustrated in Figure 1–1. The majority (76.4%) were from the North American continent (Canada, United States). A total of 86% were from countries where the predominant language was English (Australia, Canada, United Kingdom, United States), similar to findings from a survey of LSLS Cert AVTs conducted a little over a decade previously (Morrison, 2008). The global distribution of respondents, however, is more widespread than in 2008, when no representation was obtained from the European continent, Asia, or from South Africa.

Respondents were asked to report on the services they provide by selecting all that applied from a list of seven activities—providing AVT to families, providing professional development, coaching and mentoring practitioners for LSLS Cert. AVT certification, teaching at the university level, supervising university students, supervising other professionals, and engaging in research. The responses are presented in Figure 1–2. The majority of responding LSLS Cert. AVTs (84%) provide AVT to families. They also engage in multiple other activities that serve to increase knowledge about AVT to colleagues and university students.

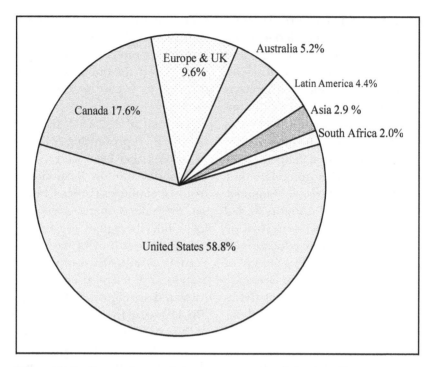

Figure 1-1. Percentage of survey respondents by location.

Over half (64%) provide professional development and 50% mentor other professionals who are working toward LSLS Cert. AVT certification.

The LSLS Cert. AVTs who provide AVT to families were asked a series of questions to identify current trends regarding their primary practice site, scheduling, and caseloads. The largest group (50%) work in medical or clinical settings that are funded privately, publicly, by universities, or by non-profit organizations. The next largest group (18%) work in public or private school settings. Another 15% engage in private practice and 13% see families in the families' homes. The remainder work in unspecified non-profit organizations or for cochlear implant manufacturers.

The average AVT session is 1 hour in duration. The majority (75%) of LSLS Cert. AVTs provide services to families weekly; 14%, bi-weekly; and the remainder report that schedules vary depending upon the needs of the families. These findings are commensurate with the practice patterns of LSLS Cert. AVTs also reported by Morrison (2008). Just over half (53.4%) of the LSLS Cert. AVTs today provide telepractice services to families.

The majority of LSLS Cert. AVTs tend to serve families with children predominantly age 6 years and younger. They reported that an average of just over half (55%) of the children are between birth and 3 years of age, and close to a third (31%) are between 4 and 6 years. The remainder of children on their caseloads (reported on average as about 25%) are older than 6 years. Children who are older than 6 years were reported to be children who were transitioning into school, progressing more slowly due to additional challenges or late identification, or they were recently implanted. Among the children who are old enough to enter early childhood classrooms, an average of 58% are enrolled in regular education settings, as opposed to special classrooms for children who are deaf or hard of hearing.

Table 1–1 shows the percentage of LSLS Cert. AVTs reporting the degrees and types of hearing loss of children whom they serve. Almost all provide AVT to children who are deaf or hard of hearing from the moderate through the profound range (90% to 100% of respondents). Close to three-quarters of the LSLS Cert AVTs serve children with mild hearing loss (73%) and 40% see children with a slight hearing loss. They see children with a variety of types of hearing loss. All reported serving chil-

dren with sensorineural hearing loss. The majority see children with auditory neuropathy spectrum disorder (ANSD), with mixed hearing loss, and with permanent conductive hearing loss. A little over one-third of respondents serve children with recurrent conductive hearing loss (e.g., recurrent otitis media with effusion). All but three respondents who see children with recurrent conductive hearing loss also see children with slight or mild degrees of hearing loss.

LSLS Cert. AVTs do not restrict their services to children whose only challenge is hearing loss. An average of 41% of the children on their caseloads have challenges additional to hearing loss. This is commensurate with the 40% prevalence of additional challenges in the general population of children who

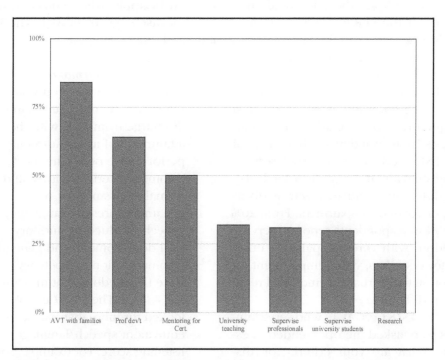

Figure 1-2. Percentage of survey respondents engaging in various professional activities.

Table 1–1. Percentage of LSLS Cert. AVTs Reporting that They Serve Children with the Indicated Degrees and Types of Hearing Loss

What degrees of hearing loss do the children on your caseload have? (Check all that apply)		What types of hearing loss do the children on your caseload have? (Check all that apply)	
Slight (15–25 dBHL)	40%	Recurrent (temporary) conductive	36%
Mild (26–55 dBHL)	73%	Permanent conductive	72%
Moderate (56–70 dBHL)	90%	Single-sided deafness	74%
Severe (71–90 dBHL)	96%	Mixed	80%
Profound (> 90 dBHL)	100%	Sensorineural	100%
		Auditory neuropathy spectrum disorder	80%

are deaf or hard of hearing in the United States (Gallaudet Research Institute, 2011). The respondents were asked to indicate the additional challenges of the children on their caseloads by selecting all that applied from a list of nine categories. The categories and responses are presented in Figure 1–3. Developmental delay and sensory integration issues were the most frequently reported additional challenges by respondents. About half of the LSLS Cert. AVTs reported serving children with attention disorder, learning differences, autism spectrum disorder, or cognitive impairment. From 20% to 40% of respondents reported serving children with cerebral palsy or other motor disorders, visual impairment, or emotional disturbance/emotional regulation difficulties.

The LSLS Cert. AVTs who serve families were asked the open-ended question "What are your criteria for 'discharge' from Auditory-Verbal Therapy?" Responses were coded according to the criteria that LSLS Cert. AVTs provided. The codes were tallied to get an idea of the predominant approaches the LSLS Cert. AVTs apply when considering a family's discharge from AVT. The following themes emerged:

■ *Informal and formal assessment.* Assessment information was most frequently cited for determining discharge from AVT, with the attainment of age-equivalent performance being the most common criteria. Informal and formal assessment of receptive and expressive language, speech production, auditory skill development, and general communication competency were the predominant measures considered. The LSLS Cert. AVTs looked for more than one age-equivalent speech/language/ listening score. For example, some required that a child maintain age-equivalent performance for

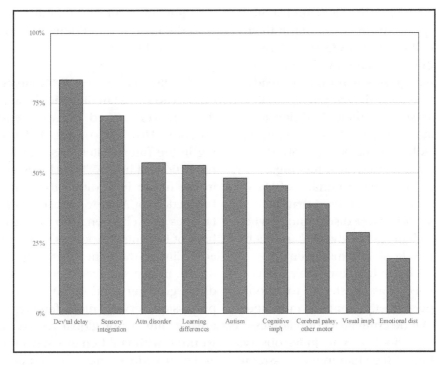

Figure 1-3. Percentage of types of additional disabilities reported by survey respondents.

more than 1 year or across two or three assessment periods. Others looked for age-equivalent performance in more than one domain (e.g., expressive language and listening skills) or required age-equivalent performance on more than one assessment within a domain (e.g., two standard-ized assessments of language, two standardized assessments of speech production). Some LSLS Cert. AVTs specified that performance be assessed using standardized instruments. A smaller collection of comments pointed to lack of progress or plateaus as indicators for discharge and a need for referral to more appropriate services. Examples included consideration

of discharge if a child obtained minimal gains over a 6-month period or failed to achieve at least 1 year's growth within 1 year's time.

▪ *Parent skill level.* Several comments pointed out that discharge from AVT is a joint decision of the LSLS Cert. AVT and the child's parents. This joint decision included assessment by the practitioner and parents themselves regarding their *readiness* for discharge. Representative comments included: when parents are familiar and comfortable using various strate-gies and advocating for their child, when parents no longer need consistent guidance, when parents are able to demonstrate the independent ability to utilize strategies that facilitate listening, speaking, and thinking in their child. One LSLS Cert. AVT put it this way: "Empowered families recognize when they are ready to reduce the frequency of AVT sessions as their child develops auditory, speech, and language skills commensurate with their peers with typical hearing."

- *School entry*. A number of LSLS Cert. AVTs indicated that AVT services were discontinued when a child was ready for enrollment in school, and management of the child's communication needs was transferred to school personnel. Comments indicated that determination of readiness for school entry includes observation of the child in the classroom and social environment as well as performance assessments in AVT. The school itself featured in determining whether a child might be discharged and services transferred to the school— respondents frequently stressed the need for verifying that appropriate support was available in the school before considering discharge.

- *Tapering off, monitoring, providing services as needed*. A few respondents reduce the frequency of AVT sessions from weekly to bi-weekly or monthly sessions prior to discharge in order to monitor the maintenance of skills when the frequency of sessions is reduced. A larger number of the respondents invite the family once or twice a year for *monitoring*. Several indicated they "leave the door open"

and are available if families feel the need for additional sessions after discharge.

Finally, all LSLS Cert. AVTs surveyed, those who serve families and those who do not, were asked the open-ended question "How do you see AVT evolving in the future?" Responses included predictions of how AVT will be practiced in the future in addition to what will be needed for AVTs to best serve future families and children who are deaf or hard of hearing. Responses were coded according to the issues that were introduced. In general, LSLS Cert. AVTs predict a growing need for AVT, with the profession serving more families in a greater number of global regions, and working with children at younger ages and with a wider range of needs. Several interconnected themes emerged:

- *Earlier identification and fitting with hearing technology*. LSLS Cert. AVTs predict that countries that have established 1-3-6 Early Hearing Detection and Intervention (EDHI) protocols— screening by 1 month of age, diagnosis by 3 months, intervention with hearing technology and family services by 6 months (JCIH, 2007)—will move to a more stringent 1-2-3 plan. Others predict that global regions that do not have 1-3-6 practices will move in that direction, and they presented a call for action: for Auditory-Verbal practitioners to assist in the efforts toward establishing more widespread early detection and intervention practices. These predictions and the call for action are accompanied by the expectation that the children served by Auditory-Verbal practitioners in the future will be even younger than today. As a consequence, Auditory-Verbal practitioners will need to be (1) more knowledgeable about infant development, (2) more skilled at developmentally based practice as opposed to a remedial "catch-up" model, and (3) better oriented to family-centered practices. Auditory-Verbal practitioners are more likely to be providing services in the families' homes to accommodate the family-focused orientation of working with infants and very young children, requiring a shift from center-based practices to home- and other family-centered environments (Morrison, 2017). Finally, the LSLS Cert. AVTs predicted that with earlier intervention in AVT, children will continue to attain levels of auditory and communication performance that will enable discharge from AVT earlier, resulting in shorter care durations and an increase in consulting/monitoring practices with families who have moved forward.

▪ *Global growth and social/linguistic/cultural diversity.* Global exposure to AVT will continue to increase with information coming from social media, online sources, and professional development provided by LSLS Cert. AVTs. In turn, global exposure will increase the demand for AVT globally. A need for greater social/linguistic/cultural diversity among practitioners and adaptation of AVT practices to best serve the variety of communities where AVT services are provided will be in tandem with a greater global presence of the LSLS Cert. AVT. In particular, there will be a need for LSLS Cert. AVTs who can serve families within various language communities and from various cultures. The LSLS Cert. AVTs surveyed also called for translation of the LSLS certification examination into more languages.

▪ *Telepractice.* The greatest number of comments regarding the evolution of AVT in the future indicated that telepractice will continue to increase. This is predicted to be due to the increase in families of infants and young children who receive home-based services as well as to the global desire for AVT in regions where there are too few or no Auditory-Verbal practitioners to serve families face-to-face. As described in Chapter 25, telepractice requires Auditory-Verbal practitioners to demonstrate additional skills to those applied in center-based practices. Several respondents predicted that telepractice will be instrumental in moving AVT forward because the interactions with the child are almost exclusively done by the parents, fostering family-centered intervention.

▪ *Expanded children's needs and interprofessional practice.* The trend toward serving more children with recurrent otitis media, slight hearing loss, and single-sided deafness will continue as outcomes demonstrate that these children benefit from intervention that supports auditory learning. More newborns will survive neonatal intensive care with hearing intervention needs. The evidence for effective intervention approaches for children with challenges in addition to hearing loss will continue to increase. Consequently, Auditory-Verbal practitioners will be applying a greater variety of strategies to meet the needs of this varied caseload. The LSLS Cert. AVTs also predicted that with a greater number of children with additional challenges on caseloads, there will be even greater need for interprofessional practice with disciplines such as occupational therapy, physical therapy, and psychotherapy, which are expert at children's developmental needs far beyond listening and spoken language.

■ *Training/increasing the number of LSLS Cert. AVTs.* With an increased number of children identified with hearing loss in the future and with a larger global demand for AVT, the need for more LSLS Cert. AVTs will continue to rise. The cohort of respondents to the survey called for increased training at the university level and for more coaches and mentors to help professionals join the global LSLS Cert. AVT community. The greater number of infants, very young children, family-centered services, increased social/linguistic/cultural diversity

in families, telepractice models, and children with additional needs will require Auditory-Verbal practitioners to re-tool to meet the future needs of families and their children who are deaf or hard of hearing. Professional development, coaching, and mentoring will continue as significantly important roles for Auditory-Verbal practitioners.

■ *Outcome research.* Numerous comments indicated a need for more evidence-based research and publication of studies in peer-reviewed journals to present evidence that supports AVT. One respondent summarized many comments well: "I hope to see our leaders and university professionals conduct more research to support the AVT, and this will only happen through methodical planning and training of new professionals."

Overall, the LSLS Cert. AVTs were hopeful and looking forward to the future of AVT. As one of the respondents put it, "We'll make the future. We must support one another in a caring and collaborative manner."

CONCLUSION

Auditory-Verbal practitioners and their allied health and educational professionals are working in partnership with parents to prepare their children who are deaf or hard of hearing to lead abundant and productive lives for today and for the future. As hearing technology and neuroscience continue to intersect to provide high-quality sound accessibility for children with hearing aids, cochlear implants, and other implantable devices, they are focusing on bringing AVT to families who desire the outcomes of listening and spoken language. Across the world, audiologists, speech-language pathologists, and teachers of children who are deaf or hard of hearing continue to seek training and education as Auditory-Verbal practitioners so that they can meet demands and face the dreams in collaboration with these families.

Through AVT, parents come to realize their children can learn to listen, learn to talk, learn to engage in robust, inspired, imaginative, and meaningful spoken conversations, and develop literacy and academic competencies comparable to their hearing peers—a reality more possible than ever before. We all strive together to advance the work of AVT and in doing so, we help eliminate barriers to equitable services for children who are deaf or hard of hearing. We value the knowledge that similarities as humans are equally as important as our cultural differences, and we welcome the timely opportunity to promote global kindness, compassion, respect, and gratitude in the spirit of community.

REFERENCES

Akhtar, N., Jipson, J., & Callanan, M. A. (2001). Learning words through overhearing. *Child Development, 72,* 416–430.

Alexander Graham Bell Academy for Listening and Spoken Language (2017). *Listening and Spoken Language Specialist Certified Auditory-Verbal Therapist (LSLS Cert. AVT®) Application Packet.* Retrieved May 22, 2019 from: https://agbellacad emy.org/wp-content/uploads/2018/10 /Certification-Handbook-1.pdf

A. G. Bell Association for the Deaf (2019). *Recommended protocol for audiological assessment, hearing aid and cochlear implant evaluation, and gollow-up.* Retrieved July 6, 2019 from https://www .agbell.org/Advocacy/Alexander-Gra ham-Bell-Associations-Recommended -Protocol-for-Audiological-Assessment -Hearing-Aid-and-Cochlear-Implant-Evalu ation-and-Follow-up

American Cochlear Implant Alliance (2015). *Position paper: Pediatric habilitation following cochlear implantation.* Retrieved July 6, 2019 from https://c.ymcdn.com /sites/acialliance.site-ym.com/resource /resmgr/Docs/ACI_Paper_Pediatric_Re hab.pdf

Auditory-Verbal International, Inc. (1994). *Auditory-verbal international principles and rules of ethics.* Washington, DC: AVI.

Auditory-Verbal International, Inc. (2003). *Auditory-verbal international standardized curriculum.* Washington, DC: AVI.

Auditory-Verbal Network, Inc. (1988). A parent's guide to auditory-verbal therapy. *Auditory-Verbal Network Newsletter, 5*(1), 1–4.

Beebe, H. (1953). *A guide to help the severely hard of hearing child.* New York, NY: Karger.

Bellis, T. J. (2011). *Assessment and management of central auditory processing disorders in the educational setting: From science to practice.* Clifton Park, NY: Delmar Learning.

Caleffe-Schenck, N. (1992). The auditory-verbal method: Description of a training program for audiologists, speech language pathologists, and teachers of children with hearing loss. *The Volta Review, 94*(1), 65–68.

Ching, T. Y., Dillon, H., Leigh, G., & Cupples, L. (2017). Learning from the longitudinal outcomes of children with hearing impairment (LOCHI) study: Summary of 5-year findings and implications. *International*

Journal of Audiology, 57 (suppl. 2), S105–S111.

Cole, E. B., & Flexer, C. A. (2011). *Children with hearing loss: Developing listening and talking, birth to six.* San Diego, CA: Plural Publishing.

Constantinescu-Sharpe, G., Phillips, R. L., Davis, A., Dornan, D., & Hogan, A. (2017). Social inclusion for children with hearing loss in listening and spoken language early intervention: An exploratory study. *BMC Pediatrics, 17*(1), 74.

Cowan, R. S., Edwards, B., & Ching, T. Y. (2018). Longitudinal outcomes of children with hearing impairment (LOCHI): 5-year data. *International Journal of Audiology, 57* (suppl. 2), S1–S2.

Dawes, L. (2014). *100 Years of deaf education and audiology at the University of Manchester.* Manchester, UK: University of Manchester Press. Retrieved July 6, 2019 from http://documents.manchester.ac.uk/display.aspx?DocID=23262

Dettman, S., Wall, E., Constantinescu, G., & Dowell, R. (2013). Communication outcomes for groups of children enrolled in auditory-verbal, aural-oral and bilingual-bicultural early intervention programs. *Otology & Neurotology, 34*, 451–459.

Dornan, D., Hickson, L., Murdoch, B., Houston, T., & Constantinescu, G. (2010). Is auditory-verbal therapy effective for children with hearing loss? *The Volta Review, 110*, 361–387.

Duncan, J., & Rhoades, E. A. (2017). Introduction to auditory-verbal practice. In E. A. Rhoades & J. Duncan (Eds.), *Auditory-verbal practice: Family centered early intervention* (pp. 5–19). Springfield, IL: Charles C. Thomas.

Engum, S. A., & Jeffries, P. R. (2012). Interdisciplinary collisions: Bringing healthcare professionals together. *Collegian, 19*(3), 145–151.

Ernst, M. (2012). What is an auditory-verbal treatment plan? In Estabrooks, W. (Ed.), *101 Frequently asked questions about auditory-verbal practice* (pp. 334–337). Washington, DC: A. G. Bell.

Estabrooks, W., MacIver-Lux, K., & Rhoades, E. (2016). *Auditory-verbal therapy for children with hearing loss and their families, and the practitioners who guide them.* San Diego, CA: Plural Publishing.

Fulcher, A., Purchell, A. A., Baker, E., & Munro, N. (2012). Listen up: Children with early identified hearing loss achieve age-appropriate speech/language outcomes by 3 years of age. *International Journal of Pediatric Otorhinolaryngology, 76*(12), 1785–1794.

Fuller, E. A., & Kaiser, A. P. (2019). The effects of early intervention on social communication outcomes for children with autism spectrum disorder: A meta-analysis. *Journal of Autism and Developmental Disorders*, 1–18.

Gallaudet Research Institute. (2011). *Regional and national summary report of data from the 2009–2010 annual survey of deaf and hard of hearing children and youth.* Retrieved June 9, 2019, from http://research.gallaudet.edu/Demographics/2010_National_Summary.pdf

Geers, A. E., Mitchell, C. M., Warner-Czyz, A., Wang, N. Y., Eisenberg, L. S., & CDaCI Investigative Team. (2017). Early sign language exposure and cochlear implantation benefits. *Pediatrics, 140*(1), e20163489.

Geers, A. E., Nicholas, J., Tobey, E., & Davidson, L. (2016). Persistent language delay versus late language emergence in children with early cochlear implantation. *Journal of Speech, Language, and Hearing Research, 59*(1), 155–170.

Goldberg, D. (1993). Auditory-verbal philosophy: A tutorial. *The Volta Review, 95*(3), 181–186.

Goldberg, D. M., & Flexer, C. (2012) What is the history of Auditory-Verbal practice? In W. Estabrooks (Ed.), *101 Frequently asked questions about Auditory-Verbal practice.* (pp. 6–9). Washington, DC: A. G. Bell.

Goldberg, D. M., & Talbot, P. J. (1993). The Larry Jarret House Program at the Helen Beebe Speech and Hearing Center. *The Volta Review, 95*(5), 91–96.

Goldblat, E., & Pinto, O. Y. (2017). Academic outcomes of adolescents and young adults with hearing loss who received auditory-verbal therapy. *Deafness & Education International, 19*(3–4), 126–133.

Goldstein, M. (1939). *The acoustic method for training the deaf and hearing impaired child.* St. Louis, MO: Laryngoscope Press.

Graham, F., Rodger, S., & Ziviani, J. (2009). Coaching parents to enable children's participation: An approach for working with parents and their children. *Australian Occupational Therapy Journal, 56*(1), 16–23.

Griffiths, C. (1964). The auditory approach for preschool deaf children. *The Volta Review, 66*(7), 387–397.

Griffiths, C. (1979). *Proceedings of the international conference on auditory techniques.* Pasadena, CA: HEAR Center.

Griffiths, C. (1991). *Hear: A four letter word.* Laguna Hills, CA: Wide Range Press

Griffiths, C., Horton, H. B., Stuwart, H., Gentenbein, A., Ling, D., & Northcott, W. H. (1973). The auditory approach. *The Volta Review, 75*(6), 344–372.

Hirsh, I. (1980). Psychological aspects of early auditory education. *Journal of the Royal Society of Medicine, 73,* 611–616.

Huizing, E. H. (2013). Hendrik Cornelis Huizing. *Audinews, the Newsletter of the International Society of Audiology, 13*(2), 1–2.

Joint Committee on Infant Hearing (JCIH). (2007). Year 2007 position statement: Principles and guidelines for early hearing detection and intervention programs. *Pediatrics, 120*(4), 898–921.

Joint Committee on Infant Hearing (JCIH). (2019). Year 2019 position statement: Principles and guidelines for early hearing detection and intervention programs. *Journal of Early Hearing Detection and Intervention, 4*(2), 1–44. doi: 10.15142 /fptk-b748

Kaipa, R., & Danser, M. L. (2016). Efficacy of auditory-verbal therapy in children with hearing impairment: A systematic review from 1993–2015. *International Journal of Pediatric Otorhinolaryngology, 86,* 124–134.

Kaiser, A. P., & Hancock, T. B. (2003). Teaching parents new skills to support their young children's development. *Infants & Young Children, 16*(1), 9–21.

Kaiser, A. P., & Roberts, M. Y. (2013). Parent-implemented enhanced milieu teaching with preschool children who have intellectual disabilities. *Journal of Speech, Language, and Hearing Research, 56*(1), 295–309.

Lake, S. B. (2001). The history of AVI. *The Listener,* 72–75.

Langereis, M., & Vermeulen, A. (2015). School performance and wellbeing of children with CI in different communicative-educational environments. *International Journal of Pediatric Otorhinolaryngology, 79*(6), 834–839.

Leffel, B. S., & Suskind, D. (2013). Parent-directed approaches to enrich the early language environments of children living in poverty. *Seminars in Speech and Language, 34*(4), 267–277.

Li, B., Soli, S. D., Zheng, Y., Li, G., & Meng, Z. (2014). Development of Mandarin spoken language after pediatric cochlear implantation. *International Journal of Pediatric Otorhinolaryngology, 78*(7), 1000–1009.

Liang, D., Xiao, Y., Feng, Y., & Yan, Y. (2014). The role of auditory feedback in speech production: Implications for speech perception in the hearing impaired. *2014 International Symposium on Integrated Circuits (ISIC).*

Ling, D. (1976, 2002). *Speech and the hearing-impaired child.* Washington, DC: A. G. Bell.

Ling, D. (1989). *Foundations of spoken language for hearing-impaired children.* Washington, DC: Alexander Graham Bell Association for the Deaf.

Ling, D. (1993). Auditory-verbal options for children with hearing impairment: Helping to pioneer an applied science. *The Volta Review, 95,* 187–196.

Ling, D., & Ling, A. H. (1978). *Aural habilitation: The foundations of verbal learning.*

Washington, DC: Alexander Graham Bell Association for the Deaf.

Marlowe, J. A. (1993). Audiological assessment and management in the auditory-verbal approach. *The Volta Review, 95,* 205–215.

Mashburn, A. J., Pianta, R. C., Hamre, B. K., Downer, J. T., Barbarin, O. A., Bryant, D., ... Howes, C. (2008). Measures of classroom quality in prekindergarten and children's development of academic, language, and social skills. *Child Development, 79*(3), 732–749.

McCreery, R. W., Walker, E. A., Spratford, M., Lewis, D., & Brennan, M. (2019). Auditory, cognitive, and linguistic factors predict speech recognition in adverse listening conditions for children with hearing loss. *Frontiers in Neuroscience, 13,* 1093. doi: 10.3389/fnins.2019.01093

Moeller, M. P., Carr, G., Seaver, L., Stredler-Brown, A., & Holzinger, D. (2013). Best practices in family-centered early intervention for children who are deaf or hard of hearing: An international consensus statement. *Journal of Deaf Studies and Deaf Education, 18*(4), 429–445.

Morrison, H. M. (2008). Auditory-verbal therapy: Principles, practices, outcomes. *Educational Audiology Review,* Fall, 22–26.

Morrison, H. M. (2017). Home visits. In E. Rhoades & J. Duncan (Eds.), *Auditory-verbal practice: Toward a family-centered approach* (pp. 266–285). New York, NY: Charles C. Thomas.

National Research Council and Institute of Medicine (2000). From neurons to neighborhoods: The science of early childhood development. In J. Shonkoff & D. Phillips (Eds.), *Board on children, youth, and families, commission on behavioral and social sciences and education.* Washington, DC: National Academies Press.

Percy-Smith, L., Cayé-Thomasen, P., Gudman, M., Jensen, J. H., & Thomsen, J. (2018). Self-esteem and social well-being of children with cochlear implant compared to normal-hearing children. *International Journal of Pediatric Otorhinolaryngology, 72*(7), 1113–1120.

Pollack, D. (1964). Acoupedics: A unisensory approach to auditory training. *The Volta Review,* September, 400–409.

Pollack, D. (1970). *Educational audiology for the limited hearing infant.* Springfield, IL: Charles C. Thomas.

Pollack, D. (1985). *Educational audiology for the limited hearing infant and preschooler.* Springfield, IL: Charles C. Thomas.

Pollack, D. (1993). Reflections of a pioneer. *The Volta Review, 95,* 197–204.

Pollack, D., & Ernst, M. (1973). Learning to listen in an integrated preschool. *The Volta Review,* 359–367.

Pollack, D., Goldberg, D., & Caleffe-Schenck, N. (1997). *Educational audiology for the limited hearing infant and preschooler.* Springfield, IL: Charles C. Thomas.

Potter, T. M. (2015). Partnership—imaging a new model in health care. *Journal of Radiology Nursing, 34*(2), 57–62.

Rhoades, E. A. (2001). Language progress with an auditory-verbal approach for young children with hearing loss. *International Pediatrics, 16*(1), 41–47.

Roberts, M. Y., Curtis, P. R., Sone, B. J., & Hampton, L. H. (2019). Association of parent training with child language development. *JAMA Pediatrics, 173*(7), 671–680. doi: 10.1001/jamapediatrics.2019.1197

Robertson, L. (2014). *Literacy and deafness: Listening and spoken language.* San Diego, CA: Plural Publishing.

Ruben, R. J. (2018). Language development in the pediatric cochlear implant patient. *Laryngoscope Investigative Otolaryngology, 3*(3), 209–213.

Scheerer, N. E., & Jones, J. A. (2018). The role of auditory feedback at vocalization onset and mid utterance. *Frontiers in Psychology, 9.*

Sharma, A., Glick, H., Campbell, J., Torres, J., Dorman, M., & Zeitler, D. M. (2016). Cortical plasticity and reorganization in pediatric single-sided deafness pre- and postcochlear implantation: A case study. *Otology & Neurotology, 37,* e26–e34.

Staab, W. (2017). From the audimeter to the audiometer. *Canadian Audiologist, 4*(3), 1–5.

Suskind, D. (2016). *Thirty million words: Building a child's brain: Tune in, talk more, take turns.* New York, NY: Dutton Books.

Suskind, D., & Leffel, K. (2013). Parent-directed approaches to enrich the early language environments of children living in poverty. *Seminars in Speech and Language, 34*(04), 267–278.

Tomblin, J. B., Oleson, J. J., Ambrose, S. E., Walker, E., & Moeller, M. P. (2014). The influence of hearing aids on the speech and language development of children with hearing loss. *JAMA Otolaryngology–Head & Neck Surgery, 140*(5), 403.

Turnbull, M. (2005). The life and times of Doreen Pollack. *The Listener,* 76–78.

Urbantschitsch, V. (1895). *Auditory training for deaf mutism and acquired deafness.* Washington, DC: A. G. Bell. Translated by Silverman, S. R. (1982).

Vygotsky, L. S., & Cole, M. (1981). *Mind in society: The development of higher psychological processes.* Cambridge, MA: Harvard University Press.

Walker, E. A., Holte, L., McCreery, R. W., Spratford, M., Page, T., & Moeller, M. P. (2015). The influence of hearing aid use on outcomes of children with mild hearing loss. *Journal of Speech, Language, and Hearing Research, 58*(5), 1611–1625.

Walker, E. A., Redfern, A., & Oleson, J. J. (2019). Linear mixed-model analysis to examine longitudinal trajectories in vocabulary depth and breadth in children who are hard of hearing. *Journal of Speech, Language, and Hearing Research, 62*(3), 525–542.

Warner-Czyz, A. D., Loy, B., Pourchot, H., White, T., & Cokely, E. (2018). Effect of hearing loss on peer victimization in school-age children. *Exceptional Children, 84*(3), 280–297.

Whetnall, E., & Fry, D. B. (1954). The auditory approach in the training of deaf children. *Lancet 266*(6812), 583–587.

Wiseman, K. B., & Warner-Czyz, A. D. (2018). Inconsistent device use in pediatric cochlear implant users: Prevalence and risk factors. *Cochlear Implants International, 19*(3), 131–141.

Yoshinaga-Itano, C. (2003). From screening to early identification and intervention: Discovering predictors to successful outcomes for children with significant hearing loss. *Journal of Deaf Studies and Deaf Education, 8*(1), 11–30.

Yoshinaga-Itano et al. (2017). Early hearing detection and vocabulary of children with hearing loss. *Pediatrics,* Epub August 2017, Retrieved from https://pediatrics.aappublications.org/content/140/2/e20162964

Appendix 1-A

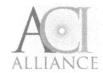

AMERICAN COCHLEAR IMPLANT ALLIANCE

Research. Advocacy. Awareness.

Position Paper: Pediatric Habilitation Following Cochlear Implantation

ABOUT US

The American Cochlear Implant Alliance (ACI Alliance) is a non-profit, 501(c)3 whose mission is to advance the gift of hearing by cochlear implantable prosthetic hearing implants through research, advocacy and awareness. The membership includes those who provide intervention (e.g., ENT surgeons, audiologists, speech-language pathologists), other professionals on implant teams (e.g., educators, psychologists, researchers), parents of children with cochlear implants, and other advocates. For more information: **www.acialliance.org.**

This document defines appropriate speech/language habilitation services for children following cochlear implantation. It provides a rationale based upon state-of-the-art research and clinical findings. Speech-language habilitation for children after cochlear implantation falls under the definition of "habilitative services" crafted in 2010 by the National Association of Insurance Commissioners. It defines habilitation, in part, as:

"Health care services that help a person keep, learn, or improve skills and functioning for daily living. Examples include therapy for a child who isn't walking or talking at the expected age."

RATIONALE

Recommendations are not based upon a single factor; but rather on evidence from five domains of knowledge and practice that reinforce one another and provide a compelling rationale. These are:

1. Independent research studies of children with cochlear implants have documented that, on average, these children receive one to two (1)-hour speech/language habilitation sessions per week (Dettman et al., 2013; Dornan et al., 2010; Rhoades, 2001). These findings apply to children who develop spoken language in synchrony with their hearing peers as well as those who demonstrate "catch up" growth. Domain: Clinical Outcomes Research

2. When a child with hearing loss demonstrates a delay in spoken language relative to his/her chronological age, the amount of habilitation time needed to close the gap is directly proportional to the delay. In other words, if a child receives amplification at 18 months, clinical experience suggests that it takes about three years of habilitation to achieve speech and language skills equivalent to a hearing peer (Flexer and Richards, 1998). Domain: Clinical Management Reports

3. Deafness causes a child's brain to re-organize in the absence of consistent auditory input. Without sound, areas of the brain designated as auditory centers are assigned to other sensory modalities, such as vision or touch. After stimulation of the auditory cortex of the brain via cochlear implants, there is urgency in providing rich and consistent auditory-based habilitation. Only limited time is available within the sensitive period of cortical development to intervene with habilitation (Gordon et.al.,2011; Kral, 2013; 2011; Sharma, Nash, & Dorman, 2009; Sharma & Campbell, 2011). Domain: Neuroplasticity Research

4. To achieve maximum benefit from cochlear implants, children need ongoing, consistent habilitation, rather than episodic services occurring as a result of a limited number of sessions allowed in a given benefit year. Experts in pediatric communication endorse the notion that professionals must use evidence and clinical decision making to individualize recommendations for each child (Bailes, Reder, & Burch, 2008). Major changes occur in children's communication skills over a period of four years—the last 2 years involve the most "catch up growth" (Lin, Niparko, & Francis 2009.). Domain: Habilitation Best Practices

5. When analyzed over a lifetime, children who are denied the benefits of cochlear implantation have demonstrated a dramatically disproportionate shortfall in quality of life relative to other disease states (Lindemark, Norheim, & Johansson, 2014). The negative economic impact of lifelong hearing loss, referred to as "societal cost of deafness," is reduced dramatically when interventions such as cochlear implants and appropriate follow-up habilitation are provided (Mohr et al., 2000; Lin, Niparko & Francis, 2009). The savings to society may be as high as one million dollars over the lifetime of an individual born with severe/profound hearing loss (Mohr et al., 2000). Domain: Health Economics Research

RECOMMENDED HABILITATION STANDARD

Based upon the published evidence reviewed above, 50 to 100 (1) hour speech/language habilitation sessions are recommended per year for pediatric cochlear implant users. Helping a child learn to understand and utilize the hearing benefit provided by a cochlear implant is a complex process that requires expertise and specialized training. Because of this, speech/language habilitation should be provided by a professional who is knowledgeable about the hearing and listening needs of the child with a cochlear implant. In order to obtain optimal outcomes, such habilitation typically involves provision of service and coordination by all professionals involved in a child's care. As each child is unique, health care providers will make individual recommendations as part of their management of the child. Some children may require fewer habilitation sessions, while others may require more.

REFERENCES

Bailes, A.F., Reder. R., & Burch. C. (2008). Development of guidelines for determining frequency of therapy services in a pediatric medical setting. *Pediatric Physical Therapy*. Summer; 20(2): 194-8.

Dornan D., Hickson, L, Murdoch, B., Houston, K.T. & Constantinescu, G. (2010). Is auditory-verbal therapy effective for children with hearing loss? *Volta Review*, 110 (3),361-387.

Dettman, S., Wall, E., Constantinescu, G., & Dowell, R. (2013). Communication outcomes for groups of children enrolled in auditory-verbal, aural-oral and bilingual-bicultural early intervention programs. *Otology & Neurotology*, 34, 451-459.

Flexer, C, & Richards, C. (1998). *We can hear and speak! The power of auditory-verbal communication for children who are deaf or hard of hearing*. Washington, DC: Alexander Graham Bell Association for the Deaf and Hard of Hearing.

Glossary of Health Insurance and Medical Terms. http://www.naic.org/documents/committees_b_consumer_information_ppaca_glossary.pdf

Gordon, K., Wong. D., Valero, J., Jewell, S., Yoo, P. & Papsin, B. (2011).Use it or lose it? Lessons learned from the developing brains of children who are deaf and use cochlear implants to hear. Brain Topography 24 (3-4), 204-219.

Kral, A. (2013). Auditory critical periods. A review from system's perspective. *Neuroscience*. 247, 117-133.

Lin, L.M., Niparko, J.K., & Francis, H.W. (2009). Outcomes in cochlear implantation assessment of quality of life impact and economic evaluation of the benefits of the CI in relation to costs. In Niparko, Kirk, & Robbins (Eds.), *Cochlear implants principles and practices*, (2nd ed.). Philadelphia: Lippincott Williams & Wilkins.

Lindemark, F., Norheim, O.F., & Johansson, K.A. (2014). Making use of equity sensitive QALYs: A case study on identifying the worse off across diseases. *Cost Effectiveness and Resource Allocation* 2014, 12:16

Mohr, P.E., Feldman, J.J., Dunbar J.L., Niparko, J.K., Robbins, A.M., Rittenhouse, R.K., & Skinner, M.W. (2000). The societal cost of severe to profound hearing loss in the United States. *International Journal of Technology Assessment in Health Care*, 16 (4), 1120-1135.

Niparko, J. (Ed.). (2009). Cochlear implants: Principles and practices, (2nd ed.). Philadelphia: Lippincott Williams & Wilkins.
Rhoades, E.A. (2001). Language progress with an auditory-verbal approach for young children with hearing loss. *International Pediatrics*, 16(1), 1-7.

Sharma, A., & Campbell, J. (2011). A sensitive period for cochlear implantation in deaf children. *Journal of Maternal, Fetal. Neonatal Medicine*, 24 (Suppl 1), 151-153.

Sharma A., Nash, A. A., & Dorman, M. (2009). Cortical development, plasticity, and re-organization in children with cochlear implants. *Journal of Communication Disorders* 42 (4), 272-9.

Authored by: Hannah R. Eskridge, MSP, CCC-SLP, LSLS Cert. AVT, Amy McConkey Robbins, MS, CCC-SLP, LSLS Cert. AVT, Kathryn Wilson, MA, CCC-SLP, LSLS Cert. AVT, Lindsay Zombek, MS, CCC-SLP, LSLS Cert. AVT

Approved by the Board of Directors, American Cochlear Implant Alliance, July 27, 2015

ACI ALLIANCE • P.O. BOX 103 • McLEAN, VA 22101-0103 • WWW.ACIALLIANCE.ORG • 703.534.6146

PEDS AUG15

2

AUDITORY BRAIN DEVELOPMENT AND AUDITORY-VERBAL THERAPY

Carol Flexer and Jace Wolfe

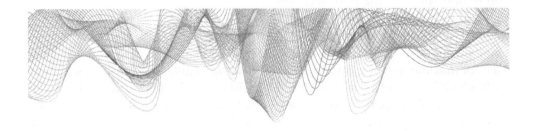

INTRODUCTION

Childhood hearing loss is a serious and relatively common condition. About 12,000 new babies with hearing loss are identified every year in the United States alone, according to the National Institute on Deafness and Other Communication Disorders. In addition, estimates are that in the same year, another 4,000 to 6,000 infants and young children between birth and 3 years of age who passed the newborn hearing screening test acquire late-onset hearing loss. The total population of new babies and toddlers identified with hearing loss, therefore, is about 16,000 to 18,000 per year. The problem is that hearing loss caused by damage or blockage in the outer, middle, or inner ear keeps auditory/linguistic information from reaching the child's brain, where actual hearing occurs.

In recent years, there has been an explosion of information and technology about testing for and managing hearing loss in infants and children, thereby enhancing their opportunities for auditory brain access that create neural pathways for spoken language, literacy, and social connections. What has happened in the field of hearing loss is truly revolutionary as we implement brain-based science. The historical and ongoing success of Auditory-Verbal Therapy (AVT) in attaining age-appropriate spoken communication outcomes has been due to the correct application of neural development principles—even though the specific neurological principles weren't known years ago, nor was the brain directly referred to early on.

So, why has the ecology of hearing loss changed? Newborn infant hearing screening programs, new hearing aid and remote microphone (RM) technologies, and cochlear implants have permitted critical brain centers access to auditory-linguistic information during times of maximum neuroplasticity. This early identification of hearing loss has allowed us to fit amplification technologies and cochlear implants on very young babies. We can now stimulate auditory brain centers that could not be reached with previous, less effective generations of amplification technologies. Family-focused auditory language enrichment can be provided during critical periods of maximum brain neural plasticity—the first few months and years of life.

Therefore, the purpose of this chapter is to discuss hearing loss and AVT from a brain-based perspective. Topics include definitions of terminology used by AV practitioners (practitioners), a detailed overview of auditory neural anatomy and physiology, discussions of recent outcomes research, and implications for current practices in AVT.

DEFINITIONS OF TERMINOLOGY USED BY AV PRACTITIONERS

Sound

Sound is an event, not a label (Boothroyd, 2019). For example, you don't hear Daddy if he is not moving. Daddy is heard in action, such as walking, talking, and singing. An action or an event creates vibrations. Vibrations are picked up by the "ear doorway," sent to the brain as energy for neural coding, and then perceived as information.

Five Senses

Discussion of the five human senses (hearing, sight, smell, taste, touch) can assist in developing a context for understanding hearing loss, beginning with the brain (Cole & Flexer, 2020). The brain is completely encased in bone with no direct access to the world. So, how does the brain control all aspects of the body's internal and external function? Our remarkable sensory organs capture different types of raw information from the environment and transform that raw data into chemoelectric and neuroelectric impulses that can be read by the brain. The sense organs are portals to the brain for environmental information. Consider the following examples:

Nose

The nose is the doorway to the brain for the sense of smell. The nose picks up olfactory molecules and changes those molecules into chemoelectric and neuroelectric impulses that can be processed by the brain. Knowing the meaning of the smell occurs in the brain, not in the nose. For example, when we sniff and smell a chocolate chip cookie, the nose doesn't know it's a cookie. The nose just randomly picks up environmental olfactory data. The brain receives this olfactory information, and through exposure, practice, and experience that include connecting that olfactory data to other parts of the brain, we come up with, "Oh, that's a cookie." A baby's dirty diaper is another example. Does the nose know a particular smell indicates a soiled diaper? Of course not. It is the brain that knows the baby has a diaper that needs changing because those olfactory molecules have been linked to the environmental exposure and experience of diapers.

Eyes

Adding another example, the eye is the portal to the brain for optic wavelengths, but knowing the meaning of what we see occurs in the brain. Knowing the visual image is a dog or a chair doesn't occur in the eye; the brain knows and learns the meaning of the visual event through exposure, practice, experience, and language. Seeing, like smelling, occurs in the brain.

Ears

What about the auditory doorway? The ear is the doorway to the brain for sound, for spoken language information, for talking, and for reading. Vibratory data are picked up by the ear, but understanding the meaning of those vibrations occurs in the brain. The ear doesn't know that particular vibrations

mean "Mommy" or "doorbell." Learning, and thus knowing, the meaning of auditory events occurs in the brain, not in the ear. Indeed, sound processing is one of the most computationally demanding tasks the nervous system has to perform (Kraus & White-Schwoch, 2019). The task relies on the exquisite timing of the auditory system, which responds to input more than 1,000 times faster than the photoreceptors in the visual system. Humans can hear faster than they can see, taste, smell, or feel.

Hearing Loss

Hearing loss can be thought of as a doorway problem (Cole & Flexer, 2020). Whether it's wax in the ears, fluid in the ears, or sensorineural hearing loss, there is some type and amount of obstruction in the ear doorway that prevents auditory environmental data from reaching the brain, where learning the meaning of that auditory information occurs. A small doorway obstruction might be labeled hard of hearing. A complete doorway obstruction might be called deaf. If auditory information does not reach the brain in sufficient quantity and quality, neural connections will not develop well, and the child's spoken language, literacy, and knowledge will be limited (Kral, 2013; Kral, Kronenberger, Pisoni, & O'Donoghue, 2016; Kral & Lenarz, 2015).

Purpose of Hearing Technology

Hearing aids and cochlear implants break through the doorway to allow access, stimulation, and development of auditory neural pathways. The choice of technology for a particular child who is deaf or hard of hearing depends on the nature of the doorway problem. The only purpose of these technologies and others such as RMs and classroom audio distribution systems is to capture auditory information from the environment, breach the doorway, and deliver auditory information to the brain for learning—there is no other purpose. If a child has a doorway problem and isn't wearing his or her technology, the brain is being deprived of auditory information—of knowledge. We can think of auditory technologies as brain access devices, not as ear devices.

Hearing and Listening

There is a distinction between hearing and listening. Hearing is acoustic access of auditory information to the brain. For children who are deaf or hard of hearing, hearing includes improving the signal-to-noise ratio by managing the environment and utilizing hearing technologies. Listening, on the other hand, is when the individual attends to acoustic events with intentionality. Sequencing is important. *Hearing (auditory information)* must be made available to the brain before *listening* can be learned and understanding developed. That is, parents and practitioners can focus on developing the child's listening skills, strategies, and choices only after the pediatric audiologist channels acoustic information to the brain by fitting and programming technologies—not before.

New Context for the Word *Deaf*

Today, hearing aids, cochlear implants, and RM technologies can allow the brains of infants and children with even the most profound hearing loss/deafness to access the entire speech spectrum. There is no degree of hearing loss that prohibits the brain's access to auditory information if cochlear implants are available. Degree of hearing loss as a limiting factor in auditory acuity is now an "old" acoustic conversation. That is, when one uses the word *deaf*, the implication is that one's brain has no access to auditory information, period. The word *deaf* in 1970, in 1980, or even in 1990, occurred in a very different context than the word *deaf* as used today. Today's child who is deaf (closed doorway) but who is given appropriate hearing aids or cochlear implants early in life can actually receive enough auditory information to perceive and understand spoken language—if the device is programmed well, if it is worn at least 10 hours per day (12 hours is better), and if the child is in an auditory and spoken language enriched environment (Ching, Dillon, Leigh, & Cupples, 2018; McCreery et al., 2015). This means that his or her brain can be developed with meaningful sound—that is, with auditory-linguistic information. That child is deaf without his or her hearing technologies to breach the doorway but certainly does not function as deaf in the 1970, 1980, or 1990 sense, because the child has developed a hearing and listening brain. Perhaps we need some new words because the context has changed.

OVERVIEW OF AUDITORY ANATOMY AND PHYSIOLOGY

The human auditory system may be roughly categorized into two sections, the peripheral and the central auditory nervous systems. The peripheral auditory system comprises the external ear (the auricle and external auditory meatus), the middle ear (the middle ear space, middle ear ossicles and muscles, and Eustachian tube), the inner ear (cochlea), and the cochlear nerve. Figure 2–1 provides a visual representation of the peripheral auditory system.

The primary function of the peripheral auditory system is to deliver auditory information to the central auditory nervous system. The external ear serves to collect sound, in the form of vibrations, and deliver it to the tympanic membrane. The middle ear converts

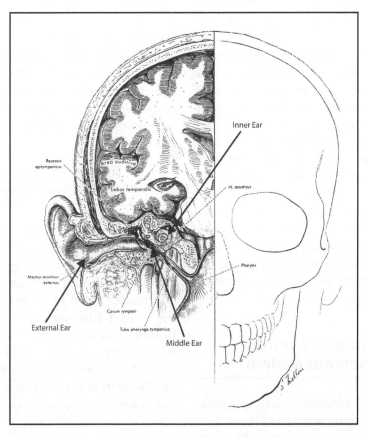

Figure 2–1. An illustration of the peripheral auditory system within the temporal bone of the skull. (Based on Melloni, 1957) Modified from *Hearing: Anatomy, Physiology, and Disorders of the Auditory System, Third Edition.* Copyright © 2013 Plural Publishing, Inc. All rights reserved.

acoustic energy into mechanical energy and efficiently delivers the mechanical energy to the cochlea. The inner ear converts the mechanical energy into neuro-chemical signals that elicit neuroelectric responses in the cochlear nerve. The cochlear nerve then delivers the neuro-electric potentials to the central auditory nervous system.

The structure and function of the peripheral auditory system is fascinatingly intricate, complex, and sophisticated. However, the peripheral auditory system is not ultimately responsible for our ability to perceive and then to understand sound. The peripheral auditory system does not allow sound to come to life and possess higher-order meaning. On its own, the peripheral auditory system does not allow us to understand speech and other environmental sounds, enjoy music, determine the origin of sound, or make sense of the acoustic signals that surround every minute of our day. Instead, our ability to perceive, experience, understand, and enjoy the sounds of life is governed by the processing that takes place within the central auditory nervous system. Again, we listen with our brains. The ears are simply the doorway to the brain for auditory information.

Central Auditory Nervous System

The central auditory system comprises several components (see Figure 2–2). The cochlear nerve carries auditory signals to the cochlear nucleus, a group of auditory neurons that reside in the pons of the brainstem. The auditory nervous system pathway extends upward from the cochlear nuclei through a group of auditory fibers known as the lateral lemnisci within the pons. The axonal fibers of the lateral lemnisci terminate at the inferior colliculi, a group of auditory neurons in the midbrain of the brainstem. Then, the auditory pathway extends to the medial geniculate bodies, a group of auditory neurons in the thalamus. Finally, the auditory signals are transmitted from the thalamus to the auditory cortex within the brain. The auditory structures within the brainstem and thalamus play several important roles, including transmission of auditory information to the brain, localization, refinement and coding of sound so that neural messages are enhanced for optimal processing by the auditory cortices, etc. However, the vast majority of processing that is responsible for our comprehension of sound takes place within the brain.

Primer on Basic Brain Anatomy

Practitioners and educators who work with children who are deaf or hard of hearing should possess a good understanding of how the brain processes and makes sense of sound as well as the impact that untreated congenital hearing loss has on the brain's ability to derive meaning from sound. A basic tutorial on brain anatomy helps to lay the foundation for a discussion of how the brain processes sound.

Basic Brain Anatomy

The brain is divided into two halves called cerebral hemispheres. The frontal lobe is the largest lobe of the brain and is responsible for governing a variety of

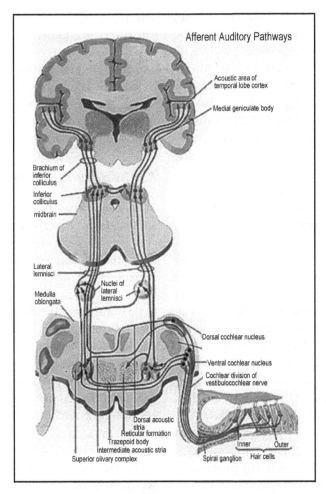

Figure 2-2. A visual representation of the auditory nervous system from the cochlea to the auditory cortex (as illustrated by Frank Netter). From Hall (1992), *Handbook of Auditory Evoked Responses* (p. 4). Copyright 1992. Reprinted with permission.

important functions. The frontal lobe serves many cognitive functions, including higher-order thinking, executive function, reasoning, intelligence, decision making, problem solving, impulse control, abstract thinking, formation of memories, emotional expression and regulation, managing attention, regulation of personality, etc. (see Andreatta, 2020, for overview). Also, the inferior prefrontal cortex, which includes Broca's region, has been shown to play an important role in speech production, speech perception, and reading. When an individual suffers an injury to Broca's region (e.g., a stroke), she/he often experiences difficulty producing intelligible speech. Broca's region has also been shown to play an important role in phonemic awareness (i.e., an understanding of the sound-to-letter relationship; the "B" says / buh / and the "D" says /duh /). Additionally, the posterior portion of the frontal lobe houses the motor cortex and is responsible for regulating motor function across the body, including speech movements.

The parietal lobe contains the primary sensory cortex and is responsible for somatosensory sensation (i.e., the sense of touch, tactile sensation, pain, etc.). The parietal cortex also plays a role in synthesizing and integrating the input from all of our sensory systems. Furthermore, the parietal lobe most likely contributes to higher-order cognitive functions (but to a much lesser extent than the frontal lobe), such as attention, memory, etc. The occipital lobe is located at the back of the brain. The primary function of the occipital lobe is to process visual information.

The temporal lobe is located below and slightly behind the frontal lobe, below the parietal lobe, and in front of the occipital lobe. The temporal lobe is primarily responsible for processing auditory stimuli. However, it is important to recognize that auditory stimuli are also processed in regions outside the temporal lobe.

Primary Auditory Cortex

The auditory cortex may be divided into two regions, the primary auditory cortex and the secondary auditory cortex (Moore, 2007). The primary auditory cortex cannot be seen well from a surface view of the brain. However, when parts of the frontal and parietal lobes are removed, the primary auditory cortex, which resides within a ridge of brain tissue (i.e., gyrus) known as Heschl's gyrus, may be viewed clearly.

The main function of the primary auditory cortex likely involves the processing and analysis of the acoustical features/characteristics (e.g., spectral/ frequency/pitch, temporal, and intensity properties) that represent the infinite number of sounds to which we are exposed on a daily basis.

Secondary Auditory Cortex

The secondary auditory cortex is not as well defined as the primary auditory cortex. The secondary auditory cortex is thought to consist of several gyri that surround the primary auditory cortex like a belt. Structures that are thought to be comprised by the secondary auditory cortex include the superior temporal gyrus, supramarginal gyrus, angular gyrus, planum temporale, insula, medial temporal gyrus, inferior temporal gyrus, the inferior pre-central and post-central gyri, and the posterior-inferior frontal gyrus. Of note, Wernicke's area (Brodmann area #42) resides within the secondary auditory cortex. An injury to Wernicke's area, such as a stroke, typically results in the affected individual's inability to comprehend speech.

The secondary auditory cortex most likely serves two primary purposes, (1) as a "launching pad" that distributes auditory information from the auditory cortex to the rest of the brain, and (2) to provide feedback from higher-order areas of the brain (e.g., frontal lobe, parietal lobe) back to primary auditory cortex to optimize the latter's ability to analyze ("tune in") to the most relevant properties of the auditory signal (i.e., signal of interest) and inhibit ("tune out") the less important parts of the auditory stimulus (i.e., the "competing noise").

Intrahemispheric Fiber Tracts

Information processed within the auditory pathway does not simply terminate within the auditory cortices. Instead, auditory information is distributed throughout the rest of the brain so that it can be integrated with the information from other sensory systems and can "come to life" and process higher-order meaning. Intrahemispheric fiber tracts deliver information from one area within one hemisphere of the brain to another area within the same hemisphere. For instance, the arcuate fasciculus is an important intrahemispheric tract that transmits auditory information from the secondary auditory cortex to the frontal lobe. Intrahemispheric fiber tracts allow for the formation of broad and complex neural networks, which allow neural information to be processed across the entire brain. Of note, intrahemispheric tracts should not be confused with interhemispheric tracts, which are fibers that deliver information between the two hemispheres of the brain (i.e., the corpus callosum).

Conscious Thought Represented as Patterns of Neural Activities

Kyle Kai-How Farh, M.D. (2019), states, "Everything that comes into our minds reduces to patterns of neural activities." In other words, every sensory stimulus we encounter elicits its own unique response from a unique set of neurons across the brain. With regard to the auditory system, every specific and unique sound we perceive is associated with its own similarly specific and unique pattern of firing neurons that are stimulated by and respond to the sound we perceive. Figure 2–3 provides an elementary and grossly oversimplified illustration of the pattern of neural activities (i.e., neuronal responses) that may occur throughout the brain when a listener hears the word "blue" in a conversation. In this example, the stars are intended to represent specific neurons that respond to the word "blue." As shown, a robust neuronal response is seen in the primary and secondary auditory cortices, but neurons also fire in higher-order areas such as the parietal lobe and especially in the frontal lobe.

The neurons firing in the primary auditory cortex are likely processing the acoustical information in the individual elements (/buh/, /luh/, /oo/) that make up the word "blue." The neurons firing in the secondary auditory cortex are most likely involved in the processing that is necessary to perceive the word (i.e., a single auditory unit) "blue" from the individual acoustic phonemes that make up the word. The firing of neurons in the frontal lobe as well as the parietal lobe and occipital lobes allows the sound to come to life and take on a higher-order meaning. The activity in the frontal lobe is what allows the listener to determine whether she/he likes or dislikes the color blue. The responses in the inferior prefrontal cortex facilitates awareness of the phonemic units of blue, which supports the ability to read the word blue when the letters are seen in print and say the word blue when speaking. Activity in neurons in and around the occipital lobe allows the listener to see the color blue in her/his mind's eye. Activity across the brain allows the listener to derive meaning from

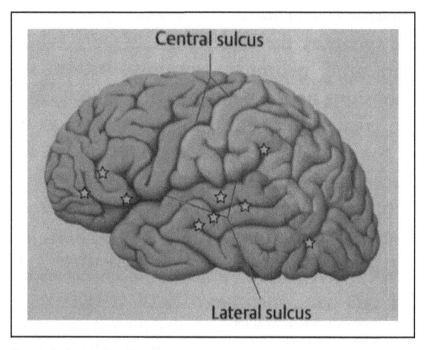

Figure 2–3. An oversimplified visual representation of neurons responding to the word "blue" when spoken in a conversation. The stars are intended to represent neural activity. From S. C. Bhatnagar, *Neuroscience for the Study of Communicative Disorders, Second Edition.* Lippincott Williams & Wilkins (2001).

the word blue. Hearing the word blue in conversation may cause the listener to think of a lake, the Cookie Monster, an afternoon sky on a sunny day, or a sad and depressing disposition. Responses within the frontal lobe and other centers of the brain that are involved in processing and regulating emotions, memories, and opinions may cause the listener to have a wide range of thoughts, including, "Who would wear blue lipstick?", "I love the color blue," or "I need to visit my grandmother because she has been blue lately!"

The more compelling, meaningful, or provocative a conversation, the more likely it is that a more robust pattern of neural activity will be elicited in response to the stimulus. Figure 2–4 provides a contrived example of the pattern of neural firings that may occur when a listener hears a chef talk about the best way to perfectly prepare fajitas. As shown, a larger number of neurons respond in this scenario compared with the response to the word blue. When hearing the sound of the sizzling fajita chicken, the listener can likely close her/his eyes and see an image of fajitas on a serving tray in her/his mind's eye. The engagement of higher-order areas of the brain may cause the listener's stomach to grumble because she/he begins to think about how much she/he would like to eat fajitas for lunch. However, frontal lobe activity may also cause the listener to think that she/he should go easy on the cheese and sour

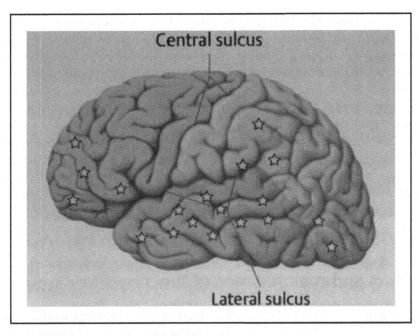

Figure 2-4. An oversimplified visual representation of neurons responding to a lesson on making the perfect fajita as it sizzles in a frying pan. The stars are intended to represent neural activity. From S. C. Bhatnagar, *Neuroscience for the Study of Communicative Disorders, Second Edition.* Lippincott Williams & Wilkins (2001).

cream in order to comply with her/his Weight Watchers diet plan.

Of note, the pattern of neural responses seen in the two scenarios above are unique. As Dr. Farh said, "Everything that comes into our minds reduces to a pattern of neural activities." These patterns of neural firings to "blue" and "sizzling fajitas" are uniquely associated with each of the individual auditory objects. Similarly, every sound we encounter evokes its own unique pattern of neural activities.

Neural Networks

Neural circuits, synaptogenesis, and neural networks describe the manner in which groups of neurons work together to convert sensory stimuli into complex perceptions and thoughts. **Neural circuits** describe groups of neurons that are interconnected through numerous synapses to execute a particular function (e.g., process the acoustical features that make up a speech token, decode the acoustical features into auditory objects). A synapse is the functional connection that exists between two neurons. Synaptogenesis refers to development of synapses (i.e., the development of functional connections between neurons). Synaptogenesis establishes the connections that serve as the foundation from which neural circuits are formed. Synaptogenesis is particularly prevalent during the first few years of a child's life. Strong synapses are formed between neurons that are frequently stimulated during the early years of life. Neurons that are not stimulated may be eliminated through a process called **pruning**.

Neural networks comprise a number of neural circuits that are interconnected via synapses and intrahemispheric fiber tracts. Consistent with Kai-How Farh's premise that "everything that comes into our minds reduces to a pattern of neural activities," neural networks manifest through a pattern of neural firings that occur across the different functional centers of the brain as we process sensory stimuli into perceptual thought.

The Connectome

The concept of neural networks may be expanded further to include the concept of a neural connectome. Kral et al. (2016) define a **connectome** as a "network map of effective synaptic connections and neural projections that comprise a nervous system and shape its global communication and integrative functions." Kral and colleagues make a compelling case that the development of the brain's connectome is dependent on the sensory stimulation children receive during their first two to three years of life. When auditory deprivation occurs during the critical period of listening and spoken language development, the auditory neural circuits and networks that contribute to the formation of the connectome develop atypically and form atypical connections throughout the brain. This atypical development of the connectome negatively affects both auditory and non-auditory func-

tions. For instance, auditory deprivation may lead to more robust connections within and across other sensory systems that are intact during the critical period of development, causing reorganization and weakening of the areas of the brain that are typically associated with processing the input from the impaired sensory system, and a potential for cross-modal reorganization occurs (e.g., use of the secondary auditory cortex to process visual and/or somatosensory information rather than auditory information).

The reorganization and restructuring that occur within the areas of the brain associated with the auditory deprivation (e.g., changes in the auditory cortices in the case of congenital hearing loss) as well as other areas of the brain are likely to lead to a disruption in developmental processes beyond those associated with auditory function. As a result, unmanaged congenital hearing loss threatens not only listening and spoken language development, but subsequently also the development of numerous other non-auditory functions, including cognition.

Figure 2–5 provides a visual representation (adapted from Kral et al., 2016) of the auditory component of the brain's connectome. The proposed "connectome model of deafness" illustrates the manner in which the development of neural circuits extending from and to the auditory cortices may potentially influence the development of a variety of higher-order tasks that are mediated in other brain areas, including but not limited to executive function, sensory integration, working memory, attention, motor planning, sequence processing, object identification and concept formation, social pragmatics, etc.

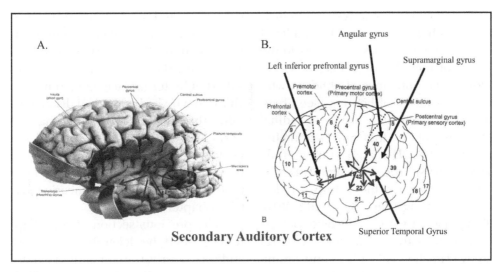

Figure 2-5. An illustration of the auditory component of the brain's connectome. From S. C. Bhatnagar, *Neuroscience for the Study of Communicative Disorders, Second Edition.* Lippincott Williams & Wilkins (2001).

Executive Function

Executive function (see Chapter 14) refers to the mental processes that enable individuals to plan and undertake volitional activities, focus attention, follow instructions, and successfully execute multiple tasks in sequence or in tandem (Barkley, 2012). Publications have shown deficits in executive function of children who are deaf or hard of hearing (Botting et al., 2017; Figueras, Edwards, & Langdon, 2008). Research with children who are deaf or hard of hearing has also shown an increased incidence of sensory processing disorder (Allen & Casey, 2017), delays in working memory (Nittrouer, Caldwell-Tarr, Low, & Lowenstein, 2017), and potential deficits in domains that influence social pragmatics, such as Theory of Mind (Netten et al., 2017). In short, the work reviewed above and numerous other research studies have indicated that congenital hearing loss has a cascading effect that extends beyond delays in spoken communication. Auditory deprivation during the critical period of language development impairs the growth of auditory neural circuits and networks, resulting in disruption of the neural connectome that supports listening and spoken language development and a number of other cognitive and behavioral functions. Congenital hearing loss truly is a neurodevelopmental emergency.

SUMMARY OF KEY STUDIES ABOUT THE IMPORTANCE OF EARLY AUDITORY BRAIN DEVELOPMENT ON LISTENING AND SPOKEN LANGUAGE OUTCOMES

The importance of providing children who are deaf or hard of hearing with early and consistent access to intelligible speech is reflected in the results of brain imaging studies as well as in the results of a number of recent studies exploring the outcomes of children who are deaf or hard of hearing (see Chapter 3). In particular, the Longitudinal Outcomes of Children with Hearing Impairment (LOCHI) study (Ching et al., 2013, 2018), the Childhood Development after Cochlear Implantation (CDaCI) study (Niparko et al., 2010; Tobey et al., 2013), the Outcomes of Children with Hearing Impairment (OCHL) study (Moeller et al., 2015), and a number of studies published by researchers from Melbourne, Australia have all provided impressive data that illustrate the vital importance of the early provision of hearing technology for children who are deaf or hard of hearing. In short, the latest research on the impact of age at implantation on the outcomes of children with congenital severe to profound hearing loss suggests that age-appropriate listening and spoken language outcomes are **probable** when children who are deaf or hard of hearing receive their cochlear implants prior to 12 months of age (Ching et al., 2018; Dettman et al., 2016; Hoff et al., 2019; Leigh et al., 2016). For instance, Dettman et al. (2016) reported that 81% of children implanted prior to 12 months of age had achieved typical vocabulary development when measured at 5 to 6 years old, whereas only 52% achieved typical vocabulary development when implanted between 13 to 18 months of age. Similarly, Hoff et al. (2019) reported that 88% of children implanted prior to 12 months communicated exclusively through listening and spoken language, whereas only 48% of children implanted between 13 and 37 months

communicated solely through the use of listening and spoken communication. Of note, the LOCHI researchers also found that early implantation resulted in better language outcomes for children who had additional disabilities other than hearing loss, a finding that particularly highlights the critical importance of early brain access to sound for children who are dealing with multiple challenges aside from hearing loss (see Chapter 22).

The previous section of this chapter described the deleterious impact of auditory deprivation on auditory brain development. The Dettman and Hoff studies highlight the detrimental impact of auditory deprivation on listening and spoken language outcomes. However, these studies also provide good news. When pediatric audiologists provide early brain access to intelligible speech by the appropriate fitting of hearing technologies and practitioners coach caregivers to create a language-rich listening environment, age-appropriate listening and spoken language outcomes aren't just possible, they are probable! Table 2–1 provides a brief summary of some recent studies exploring the impact of early intervention for children who are deaf or hard of hearing.

FAMILY-FOCUSED LANGUAGE ENRICHMENT: A CRITICAL VARIABLE FOR OUTCOME SUCCESS

The prompt and early provision of appropriately selected and fitted hearing technology is the first step toward ensuring optimal auditory brain devel-

Table 2–1. Summary of Studies Exploring the Effect of Age at Implantation on Listening and Spoken Language Outcomes

Study	Characteristics	Findings
Ching et al., 2013, *Ear and Hearing*	• 451 children with hearing loss who received hearing aid or CI prior to 3 years of age • Evaluated listening and spoken language outcomes at 3 years of age • 134 children with CIs	• Children implanted prior to 12 months achieved better language outcomes • Language aptitude decreased approximately ½ standard deviation for every 6-month delay in implantation after 6 months of age
Ching et al., 2018, *International Journal of Audiology*	• Evaluated listening and spoken language outcomes at 3 years of age • *n* = 39 children • 37% of children had additional disabilities other than hearing loss	• Children fitted with hearing aids at an early age achieved better language outcomes than children fitted at later ages • Children implanted prior to 12 months achieved better language outcomes • Language aptitude decreased approximately ½ standard deviation for every 6-month delay in implantation after 6 months of age • Children with additional disabilities achieved better outcomes when implanted at earlier ages
Dettman et al., 2016, *Otology and Neurotology*	• 403 children with CIs • Received CI prior to 6 years of age • Congenital severe to profound bilateral hearing loss • 151 children implanted before 12 months old • Evaluated listening and spoken language outcomes at school-age entry	• Children implanted before 12 months of age achieved better language, vocabulary, speech perception, and speech production than children implanted after 12 months • 81% of children implanted before 12 months achieved normal vocabulary development

continues

Table 2–1. *continued*

Study	Characteristics	Findings
Leigh et al., 2016, *International Journal of Audiology*	• 78 children with CIs and 62 children with hearing aids • Received CIs prior to 3 year of age • Identify optimal age at implantation • Define audiometric criteria to identify infants who need CIs	• Extent of language delay roughly corresponded to age at implantation • Children implanted at 6 months of age had little to no language delay • Children implanted prior to 12 months old had better language outcomes • Age at implantation explained 67% of variance in language outcomes • 75% of children with CIs achieved better aided word recognition than children who used hearing aids and had pure tone average of 60 dB HL or worse
Chu et al., 2016	• 165 children who received CI before 7 years of age	• Children who received CI before 12 months of age achieved better language outcomes • Children who received CI before 12 months of age needed less language therapy than children implanted after 12 months of age
CdaCI Niparko et al., 2010, *Journal American Medical Association* Tobey et al., 2013, *International Journal of Audiology*	• Multiple-center study evaluating language outcomes of 188 children with CIs • Received CI prior to 5 years of age	• Earlier age at implantation associated with better language outcomes
Hoff et al., 2019, *Otology and Neurotology*	• 219 children with CIs • 39 received CI before 12 months • 180 received CI after 12 months	• 88.2% of children implanted prior to 12 months communicate solely via spoken language • 48.2% of children implanted after 12 months communicated solely via spoken language • No increase in medical complications

Note: CDaCI = Childhood Development after Cochlear Implantation; CI = cochlear implant.

opment and listening and spoken language outcomes for children who are deaf or hard of hearing. After receiving hearing aids and/or cochlear implants, children who are deaf or hard of hearing must have access to an environment that is replete with intelligible and elaborate spoken language. The LOCHI, CDaCI, OCHL, and Melbourne studies have also identified a variety of factors other than the early provision of hearing technology that influence the outcomes achieved by children who are deaf or hard of hearing. Three of these factors will be discussed here.

Factor One: The Spoken Word Is the Nutrition that Grows the Auditory Brain

Several studies have explored the impact of the type of intervention (e.g., communication mode) provided to a child on the outcomes achieved by children who are deaf or hard of hearing. The LOCHI study examined language outcomes measured at 3 and 5 years of age for children using cochlear implants and hearing aids and found better language outcomes for children who communicated solely through listening and spoken language compared with children who used sign language (Ching et al., 2013, 2018).

Researchers from the University of Melbourne reported that median language outcomes of school-age children who communicated exclusively via listening and spoken language were almost one standard deviation better than those of children who communicated via the added use of sign to spoken language (Chu et al., 2016). Likewise, Dettman et al. (2013) found significantly

better open-set speech recognition in children who received intervention in AVT programs relative to children who received intervention from other listening and spoken language programs. Additionally, the speech recognition of the children in these programs was significantly better than that of children who received intervention in programs that encouraged the use of sign and spoken language.

The CDaCI also explored the effect of communication mode on the spoken language and reading comprehension outcomes of children with cochlear implants (Geers et al., 2017). Specifically, Geers and colleagues examined outcomes for children whose families communicated solely via listening and spoken language, children whose families used sign language prior to cochlear implantation and for no more than 12 months thereafter (i.e., short-term use), and children whose families used sign language prior to implantation and for at least 36 months thereafter. Spoken language and reading comprehension skills were significantly better for the children who communicated exclusively with listening and spoken language compared with the children in the short- and long-term sign language groups. Specifically, only 23% of the children in the listening and spoken language group had reading comprehension delays, whereas over 50% of the children in the sign language groups exhibited delays in reading comprehension.

Taken collectively, the results of the LOCHI, Melbourne, and CDaCI studies indicate that better language, auditory, and literacy outcomes are achieved by children who are deaf or hard of hearing when their caregivers and educators focus on maximizing an auditorily focused language-rich listening environment teeming with intelligible spoken language. These findings of the LOCHI, Melbourne, and CDaCI studies should not come as a surprise when considered within the context of auditory brain development. Developments of the auditory areas of the brain, neural networks, the neural connectome, and synaptogenesis are all optimized by early, rich, and frequent auditory stimulation. Intelligible speech is the optimal fertilizer to grow the auditory brain. An intervention approach, specifically AVT, that facilitates the family's and interventionists' collective focus on optimizing a child's exposure to a robust model of audition-centered language is the most effective method to achieve optimal auditory brain development and listening and spoken language outcomes for children who are deaf or hard of hearing.

Factor Two: Mom and Dad Matter!

The LOCHI, CDaCI, OCHL, and Melbourne studies have identified several other family-specific factors that impact the outcomes of children who are deaf or hard of hearing. The OCHL researchers reported that better outcomes were found for children whose caregivers communicated with the use of high-quality, rich, complex, and expansive spoken utterances compared with those whose caregivers communicated with simpler direct utterances (Ambrose et al., 2015). The OCHL researchers concluded that some caregivers may need more coaching and "support to provide their children with optimal language learning environments."

Similarly, Melbourne researchers found better language outcomes for children whose families had higher levels of involvement in the child's intervention. Moreover, the LOCHI and CDaCI studies found better language outcomes for children whose families had higher socioeconomic levels and whose mothers had higher educational levels (Ching et al., 2013, 2018; Eisenberg et al., 2016; Markman et al., 2011; Niparko et al., 2010).

Factor Three: Eyes Open, Ears (Brains) On

It has been established that we listen with the brain, the ears are the doorway to the brain for auditory information (Flexer, 2017), and hearing loss blocks sound from entering the doorway. Hearing aids and cochlear implants are the keys that allow sound to access the brains of children who are deaf or hard of hearing, and without full-time use of hearing aids and/or cochlear implants, children who are deaf or hard of hearing will experience at least some extent of auditory deprivation that will potentially lead to irreparable changes in brain development and poorer listening and spoken language skills.

Tomblin et al. (2015) examined the effect of hearing aid wear time on the language outcomes of children with mild to severe hearing loss. Children who used their hearing aids for more than 10 hours per day had age-appropriate language outcomes, whereas children who used their hearing aids for less than 10 hours per day had language outcomes that were approximately 1/2 standard deviation poorer than those who used their hearing aids for greater than

10 hours. The poorer outcomes of the children who had less daily wear time are most likely due to auditory deprivation associated with insufficient audibility without the use of hearing aids.

Guerzoni and Cuda (2017) examined the impact of cochlear implant wear time on the auditory, linguistic, and social development of children who received cochlear implants during their first 2 years of life. Better auditory and linguistic skills were observed in children whose data logging records indicated more hours of exposure to speech while using the cochlear implant. Indeed, one would expect the consequences of infrequent use of a cochlear implant to be even greater than those of infrequent hearing aid use given the probability that children with cochlear implants are more likely to have greater levels of hearing loss, and consequently be unable to experience sufficient stimulation of the auditory areas of the brain without the use of hearing technology.

BRAIN IMPLICATIONS FOR CURRENT AVT

Practitioners have always followed brain-based principles in a family-focused approach, even before the strategies used across most AVT programs were authenticated by scientific research. As detailed in the white paper "Start with the Brain and Connect the Dots" on the Hearing First website, the Logic Chain is a model that summarizes what we know, at this point in time, about the foundational components necessary to create a listening, speaking, and reading brain—components that are critical to AVT

(Flexer, 2017). The Logic Chain represents a system of foundational structures that must ALL be in place to optimize the attainment of age-appropriate listening, spoken language, and literacy skills, if that is the family's desired outcome. No link can be skipped.

Components of the Logic Chain that optimize AVT as discussed in this chapter include: Brain Development, General Infant/Child Language Development in the Family's Home Language, Early and Consistent Use of Hearing Technologies, Family-Focused Early Intervention following the principles of AVT, and Early Intervention for Literacy Development.

Practical Applications for AVT

Conversations with families and colleagues about AVT and the brain can be practical and logical (Cole & Flexer, 2020) (see Chapter 1). Below are some suggestions for a conversational sequence:

- Establish, through counseling, that the family has listening and spoken language as desired outcomes for their child.
- Then, from the very start of AVT, discuss the concept that we hear, listen, and understand auditory information with the brain; the ears are the way in.
- Next, describe hearing loss as a doorway problem.
- Then, emphasize that the only purpose of hearing technologies is to break through the doorway to deliver auditory information to the brain for neural integration and for the growth of knowledge.

- Stress that hearing technologies must be fit for maximum audibility; they must ensure that every speech sound reaches the brain at soft conversational levels.

- Next, it is imperative that hearing technologies are fit as early as possible in the first weeks of life and worn every waking moment for at least 10 to 12 hours per day . . . eyes open, technology on, in order to reduce auditory neural deprivation.

- Critically, the child with a doorway problem must be in an enriched, family-focused auditory-linguistic environment like AVT; the brain requires a great deal of auditory practice and auditory information—auditory-verbal nutrition—in order to grow and integrate neural connections for the development of knowledge.

- Finally, it is suggested that practitioners refer repeatedly to the family's stated desired outcome when explaining the reason for recommendations. For example, one can explain to the family that to increase the probability of attaining the family's desired outcome of listening and spoken language for their child, the child's technology (e.g., hearing aids, cochlear implants) must be worn at least 10 to 12 hours per day in order to develop the auditory brain.

It is recommended that practitioners include ongoing, embedded "Brain Conversations" with the child and family as part of every AVT session. Use the word "brain" many times during a session. For example, when talking about the child's technology, instead of saying, "Put on your ears" when we put hearing aids and cochlear implants on the child, we can say, "Put on your brain." If the family arrives to an AVT session with the hearing devices in the mother's purse, we might say something like, "Oh no, your child's brain is in your purse!" Or, when the child arrives at school wearing devices that are functioning well, we can offer a reinforcing comment to the child, such as, "Good for you! Your brain is being fed with rich auditory information and is growing strong with knowledge." Even a very young child who is deaf or hard of hearing can learn the importance of growing his or her brain.

CONCLUSION

The changing context of early developmental research and technology has transformed conversations about hearing loss. Historically, conversations about hearing loss have focused on the ear. But, due to neurobiological research, today's conversations, such as we have had in this chapter about human sensory input, focus on the brain. Strategies used in AVT (see Chapter 15), can now be described from a neurological perspective, and practitioners can offer scientific evidence-based reasons for family-focused recommendations.

When listening and spoken language (LSL) are desired outcomes expressed by the family, then the child's auditory brain centers must be developed through the use of hearing devices and thoughtful, nurturing AVT using family-focused, evidence-based intervention strategies. Getting complete auditory information through the doorway to the brain, all day, every day, impacts every area of a child's life, including language and speech development, social skills, and future academic and life success. Practitioners are, indeed, developing "a brain that listens and learns"!

In summary, early fitting of hearing aids and cochlear implants is not entirely sufficient. A child with hearing loss must also be exposed to a robust audition-based model of language such as AVT, which floods the child's brain with rich, intelligible, and meaningful speech. A child's caregivers are the best language models (see Chapters 1 and 16). To optimize auditory brain development and listening and spoken language outcomes, families of children who are deaf or hard of hearing who desire listening and spoken language outcomes can benefit greatly from brain-based AVT.

REFERENCES

Allen, S., & Casey, J. (2017). Developmental coordination disorders and sensory processing and integration: incidence, associations, and co-morbidities. *British Journal of Occupational Therapy, 80*(9), 549–557.

Ambrose, S. E., Walker, E. A., Unflat-Berry, L. M., Oleson, J. J., & Moeller, M. P. (2015). Quantity and quality of caregivers' linguistic input to 18-month and 3-year-old children who are hard of hearing. *Ear and Hearing, 36*(suppl. 1), 48S–59S.

Andreatta, R. D. (2020). *Neuroscience fundamentals for communication sciences and disorders*. San Diego, CA: Plural Publishing.

Barkley, R. A. (2012). *Executive functions: What they are, how they work, and why they evolved*. New York, NY: Guilford Press.

Bhatnagar, S. C. (2002). *Neuroscience for the study of communicative disorders* (2nd ed.). Philadelphia, PA: Lippincott Williams & Wilkins.

Boothroyd, A. (2019). The acoustic speech signal. In J. R. Madell, C. Flexer, J. Wolfe, & E. C. Schafer (Eds.), *Pediatric audiology: Diagnosis, technology, and management* (3rd ed., pp. 207–214). New York, NY: Thieme Medical Publishers.

Botting, N., Jones, A., Marshall, C., Denmark, T., Atkinson, J., & Morgan, G. (2017). Nonverbal executive function is mediated by language: A study of deaf and hearing children. *Child Development, 88*(5), 1689–1700.

Ching, T. Y. C., Dillon, H., Leigh, G., & Cupples. L. (2018). Learning from the longitudinal outcomes of children with hearing impairment (LOCHI) study: Summary of 5-year findings and implications. *International Journal of Audiology, 57*(S-2), S-105–S-111.

Ching, T. Y., Dillon, H., Marnane, V., Hou, S., Day, J., Seeto, M., . . . Yeh, A. (2013). Outcomes of early- and late-identified children at 3 years of age: Findings from a prospective population-based study. *Ear and Hearing, 34*(5), 535–552.

Chu, C., Choo, D., Dettman, S., Leigh, J., Traeger, G., Lettieri, S., . . . Dowell, D. (2016). *Early intervention and communication development in children using cochlear implants: The impact of service delivery practices and family factors*. Podium presentation at the Audiology Australia National Conference 2016, May 22–25, Melbourne, Australia.

Cole, E., & Flexer, C. (2020). *Children with hearing loss: Developing listening and talking birth to six* (4th ed.). San Diego, CA: Plural Publishing.

Dettman, S. J., Dowell, R. C., Choo, D., Arnott, W., Abrahams, Y., Davis, A., . . .

Briggs, R. S. (2016). Long-term communication outcomes for children receiving cochlear implants younger than 12 months: A multicenter study. *Otology & Neurotology, 37*(2), e82–e95.

Dettman, S., Wall, E., Constantinescu, G., & Dowell, R. (2013). Communication outcomes for groups of children using cochlear implants enrolled in auditory-verbal, aural-oral, and bilingual-bicultural early intervention programs. *Otology & Neurotology, 34*, 451–459.

Eisenberg, L. S., Fisher, L. M., Johnson, K. C., Ganguly, D. H., Grace, T., Niparko, J. K., & CDaCI Investigative Team. (2016). Sentence recognition in quiet and noise by pediatric cochlear implant users: Relationships to spoken language. *Otology & Neurotology, 37*(2), e75–e81.

Farh, K. H. (2019). Personal communication. April 24, 2019.

Figueras, B., Edwards, L., & Langdon, D. (2008). Executive function and language in deaf children. *Deaf Studies and Deaf Education, 13*(3), 362–377.

Flexer, C. (2017). *Start with the brain and connect the dots.* Retrieved on July 26, 2019 from https://hearingfirst.org/down loadables/logic-chain

Geers, A. E., Mitchell, C. M., Warner-Czyz, A., Wang, N. Y., Eisenberg, L. S., & CDaCI Investigative Team. (2017). Early sign language exposure and cochlear implantation benefits. *Pediatrics, 140*(1), e20163489.

Guerzoni, L., & Cuda, D. (2017). Speech processor data logging helps in predicting early linguistic outcomes in implanted children. *International Journal Pediatric Otorhinolaryngology, 101*, 81–86.

Hoff, S., Ryan, M., Thomas, D., Tournis, E., Kenny, H., Hajduk, J., & Young, N. M. (2019). Safety and effectiveness of cochlear implantation of young children, including those with complicating conditions. *Otology & Neurotology, 40*, 454–463.

Kral, A. (2013). Auditory critical periods: A review from system's perspective. *Neuroscience, 247*, 117–133.

Kral, A., Kronenberger, W. G., Pisoni, D. B., & O'Donoghue, G. M. (2016). Neurocognitive factors in sensory restoration of early deafness: A connectome model. *The Lancet Neurology, 15*(6), 610–621.

Kral, A., & Lenarz, T. (2015). How the brain learns to listen: Deafness and the bionic ear. *E-Neuroforum, 6*(1), 21–28.

Kraus, N., & White-Schwoch, T. (2019). Auditory neurophysiology of reading impairment: Theory and management. In J. R. Madell, C. Flexer, J. Wolfe, & E. C. Schafer (Eds.), *Pediatric audiology: Diagnosis, technology, and management* (3rd ed., pp. 163–172). New York, NY: Thieme Medical Publishers.

Leigh, J. R., Dettman, S. J., & Dowell, R. C. (2016). Evidence-based guidelines for recommending cochlear implantation for young children: Audiological criteria and optimizing age at implantation. *International Journal of Audiology, 55*, S9–S18.

Markman, T. M., Quittner, A. L., Eisenberg, L. S., Tobey, E. A., Thal, D., Niparko, J. K., . . . CDaCI Investigative Team. (2011). Language development after cochlear implantation: An epigenetic model. *Journal of Neurodevelopmental Disorders, 3*, 388–404.

McCreery, R. W., Walker, E. A., Spratford, M., Bentler, R., Holte, L., Roush, P. . . . Moeller, M. P. (2015). Longitudinal predictors of aided speech audibility in infants and children. *Ear and Hearing, 36*, 24S–37S.

Moeller, M. P., Tomblin, J. B., & OCHL Collaboration. (2015). Epilogue: Conclusions and implications for research and practice. *Ear and Hearing, 36*(suppl. 1): 92S–98S.

Moller, A. R. (2013). *Hearing: Anatomy, physiology, and disorders of the auditory system* (3rd ed.). San Diego, CA: Plural Publishing.

Moore, D. (2007). Auditory cortex 2006—The listening brain. *Hearing Research, 229*, 1–2.

Netten, A. P., Rieffe, C., Soede, W., Dirks, E., Korver, A. M. H., Konings, S., . . . DECIBEL

Collaborative Study Group. (2017). Can you hear what I think? Theory of mind in young children with moderate hearing loss. *Ear and Hearing, 38*(5), 588–597.

Niparko, J. K., Tobey, E. A., Thal, D. J., Eisenberg, L. S., Wang, N. Y., Quittner, A. L., . . . CDaCI Investigative Team. (2010). Spoken language development in children following cochlear implantation. *Journal of the American Medical Association, 303*(15), 1498–1506.

Nittrouer, S., Caldwell-Tarr, A., Low, K. E., & Lowenstein, J. H. (2017). Verbal working memory in children with cochlear implants. *Journal of Speech, Language, and Hearing Research, 60*(11), 3342–3364. doi:10.1044/2017_JSLHR-H-16-0474

Tharpe, A. M., & Seewald, R. (2017). *Comprehensive handbook of pediatric audiology* (2nd ed.). San Diego, CA: Plural Publishing.

Tobey, E. A., Thal, D., Niparko, J. K., Eisenberg, L. S., Quittner, A. L., Wang, N-Y., & CDaCI Team (2013). Influence of implantation age on school-age language performance in pediatric cochlear implant users. *International Journal of Audiology, 52*(4), 219–229.

Tomblin, J. B., Harrison, M., Ambrose, S. E., Walker, E. A., Oleson, J. J., & Moeller, M. P. (2015). Language outcomes in young children with mild to severe hearing loss. *Ear and Hearing, 36*(suppl. 1), 76S–91S.

3

EVALUATING THE RESEARCH EXAMINING OUTCOMES OF AUDITORY-VERBAL THERAPY: MOVING FROM EVIDENCE-BASED TO EVIDENCE-INFORMED PRACTICE

Alice Eriks-Brophy, Hillary Ganek,
and Glynnis DuBois

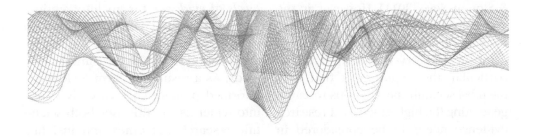

Evidence-based practice (EBP) is defined as the "conscientious, explicit, and judicious use of current best evidence in making decisions about the care of individual patients" (Sackett et al., 1997, p. 3). The goal of EBP is to enhance our knowledge of the effectiveness of existing clinical practices by gathering outcome data related to specific clinical intervention approaches (Dollaghan, 2004). The primary benefits of EBP are that it permits practitioners to plan for clinical practice and to develop new and improved models and approaches to intervention and service delivery based on solid evidence supporting these decisions. We turn to research to inform our daily practice based on what we have determined to be the most effective intervention strategies. Constant upgrading of current practices in light of compelling research evidence is expected to lead to improved outcomes for our clients. EBP also allows us to demonstrate to those outside our discipline that what we do works and is therefore worth doing. Finally, EBP enables us to make links with other fields, resulting in new applications of knowledge and new treatment approaches, thus continually advancing our discipline.

The concept of evidence-based practice has long governed and directed audiology, speech-language pathology, and other disciplines in medicine and rehabilitation. The first version of this chapter explored the existing state of EBP within Auditory-Verbal Therapy (AVT) as well as the introduction of evidence-informed practice (EIP) (Nevo & Slonim-Nevo, 2011). However, in the years since these volumes were originally published, advances have been made in Auditory-Verbal research. In particular, the requirement that only the most scientifically rigorous research generating the highest levels of research evidence needs to be considered in order to support any given intervention approach has been called into question (Eriks-Brophy, Ganek, & DuBois, 2016; Nevo & Slonim-Nevo, 2011). As Auditory-Verbal practitioners (practitioners) have an obligation not only to consider the existing evidence that our intervention methods and strategies work, but also to find the flexibility

to support all of our families based on an informed understanding of listening and spoken language intervention and practice. Auditory-Verbal Therapy must be individualized to best accommodate the needs of each individual family (AG Bell, 2007). The principles of AVT lead practitioners to regularly adjust or modify existing AVT strategies and procedures to fit the needs of any individual family (see Chapters 1 and 15). However, a strict EBP approach limits the consideration and value given to studies investigating the ways in which unique cases influence intervention outcomes, often disregarding or dismissing these studies altogether (Rubin, 2007). Furthermore, it has become apparent that the level of evidence assigned to an intervention outcome study may obscure issues related to the quality of the research methodology and its reported results, as will be discussed in more detail below (Straus, Glaszious, Richardson, & Haynes, 2011).

Practitioners and researchers alike have therefore begun to move away from strict definitions of EBP, recognizing the importance of considering *all levels of evidence* for an intervention approach as the basis upon which to identify and evaluate the best possible intervention strategies for clinical caseloads. As a result, the term "evidence-informed practice" has recently come into wider usage. EIP uses both scientific research outcomes and insights from practitioners and their clients (active recipients of AVT) to form the basis for decisions regarding therapy while still maintaining a critical stance toward the evidence provided from each source of data, resulting in a more comprehensive and inclusive approach to the evaluation of therapy outcomes (Nevo & Slonim-Nevo, 2011). Nevo and

Slonim-Nevo (2011, p. 1178) define EIP as research based, but with room for "constructive and imaginative judgment and knowledge of practitioners and clients." They state that research findings alone should not override, take precedence over, or negate clinical experience or the experiences, knowledge, and values of the clients (families) we serve. In particular, the EIP philosophy challenges the current dependency and priority given to randomized controlled trials (RCTs) in existing frameworks of EBP and argues that the undervalued lower levels of evidence should be, in some cases, considered alongside higher level evidence (Clarke et al., 2013; Howick, 2011). In fact, Clarke et al. (2013) argue that strong evidence obtained through studies at lower levels of the evidence hierarchy can sometimes override evidence obtained through statistically controlled studies that are higher up in the hierarchy, including RCTs.

As its name implies, EIP allows for a more flexible method of assessing practice through the inclusion of complementary converging evidence at all levels of the hierarchy, including the practical experience of practitioners and the needs and wishes of clients, to add to the support base for a particular practice. Although EIP is still research supported, it does not rely exclusively on a defined hierarchy or framework for assessing outcomes. Instead, EIP includes all available outcome data in order to better inform decision making (Nevo & Slonim-Nevo, 2011). Encouraging practitioners to take a broad yet critical view of available information in light of their own experience and that of their clients ultimately allows for a greater number of alternatives to be generated that might be used to inform clinical practice.

According to Nevo and Slonim-Nevo (2011, p. 1178), "practice is as much art as it is science, and as much a dialogue as it is an application of empirical findings to clients' unique characteristics and context" (see Chapter 17).

Critically evaluating research outcomes obtained from diverse sources of evidence is an important part of clinical practice. However, developing the skill set to be able to synthesize many ideas and strategies into a well-supported set of therapeutic practices can be challenging, as well as very time consuming. As a practitioner, one must use his or her clinical expertise to be able to quickly identify available information, its utility in a particular situation and with a particular client, and then determine an appropriate course of action (Gambrill, 2007). Stated succinctly, "(e)vidence-informed practice describes a philosophy and an evolving process designed to help practitioners gain needed information and to become lifelong learners. The uncertainty in making decisions is highlighted, efforts to decrease it are made, and clients are involved as informed participants" (Gambrill, 2007, p. 458).

NEW OUTCOME EVIDENCE IN SUPPORT OF AVT

This chapter investigates and evaluates new research that has documented outcomes in AVT over the last 18 years. Like the earlier version of this chapter (Eriks-Brophy et al., 2016), this is guided by the same three primary objectives. The first is to incorporate an EIP perspective into the review of the existing evidence base supporting AVT outcomes. The second is to locate any new research articles on the topic of outcomes of AVT that have been published in peer-reviewed journals since 2016. The third is to update the evaluative framework on the basis of which the scientific merits of these new articles could be judged.

Meeting each of these objectives required methodological decisions in order to reach a consensus among the authors both on which articles to include in the review and on the level of evidence each of these articles represented. Although the search strategy did not adhere to the strict standards to which systematic reviews are typically held, a transparent search methodology was devised to ensure that as much of the currently published research as possible would be located.

We began by compiling a list of key words from several AV-related outcome studies we had already located. After we shortened the list to better serve our research objective, we used specific search terms to look for new articles. The list of search terms used in the review is presented in Table 3–1.

The most relevant databases were chosen in order to maximize the chances of capturing publications in both medical and education-related journals. These databases were Medline, PsychINFO, ERIC, and Google Scholar. In order to be included in the review, all articles were required to meet the following criteria:

- a publication date after 2016 unless not reported in the previous (2016) version of this chapter;
- an explicit statement that the children received AVT, as opposed

to other forms of intervention; and

- documented outcomes in the domains of speech, language, listening, literacy, and/or social-emotional development.

Studies were excluded if participants receiving different types of intervention were grouped together as part of a single cohort. No qualitative studies or studies examining parent outcomes were included.

A total of 15 new articles were retrieved following this protocol. Two of the authors independently extracted study information and evaluated the study design and the quality of the research methodology. Following this, the two authors met to ensure their judgments were aligned and accurate. The studies were then grouped according to their levels of evidence following the definitions contained in the levels of evidence of the Oxford Centre for Evidence-Based Medicine (2011, hereafter OCEBM), an internationally accepted frame of reference for the evaluation of clinical research evidence. During discussions between the two authors, decisions were made regarding how to rank the studies reviewed in order to maintain consistency. A consensus was reached for all included studies. Research in which all participants received AVT but in which AVT intervention effects were not the specific focus of investigation was separated into an independent category.

The OCEBM (2011) levels of evidence uses the methodology from an individual study to determine its place on the hierarchy, with further rankings being possible, based on the overall quality of the research. There are five levels or steps of evidence, with spe-

Table 3–1. List of Search Terms Used in Locating AVT Outcomes Research

Search Terms	
Speech	Intervention
Speech perception	Early intervention (support)
Speech production measurement	Preschool
Speech recognition assessment	Auditory-oral
Comprehension	Treatment/long-term/clinical outcomes
Vocabulary	Verbal learning
Language	Infants
Language development	Children and youth/toddler, pre-school, preschool
Language development disorders—rehabilitation speech and language	Parents and parenting
(Spoken) language outcomes	Reading comprehension
Hearing impairments/hearing impaired	AVT
Deaf/deafness—rehabilitation	Listening
Prelingual deafness	Speech therapy
Hearing aids	Speech-language pathology
Hearing	Language therapy
Pediatric cochlear implants	Audition
Acoustic analysis	Communication methods
Auditory-verbal (therapy)	

cific methodological parameters provided for ranking the scientific rigor of research at each level. In order to aid in decision making, a glossary is also available defining each of these research methodologies. The levels of evidence available through the OCEBM vary depending on the specific question the research review is attempting to answer. Thus, levels of evidence for ranking studies examining questions related to prognosis or diagnosis differ somewhat from those used in examining intervention outcomes. The five levels of evidence from the OCEBM (2011) are summarized in Table 3–2, with Level 1 being considered the strongest evidence supporting a particular research question and Level 5 being considered the weakest evidence. For the purposes of this review, the evidence levels associated with the evaluation of intervention outcomes formulated in the hierarchy as "Does this intervention help?" were used in organizing and representing relevant research articles.

Table 3–2. Oxford Centre for Evidence-Based Medicine 2011 Levels of Evidence

Question	Step 1 (Level 1*)	Step 2 (Level 2*)	Step 3 (Level 3*)	Step 4 (Level 4*)	Step 5 (Level 5)
How common is the problem?	Local and current random sample surveys (or censuses)	Systematic review of surveys that allow matching to local circumstances*‡	Local non-random sample*‡	Case series*‡	n/a
Is this diagnostic or monitoring test accurate? (Diagnosis)	Systematic review of cross sectional studies with consistently applied reference standard and blinding	Individual cross-sectional studies with consistently applied reference standard and blinding	Non-consecutive studies, or studies without consistently applied reference standards*‡	Case-control studies, or "poor or non-independent reference standard*‡	Mechanism-based reasoning
What will happen if we do not add a therapy? (Prognosis)	Systematic review of inception cohort studies	Inception cohort studies	Cohort study or control arm of randomized trial*	Case-series or case-control studies, or poor quality prognostic cohort study*‡	n/a
Does this intervention help? (Treatment Benefits)	Systematic review of randomized trials or n-of-1 trials	Randomized trial or observational study with dramatic effect	Non-randomized controlled cohort/follow-up study*‡	Case-series, case-control studies, or historically controlled studies*‡	Mechanism-based reasoning

	Level 1	Level 2	Level 3	Level 4	Level 5
What are the COMMON harms? (Treatment Harms)	Systematic review of randomized trials, systematic review of nested case-control studies, n-of-1 trial with the patient you are raising the question about, or observational study with dramatic effect	Individual randomized trial or (exceptionally) observational study with dramatic effect	Non-randomized controlled cohort/follow-up study (post-marketing surveillance) provided there are sufficient numbers to rule out a common harm. (For long-term harms the duration of follow-up must be sufficient.)**	Case-series, case-control, or historically controlled studies**	Mechanism-based reasoning
What are the RARE harms? (Treatment Harms)	Systematic review of randomized trials or n-of-1 trial	Randomized trial or (exceptionally) observational study with dramatic effect	Non-randomized controlled cohort/follow-up study**	Case-series, case-control, or historically controlled studies**	Mechanism-based reasoning
Is this (early detection) test worthwhile? (Screening)	Systematic review of randomized trials	Randomized trial	Non-randomized controlled cohort/follow-up study**	Case-series, case-control, or historically controlled studies**	Mechanism-based reasoning

Notes:

*Level may be graded down on the basis of study quality, imprecision, indirectness (study PICO does not match questions PICO), because of inconsistency between studies, or because the absolute effect size is very small; Level may be graded up if there is a large or very large effect size.

**As always, a systematic review is generally better than an individual study.

Source:

OCEBM Levels of Evidence Working Group.* "The Oxford 2011 Levels of Evidence." Oxford Centre for Evidence-Based Medicine. http://www.cebm.net/index.aspx?o=5653. Creative Commons License 4.0.

* OCEBM Table of Evidence Working Group = Jeremy Howick, Iain Chalmers (James Lind Library), Paul Glasziou, Trish Greenhalgh, Carl Heneghan, Alessandro Liberati, Ivan Moschetti, Bob Phillips, Hazel Thornton, Olive Goddard, and Mary Hodgkinson.

In the case of intervention studies, **Level 1 Evidence** consists of either a systematic review or an n-of-1 study. These two research methodologies are considered to constitute the highest level of evidence in assessing intervention efficacy. N-of-1 studies are single subject research paradigms in which an experimental and a control intervention are applied and then withdrawn using random allocation and a carefully implemented multiple baseline design in order to demonstrate treatment efficacy. Ideally, both the client and the practitioner should be blinded to the control versus the experimental conditions as outcomes are monitored. Intervention periods continue until evidence demonstrating that the outcomes associated with the two conditions are, or are not, different is generated (Center for Evidence-Based Medicine, 2014). An aggregated series of n-of-1 studies can also be used to prospectively document the effectiveness of a specific intervention. Systematic reviews examine peer-reviewed publications about a well-defined health-related question using a rigorous, standardized, and transparent methodology for determining which articles to include in the review. Researchers conducting systematic reviews perform extensive orderly database searches with specific search terms to ensure that no relevant study is overlooked. The individual studies are then critically appraised and synthesized, often providing a quantitative summary of the results through the application of a complex statistical procedure known as a meta-analysis (Center for Evidence-Based Medicine, 2014; Straus et al., 2011). This process minimizes the bias and random error found in individual studies (Straus et al., 2011). In many cases, only studies that consist of RCTs are included in systematic reviews. The synthesized results from a specific field of study obtained through a systematic review are perceived as contributing the highest level of evidence to justify decisions about inventions.

Level 2 Evidence in intervention studies consists of RCTs or less well controlled observational studies with very large effect sizes. In a randomized trial, participants are randomly assigned to a study or a control group and either receive or do not receive a specific experimental intervention. Again, ideally, both the participants and the practitioners who are administering intervention should be blinded to the control versus the experimental condition. Rigorous statistical comparisons between the outcomes of the two groups, which are often matched on particular variables, demonstrate the effectiveness or ineffectiveness of the applied intervention. Also included in this level of evidence are observational studies with large effect sizes. These are studies that were not well controlled methodologically but nevertheless yield a performance difference between the control and experimental groups that is significant enough that it cannot be ignored. Effect size is a way of quantifying the size of the difference between two groups and is particularly useful in evaluating the effectiveness of a specific intervention relative to a comparison. It allows us to evaluate how well an intervention works in a specific context rather than simply asking whether it works. Effect size complements statistical hypothesis testing by emphasizing the size of the difference between groups independently from sample size (Ellis, 2010).

Level 3 Evidence consists of non-randomized cohort studies in which subsets of a pre-defined population are, have been, or in the future may be exposed, not exposed, or exposed in different degrees to an intervention that is hypothesized to influence the probability of a certain outcome. Cohort studies typically conduct observations of large numbers of participants over a long period of time, often many years. Outcomes across participant groups are compared as a function of differences in exposure levels to a specific intervention (Center for Evidence-Based Medicine, 2014). A non-random sample is a population that has been defined through a non-random method where some members of the overall population have no chance of being selected to participate in the study. As there was no available definition in the glossary, for the purposes of this review a non-randomized controlled cohort study was defined as a study that included a comparison group but lacked randomization in the selection of participants. Any studies that did not contain a comparison group were ranked as case series studies (Level 4 Evidence) as this glossary definition was deemed to be best suited to their methodology.

Level 4 Evidence consists of case series, case-control studies, or historically controlled studies. A case series is defined as consisting of a series of case reports involving participants who were exposed to a similar intervention. Such case series reports typically contain detailed information about individual participants including demographics such as age, sex (gender), ethnic origin as well as information on diagnosis, intervention, response to and follow-up after intervention (Center

for Evidence-Based Medicine, 2014). A case-control study compares participants who have a disease or outcome of interest (cases) with patients who do not have the disease or outcome (controls) using retrospective observations in order to determine the relationship between any given risk factor and the disease in question (Center for Evidence-Based Medicine, 2014). In a historically controlled study, data are collected from control subjects who are recruited prior to the beginning of the study, while data from the experimental group are collected prospectively (Center for Evidence-Based Medicine, 2014).

Level 5 Evidence consists of mechanism-based reasoning, a form of inferential thinking through which a logical chain or link is made between a specific intervention and a treatment outcome through relevant mechanisms (Howick, 2011). Illari and Williamson (2012, p. 120) define a mechanism as consisting of "entities and activities organised in such a way that they are responsible for the phenomenon." Evidence of mechanisms is typically obtained through laboratory or statistical studies and relies on clinical expertise and observation in the linking of an intervention to participant outcomes. Practitioners and many others have used mechanism-based reasoning to defend their interventions for many years.

Demographic information from the 43 articles retained for inclusion in this review along with their evidence level ranking from the OCEBM (2011) is provided in Table 3–3. This information was synthesized based on a thorough analysis of the methodology and outcomes of each of the included articles. The authors ranked 2 studies as

Table 3-3. Demographics

Level 3			
Authors	**Age Range**	**Gender**	**SES**
Dettman, S., Wall, E., Constantinescu, G., & Dowell, R. (2013). Communication outcomes for groups of children using cochlear implants enrolled in auditory-verbal, aural-oral, and bilingual-bicultural early intervention programs. *Otology & Neurotology, 34,* 451–459.	AV: 6.2 years AO: 4.9 years BB: 4.9 years	All male	Not Reported
Dornan, D., Hickson, L., Murdoch, B., Houston, T., & Constantinescu, G. (2010). Is auditory-verbal therapy effective for children with hearing loss? *The Volta Review, 110*(3), 361–387.	AV: 96.26 months (SD = 15.32) TD: 87.84 months (SD = 16.68)	14 male 5 female in each group	HL: Professional: 14% Manager: 43% Trade: 29% TD: Professional: 65% Manager: 15% Trade: 5% Both groups had 18 parents with higher education
Dornan, D., Hickson, L, Murdoch, B., & Houston, T. (2009). Longitudinal study of speech perception, speech, and language for children with hearing loss in an auditory-verbal therapy program. *The Volta Review, 109*(2–3), 61–85.	AV: 68.4 months TD: 57.42 months	18 male 7 female in each group	High SES

Level 3				
Age at Dx	Technology	Length of Time with Technology	Length of Time with AVT	Language
Not Reported	HAs followed by CIs	AV: 4.2 years AO: 3.3 years BB: 3.1 years	Not Reported	Australian English & AUSLAN
22.29 months (SD = 11.82)	6 bilateral CI 1 unilateral CI 6 HA and CI 1 unilateral HA 5 bilateral HA	Not reported	70 months (SD = 16.34)	Australian English
24.6 months	2 CI only 12 HA and CI 1 unilateral HA 10 bilateral HA	Not reported	41 months (SD = 16.34)	Australian English

continues

Table 3–3. *continued*

Level 3			
Authors	**Age Range**	**Gender**	**SES**
Dornan, D., Hickson, L., Murdoch, B., & Houston, T. (2007). Outcomes of an auditory-verbal program for children with hearing loss: A comparative study with a matched group of children with normal hearing. *The Volta Review, 107*(1), 37–54.	AV: 3.79 years (SD = 1.25) TD: 2.97 years (SD = 13 months)	21 male 8 female in each group	High SES
Eriks-Brophy, A., Gibson, S., & Tucker, S. (2013). Articulatory error patterns and phonological process use of preschool children with and without hearing loss. *The Volta Review, 113*(2), 87–12.	HL: 52.3 months TD: 52.1 months	Not reported	Not reported but: HL: 17.8 years of education (SD = 2.3) TD: 18.11 years of education (SD = 2.5)
*Goldblat, E. & Pinto, O. (2017). Academic outcomes of adolescents and young adults with hearing loss who received auditory-verbal therapy. *Deafness & Education International, 19*(3–4), 126–133.	18–29 years	AV: 13 male 13 female Non-AV: 13 male 13 female	AV: maternal education 31% non-academic Non-AV: 58% non-academic
Hogan, S., Stokes, J., & Weller, I. (2010). Language outcomes for children of low-income families enrolled in auditory verbal therapy. *Deafness & Education International, 12*(4), 204–216.	28.33 months at entry (range: 5–42 months)	Not reported	Low income (less than 30,000 British pounds/ year)

Level 3				
Age at Dx	Technology	Length of Time with Technology	Length of Time with AVT	Language
24.6 months	14 CI 15 HA (2 children with HAs received CIs during the study)	Not reported	20 months	Australian English
14 months (SD = 8.6)	15 unilateral CI 10 bilateral HA	30.1 months (SD = 13.9)	34.8 months (SD = 8.5)	Canadian English 25% of the participants spoke a second language
Not reported	AV: HA 6 CI: 20 Non-AV: HA 9 CI: 15 No device: 2	AV: 4.55 (SD = 4.5) Non-AV: 9.5 (SD = 7.71)	3 years	Hebrew
2.75 months (range: 1–9 months)	4 bilateral CI 2 unilateral CI 1 HA followed by CI 6 HA	Not reported	At least 12 months	Not reported

continues

Table 3-3. *continued*

Level 3			
Authors	**Age Range**	**Gender**	**SES**
*Lim, S. (2017). The effects of early auditory-based intervention on adult bilateral cochlear implant outcomes. *Cochlear Implants International, 18*(5), 256–265.	36 years (SD = 21.1; range: 18–67 years)	4 male 6 female	Not reported
*Percy-Smith, L., Hall-strom, M., Josvassen, J., Mikkelsen, J., Nissen, L., Dieleman, E., & Caye-Thomasen, P. (2018). Differences and similarities in early vocabulary development between children with hearing aids and children with cochlear implant enrolled in 3-year auditory verbal intervention. *International Journal of Pediatric Otorhinolaryngology, 108*, 67–72.	Birth to 4	CI: 20 male 16 female HA: 14 male 5 female TD: Not reported	Maternal education CI: 5% < 13 years HA: 1% < 13 years
*Percy-Smith, L., Tonning, T., Josvassen, J., Mikkelsen, J., Nissen, L., Dieleman, E., Hallstrom, M., & Caye-Thomasen, P. (2017). Auditory verbal habilitation is associated with improved outcome for children with cochlear implant. *Cochlear Implants International, 19*(1), 38–45.	AV: 49 months Non-AV: 47 months	AV: 17 male 14 female Non-AV: 42 male 52 female	Maternal education AV: 8 < 13 years Non-AV: 27 < 13 years

Level 3				
Age at Dx	Technology	Length of Time with Technology	Length of Time with AVT	Language
9 at birth 1 at 10 years old	All CI	17–65 years	Not reported	Not reported
Median: CI: 6 months HA: 6 months	CI: 36 HA: 19	Not reported	3 years	Danish
Birth	All CI	Median AV: 29.5 months Non-AV: 21 months	2 years	Danish

continues

Table 3-3. *continued*

Level 3			
Authors	**Age Range**	**Gender**	**SES**
Robertson, L., Dow, G., & Hainzinger, S. (2006). Story retelling patterns among children with and without hearing loss: effects of repeated practice and parent-child attunement. *The Volta Review, 106*(2), 147–170.	HL: 4;9 months (range: 3–6 months) TD: 4;7 months (range: 3–5 months)	AV: 6 male 4 female TD: 6 male 5 female	Not reported
*Tejeda-Franco, C., Valadez-Jimenez, V., Hernandez-Lopez, X., Ysunza, P., Mena-Ramirez, M., Garcia-Zalapa, R., & Miranda-Duarte, A. (2018). Hearing aid use and auditory verbal therapy improve voice quality of deaf children. *Journal of Voice*, 1–5.	2–5 years	HL: 11 males 8 females TD: 11 male 8 female	Not reported
*Thomas, E. & Zwolan, T. (2019). Communication mode and speech and language outcomes of young cochlear implant recipients: A comparison of auditory-verbal, oral communication, and total communication. *Otology & Neurotology, 40*, 1–9.	AV: 19.74 months OC: 32.29 months TC: 40.9 months	AV: 16 females 23 males OC: 60 females 47 males TC: 35 females 22 males	% with Medicaid insurance AV: 10% OC: 23% TC: 38%

Level 3				
Age at Dx	Technology	Length of Time with Technology	Length of Time with AVT	Language
Not reported	3 CI 7 HA	1.6–4.8 years	Not reported	Not reported
Not reported	All hearing aids	Not reported	1 year	Mexican Spanish
Not reported	All CI	Not reported	2–7 years	Not reported

continues

Table 3–3. *continued*

Level 3			
Authors	**Age Range**	**Gender**	**SES**
Yanbay, E., Hickson, L., Scarinci, N., Constantinescu, G., & Dettman, S. (2014). Language outcomes for children with cochlear implants enrolled in different communication programs. *Cochlear Implants International, 15*(3), 121–135.	AV: 3.64 years (SD = 1.16) AO: 4.6 years (SD = 1.47) SS: 4.31 (SD = 1.68)	AV: 8 male 10 female AO: 7 male 7 female SS: 4 male 6 female	AV: 8 low to mid 6 high AO: 8 low to mid 10 high SS: 7 low to mid 3 high
Level 4			
Authors	**Age Range**	**Gender**	**SES**
*Dieleman, E., Percy-Smith, L., & Caye-Thomasen, P. (2019). Language outcome in children with congenital hearing impairment: The influence of etiology. *International Journal of Pediatric Otorhinolaryngology, 117*, 37–44.	Birth–4 years at the start	33 male 20 female	Not reported
Eriks-Brophy, A., Durieux-Smith, A., Olds, J., Fitzpatrick, E., Duquette, C., & Whittingham, J. (2012). Communication, academic, and social skills of young adults with hearing loss. *The Volta Review, 112*(1), 5–35.	18.6 years (range: 14–30 years)	Not reported	Not reported but 73.9% of mothers had postsecondary educations

Level 3				
Age at Dx	**Technology**	**Length of Time with Technology**	**Length of Time with AVT**	**Language**
AV: 0.34 years (SD = 0.44) AO: 0.42 years (SD = 0.38) SS: 0.68 years (SD = 0.67)	All CI	PPVT: AV: 3.66 years (SD = 0.95) AO: 3.70 years (SD = 1.13) SS: 3.14 years (SD = 1.08) PLS-4 AV: 2.59 years (SD = 0.97) AO: 3.55 years (SD = 1.34) SS: 2.72 years (SD = 1.59)	PPVT: 4.05 years (SD = 1.18) PLS-4 2.92 years (SD = 1.01)	Australian English

Level 4				
Age at Dx	**Technology**	**Length of Time with Technology**	**Length of Time with AVT**	**Language**
6 months (range: birth–34 months)	CI: 34 HA: 16 BAHA: 3	Not reported	3 years	Danish
Not reported	All HA	Not reported	25 months (SD = 6.9)	Canadian English

continues

Table 3-3. *continued*

Level 4			
Authors	**Age Range**	**Gender**	**SES**
Fairgray, E., Purdy, S., & Smart, J. (2010). Effects of auditory-verbal therapy for school-aged children with hearing loss: an exploratory study. *The Volta Review, 110*(3), 407–433.	9.8 years (range: 5.5–17.7 years)	2 male 5 female	Not reported
Harris, L. (2014). *Social-emotional development in children with hearing loss.* (Unpublished master's thesis). University of Kentucky: Lexington.	3–6.6 years	Children: 3 male 2 female Caregivers: 1 male 4 female	Not reported but caregiver education level: 1 high school diploma 3 bachelor's degree 1 master's degree
*Hitchins, A. & Hogan, S. (2018). Outcomes of early intervention for deaf children with additional needs following an Auditory Verbal approach to communication. *International Journal of Pediatric Otorhinolaryngology, 115*, 125–132.	<5 years to start	Not reported	Not reported
Hogan, S., Stokes, J., White, C., Tyszkiewicz, E., & Woolgar, A. (2008). An evaluation of auditory verbal therapy using the rate of early language development as an outcome measure. *Deafness and Education International, 10*(3), 143–167.	23 months at entry (range 5–56 months)	Not reported	Not reported

Level 4				
Age at Dx	Technology	Length of Time with Technology	Length of Time with AVT	Language
1.9 years (range: 11 months– 2.5 years)	2 bilateral CI 3 unilateral CI 2 bilateral HA	Not reported	Not reported	Not reported
9.6 months (range: birth– 24 months)	2 bilateral CI 2 bilateral HA 1 unilateral HA	Not reported	Not reported	Not reported
6.5 months (SD = 8.7)	33 bilateral HA 19 bimodal 72 bilateral CI 1 BAHA	CI: 12.4 months HA: 23.4 months	>2 years	British English
12 months (range: 1–47 months)	5 bilateral CI 18 unilateral CI 14 bilateral HA	Not reported	89% of participants received less than 3 years of AVT 62% of participants received less than 2 years of AVT (range: 13–60 months)	Not reported

continues

Table 3–3. *continued*

Level 4			
Authors	**Age Range**	**Gender**	**SES**
*Kim, L., Wisely, E., & Lucius, S. (2016). Positive outcomes and surgical strategies for bilateral cochlear implantation in a child with X-linked deafness. *Annals of Otology, Rhinology, & Laryngology, 125*(2), 173–176.	6 months	1 male	Not reported
*Lim, S., Goldberg, D., & Flexer, C. (2018). Auditory-Verbal Graduates—25 years later: outcome survey of the clinical effectiveness of the listening and spoken language approach for young children with hearing loss. *The Volta Review, 118*(1.2), 5–40.	18–79 years	73 male 132 female	Not reported
*Necula,V., Cosgarea, M., Maniu, A. (2018). Effects of family environment features on cochlear-implanted children. *European Archives of Oto-Rhino-Laryngology, 275*(9), 2209–2217.	8 years (Range: <18)	40 male 18 female	69% of caregivers had higher education
Sahil, A. & Belgin, E. (2011). Researching auditory perception performance of children using cochlear implants and being trained by an auditory-verbal therapy. *The Journal of International Advanced Otology, 7*(3), 385–390.	44 months (SD = 5.2)	9 male 6 female	Not reported

Level 4				
Age at Dx	Technology	Length of Time with Technology	Length of Time with AVT	Language
Birth	CI	26 months	>24 months	English
1.6 years (SD = 1.2)	77 bilateral CI 77 unilateral CI 77 bimodal 43 HA 2 Other	Not reported	8.8 years	English
16.7 months (SD = 11)	All CI	57.1 months (SD = 40.2)	Not reported	Romanian
14 months (SD = 5.4)	All CI	18 months (SD = 4.8)	15 months (SD = 3.7)	Not reported

continues

Table 3-3. *continued*

Level 4			
Authors	**Age Range**	**Gender**	**SES**
*Sharma, S., Bhatia, K., Singh, S., Lahiri, A., Aggarwal, A. (2017). Impact of socioeconomic factors on paediatric cochlear implant outcomes. International *Journal of Pediatric Otorhinolaryngology, 102*, 90–97.	<4 years at implantation	Not reported	High School: 41 Bachelors: 110 Grad School: 29
Von Muenster, K. & Baker, E. (2014). Oral communicating children using a cochlear implant: Good reading outcomes are linked to better language and phonological processing abilities. *International Journal of Pediatric Otorhinolaryngology, 78*(3), 433–444.	At reading and phonological processing testing: 8.75 years (SD = 2.05) At speech perception, speech and language testing: 8.74 years (SD = 2.15)	23 male 24 female	Not reported
Warner-Czyz, A., Davis, B., & Morrison, H. (2005). Production accuracy in a young cochlear implant recipient. *The Volta Review, 105*(1), 5–25.	One participant from 13–32 months	1 female	Not reported
Wong, S., Scarinci, N., Hickson, L., Rose, T., & Constantinescu, G. (2013). Bilateral cochlear implants in children: A preliminary study of language and speech perception outcomes. *The Australian and New Zealand Journal of Audiology, 33*(1), 48–68.	9.9 years (SD = 3.8)	11 males 11 females	Not reported

Level 4				
Age at Dx	Technology	Length of Time with Technology	Length of Time with AVT	Language
Not reported	All CI	Testing completed at 3, 6, 9, and 12 months post-CI	24 months	Not reported
Not reported	All CI	5.37 years (SD = 1.93)	At least 6 to 12 months	Australian English
12 months of age	HA followed by CI	12 months with HA 8 months with CI	19 months	American English
At birth	All sequential bilateral CI	7.9 years from first CI (range: 2;2 to 14;2)	Not reported	Australian English

continues

Table 3-3. *continued*

Level 4			
Authors	**Age Range**	**Gender**	**SES**
Wood, Jackson, C., & Schatschneider, C. (2014). Rate of language growth in children with hearing loss in an auditory-verbal early intervention program. *American Annuals of the Deaf, 158*(5), 539–554.	3 months– 6.5 years	12 male 12 female	Not reported
NON-AVT			
Authors	**Age Range**	**Gender**	**SES**
Allegro, J., Papsin, B., Harrison, R., & Campisi, P. (2010). Acoustic analysis of voice in cochlear implant recipients with post-meningitic hearing loss. *Cochlear Implants International, 11*(2), 100–116.	7.2 years (range: 2.1–11.1 years)	3 male 7 female	Not reported
Bakhshaee, M., Ghasemi, M., Shakeri, M., Razmara, N., Tayarani, H., & Tale, M. (2007). Speech development in children after cochlear implantation. *Ear Archives of Otorhinolaryngology, 264*, 1263–1266.	Not reported	Not reported	Not reported

Level 4				
Age at Dx	**Technology**	**Length of Time with Technology**	**Length of Time with AVT**	**Language**
10.75 months (range birth–36 months)	11 CI 13 HA	Not reported	Not reported	American English

NON-AVT				
Age at Dx	**Technology**	**Length of Time with Technology**	**Length of Time with AVT**	**Language**
18 months (range: 4 days–5 years)	All unilateral CI	58 months (range: 21–95 months)	Not reported	Not reported
2.05 years (SD = 6.17)	All CI	5 years	Not reported	Not reported

continues

Table 3-3. *continued*

NON-AVT			
Authors	**Age Range**	**Gender**	**SES**
*Baungaard, L., Sandvej, M., Kroijer, J., Hestbaek, M., Samar, C., Percy-Smith, L., & Caye-Thomasen, P. (2019). Auditory verbal skills training is a new approach in adult cochlear implant rehabilitation. *Danish Medical Journal, 66*(3), A5535.	AV: 69.5 years Non-AV: 72 years	AV: 5 male 5 female Non-AV: 3 male 4 female	Not reported
*Chen, P. & Liu, T. (2017). A pilot study of telepractice for teaching listening and spoken language to Mandarin-speaking children with congenital hearing loss. *Deafness & Education International, 19*(3–4), 134–143.	AV: 58.2 months (SD = 6.11) eAV: 60.6 months (SD = 5.05)	AV: 3 male 2 female eAV: 1 male 4 female	Maternal education AV: 16.4 years education (SD = .89) eAV: 14.4 years education (SD = 2.19)
Easterbrooks, S. & O'Rourke, C. (2001). Gender differences in response to auditory-verbal intervention in children who are deaf or hard of hearing. *American Annals of the Deaf, 146*(4), 309–319.	Not reported	28 male 42 female	Affluent, highly educated mothers

NON-AVT				
Age at Dx	Technology	Length of Time with Technology	Length of Time with AVT	Language
Not reported	All CI	Not reported	10 sessions	Danish
Not reported	AV: 4 bilateral HAs 1 bimodal eAV: 4 bilateral HAs 1 bimodal	AV: 52.8 months (SD = 5.53) eAV: 55.4 months (SD = 5)	2 years	Not reported
Not reported	Not reported	Not reported	Males: 39 months (SD = 25.1) Females: 51.6 months (SD = 26.6)	Not reported

continues

Table 3–3. *continued*

NON-AVT			
Authors	**Age Range**	**Gender**	**SES**
*Fulcher, A., Purcell, A., Baker, E., & Munro, N. (2015). Factors influencing speech and language outcomes of children with early identified severe/profound hearing loss: Clinician-identified facilitators and barriers. International *Journal of Speech-Language Pathology, 17*(3), 325–333.	N/A	N/A	N/A
Fulcher, A., Purcell, A., Baker, E., & Munro, N. (2012). Listen up: Children with early identified hearing loss achieve age-appropriate speech/language outcomes by 3 years-of-age. *International Journal of Pediatric Otorhinolaryngology, 76*, 1785–1794.	Assessed at 3, 4, & 5 years old	Early ID'd: 29 male; 16 female Late ID'd: 27 male 22 female	Early ID'd: 9 lower 32 middle 4 upper middle Late ID'd: 16 lower 32 middle 1 upper middle

NON-AVT				
Age at Dx	Technology	Length of Time with Technology	Length of Time with AVT	Language
N/A	N/A	N/A	N/A	English
Early ID'd: Severe/profound: 8.4 weeks (SD = 8.7) Mild/moderate: 7.2 weeks (SD = 5.3) Late ID'd: Severe/profound: 92.1 weeks (SD = 25.6) Mild/moderate: 114.4 weeks (SD = 45.8)	Not reported	Not reported	Not reported	Not reported

continues

89

Table 3-3. *continued*

NON-AVT			
Authors	**Age Range**	**Gender**	**SES**
Lew, J., Purcell, A., Doble, M., & Lim, L. (2014). Hear here: Children with hearing loss learn words by listening. *International Journal of Pediatric Otorhinolaryngology, 78*, 1716–1725.	2 years, 8 months (range: 2.6–3.1)	Not reported	Not reported
Moog, J. & Geers, A. (2010). Early educational placement and later language outcomes for children with cochlear implants. *Otology & Neurotology, 31*, 1315–1319.	5 years, 10 months (SD = 6 months)	Not reported	Not reported but the mean highest educational level completed by either parent was close to completion of a 4-year college program.
Morrison, H. (2011). Coarticulation in early vocalizations by children with hearing loss: A locus perspective. *Clinical Linguistics & Phonetics, 26*(3), 288–309.	11–50 months longitudinally	2 male 1 female	Middle Class families with all adults having a university degree
Pundir, M., Nagarkar, A., & Panda, N. (2007). Intervention strategies in children with cochlear implants having attention deficit hyperactivity disorder. *International Journal of Pediatric Otorhinolaryngology, 71*, 985–988.	6 & 7 years	1 male 1 female	Not reported

NON-AVT				
Age at Dx	Technology	Length of Time with Technology	Length of Time with AVT	Language
Not reported	1 bilateral CI 2 bilateral HA	Not reported	Not reported	English but may have had some exposure to other languages
2 months (SD = 5)	All CI	3 years, 7 months (SD = 10 months)	Not reported	Not reported
1.33 months (range: 1–2 months)	2 CI 1 HA	7–32 months longitudinally (corrected for cochlear implantation)	Not reported	American English
1.5 years	Both CI	Male: 4.5 years with HA 9 months with CI Female: 5 years with HA 9 months with CI	9 months	Not reported

continues

Table 3–3. *continued*

NON-AVT			
Authors	**Age Range**	**Gender**	**SES**
Wolfe, J., Baker, S., Caraway, T., Kasulis, H., Mears, A., Smith, J., Swim, L., & Wood, M. (2007). 1-Year postactivation results for sequentially implanted bilateral cochlear implant users. *Otology & Neurotology, 28*(5), 589–596.	Not reported	Not reported	Not reported

Note: *Article added since the last publication of this chapter.

NON-AVT				
Age at Dx	Technology	Length of Time with Technology	Length of Time with AVT	Language
Not reported	All bilateral CI	Not reported	Not reported	Not reported

representing Level 1 evidence related to AVT, no studies were ranked as contributing Level 2 evidence, 14 studies were found to represent Level 3 evidence, and 15 studies were classified as Level 4 studies. No studies representing Level 5 evidence were located for inclusion in the review; however, there were 12 articles that were categorized as non-AVT studies that were considered to be of interest to the review and have therefore been included in a separate section.

In light of the considerations around EIP, as previously discussed, the OCEBM 2011 Levels of Evidence were used in organizing and synthesizing the most recent AV research rather than as a strict evaluative tool for classifying the quality of the existing research in AVT. As discussed above, lower levels of evidence may still provide important support in favor of an intervention approach as long as the quality of the research receives appropriate critical appraisal and any areas of potential bias are clearly identified. The importance of evaluating not only the level of evidence a study provides but also the quality of this evidence is discussed in further detail below.

Level 1 Evidence

Two systematic reviews that examined the effectiveness of AVT were identified in this update from the 2016 chapter. The Cochrane Collaboration is a nonprofit organization dedicated to conducting and transmitting the results of systematic reviews, compiling medical research evidence in many domains to aid health workers in their clinical decision making. In this systematic review,

Brennan-Jones et al. (2014) searched 18 databases using a comprehensive set of search terms. The investigation yielded 2,233 titles that were then reviewed for inclusion based on the following criteria: (1) the study had to consist of an RCT), (2) the pediatric participants with bilateral moderate to profound hearing loss had to be enrolled in AVT that was provided by a Listening and Spoken Language Specialist (LSLS) Certified AVT, and (3) language level or rate of language growth had to be the primary outcome measure. Thirteen studies were judged to have fulfilled the review inclusion requirements, while none of the remaining papers were RCTs and were therefore excluded from the systematic review. Also, as none of the studies used randomization or blinding of the outcome assessors, the risk of biases was problematic when assessing primarily subjective outcome measures. Therefore, due to the lack of well-controlled studies reviewed, the authors were unable to draw any conclusions regarding the potential positive effects of AVT intervention (Brennan-Jones et al., 2014).

Kaipa and Danser (2016) also conducted a systematic review in which they engaged the use of the guidelines of Preferred Reporting Items for Systematic reviews and Meta-Analyses (PRISMA) (Liberati et al., 2009). Their search of six databases with a more directive set of search terms yielded 1,251 articles. All the studies included in Kaipa and Danser's (2016) review involved children between 2 and 17 years of age, discussed the effects of AVT on language development, speech perception, and/or mainstreaming, and were published in English. After the criteria were applied, 14 studies remained for analysis. The Critical Appraisal of Treatment Evidence

(CATE) checklist (Kaipa & Peterson, 2016) was used to evaluate the quality of the articles. Under Kaipa and Danser's (2016) criteria, non-RCT studies were included for analysis. While the systematic review found that AVT can help children who are deaf or hard of hearing to improve language, speech perception, and mainstreaming outcomes, the authors also admit that there is limited evidence and more well-controlled studies are necessary to confirm the results.

In a follow-up article to the Brennan-Jones et al. (2014) systematic review, the authors reiterated the importance of research generally and RCTs specifically within communication interventions for families of children who are deaf or hard of hearing. They stated that AVT was well suited for higher levels of investigation in part because of the clarity with which AVT is defined (i.e., AG Bell, 2007; Principles of Auditory-Verbal Therapy; White & Brennan-Jones, 2014). White and Brennan-Jones (2014) propose a large-scale multicenter RCT investigation of AVT as the next step toward proving AV efficacy. However, while such an RCT might be possible, a number of factors make it difficult to execute in AV practice. First and most importantly, since AV practice is dependent on parental choice and involvement, assigning a family to an intervention approach rather than allowing the family to make their own informed decisions concerning their child's intervention goes against the basic principles of AVT. Furthermore, it would be near to impossible to blind a family or a practitioner to the type of intervention being received or provided. As parent engagement and active involvement is key to AVT, it would be difficult to disguise most caregiver-focused AVT strategies. Finally, Auditory-Verbal researchers have not yet reached a consensus about which outcomes to measure and how to best accomplish them. Deciding whether speech, language, or socio-emotional factors, or some combination of these are the best measure of AV outcomes and those assessment tools that might best represent such outcomes is also a point of continuing debate. Finally, and perhaps most importantly, randomly assigning children to an intervention or non-intervention control group could potentially delay or limit access to intervention for children in the control group, which might have a significant disruptive effect on their listening and spoken language development (Stewart-Brown et al., 2011).

Level 2 Evidence

No published articles representing this level of evidence were identified in the review. The reasons for this are analogous to the arguments presented above regarding the difficulties associated with random assignment of children to AVT and non-AVT intervention groups. Furthermore, as none of the retrieved studies reported effect size, no observational research could be included at this evidence level.

Level 3 Evidence

Fourteen studies, an increase of 88% since the 2016 publication, ranked as providing Level 3 evidence in favor of AVT. These studies are presented in Table 3–4. All of the studies were ranked as representing non-randomized control studies as defined above. Sample

Table 3–4. Quality of Evidence: Level 3 Table

LEVEL 3				
Authors	**N**	**Comparison Groups**	**Matching**	**Sample Pool**
Dettman, S., Wall, E., Constantinescu, G., & Dowell, R. (2013). Communication outcomes for groups of children using cochlear implants enrolled in auditory-verbal, aural-oral, and bilingual-bicultural early intervention programs. *Otology & Neurotology, 34,* 451–459.	AV: 8 AO: 23 BB: 8	AV, AO, & BB Retrospective data	Retrospective matching Age at implant Age at hearing aid fitting test age device experience at the time of Ax	Multi-site
Dornan, D., Hickson, L., Murdoch, B., Houston, T., & Constantinescu, G. (2010). Is auditory-verbal therapy effective for children with hearing loss? *The Volta Review, 110*(3), 361–387.	19 in each group	AV & TD	Total language age Receptive vocab Gender SES	1 site
Dornan, D., Hickson, L, Murdoch, B., Houston, T. (2009). Longitudinal study of speech perception, speech, and language for children with hearing loss in an auditory-verbal therapy program. *The Volta Review, 109*(2–3), 61–85.	25 in each group	AV & TD	Total language age Receptive vocab Gender SES	1 site

LEVEL 3			
Study Design	**Tests**	**Stats**	**Findings**
Prospective	PPVT, CNC, & BKB wordlists	ANOVA, correlations, & descriptive statistics	Three years post cochlear implantation, children in AVT and auditory-oral intervention programs outperformed children in bilingual-bicultural programs on speech perception and receptive vocabulary assessments.
Prospective	PLS-4, CELF-3, PPVT-3, GFTA-2, Reading Progress Test (RPT), I Can Do Maths, Progressive Achievement Tests in Mathematics, & Insight (self-esteem test: parent report)	Wilcoxon signed rank test, Mann Whitney Test & descriptive statistics	Children in AVT for 50 months had speech, language and self-esteem levels similar to their typically developing peers and comparable reading and math scores.
Prospective	PLOTT Manchester junior words, PBK, CNC, BKB wordlist, PLS-4, CELF-3, PPVT-3, GFTA2, & CASALA	Wilcoxon signed rank test, t-test, ANOVA, descriptive statistics	Over 21 months, children in AVT improved their live-voice speech perception, language and speech scores significantly and similarly to typically developing peers. While both groups were in the normal range for receptive vocabulary development, the typically developing group did outperform the children in AVT.

continues

Table 3–4. *continued*

LEVEL 3				
Authors	**N**	**Comparison Groups**	**Matching**	**Sample Pool**
Dornan, D., Hickson, L., Murdoch, B., & Houston, T. (2007). Outcomes of an auditory-verbal program for children with hearing loss: A comparative study with a matched group of children with normal hearing. *The Volta Review, 107*(1), 37–54.	29 in both groups	AV & TD	Total language age Receptive vocab Gender SES	1 site
Eriks-Brophy, A., Gibson, S., & Tucker. S. (2013). Articulatory error patterns and phonological process use of preschool children with and without hearing loss. *The Volta Review, 113*(2), 87–12.	AV: 25 TD: 35	AV & TD	Age, Family structure, Home language, Parental education	Multi-site
*Goldblat, E. & Pinto, O. (2017). Academic outcomes of adolescents and young adults with hearing loss who received auditory-verbal therapy. *Deafness & Education International, 19*(3–4), 126–133.	AV: 26 Non-AV: 26	AV & Non-AV	Year of birth; gender, residence, and parental income	Multi-site
Hogan, S., Stokes, J., & Weller, I. (2010). Language outcomes for children of low-income families enrolled in auditory verbal therapy. *Deafness & Education International, 12*(4), 204–216.	Low SES AV: 12 AV: 37 (collected in Hogan et al., 2008)	Low SES in AV & the subjects in Hogan et al., 2008	No matching	Multi-site

LEVEL 3			
Study Design	**Tests**	**Stats**	**Findings**
Prospective	PPVT-3, PLS-4 or CELF-3, & GFTA-2	t-test, mixed model analysis, & descriptive statistics	Children enrolled in AVT performed similarly to typically developing peers on speech and language assessments.
Prospective	GFTA-2 & KLPA-2	t-test, descriptive statistics, & correlation	Typically developing children outperformed children in AVT on articulation and phonologic processing assessments. However, the children in AVT did have phonologic processing systems that resembled their peers' and most demonstrated at least 12 months progress in 12 months' time.
Prospective	Questionnaire	Pearson correlations; descriptive statistics; logistic regression; t-tests;	AVT correlated with Hebrew, literature, and academic grades and matriculation, which were significantly different from Non-AVT group results. There was a positive correlation between AVT and father's education level.
Prospective	RLD (rate of language delivery) calculated using PLS-4 (UK) scores Ax done every 6 months	Mann, Whitney, t-test, & descriptive statistics	SES did not play a role in spoken language outcomes for children in AVT.

continues

Table 3–4. *continued*

LEVEL 3				
Authors	**N**	**Comparison Groups**	**Matching**	**Sample Pool**
*Lim, S. (2017). The effects of early auditory-based intervention on adult bilateral cochlear implant outcomes. *Cochlear Implants International, 18*(5), 256–265.	AV: 5 AO: 5	AV & AO	Not reported	Multi-site
*Percy-Smith, L., Hallstrom, M., Josvassen, J., Mikkelsen, J., Nissen, L., Dieleman, E., & Caye-Thomasen, P. (2018). Differences and similarities in early vocabulary development between children with hearing aids and children with cochlear implant enrolled in 3-year auditory verbal intervention. *International Journal of Pediatric Otorhinolaryngology, 108*, 67–72.	CI; 36 HA: 19 TD: 59	CI, HA, & TD	Gender and age	2 sites
*Percy-Smith, L., Tonning, T., Josvassen, J., Mikkelsen, J., Nissen, L., Dieleman, E., Hallstrom, M., & Caye-Thomasen, P. (2017). Auditory verbal habilitation is associated with improved outcome for children with cochlear implant. *Cochlear Implants International, 19*(1), 38–45.	AV: 36 Non-AV: 94	AV & Non-AV	Not reported	Multi-site

LEVEL 3			
Study Design	**Tests**	**Stats**	**Findings**
Prospective	BKB-SIN	Independent t-tests; Descriptive statistics	AV group had better listening skills in noise but the difference was not significant
Prospective	PPVT; Reynell; Viborgmaterialet	Descriptive statistics; t-tests	While the TD group did best, there was no difference between the two groups with hearing loss. All families continued with AVT indicating that they found it relevant
Retrospective	PPVT; Reynell; Viborgmaterialet	Fisher's exact tests; logistic regression; odds ratio testing	Children in AV group outperformed their peers in non-AV intervention

continues

Table 3–4. *continued*

LEVEL 3				
Authors	**N**	**Comparison Groups**	**Matching**	**Sample Pool**
Robertson, L., Dow, G., & Hainzinger, S. (2006). Story retelling patterns among children with and without hearing loss: Effects of repeated practice and parent-child attunement. *The Volta Review, 106*(2), 147–170.	AV: 10 TD: 11	AV & TD	No matching	1 site
*Tejeda-Franco, C., Valadez-Jimenez, V., Hernandez-Lopez, X., Ysunza, P., Mena-Ramirez, M., Garcia-Zalapa, R., & Miranda-Duarte, A. (2018). Hearing aid use and auditory verbal therapy improve voice quality of deaf children. *Journal of Voice*, 1–5.	HA: 19 TD: 19	HA & TD	Gender and age range	2 sites
*Thomas, E. & Zwolan, T. (2019). Communication mode and speech and language outcomes of young cochlear implant recipients: A comparison of auditory-verbal, oral communication, and total communication. *Otology & Neurotology, 40*, 1–9.	AV: 39 OC: 107 TC: 57	AV, OC, & TC	No matching	1 site
Yanbay, E., Hickson, L., Scarinci, N., Constantinescu, G., & Dettman, S. (2014). Language outcomes for children with cochlear implants enrolled in different communication programs. *Cochlear Implants International, 15*(3), 121–135	AV: 18 AO: 14 SS: 10	AV, AO, SS Retrospective data	No matching	1 site

Note: *Article added since the last publication of this chapter.

LEVEL 3			
Study Design	**Tests**	**Stats**	**Findings**
Prospective	PPVT-3 , transcripts coded for memory tasks	Descriptive statistics, t-test, ANCOVA	Children with hearing loss benefit from shared reading activities and memory for the text was improved when the parents were more directed to the child's listening needs.
Prospective	Fundamental frequency (F0); shimmer; jitter	Two-tailed paired student t-tests	Fundamental frequency increased after AVT and jitter and shimmer improved but were still below the typically hearing group
Prospective	PPVT; EVT; WJ-3 & 4; GFTA; AAPS-3	Descriptive statistics; ANOVA; linear mixed-effects model	All groups demonstrated improvements over time. The AV group had significantly higher scores than participants in the other groups.
Retrospective	PPVT, PLS4, FPRS (family participation rating scale)	ANCOVA, t-test, Pearson correlation	Regardless of communication option, children with hearing loss who were diagnosed early and have parents who are highly involved produce higher language scores than those who do not.

Table 3-5. Test Measures (Alphabetical Order) Used in Research Studies

AAPS-3	Arizona Articulation Proficiency Scale—Third Edition	Fudala, J. *Arizona Articulation Proficiency Scale, Third Revision*. Los Angeles, CA: Western Psychological Services; 2000.
ACAP-A	Assessment of Children's Articulation and Phonology	James, D. (1995). *Assessment of Children's Articulation and Phonology*. South Australia: Flinders University.
BASC-2	Behavioral and Emotional Screening System, Second Edition	Kamphaus, R., & Reynolds, C. (2007). *Behavioral & Emotional Screening System Manual*. Bloomington, MN: NCS Pearson, Inc.
BKB	Bamford-Kowal-Bench	Bench J, Bamford J. *Speech-Hearing Tests & the Spoken Language of Hearing-Impaired Children*. London, UK: Academic Press, 1979.
BKB/A	Bamford-Kowal-Bench/Australian	Bench, R., Doyle, J., & Greenwood, K. (1987). A standardization of the BKB/A sentence test for children in comparison with the NAL-CID sentence test and CAL-PBM word test. *Australian Journal of Audiology, 9*, 39–48.
BKB-SIN	Bamford-Kowal-Bench Speech in Noise Test	Etymotic Research Labs. (2005). *BKB-SIN™ Speech-in-Noise Test Version 1.03*. [CD] Elk Grove Village, IL: Etymotic Research.
CAP	Categories of Auditory Performance	Archbold, S., Lutman, M., & Marshall, D. (1995) Categories of Auditory Performance. *The Annals of Otology, Rhinology & Laryngology Supplement 166*, 312–314.
CASALA	Computer Aided Speech and Language Analysis	Serry, A., Dorman, M., & Kral, A. (1997). Computer-Aided Speech and Language Analysis. *Australian Communication Quarterly* (Spring), 27–28.
CELF-3	Clinical Evaluation of Language Fundamentals, Third Edition	Semel, E., Wiig., E., & Secord, W. (1995). *Clinical Evaluation of Language Fundamentals, Third Edition*. San Antonio, TX: The Psychological Corporation.

Table 3–5. *continued*

CELF-4	Clinical Evaluation of Language Fundamentals, Fourth Edition	Semel, E., Wiig., E., & Secord, W. (2003). *Clinical Evaluation of Language Fundamentals, Fourth Edition*. San Antonio, TX: The Psychological Corporation.
CELF-P	Clinical Evaluation of Language Fundamentals–Preschool	Wiig, E., Secord, W., & Semel, E. (1992). *Clinical Evaluation of Language Fundamentals–Preschool*. San Antonio, TX: The Psychological Corporation.
CNC	Consonant–nucleus–consonant word lists	Peterson, G., Lehiste, I. (1962). Revised CNC word lists for auditory tests. *Journal of Hearing and Speech Disorders*, 27: 67Y70.
CTOPP	Comprehensive Test of Phonological Processing	Wagner, R., Torgesen, J., & Rashotte, C. (1999). *Comprehensive Test of Phonological Processing*. Austin, TX: Pro-Ed, Inc.
EOWPVT	Expressive One-Word Picture Vocabulary Test	Gardner, M. (2000). *Expressive One-Word Picture Vocabulary Test*. Novato, CA: Academic Therapy Publications.
ESP	Early Speech Perception	Moog, J., & Geers, A. (1990). *Early Speech Perception (ESP) Test*. St. Louis, MO: Central Institute for the Deaf.
EVT-2	Expressive Vocabulary Test	Williams, K. (2007). *Expressive Vocabulary Test Manual, Second Edition*. Minneapolis, MN: NCS Pearson, Inc.
FES	Family Environment Scale	Moos, R., Insel, P., & Humphrey, B. (1974). *Preliminary manual for Family Environment Scale, Work Environment Scale, Group Environment Scale*. Palo Alto, CA: Consulting Psychologists Press.
FPRS	Family Participation Rating Scale	Moeller M. (2000). Early intervention and language development in children who are deaf and hard of hearing. *Pediatrics, 106*(3): 1–9.
GFTA-2	Goldman-Fristoe Test of Articulation, Second Edition	Goldman, R. & Fristoe, M. (2001). *Goldman-Fristoe Test of Articulation – Second Edition*. Shoreview, MN: American Guidance Service.

continues

Table 3–5. *continued*

HAPP-3	Hodson Assessment of Phonological Patterns, Third Edition	Hodson, B. (2004). *HAPP-3 Hodson Assessment of Phonological Patterns, Third Edition*. Austin, TX: Pro-Ed.
I Can Do Maths	I Can Do Maths	Doig, B., & de Lemnos, M. (2000). *I Can Do Maths*. Melbourne, Australia: ACER Press.
Insight	Insight	Morris, E. (2003). *Insight*. London, UK: Nfer Nelson.
Integrated Scales of Language Development	Integrated Scales of Language Development	Cochlear Ltd. (2003). *Integrated Scales of Language Development*. Listen, Learn, & Talk. Cochlear Ltd.
IT-MAIS	Infant-Toddler Meaningful Auditory Integration Scale	Zimmerman-Phillips, S., Robbins, A., & Osberger, M. (2001). *Infant-Toddler Meaningful Auditory Integration Scale*. Sylmar, CA: Advanced Bionics Corp.
KLPA-2	Khan-Lewis Phonological Analysis, Second Edition	Kahn, L. & Lewis, N. (2002). *Khan-Lewis Phonological Analysis, Second Edition*. Circle Pines, MN: American Guidance Systems.
Ling 5	Ling 5	Ling D. (1989). *Foundations of Spoken Language for Hearing-Impaired Children*. Washington DC: Alexander Graham Bell Association for the Deaf.
LIP	Listening Process Profile	Archold, S. (1994). Monitoring progress in children at the preverbal stage. In McCormick B., et al. (Eds), *Cochlear implants for young children* (pp. 197–213). London, UK: Whurr.
Leiter-R	Leiter International Performance Scale–Revised	Roid, G. & Miller, L. (1997). *Leiter-R Parent Rating Scale*. Wood Dale, IL: Stoelting.
LNT	Lexical Neighborhood Test	Kirk, K., Pisoni, D., & Osberger, M. (1995). Lexical effects on spoken word recognition by pediatric cohlear implant users. *Ear and Hearing, 16*, 470–481.

Table 3–5. *continued*

MAIS	Meaningful Auditory Integration Scale	Robbins, A., Renshaw, J., & Berry, S. (1991). Evaluating meaningful integration in profoundly hearing-impaired children. *American Journal of Otolaryngology, 12*(suppl.), 144–150.
MCDI	MacArthur-Bates Communicative Inventories	Fenson, L., Dale, P., Reznick, J., Thal, D., Bates, E., Hartung, J., Pethick, S., & Reilly, J. (1993). *MacArthur Communicative Inventories: User's Guide and Technical Manual.* San Diego, CA: Singular Publishing.
MDVP	Multi-Dimensional Voice Program	Kay Elemetrics Corp. (1999). *Multi–Dimensional Voice Program Software* instruction manual.
MLNT	Multisyllabic Lexical Neighborhood Test	Kirk, K., Pisoni, D., & Osberger, M. (1995). Lexical effects on spoken word recognition by pediatric cochlear implant users. *Ear and Hearing, 16,* 470–481.
MTP	Monosyllable, Prochee and Polysyllable Test	Erber, N. & Alencewicz, C. (1976). Audiological evaluation of deaf children. *Journal of Speech and Hearing Disorders, 41,* 256–267.
Neale-3	Neale Analysis of Reading Ability, Third Edition	Neale, M. (1999). *Neale Analysis of Reading Ability.* Melbourne, Vic: Australian Council of Educational Research Ltd.
NZAT	New Zealand Articulation Test	Moyle, J. (2005). The New Zealand Articulation Test Norms Project. *New Zealand Journal of Speech-Language Therapy, 60,* 61–75.
PAT Maths	Progressive Achievement Tests in Mathematics, Third Edition	Australian Council of Education Research. (2005). *Progressive Achievement Tests in Mathematics, Third Edition.,* Melbourne, Australia: ACER Press.
PBK/ Manchester Junior Words	Phonetically Balanced Kindergarten lists	Watson, T. (1957). Speech audiometry for children. In A. W. G. Ewing (Ed.), *Educational guidance and the deaf child* (pp. 278–296). Manchester, UK: The University Press.

continues

Table 3-5. *continued*

PIPPS	Penn Interactive Peer Play Scale	McWayne, C., Sekino, Y., Hampton, G., & Fantuzzo, J. (2007). *Penn Interactive Peer Play Scale Manual.* Philadelphia, PA: John Fantuzzo.
Plott Test Battery	The PLOTT test	Plant, G., & Westcott, S. (1983). *The PLOTT test.* Chatswood, Australia: National Acoustic Laboratories.
PLS-3 (UK)	Preschool Language Scale, Third Edition (UK Adaptation)	Zimmerman, I., Steiner, V., Pond, R., Boucher, J., and Lewis, V. (1991). *Preschool Language Scales, Third Edition* (UK Adaptation). The Psychological Corporation, London
PLS-4	Preschool Language Scale, Fourth Edition	Zimmerman, I., Steiner, V., & Pond, R. (2002). *Preschool Language Scale, Fourth Edition.* San Antonio, TX: The Psychological Corporation.
PLS-5	Preschool Language Scale, Fifth Edition	Zimmer, I., Steiner, V., & Pond, R. (2011). Preschool Language Scale, Fifth Edition. Bloomington, MN: Pearson/PsychCorp.
PPVT-3	Peabody Picture Vocabulary Test, Third Edition	Dunn, L. & Dunn, D. (1997). *Peabody picture vocabulary test, Third Edition.* Circle Pines, MN: American Guidance Service.
PPVT-4	Peabody Picture Vocabulary Test, Fourth Edition	Dunn L. & Dunn D. *Peabody Picture Vocabulary Test, Fourth Edition.* Circle Pines, MN: American Guidance Service, 2007.
QUIL	Queensland Inventory of Literacy	Dodd, B., Holm, S. Oerlemans, M., & McCormick, M. (1996). *Queensland Inventory of Literacy.* Queensland, Australia: University of Queensland.
Reading Progress Tests	Reading Progress Tests	Vincent, D., Crumpler, M., & Mare, M. (1997). *Reading Progress Tests.* Berkshire, UK: Nfer Nelson.
Reynell	Reynell Developmental Language Scales	J.K. Reynell, Huntley, M. (1985). *Reynell Developmental Language Scales, Revised Second Edition*, NFER-Nelson Publishing Company Ltd, Windsor, UK.

Table 3-5. *continued*

Rossetti Infant-Toddler Language Scale	Rossetti Infant-Toddler Language Scale	Rossetti, L. (1990). *The Rossetti Infant-Toddler Language Scale*. East Moline, IL: Linguisystems.
SCBE	Social Competence and Behavior Evaluation	LaFreniere, P. & Dumas, J. (1995). *Social Competence and Behavior Evaluation: Preschool Edition Manual*. Los Angeles, CA: Western Psychological Services.
SDQ-2	Self-Description Questionnaire, Second Edition	Marsh, H. (1990). *Self-Description Questionnaire II: Manual*. New South Wales, Australia: University of Western Sydney, Macarthur Faculty of Education Publication Unit.
SDQ-3	Self-Description Questionnaire, Third Edition	Marsh, H. (1992). *Self-Description Questionnaire III: Manual*. New South Wales, Australia: University of Western Sydney, Macarthur Faculty of Education Publication Unit.
SIR	The Speech Intelligibility Rating	Cox, R., & McDaniel, D. (1989). Development of the Speech Intelligibility Rating (SIR) test for hearing aid comparisons. *Journal of Speech and Hearing Research, 32*(2), 347–352.
SPEAK-probes	Speech Perception Education and Assessment Kit–Probes	Boothroyd, A. (1978). Speech perception and sensorineural hearing loss, in: M. Ross & T. Giolas (Eds.). *Auditory management of hearing-impaired children* (pp. 117–144). Baltimore, MD: University Park Press.
SPINE	SPeech INtelligibility Evaluation	Monsen, R., Moog, J., & Geers, A. (1988). *CID Picture SPINE (SPeech INtelligibility Evaluation)*. St. Louis, MO: Central Institute for the Deaf.
TOWRE	Test of Word Reading Efficiency	Wagner, R., Torgesen, J., & Rashotte, C. (1999). *Test of Word Reading Efficiency*. Austin, TX: Pro-Ed, Inc.
Viborgmaterialet	Viborgmaterialet	Pedersen, E., Kjøge, G. (2005). Viborgmaterialet. Herning. Specialpædagogisk Forlag,
Wechsler Preschool and Primary Scale of Intelligence	Wechsler Preschool and Primary Scale of Intelligence	Wechsler, D. (2002). *Wechsler Preschool and Primary Scale of Intelligence*. San Antonio, TX: Psychological Corporation.

continues

Table 3–5. *continued*

WIAT-2	Wechsler Individual Achievement Test, Second Edition	Wechsler, D. (1992) *Wechsler Individual Achievement Test, Second Edition.* San Antonio, TX: Harcourt Assessment.
WIAT-2 (Australian)	Wechsler Individual Achievement Test, Second Edition (Australian Adaptation)	Pearson PsychCorp. (2007). *Wechsler Individual Achievement Test, Second edition Australian Standardised Edition.* Sydney, NSW: NCS Pearson Ltd.
WJ-3	Woodcock Johnson Tests of Achievement III	Wendling, B., Schrank, F., & Schmitt, A. *Educational Interventions Related to the Woodcock-Johnson III Tests of Achievement (Assessment Service Bulletin No. 8).* Rolling Meadows, IL: Riverside Publishing; 2014.
WJ-4	Woodcock Johnson Tests of Achievement IV	Schrank, F., Mather, N., & McGrew, K. *Woodcock-Johnson IV Tests of Achievement.* Rolling Meadows, IL: Riverside; 2014.
WRAT-3	Wide Range Achievement Test, Third Edition	Jastak, J. & Wilkinson, G. (1993). *Wide Range Achievement Test, Third Edition.* Wilmington, DE: Wide Range Publishers.

sizes ranged from 10 to 203 participants, with some studies attempting to match the control and the experimental groups, in some cases retrospectively. The sample size of some of the new studies more than double the largest studies found just three years ago. In most cases the control groups consisted of children with typical hearing, but four of the six new studies deemed Level 3 research include a group of participants with hearing loss who received an intervention other than AVT. The majority of studies involved the administration of various standardized measures of articulation and language to both groups of children, comparing their performance using statistical analyses that ranged from descriptive statistics to mixed model analyses. Some of the studies were based on retrospective data obtained from the children's case files, while others were longitudinal in nature. Two of the newly added studies gathered data from adults who had received AVT as children. In most studies a convenience sample of children enrolled in AVT at a specific intervention center providing AVT intervention formed the experimental group. All but one of the new studies in Level 3 recruited participants from two or more centers. A complete list of the test measures (in alphabetical order according to test acronym) and their authors is provided in Table 3–5 and Appendix 3–A.

Level 4 Evidence

Of the research evaluated in this review, 15 articles were ranked as representing Level 4 evidence in favor of AVT, including 6 articles from the past three years. These articles are summarized in Table 3–6. Samples size ranged from 1 to 180, with several of the studies representing small case studies of individual children. None of the studies had a control group and most consisted of convenience samples of children enrolled in AVT at various intervention centers. In many of the studies, children were administered standardized tests and their performance was compared with the test norms using chronological and/or hearing age. Some studies had no statistical analyses while others reported t-tests, analyses of variance (ANOVAs), and correlational findings. A number of the studies were retrospective in nature.

Level 5 Evidence

Although some practitioners have historically used this form of evidence to support their practice, the authors here did not identify any studies at this evidence level.

NON-AVT OUTCOME RESEARCH

Twelve articles, including three added since the last publication of this chapter,

were identified in the review that utilized participants enrolled in AVT as an inclusion criterion to examine outcomes not directly related to AVT. These articles are summarized in Table 3–7 as the findings are of considerable interest to the field, although they do not specifically constitute AVT outcome research. The included studies examined variables such as age of diagnosis and age of cochlear implantation, speech perception and coarticulation abilities, gender differences, the impact of educational placement on speech and language outcomes, adult populations, and the impact of concomitant disorders in addition to hearing loss on various domains of communication outcome. Some of the studies represented relatively high levels of evidence, including one multiple baseline across participants design with each participant serving as his or her own control, which constitutes Level 1 research evidence. In some cases, random assignment to intervention groups was possible as the focus of the studies was not AVT per se. Statistical analyses varied, ranging from descriptive to linear regressions and mixed model analyses.

EVALUATING RESEARCH QUALITY

While rankings of research evidence levels as described above provide important information to evaluate the scientific rigor of research findings, a number of other important variables should also be taken into account when determining the quality of research contributing to the understanding of intervention efficacy. While two

Table 3-6. Quality of Evidence: Level 4 Table

LEVEL 4				
Authors	**N**	**Comparison Groups**	**Matching**	**Sample Pool**
*Dieleman, E., Percy-Smith, L., & Caye-Thomasen, P. (2019). Language outcome in children with congenital hearing impairment: The influence of etiology. *International Journal of Pediatric Otorhinolaryngology*, *117*, 37–44.	53	N/A	N/A	2 sites
Eriks-Brophy, A., Durieux-Smith, A., Olds, J., Fitzpatrick, E., Duquette, C., & Whittingham, J. (2012). Communication, academic, and social skills of young adults with hearing loss. *The Volta Review, 112*(1), 5–35.	43 24 of those in phase 2	N/A	N/A	1 site
Fairgray, E., Purdy, S., & Smart, J. (2010). Effects of auditory-verbal therapy for school-aged children with hearing loss: an exploratory study. *The Volta Review, 110*(3), 407–433.	7	N/A	N/A	Multi-site

LEVEL 4			
Study Design	**Tests**	**Stats**	**Findings**
Retrospective	PPVT, Reynell, Viborgmaterialet	Chi-square; Fisher's exact; Kruskal-Wallis; McNemar Test; logistic regression	There was no difference in outcome over three years between etiology groups. Parents didn't always know the etiology of their child's hearing loss.
Prospective	Questionnaire based on Goldberg & Flexer 1993, PPVT-R, CID SPINE, WIAT: academic function oral language skills and academic achievement, WRAT-3, & SDQ: Self perception	t-test, ANOVA, chi-square, & descriptive statistics	People who received AVT in childhood and were supported throughout their school years were successful in mainstream environments. They also performed comparably to their typically hearing peers on communication and self-perception assessments as well as in academic achievement.
Prospective	Australian CELF-4, HAPP-3, NZAT, WIAT- II: Word Reading, Pseudoword Decoding, and reading comprehension, & LNT speech in noise recorded with NZ female speaker	Wilcoxon Matched Pairs, descriptive statistics	After 20 weeks of AVT, children showed improvement on speech perception, speech production, and receptive language measures. There was less improvement shown in the area of reading.

continues

Table 3–6. *continued*

LEVEL 4				
Authors	**N**	**Comparison Groups**	**Matching**	**Sample Pool**
Harris, L. (2014). *Social-emotional development in children with hearing loss*. (Unpublished master's thesis). University of Kentucky: Lexington.	5	N/A	N/A	1 site
*Hitchins, A. & Hogan, S. (2018). Outcomes of early intervention for deaf children with additional needs following an Auditory Verbal approach to communication. *International Journal of Pediatric Otorhinolaryngology, 115*, 125–132.	129	N/A	N/A	1 site
Hogan, S., Stokes, J., White, C., Tyszkiewicz, E., & Woolgar, A. (2008). An evaluation of auditory verbal therapy using the rate of early language development as an outcome measure. *Deafness and Education International, 10*(3), 143–167.	37	N/A	N/A	1 site

LEVEL 4			
Study Design	**Tests**	**Stats**	**Findings**
Prospective	Penn Interactive Peer Play Scale (PIPPS) (McWayne, Sekino, Hampton, & Fantuzzo, 2007), the Social Competence and Behaviour Evaluation-Preschool Edition (SCBE) (LaFreniere & Dumas, 1995), and the Behaviour Assessment System for Children- Second Edition (BASC-2) (Kamphaus & Reynolds, 2007) PPVT-4, EVT-2 and GFTA-2 scores taken retrospectively	N/A	Using psychosocial scales of social-emotional development, only one of the five participants appeared to demonstrate problems in this area.
Retrospective	RLD (rate of language delivery) calculated using PLS-4 and 5 (UK) scores	z-scores; Pearson correlation; one-way ANOVA	79% of the participants achieved age appropriate language. Children with developmental delay showed slower language learning.
Prospective	RLD (rate of language delivery) calculated using PLS-3 (UK) scores	Kolmogorov-Smirnov tests, t-test, & descriptive statistics	AVT improved rate of language development regardless of the child's age or hearing technology.

continues

Table 3–6. *continued*

LEVEL 4				
Authors	**N**	**Comparison Groups**	**Matching**	**Sample Pool**
*Kim, L., Wisely, E., & Lucius, S. (2016). Positive outcomes and surgical strategies for bilateral cochlear implantation in a child with X-linked deafness. *Annals of Otology, Rhinology, & Laryngology, 125*(2), 173–176.	1	N/A	N/A	1 site
*Lim, S., Goldberg, D., & Flexer, C. (2018). Auditory-Verbal Graduates—25 years later: Outcome survey of the clinical effectiveness of the listening and spoken language approach for young children with hearing loss. *The Volta Review, 118*(1.2), 5–40.	207	N/A	N/A	16 countries
*Necula,V., Cosgarea, M., & Maniu, A. (2018). Effects of family environment features on cochlear-implanted children. *European Archives of Oto-Rhino-Laryngology, 275*(9), 2209–2217.	58	N/A	N/A	1 site

LEVEL 4			
Study Design	Tests	Stats	Findings
Prospective	Auditory Learning Guide; REEL-3; PLS-5	Raw data	A combination of CI and AVT can lead to age appropriate language development in kids with X-linked deafness.
Prospective	Questionnaire (70 questions) looking at: demographics, hearing loss, technology, AVT, additional disabilities, education/occupation, languages spoken and community involvement, and a final question "Would you do AVT again if you had to do it all again?"	Percentages for each area of interest from questionnaire	Children with hearing loss grow up listening and talking in typical school, university, and living environments. They integrate into mainstream society. 76% wearing CIs in this study compared to 16% in 2001 study. This study had participants from 16 countries (1993 and 2001 studies were only from US and Canada). Comment on the potential of children with HL to learn other languages.
Prospective	FES questionnaire; CAP; SIR	Descriptive statistics	Families of children with CIs had high scores on cohesion and organization.

continues

Table 3–6. *continued*

LEVEL 4				
Authors	**N**	**Comparison Groups**	**Matching**	**Sample Pool**
Sahli, A. & Belgin, E. (2011). Researching auditory perception performance of children using cochlear implants and being trained by an auditory-verbal therapy. *The Journal of International Advanced Otology, 7*(3), 385–390.	15	N/A	N/A	1 site
*Sharma, S., Bhatia, K., Singh, S., Lahiri, A., & Aggarwal, A. (2017). Impact of socioeconomic factors on paediatric cochlear implant outcomes. *International Journal of Pediatric Otorhinolaryngology, 102*, 90–97.	180	N/A	N/A	1 site

LEVEL 4			
Study Design	**Tests**	**Stats**	**Findings**
Prospective	IT MAIS/MAIS, LIP, Ling 5 sound test, MTP	Mann-Whitney U-test, & descriptive statistics	A combination of cochlear implants and AVT improves auditory perception skills in children with hearing loss.
Prospective	CAP; MAIS; SIR	Descriptive statistics; Pearson correlation	Regardless of SES, children with hearing loss do well if they receive their CIs early and attend AV therapy.

continues

Table 3-6. *continued*

LEVEL 4				
Authors	**N**	**Comparison Groups**	**Matching**	**Sample Pool**
Von Muenster, K. & Baker, E. (2014). Oral communicating children using a cochlear implant: Good reading outcomes are linked to better language and phonological processing abilities. *International Journal of Pediatric Otorhinolaryngology, 78*(3), 433–444.	47	N/A	N/A	1 site
Warner-Czyz, A., Davis, B., & Morrison, H. (2005). Production accuracy in a young cochlear implant recipient. *The Volta Review, 105*(1), 5–25.	1	N/A	N/A	1 site

LEVEL 4			
Study Design	**Tests**	**Stats**	**Findings**
Prospective	Sight word reading- TOWRE Sight word reading of non-words- QUIL Passage reading- Neal-3 Reading comprehension- Neal-3 Words level- CNC Sentence level-BKB PPVT 3 Receptive/ expressive language- CELF 3 or CELF preschool Production of mono, di, and polysyllabic words-ACAP-A Phonological awareness, Phonological working memory, Phonological retrieval-CTOPP	Pearson Product Moment Correlation & Principal Component Analysis	Children with hearing loss who have higher language and phonologic processing skills have better reading outcomes.
Prospective	Rosetti Infant Toddler Language Scale	Descriptive statistics	A child who received a cochlear implant at 24 months showed an increase in her phonetic inventory over a four month period.

continues

Table 3-6. *continued*

LEVEL 4				
Authors	**N**	**Comparison Groups**	**Matching**	**Sample Pool**
Wong, S., Scarinci, N., Hickson, L., Rose, T., & Constantinescu, G. (2013). Bilateral cochlear implants in children: A preliminary study of language and speech perception outcomes. *The Australian and New Zealand Journal of Audiology, 33*(1), 48–68.	21	N/A	N/A	1 site
Wood, Jackson, C. & Schatschneider, C. (2014). Rate of language growth in children with hearing loss in an auditory-verbal early intervention program. *American Annuals of the Deaf, 158*(5), 539–554.	24	N/A	N/A	1 site

Note: *Article added since the last publication of this chapter.

LEVEL 4			
Study Design	**Tests**	**Stats**	**Findings**
Prospective	Plott battery tests, CNC test, Manchester Junior Words Test, BKB Sentences, PPVT-3, PLS-4, CELF-P, CELF-3, & CELF-4	Descriptive statistics, & Wilcoxon signed- rank test	Bilateral cochlear implantation did not seem to affect spoken language or receptive vocabulary scores but some of the children did improve in the area of speech perception.
Retrospective	PLS-4 (retrospectively)	Mixed Model Analysis (hierarchal linear modeling) & descriptive statistics	Over a six-month period, children in AVT did not demonstrate an improvement in standard language scores. However, the longer the child had been enrolled in AVT, the better they performed; indicating the impact of AVT on language development.

Table 3-7. Quality of Evidence: Non-AVT Outcomes Table

Non-AVT Outcome Studies				
Author	**N**	**Comparison Groups**	**Matching**	**Sample Pool**
Allegro, J., Papsin, B., Harrison, R., & Campisi, P. (2010). Acoustic analysis of voice in cochlear implant recipients with post-meningitic hearing loss. *Cochlear Implants International, 11*(2), 100–116.	10	N/A	N/A	1 site
Bakhshaee, M., Ghasemi, M., Shakeri, M., Razmara, N., Tayarani, H., & Tale, M. (2007). Speech development in children after cochlear implantation. *Ear Archives of Otorhinolaryngology, 264*, 1263–1266.	47	N/A	N/A	1 site
*Baungaard, L., Sandvej, M., Kroijer, J., Hestbaek, M., Samar, C., Percy-Smith, L., & Caye-Thomasen, P. (2019). Auditory verbal skills training is a new approach in adult cochlear implant rehabilitation. *Danish Medical Journal, 66*(3), A5535.	AVST: 10 Non-AVST: 7	AVST & Non-AVST	Not reported	1 site
*Chen, P. & Liu, T. (2017). A pilot study of telepractice for teaching listening and spoken language to Mandarin-speaking children with congenital hearing loss. *Deafness & Education International, 19*(3-4), 134–143.	AV: 5 eAV: 5	AV & eAV	Hearing level; age; duration in AVT; age at fitting	1 site

Non-AVT Outcome Studies			
Study Design	**Tests**	**Stats**	**Findings**
Prospective	Multidimensional Voice program	Descriptive statistics & trend analysis	After meningitis, children who had aided residual hearing, received a cochlear implant, attended AVT, and did not have cochlear ossification had better long-term control of vocal frequency and amplitude.
Prospective	Speech Intelligibility Rating (SIR) test	Mann-Whitney U test	Subjective speech intelligibility rankings of children post cochlear implant increased significantly for three years and did not seem to plateau after five years.
Prospective	Dantale I; HINT; NCIQ	Descriptive statistics; Wilcoxon signed rank test; Mann Whitney U test	While the AVST group received more fine tuning for their CI programs, both groups improved in speech understanding and quality of life measures.
Prospective	RPLA; parent/ therapist satisfaction questionnaire	t-tests; Mann-Whitney U-tests; Descriptive statistics	No differences found between the two groups

continues

Table 3–7. *continued*

Non-AVT Outcome Studies				
Author	**N**	**Comparison Groups**	**Matching**	**Sample Pool**
Easterbrooks, S. & O'Rourke, C. (2001). Gender differences in response to auditory-verbal intervention in children who are deaf or hard of hearing. *American Annals of the Deaf, 146*(4), 309–319.	70	N/A	N/A	1 site
*Fulcher, A., Purcell, A., Baker, E., & Munro, N. (2015). Factors influencing speech and language outcomes of children with early identified severe/ profound hearing loss: Clinician-identified facilitators and barriers. International *Journal of Speech-Language Pathology, 17*(3), 325–333.	6 clinicians	N/A	N/A	1 site
Fulcher, A., Purcell, A., Baker, E., & Munro, N. (2012). Listen up: Children with early identified hearing loss achieve age-appropriate speech/language outcomes by 3 years-of-age. *International Journal of Pediatric Otorhinolaryngology, 76*, 1785–1794.	Early ID'd: 45 Late ID'd: 49	Early ID'd & Late ID'd	No matching	1 site
Lew, J., Purcell, A., Doble, M., & Lim, L. (2014). Hear here: Children with hearing loss learn words by listening. *International Journal of Pediatric Otorhinolaryngology, 78*, 1716–1725.	3	N/A	N/A	1 site

Non-AVT Outcome Studies			
Study Design	**Tests**	**Stats**	**Findings**
Prospective/ retrospective	Parent Interview & Leiter International Performance Scale, revised	Descriptive statistics & t-test	Although both boys and girls had high language scores, the girls outperformed the boys. Parents were more likely to say that their sons behave well in AVT sessions.
Prospective	Clinician interviews	Qualitative analysis	Barriers to AV treatment including living in remote areas, clinician confidence with young children and families from cultures that differ from their own.
Prospective/ retrospective	GFTA-2, PPVT-4, PLS-4	Independent t-tests, Cohen's d, ANOVA, Cohen's f, & Mann-Whitney U	Children who were early diagnosed, received amplification by three months, AVT by six months, and cochlear implants by 18 months, did not demonstrate a delay of speech and language skills by age three.
Prospective	ESP, SPEAK-probes, PPVT-4, 2500+ Words List, GFTA- 2, & CASALA Analysis	t-test & descriptive statistics	Intervention directed at listening alone improves vocabulary and speech skills without having to focus on them as specific goals.

continues

Table 3–7. *continued*

Non-AVT Outcome Studies				
Author	**N**	**Comparison Groups**	**Matching**	**Sample Pool**
Moog, J. & Geers, A. (2010). Early educational placement and later language outcomes for children with cochlear implants. *Otology & Neurotology, 31*, 1315–1319.	141	N/A	N/A	Multi-site
Morrison, H. (2011). Coarticulation in early vocalizations by children with hearing loss: A locus perspective. *Clinical Linguistics & Phonetics, 26*(3), 288–309.	3	N/A	N/A	1 site
Pundir, M., Nagarkar, A., & Panda, N. (2007). Intervention strategies in children with cochlear implants having attention deficit hyperactivity disorder. *International Journal of Pediatric Otorhinolaryngology, 71*, 985–988.	2	N/A	N/A	1 site
Wolfe, J., Baker, S., Caraway, T., Kasulis, H., Mears, A., Smith, J., Swim, L., & Wood, M. (2007). 1-Year postactivation results for sequentially implanted bilateral cochlear implant users. *Otology & Neurotology, 28*(5), 589–596.	12	N/A	N/A	1 site

Note: *Article added since the last publication of this chapter.

Non-AVT Outcome Studies			
Study Design	Tests	Stats	Findings
Prospective	PPVT, EOWPVT, & CELF-P, Wechsler preschool and primary scale of intelligence	Descriptive, ANOVA	Children with hearing loss benefit from cochlear implantation by age one and parent-focused spoken language intervention supplemented by an LSLS classroom by age two.
Prospective	Rosetti, MCDI, acoustic analysis of speech segments based on production characteristics, Locus Equation Analyses	Descriptive statistics	Children who received hearing aids by five months had anticipatory coarticulation patterns similar to typically developing peers. Anticipatory coarticulation patterns were affected by whether or not the child had acquired that syllable before or after cochlear implantation.
Prospective	Integrated Scales of Language Development	None	Two children receiving AVT did not begin to show improvements in listening, speech, and language skills until their ADHD was controlled using drugs.
Retrospective	MLNT (Multisyllabic Lexical Neighborhood Test) or ESP, speech recognition in noise	Linear, regression, correlation, & t-test	Sequential bilateral cochlear implantation improved children's ability to recognize speech in noise. Children who received their second cochlear implant before four years old did better than those who received theirs later.

studies may be ranked as representing the same evidence level, their overall quality may nevertheless differ considerably. Gradations in the overall quality of the evidence provided by the studies ranked at Levels 3 and 4 of the hierarchy can be determined by asking ourselves a series of questions related to the finer points of the methodological approaches and analyses used in a particular study. Such questions provide important information to clinicians when making EIP decisions. These questions consist of the following:

- Is the study design prospective or retrospective? Prospective designs are generally considered higher in quality than retrospective designs, as retrospective designs often rely on information obtained through file reviews as opposed to the direct administration of a selected outcome measure to a participant group.
- Are participants randomly assigned to intervention groups? While this variable is an essential one in deciding the level of evidence attributable to any study, it is also a quality indicator, as random assignment is a central component in avoiding bias. As has been discussed previously, however, randomly assigning participants to interventions such as AVT is not feasible.
- Were participants, practitioners, and those administering the outcome measures blinded to which children were contained in the intervention versus the experimental group? Unblinded

studies have a much larger chance of introducing bias both into the intervention itself as well as into the analysis of results.

- Do the participants represent a convenience sample or were they specifically recruited for the study? A recruited sample is generally considered to contain less bias than a convenience sample.
- If the study involves a comparison group, were the participants matched on relevant variables? Matched group designs are considered to contain less bias than unmatched group designs.
- If the study involves a comparison group, were both groups treated equally as part of the study design with respect to all study elements other than the intervention itself? Studies that provide equivalent exposure to all participants and that document differences in performance post intervention provide higher quality evidence in support of the intervention under review.
- What is the sample size used in the research? Studies involving larger numbers of participants are generally viewed as being less biased and more generalizable than studies with a small number of participants.
- How complete is the demographic information provided about the participant groups? Does this information contribute to understanding any group differences in the results reported in the study? Providing

adequate demographic information about participant groups can be essential, in many cases, to explaining differences in group performance following intervention.

▪ What outcome measures were used in documenting outcomes? Measures with well-known reliability and validity provide higher quality evidence than non-standardized measures.

▪ What types of outcome scores are reported? Are they standard scores obtained through the administration of a test measure or are they observations or parent reports? Outcomes reported as standard scores on a test measure are considered to be more reliable indicators of outcome than informal test measures and are also more readily analyzed using higher-level statistical analyses.

▪ What level of statistical analysis was performed on the outcome data? Is effect size reported, and, if so, what is the magnitude of the effect size? Higher-level statistical analyses that show significant differences in performance between the sample participants or achieve high effect sizes are considered to be of substantially higher quality than descriptive observations of performance.

▪ Was the intervention provided for a long enough period of time to illustrate a difference between intervention groups? The potential benefits of a particular intervention may be masked if the intervention period is too short for any effect to be demonstrated.

▪ Were any of the participants lost to follow-up or did any participants drop out of the study as it was being conducted? Was the participant dropout rate reported and discussed? Studies with many participants lost over the course of the study raise questions about possible underlying reasons why participants might choose to leave a particular study.

AREAS FOR IMPROVEMENT IN CONDUCTING AND REPORTING AVT OUTCOME RESEARCH

Since the original publication of this chapter in 2016, an impressive amount of new research has been carried out examining the outcomes of AVT for children who are deaf or hard of hearing in a variety of domains, including audition, speech, language, and social-emotional development. The existing research base has become increasingly international and has examined outcomes for children who speak languages other than English and/or who are being raised to be bilingual. The evidence levels as well as the overall quality of the existing research have increased, indicative of important advances in the scientific rigor represented by current studies examining the outcomes of AVT. Clearly the call to action put forward by our 2016 chapter may have created a concrete impact on the formulation of recent research questions and their associated methodologies.

Nevertheless, certain obstacles to conducting research into the outcomes of AVT remain. First, as discussed previously, conducting research that would demonstrate a clear cause/effect relationship between AVT and children's communication outcomes through RCTs remains problematic primarily due to issues associated with random group assignment to AVT and non-AVT interventions, as this circumvents some of the principles of AVT. Furthermore, the OCEMB (2011) now considers observational studies with large effect sizes as providing equally convincing evidence, offering AVT researchers additional design options for generating high level evidence. Nevertheless, systematic reviews and the RCT research they encompass are extremely important to EBP in AVT and are a gold standard toward which we should continue to strive. Through taking an EIP approach, we can use our critical appraisal skills to evaluate all the research to which we have access, including the lower levels of evidence that the Cochrane systematic review was forced to disregard. This information can inform our clinical and other intervention decisions and our conclusions regarding intervention outcomes, as well as use this information in developing research questions appropriate for use in eventual RCTs.

Second, the existing evidence base is difficult to integrate and summarize using a systematic review approach due to variations in the quality of evidence provided by the current studies. This point is well illustrated through the inconclusive results obtained by the systematic review on AVT conducted by Brennan-Jones et al. (2014) described previously. Third, some of the methodologies utilized in the studies reviewed do not permit sophisticated statistical analyses, which limits their potential contribution as supporting evidence for AVT outcomes. For example, none of the studies reviewed provided effect sizes for their results, a common current practice in reporting research findings, while only 2 studies from our 2016 chapter had research designs that would allow for magnitude of effect size to be calculated. However, 7 of the 15 studies added in the last three years did. This may indicate a small step toward better statistical analysis within AVT research. Fourth, the demographic information provided in the various studies differs widely, making comparisons across research studies difficult to carry out. It would be useful for researchers in AVT to come to a consensus on the demographic information to be reported for all participants in order to eventually be able to carry out systematic reviews leading to conclusive results. Consistency in reporting information, including age at diagnosis, age at amplification, hearing age, amount of time wearing technology, amount of time spent in AVT, language(s) used in the home, and socio-economic status would permit greater generalization of findings across comparable groups. Socio-economic status in particular has been identified as a potentially key variable influencing communication outcomes for children with and without communication disorders, and reporting this information in a consistent manner across studies would permit its impact to be examined more carefully in the AVT research. Fifth, there continue to be a large number of studies that use convenience samples and do not include a control group, a significant limitation to the existing evidence base. Furthermore, when a comparison group was provided, participants were generally poorly matched. There does appear to be a trend toward comparing outcomes for different groups of children who are deaf or hard of hearing, thus improving our ability to rigorously analyze intervention effects.

CONCLUSION

While this chapter has argued that all levels of evidence are informative and acceptable in the context of evidence-informed practice, including mechanism-based reasoning, it is nevertheless incumbent on researchers in AVT to conduct research of the highest possible quality. Advances in the evidence levels as well as the quality of the current research base supporting AVT outcomes illustrate that researchers are indeed taking up this challenge. Taking an EIP approach to the generation and interpretation of research studies examining the outcomes of AVT has great potential to improve AVT practice patterns and decision making, resulting in enhanced outcomes for the children and families served in AVT, and indeed will provide increased authority and credibility to the field of AVT around the world.

REFERENCES

AG Bell Academy for Listening and Spoken Language. (2007). Principles of LSLS. Retrieved September 8, 2015 from http:// www.listeningandspokenlanguage.org /AcademyDocument.aspx?id=563

Allegro, J., Papsin, B., Harrison, R., & Campisi, P. (2010). Acoustic analysis of voice in cochlear implant recipients with post-meningitic hearing loss. *Cochlear Implants International, 11*(2), 100–116.

Bakhshaee, M., Ghasemi, M., Shakeri, M., Razmara, N., Tayarani, H., & Tale, M. (2007). Speech development in children after cochlear implantation. *Ear Archives of Otorhinolaryngology, 264*, 1263–1266.

Baungaard, L., Sandvej, M., Kroijer, J., Hestbaek, M., Samar, C., Percy-Smith, L., & Caye-Thomasen, P. (2019). Auditory verbal skills training is a new approach in adult cochlear implant rehabilitation. *Danish Medical Journal, 66*(3), A5535.

Bero, L. A., Grilli, R., Grimshaw, J. M., Harvey, E., Oxman, A. D., & Thomson, M. A. (1998). Closing the gap between research and practice: An overview of systematic reviews of interventions to promote the implementation of research findings. *British Medical Journal, 317*, 465–468.

Brennan-Jones, C., White, J., Rush, R., & Law, J. (2014). Auditory-verbal therapy for promoting spoken language development in children with permanent hearing impairments. *Cochrane Database of Systematic Reviews, 3*, CD010100. doi: 10.1002/14651858.CD010100.pub2

Center for Evidence-Based Medicine. (2014). Glossary. Retrieved August 28, 2015 from http://www.cebm.net

Chen, P., & Liu, T. (2017). A pilot study of telepractice for teaching listening and spoken language to Mandarin-speaking children with congenital hearing loss. *Deafness & Education International, 19*(3–4), 134–143.

Clarke, B., Gillies, D., Illari, P., Russo, F., & Williamson, J. (2013) The evidence that evidence-based medicine omits. *Preventive Medicine, 57*(6), 745–747.

Dettman, S., Wall, E., Constantinescu, G., & Dowell, R. (2013). Communication outcomes for groups of children using cochlear implants enrolled in auditory-verbal, aural-oral, and bilingual-bicultural early intervention programs. *Otology & Neurotology, 34,* 451–459.

Dieleman, E., Percy-Smith, L., & Caye-Thomasen, P. (2019). Language outcome in children with congenital hearing impairment: The influence of etiology. *International Journal of Pediatric Otorhinolaryngology, 117,* 37–44.

Dollaghan, C. (2004). Evidence-based practice myths and realities. *ASHA Leader, 9*(7), 4–12.

Dornan, D., Hickson, L., Murdoch, B., Houston, T., & Constantinescu, G. (2010). Is auditory-verbal therapy effective for children with hearing loss? *The Volta Review, 110*(3), 361–387.

Dornan, D., Hickson, L, Murdoch, B., & Houston, T. (2009). Longitudinal study of speech perception, speech, and language for children with hearing loss in an auditory-verbal therapy program. *The Volta Review, 109*(2–3), 61–85.

Dornan, D., Hickson, L., Murdoch, B., & Houston, T. (2007). Outcomes of an auditory-verbal program for children with hearing loss: A comparative study with a matched group of children with normal hearing. *The Volta Review, 107*(1), 37–54.

Dunn, L., & Dunn, D. (2007). *Peabody Picture Vocabulary Test* (4th ed.). Circle Pines, MN: American Guidance Service.

Dunst, C., Trivette, C., & Cutspec, A. (2002). Toward an operational definition of evidence-based practices. *Centerscope, 1*(1), 1–10.

Easterbrooks, S., & O'Rourke, C. (2001). Gender differences in response to auditory-verbal intervention in children who are deaf or hard of hearing. *American Annals of the Deaf, 146*(4), 309–319.

Ellis, P. (2010). *The essential guide to effect sizes: Statistical power, meta-analysis, and the interpretation of research results.* Cambridge, UK: Cambridge University Press.

Eriks-Brophy, A., Ganek, H., & DuBois, G. (2016). Evaluating the research examining AVT outcomes: Moving from evidence-based to evidence-informed practice. In W. Estabrooks, K. T. Houston, K. MacIver-Lux, & E. Rhoades (Eds.), *Auditory-verbal therapy for young children with hearing loss and their families, and the practitioners who guide them.* San Diego, CA: Plural Publishing.

Eriks-Brophy, A., Gibson, S., & Tucker. S. (2013). Articulatory error patterns and phonological process use of preschool children with and without hearing loss. *The Volta Review, 113*(2), 87–12.

Eriks-Brophy, A., Durieux-Smith, A., Olds, J., Fitzpatrick, E., Duquette, C., & Whittingham, J. (2012). Communication, academic, and social skills of young adults with hearing loss. *The Volta Review, 112*(1), 5–35.

Fairgray, E., Purdy, S., & Smart, J. (2010). Effects of auditory-verbal therapy for school-aged children with hearing loss: An exploratory study. *The Volta Review, 110*(3), 407–433.

Fulcher, A., Purcell, A., Baker, E., & Munro, N. (2015). Factors influencing speech and language outcomes of children with early identified severe/profound hearing loss: Clinician-identified facilitators and barriers. *International Journal of Speech-Language Pathology, 17*(3), 325–333.

Fulcher, A., Purcell, A., Baker, E., & Munro, N. (2012). Listen up: Children with early identified hearing loss achieve age-appropriate speech/language outcomes by 3 years-of-age. *International Journal of Pediatric Otorhinolaryngology, 76,* 1785–1794.

Gambril, E. (2007). Views of evidence based practice: Social Workers' code of ethics and accreditation standards as guides for choice. *Journal of Social Work Education, 43*(3), 447–462.

Goldblat, E., & Pinto, O. (2017). Academic outcomes of adolescents and young adults with hearing loss who received auditory-verbal therapy. *Deafness & Education International, 19*(3–4), 126–133.

Hargrove, P. (2002). Evidence-based practice tutorial #3: Identifying the magnitude of the effect. *SIG 1 Perspectives on*

Language Learning and Education, 9(3), 34–36.

Harris, L. (2014). *Social-emotional development in children with hearing loss.* Unpublished Master's thesis. Lexington, KY: University of Kentucky.

Higgins, J., & Green, S. (2008). *Cochrane handbook for systematic reviews of interventions.* Chichester, UK: Wiley-Blackwell.

Hitchins, A., & Hogan, S. (2018). Outcomes of early intervention for deaf children with additional needs following an auditory verbal approach to communication. *International Journal of Pediatric Otorhinolaryngology, 115*, 125–132.

Hogan, S., Stokes, J., & Weller, I. (2010). Language outcomes for children of low-income families enrolled in auditory verbal therapy. *Deafness & Education International, 12*(4), 204–216.

Hogan, S., Stokes, J., White, C., Tyszkiewicz, E., & Woolgar, A. (2008). An evaluation of auditory verbal therapy using the rate of early language development as an outcome measure. *Deafness and Education International, 10*(3), 143–167.

Howick, J., Glasziou, P., & Aronson, J. (2010). Evidence-based mechanistic reasoning. *Journal of the Royal Society of Medicine, 103*, 433–441.

Howick, J. (2011). *The philosophy of evidence-based medicine.* Hoboken, NJ: Wiley-Blackwell, BMJ.

Howick, J., Chalmers, I., Glasziou, P., Greenhalgh, T., Heneghan, C., Liberati, I., . . . Hodgkinson, M. (2011). *The Oxford 2001 levels of evidence.* Oxford Centre for Evidence-Based Medicine. Retrieved August 14, 2015 from http://www.cebm.net/index.aspx?o=5653

Ilari, P., & Williamson, J. (2012). What is a mechanism? Thinking about mechanisms across the sciences. *European Journal of Philosophical Science, 2*, 119–135.

Jackson, C., & Schatschneider, C. (2014). Rate of language growth in children with hearing loss in an auditory-verbal early intervention program. *American Annals of the Deaf, 158*(5), 539–554.

Kaipa, R., & Danser, M. (2016). Efficacy of auditory-verbal therapy in children with hearing impairment: A systematic review from 1993 to 2015. *International Journal of Pediatric Otorhinolaryngology, 86*, 124–134.

Kaipa, R., & Peterson, A. (2016). A systematic review of treatment intensity in speech disorders. *International Journal of Speech-Language Pathology, 18*(6), 507–520.

Kim, L., Wisely, E., & Lucius, S. (2016). Positive outcomes and surgical strategies for bilateral cochlear implantation in a child with X-linked deafness. *Annals of Otology, Rhinology, & Laryngology, 125*(2), 173–176.

Liberati, A., Altman, D., Tetzlaff, J., Mulrow, C., Gotzsche, P., Ioannidis, J., . . . Moher, D. (2009). The PRISMA statement for reporting systematic reviews and meta-analyses of studies that evaluate health care interventions: Explanation and elaboration. *Journal of Clinical Epidemiology, 62*(10), e1–e34.

Lew, J., Purcell, A., Doble, M., & Lim, L. (2014). Hear here: Children with hearing loss learn words by listening. *International Journal of Pediatric Otorhinolaryngology, 78*, 1716–1725.

Lim, S. (2017). The effects of early auditory-based intervention on adult bilateral cochlear implant outcomes. *Cochlear Implants International, 18*(5), 256–265.

Lim, S., Goldberg, D., & Flexer, C. (2018). Auditory-verbal graduates—25 years later: Outcome survey of the clinical effectiveness of the listening and spoken language approach for young children with hearing loss. *The Volta Review, 118*(1.2), 5–40.

Lomas, J. (1991). Words without action? The production, dis-semination, and impact of consensus recommendations. *Annual Review of Public Health, 12*, 41–65.

Moog, J., & Geers, A. (2010). Early educational placement and later language outcomes for children with cochlear implants. *Otology & Neurotology, 31*, 1315–1319.

Morrison, H. (2011). Coarticulation in early vocalizations by children with hearing loss: A locus perspective. *Clinical Linguistics & Phonetics, 26*(3), 288–309.

Necula, V., Cosgarea, M., & Maniu, A. (2018). Effects of family environment features on cochlear-implanted children. *European Archives of Oto-Rhino-Laryngology, 275*(9), 2209–2217.

Nevo, I., & Slonim-Nevo, V. (2011). The myth of evidence-based practice: Towards evidence-informed practice. *British Journal of Social Work, 41*(6), 1176–1197.

Oxford Centre for Evidence-Based Medicine (OCEBM) (2011). *The Oxford 2011 levels of evidence.* Retrieved September 8, 2015 from http://www.cebm.net/index.aspx?o=5653

Oxman, A., Thomson, M., Davis, D., & Haynes, R. (1995). No magic bullets: A systematic review of 102 trials of interventions to improve professional practice. *Canadian Medical Association Journal, 153*, 1423–1431.

Percy-Smith, L., Hallstrom, M., Josvassen, J., Mikkelsen, J., Nissen, L., Dieleman, E., & Caye-Thomasen, P. (2018). Differences and similarities in early vocabulary development between children with hearing aids and children with cochlear implant enrolled in 3-year auditory verbal intervention. *International Journal of Pediatric Otorhinolaryngology, 108*, 67–72.

Percy-Smith, L., Tonning, T., Josvassen, J., Mikkelsen, J., Nissen, L., Dieleman, E., . . . Caye-Thomasen, P. (2017). Auditory-verbal habilitation is associated with improved outcome for children with cochlear implant. *Cochlear Implants International, 19*(1), 38–45.

Pundir, M., Nagarkar, A., & Panda, N. (2007). Intervention strategies in children with cochlear implants having attention deficit hyperactivity disorder. *International Journal of Pediatric Otorhinolaryngology, 71*, 985–988.

Robertson, L., Dow, G., & Hainzinger, S. (2006). Story retelling patterns among children with and without hearing loss: Effects of repeated practice and parent-child attunement. *The Volta Review, 106*(2), 147–170.

Rubin A. (2007). Improving the teaching of evidence-based practice: Introduction to the special issue. *Research on Social Work Practice, 17*, 541–547.

Sackett, D. (1997). Evidence-based medicine. *Seminars in Perinatology, 21*(1), 3–5.

Sahil, A., & Belgin, E. (2011). Researching auditory perception performance of children using cochlear implants and being trained by an auditory-verbal therapy. *Journal of International Advanced Otology, 7*(3), 385–390.

Sharma, S., Bhatia, K., Singh, S., Lahiri, A., & Aggarwal, A. (2017). Impact of socioeconomic factors on paediatric cochlear implant outcomes. *International Journal of Pediatric Otorhinolaryngology, 102*, 90–97.

Stewart-Brown, S., Anthony, R., Wilson, L., Winstanley, S., Stallard, N., Snooks, H., & Simkiss, D. (2011). Should randomized controlled trials be the "gold standard" for research on preventive interventions for children? *Journal of Children's Services, 6*(4), 228–235.

Strauss, S., Glasziou, P., Richardson, W., & Haynes, R. (2011). *Evidence-based medicine: How to practice and teach it* (4th ed.). Toronto, Ontario, Canada: Churchill Livingstone Elsevier.

Tejeda-Franco, C., Valadez-Jimenez, V., Hernandez-Lopez, X., Ysunza, P., Mena-Ramirez, M., Garcia-Zalapa, R., & Miranda-Duarte, A. (2018). Hearing aid use and auditory verbal therapy improve voice quality of deaf children. *Journal of Voice*, 1–5.

Thomas, E. & Zwolan, T. (2019). Communication mode and speech and language outcomes of young cochlear implant recipients: A comparison of auditory-verbal, oral communication, and total communication. *Otology & Neurotology, 40*, 1–9.

Von Muenster, K., & Baker, E. (2014). Oral communicating children using a cochlear implant: Good reading outcomes are linked to better language and phonological processing abilities. *International Journal of Pediatric Otorhinolaryngology, 78*(3), 433–444.

Warner-Czyz, A., Davis, B., & Morrison, H. (2005). Production accuracy in a young cochlear implant recipient. *The Volta Review, 105*(1), 5–25.

White, J., & Brennan-Jones, C. (2014). Auditory-verbal therapy: Improving the evidence-base. *Deafness & Education International, 16*(3), 125–128.

Wolfe, J., Baker, S., Caraway, T., Kasulis, H., Mears, A., Smith, J., . . . Wood, M. (2007). 1-Year postactivation results for sequentially implanted bilateral cochlear implant users. *Otology & Neurotology, 28*(5), 589–596.

Wong, S., Scarinci, N., Hickson, L., Rose, T., & Constantinescu, G. (2013). Bilateral cochlear implants in children: A preliminary study of language and speech perception outcomes. *Australian and New Zealand Journal of Audiology, 33*(1), 48–68.

Yanbay, E., Hickson, L., Scarinci, N., Constantinescu, G., & Dettman, S. (2014). Language outcomes for children with cochlear implants enrolled in different communication programs. *Cochlear Implants International, 15*(3), 121–135.

Zimmerman, I., Steiner, V., & Pond, R. (2002). *Preschool language scale* (4th ed.). San Antonio, TX: Psychological Corp.

Appendix 3-A

TEST MEASURES (ALPHABETICAL ORDER)
USED IN RESEARCH STUDIES

AAPS-3	Arizona Articulation Proficiency Scale—Third Edition	Fudala, J. *Arizona Articulation Proficiency Scale, Third Revision*. Los Angeles, CA: Western Psychological Services; 2000.
ACAP-A	Assessment of Children's Articulation and Phonology	James, D. (1995). *Assessment of Children's Articulation and Phonology*. South Australia: Flinders University.
BASC-2	Behavioral and Emotional Screening System, Second Edition	Kamphaus, R., & Reynolds, C. (2007). *Behavioral & Emotional Screening System Manual*. Bloomington, MN: NCS Pearson, Inc.
BKB	Bamford-Kowal-Bench	Bench J, Bamford J. *Speech-Hearing Tests & the Spoken Language of Hearing-Impaired Children*. London, UK: Academic Press, 1979.
BKB/A	Bamford-Kowal-Bench/ Australian	Bench, R., Doyle, J., & Greenwood, K. (1987). A standardization of the BKB/A sentence test for children in comparison with the NAL-CID sentence test and CAL-PBM word test. *Australian Journal of Audiology, 9*, 39–48.
BKB-SIN	Bamford-Kowal-Bench Speech in Noise Test	Etymotic Research Labs. (2005). *BKB-SIN™ Speech-in-Noise Test Version 1.03*. [CD] Elk Grove Village, IL: Etymotic Research.
CAP	Categories of Auditory Performance	Archbold, S., Lutman, M., & Marshall, D. (1995) Categories of Auditory Performance. *The Annals of Otology, Rhinology & Laryngology Supplement 166*, 312–314.
CASALA	Computer Aided Speech and Language Analysis	Serry, A., Dorman, M., & Kral, A. (1997). Computer-Aided Speech and Language Analysis. *Australian Communication Quarterly* (Spring), 27–28.

CELF-3	Clinical Evaluation of Language Fundamentals, Third Edition	Semel, E., Wiig., E., & Secord, W. (1995). *Clinical Evaluation of Language Fundamentals, Third Edition*. San Antonio, TX: The Psychological Corporation.
CELF-4	Clinical Evaluation of Language Fundamentals, Fourth Edition	Semel, E., Wiig., E., & Secord, W. (2003). *Clinical Evaluation of Language Fundamentals, Fourth Edition*. San Antonio, TX: The Psychological Corporation.
CELF-P	Clinical Evaluation of Language Fundamentals–Preschool	Wiig, E., Secord, W., & Semel, E. (1992). *Clinical Evaluation of Language Fundamentals–Preschool*. San Antonio, TX: The Psychological Corporation.
CNC	Consonant–nucleus–consonant word lists	Peterson, G., Lehiste, I. (1962). Revised CNC word lists for auditory tests. *Journal of Hearing and Speech Disorders*, 27: 67Y70.
CTOPP	Comprehensive Test of Phonological Processing	Wagner, R., Torgesen, J., & Rashotte, C. (1999). *Comprehensive Test of Phonological Processing*. Austin, TX: Pro-Ed, Inc.
EOWPVT	Expressive One-Word Picture Vocabulary Test	Gardner, M. (2000). *Expressive One-Word Picture Vocabulary Test*. Novato, CA: Academic Therapy Publications.
ESP	Early Speech Perception	Moog, J., & Geers, A. (1990). *Early Speech Perception (ESP) Test*. St. Louis, MO: Central Institute for the Deaf.
EVT-2	Expressive Vocabulary Test	Williams, K. (2007). *Expressive Vocabulary Test Manual, Second Edition*. Minneapolis, MN: NCS Pearson, Inc.
FES	Family Environment Scale	Moos, R., Insel, P., & Humphrey, B. (1974). *Preliminary manual for Family Environment Scale, Work Environment Scale, Group Environment Scale*. Palo Alto, CA: Consulting Psychologists Press.
FPRS	Family Participation Rating Scale	Moeller M. (2000). Early intervention and language development in children who are deaf and hard of hearing. *Pediatrics, 106*(3): 1–9.

continues

GFTA-2	Goldman-Fristoe Test of Articulation, Second Edition	Goldman, R. & Fristoe, M. (2001). *Goldman-Fristoe Test of Articulation – Second Edition*. Shoreview, MN: American Guidance Service.
HAPP-3	Hodson Assessment of Phonological Patterns, Third Edition	Hodson, B. (2004). *HAPP-3 Hodson Assessment of Phonological Patterns, Third Edition*. Austin, TX: Pro-Ed.
I Can Do Maths	I Can Do Maths	Doig, B., & de Lemnos, M. (2000). *I Can Do Maths*. Melbourne, Australia: ACER Press.
Insight	Insight	Morris, E. (2003). *Insight*. London, UK: Nfer Nelson.
Integrated Scales of Language Development	Integrated Scales of Language Development	Cochlear Ltd. (2003). *Integrated Scales of Language Development*. Listen, Learn, & Talk. Cochlear Ltd.
IT-MAIS	Infant-Toddler Meaningful Auditory Integration Scale	Zimmerman-Phillips, S., Robbins, A., & Osberger, M. (2001). *Infant-Toddler Meaningful Auditory Integration Scale*. Sylmar, CA: Advanced Bionics Corp.
KLPA-2	Khan-Lewis Phonological Analysis, Second Edition	Kahn, L. & Lewis, N. (2002). *Khan-Lewis Phonological Analysis, Second Edition*. Circle Pines, MN: American Guidance Systems.
Ling 5	Ling 5	Ling D. (1989). *Foundations of Spoken Language for Hearing-Impaired Children*. Washington DC: Alexander Graham Bell Association for the Deaf.
LIP	Listening Process Profile	Archold, S. (1994). Monitoring progress in children at the preverbal stage. In McCormick B., et al. (Eds), *Cochlear implants for young children* (pp. 197–213). London, UK: Whurr.
Leiter-R	Leiter International Performance Scale–Revised	Roid, G. & Miller, L. (1997). *Leiter-R Parent Rating Scale*. Wood Dale, IL: Stoelting.

LNT	Lexical Neighborhood Test	Kirk, K., Pisoni, D., & Osberger, M. (1995). Lexical effects on spoken word recognition by pediatric cohlear implant users. *Ear and Hearing, 16,* 470–481.
MAIS	Meaningful Auditory Integration Scale	Robbins, A., Renshaw, J., & Berry, S. (1991). Evaluating meaningful integration in profoundly hearing-impaired children. *American Journal of Otolaryngology, 12*(suppl.), 144–150.
MCDI	MacArthur-Bates Communicative Inventories	Fenson, L., Dale, P., Reznick, J., Thal, D., Bates, E., Hartung, J., Pethick, S., & Reilly, J. (1993). *MacArthur Communicative Inventories: User's Guide and Technical Manual.* San Diego, CA: Singular Publishing.
MDVP	Multi-Dimensional Voice Program	Kay Elemetrics Corp. (1999). *Multi-Dimensional Voice Program Software* instruction manual.
MLNT	Multisyllabic Lexical Neighborhood Test	Kirk, K., Pisoni, D., & Osberger, M. (1995). Lexical effects on spoken word recognition by pediatric cochlear implant users. *Ear and Hearing, 16,* 470–481.
MTP	Monosyllable, Prochee and Polysyllable Test	Erber, N. & Alencewicz, C. (1976). Audiological evaluation of deaf children. *Journal of Speech and Hearing Disorders, 41,* 256–267.
Neale-3	Neale Analysis of Reading Ability, Third Edition	Neale, M. (1999). *Neale Analysis of Reading Ability.* Melbourne, Vic: Australian Council of Educational Research Ltd.
NZAT	New Zealand Articulation Test	Moyle, J. (2005). The New Zealand Articulation Test Norms Project. *New Zealand Journal of Speech-Language Therapy, 60,* 61–75.
PAT Maths	Progressive Achievement Tests in Mathematics, Third Edition	Australian Council of Education Research. (2005). *Progressive Achievement Tests in Mathematics, Third Edition.,* Melbourne, Australia: ACER Press.

continues

PBK/ Manchester Junior Words	Phonetically Balanced Kindergarten lists	Watson, T. (1957). Speech audiometry for children. In A. W. G. Ewing (Ed.), *Educational guidance and the deaf child* (pp. 278–296). Manchester, UK: The University Press.
PIPPS	Penn Interactive Peer Play Scale	McWayne, C., Sekino, Y., Hampton, G., & Fantuzzo, J. (2007). *Penn Interactive Peer Play Scale Manual.* Philadelphia, PA: John Fantuzzo.
Plott Test Battery	The PLOTT test	Plant, G., & Westcott, S. (1983). *The PLOTT test.* Chatswood, Australia: National Acoustic Laboratories.
PLS-3 (UK)	Preschool Language Scale, Third Edition (UK Adaptation)	Zimmerman, I., Steiner, V., Pond, R., Boucher, J., and Lewis, V. (1991). *Preschool Language Scales, Third Edition* (UK Adaptation). The Psychological Corporation, London
PLS-4	Preschool Language Scale, Fourth Edition	Zimmerman, I., Steiner, V., & Pond, R. (2002). *Preschool Language Scale, Fourth Edition.* San Antonio, TX: The Psychological Corporation.
PLS-5	Preschool Language Scale, Fifth Edition	Zimmer, I., Steiner, V., & Pond, R. (2011). Preschool Language Scale, Fifth Edition. Bloomington, MN: Pearson/ PsychCorp.
PPVT-3	Peabody Picture Vocabulary Test, Third Edition	Dunn, L. & Dunn, D. (1997). *Peabody picture vocabulary test, Third Edition.* Circle Pines, MN: American Guidance Service.
PPVT-4	Peabody Picture Vocabulary Test, Fourth Edition	Dunn L. & Dunn D. *Peabody Picture Vocabulary Test, Fourth Edition.* Circle Pines, MN: American Guidance Service, 2007.
QUIL	Queensland Inventory of Literacy	Dodd, B., Holm, S. Oerlemans, M., & McCormick, M. (1996). *Queensland Inventory of Literacy.* Queensland, Australia: University of Queensland.
Reading Progress Tests	Reading Progress Tests	Vincent, D., Crumpler, M., & Mare, M. (1997). *Reading Progress Tests.* Berkshire, UK: Nfer Nelson.

Reynell	Reynell Developmental Language Scales	J.K. Reynell, Huntley, M. (1985). *Reynell Developmental Language Scales, Revised Second Edition*, NFER-Nelson Publishing Company Ltd, Windsor, UK.
Rossctti Infant-Toddler Language Scale	Rossctti Infant-Toddler Language Scale	Rossctti, L. (1990). *The Rossetti Infant-Toddler Language Scale*. East Moline, IL: Linguisystems.
SCBE	Social Competence and Behavior Evaluation	LaFreniere, P. & Dumas, J. (1995). *Social Competence and Behavior Evaluation: Preschool Edition Manual*. Los Angeles, CA: Western Psychological Services.
SDQ-2	Self-Description Questionnaire, Second Edition	Marsh, H. (1990). *Self-Description Questionnaire II: Manual*. New South Wales, Australia: University of Western Sydney, Macarthur Faculty of Education Publication Unit.
SDQ-3	Self-Description Questionnaire, Third Edition	Marsh, H. (1992). *Self-Description Questionnaire III: Manual*. New South Wales, Australia: University of Western Sydney, Macarthur Faculty of Education Publication Unit.
SIR	The Speech Intelligibility Rating	Cox, R., & McDaniel, D. (1989). Development of the Speech Intelligibility Rating (SIR) test for hearing aid comparisons. *Journal of Speech and Hearing Research, 32*(2), 347–352.
SPEAK-probes	Speech Perception Education and Assessment Kit–Probes	Boothroyd, A. (1978). Speech perception and sensorineural hearing loss, in: M. Ross & T. Giolas (Eds.). *Auditory management of hearing-impaired children* (pp. 117–144). Baltimore, MD: University Park Press.
SPINE	SPeech INtelligibility Evaluation	Monsen, R., Moog, J., & Geers, A. (1988). *CID Picture SPINE (SPeech INtelligibility Evaluation)*. St. Louis, MO: Central Institute for the Deaf.
TOWRE	Test of Word Reading Efficiency	Wagner, R., Torgesen, J., & Rashotte, C. (1999). *Test of Word Reading Efficiency*. Austin, TX: Pro-Ed, Inc.
Viborgmaterialet	Viborgmaterialet	Pedersen, E., Kjøge, G. (2005). Viborgmaterialet. Herning. Specialpædagogisk Forlag,

continues

Wechsler Preschool and Primary Scale of Intelligence	Wechsler Preschool and Primary Scale of Intelligence	Wechsler, D. (2002). *Wechsler Preschool and Primary Scale of Intelligence.* San Antonio, TX: Psychological Corporation.
WIAT-2	Wechsler Individual Achievement Test, Second Edition	Wechsler, D. (1992) *Wechsler Individual Achievement Test, Second Edition.* San Antonio, TX: Harcourt Assessment.
WIAT-2 (Australian)	Wechsler Individual Achievement Test, Second Edition (Australian Adaptation)	Pearson PsychCorp. (2007). *Wechsler Individual Achievement Test, Second edition Australian Standardised Edition.* Sydney, NSW: NCS Pearson Ltd.
WJ-3	Woodcock Johnson Tests of Achievement III	Wendling, B., Schrank, F., & Schmitt, A. *Educational Interventions Related to the Woodcock-Johnson III Tests of Achievement (Assessment Service Bulletin No. 8).* Rolling Meadows, IL: Riverside Publishing; 2014.
WJ-4	Woodcock Johnson Tests of Achievement IV	Schrank, F., Mather, N., & McGrew, K. *Woodcock-Johnson IV Tests of Achievement.* Rolling Meadows, IL: Riverside; 2014.
WRAT-3	Wide Range Achievement Test, Third Edition	Jastak, J. & Wilkinson, G. (1993). *Wide Range Achievement Test, Third Edition.* Wilmington, DE: Wide Range Publishers.

Part II

AUDIOLOGY, HEARING TECHNOLOGIES, SPEECH ACOUSTICS, AND AUDITORY-VERBAL THERAPY

4

AUDIOLOGY AND AUDITORY-VERBAL THERAPY

Carolyne Edwards

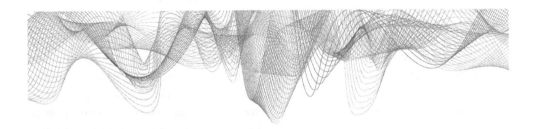

INTRODUCTION

Audiological information forms the ground from which the Auditory-Vebal practitioner (the practitioner) practices. The more fully the practitioner understands the information from the audiology clinic, the more prepared he or she will be to support, develop, and challenge the auditory skills of the child who is deaf or hard of hearing.

This chapter describes how critical information provided by the audiologist can be used by the practitioner to inform his or her work with children who are deaf or hard of hearing and support the parents' understanding of the hearing demands on their children.

Beginning with measures of hearing acuity provided by the pure tone audiogram and auditory brainstem response (ABR) testing, and measures of middle ear function that affect acuity, followed by measures of speech detection and comprehension of spoken language, this chapter describes audiological tests and their contributions to the ongoing monitoring of children's auditory skills.

OVERVIEW OF AN AUDIOLOGICAL ASSESSMENT

An audiological assessment addresses a broad spectrum of auditory issues.

Although the pure tone audiogram often attracts more attention than other audiological procedures, it is only one part of the audiological picture. The practitioner will be interested in a comprehensive audiological assessment in a clinical setting that evaluates the following:

Nature of Hearing Loss and Auditory Potential

- provision of information about auditory function
- description of current hearing levels
- description of the child's auditory potential for speech perception and auditory monitoring of the environment
- evaluation of electroacoustical functioning of amplification

Listening Skills

- description of the child's current listening skills
- measurement of changes in the child's listening skills over time
- observation of the child's attitude toward listening, communication and social interaction

Communication

- observation of communication strategies the child is currently using
- recommendations for additional strategies that would enhance child's comprehension of speech
- recommendations for alternate teaching/communication strategies when auditory limitations are present

- determination of amplification strategies to enhance the child's communication

Children and Parent(s)/Family

- evaluation of the child's and parents' acceptance of the hearing loss and the child's overall sense of self worth
- determination of need for additional counseling

THE BEGINNING: INITIAL ASSESSMENT

All audiological assessments begin with an evaluation of hearing acuity, the softest level of sound that a child can detect, using pure tone frequencies and/or speech stimuli. When the child fails to detect any one of the stimuli presented, the child is referred for a comprehensive evaluation. Where universal newborn hearing screening programs are in place, testing begins at birth.

The Pure Tone Audiogram

The pure tone audiogram is a graph indicating the softest level of speech at which the child can hear a range of frequencies that are important for the comprehension of speech. Between birth and two years of age, the audiologist may only be able to plot thresholds for a few frequencies in the better ear when testing through speakers, or if testing with insert earphones, a few frequencies in each ear. As the child gets older, thresholds at all frequencies between 250 Hz and 8000 Hz in each ear can be obtained. For newborn hearing screening and for infants, where testing cannot be completed behaviorally, ABR and otoacoustic emissions testing will elicit less specific, but baseline information.

It is this basic information that provides the starting point for understanding the child's hearing loss. Results of pure tone, ABR, or otoacoustic emissions testing can indicate:

- the presence or absence of hearing loss
- type of hearing loss
- degree of hearing loss
- hearing differences between ears

Awareness of sound is the first step in the listening domain of Auditory-Verbal Therapy (AVT). Audiological thresholds determine what is in the child's range of hearing—what is possible to detect for speech and environmental sounds and what is not. Understanding the child's auditory potential and limitations is essential to support the child's progress.

Types of Hearing Loss

Conductive Hearing Loss is the result of damage or obstruction in the outer or middle ear. By definition, bone conduction thresholds are within normal limits and a gap of 15 dB or more exists between air and bone conduction thresholds.

Sensorineural Hearing Loss is the result of damage or obstruction to the inner ear or auditory nerve. Bone conduction thresholds are poorer than 15 dB and there is no gap between air and bone conduction thresholds.

Mixed Hearing Loss is caused by a combination of damage or obstruction in the outer/middle ear and the inner ear/auditory nerve. In this case, bone conduction thresholds are poorer than 15 dB and there is a gap of 15 dB or more between the air and bone conduction thresholds. A fluctuating mixed hearing loss can result when a child experiences recurrent otitis media in conjunction with a sensorineural hearing loss.

Auditory Neuropathy Spectrum Disorder (ANSD) presents with considerable variability in auditory capacity from normal hearing to profound sensorineural hearing loss and is distinguished by particular patterns on electrophysiological testing and often disproportionately poor speech recognition abilities for the degree of hearing loss. Recent definitions of ANSD include either present otoacoustic emissions or a present cochlear microphonic in combination with either markedly abnormal or absent ABR.

Guidance for the Practitioner

- Children with permanent conductive hearing loss due to ossicular abnormalities are often identified at birth or within the first year of life. If the child is able to access amplification as soon as the hearing loss is identified, the child's auditory progress will be rapid, since amplification ensures good audibility of speech for developing understanding of language. These children do not experience any reduction in speech discrimination, since the inner ear and auditory pathways are unaffected. They are good candidates for early intervention and rarely need AVT once they reach school age.

■ Children with fluctuating mixed hearing loss due to otitis media can be at higher risk than children with sensorineural hearing loss of the same degree, since the auditory input is not stable and it is difficult to adjust amplification immediately to adapt to the reduced hearing levels when otitis media occurs and hearing levels drop.

■ Speech recognition ability varies with sensorineural hearing loss especially for children with severe hearing loss and adds equally important information to that of the pure tone audiogram. The pure tone audiogram and the speech recognition data/scores need to be viewed simultaneously in order to understand a child's auditory functioning. The audiogram is only a partial predictor of understanding of speech.

■ As ANSD continues to be better identified in the early years, we are still at the beginning stages of understanding how to adjust programming for these children. Each child has to be assessed individually in order to arrive at any conclusions regarding the child's auditory abilities and the situations that will create auditory challenges (see Chapter 22).

Degree of Hearing Loss

Because degree of hearing loss is generally based on the calculation of the pure tone average (PTA) of thresholds at 500, 1000, and 2000 Hz, it can only be regarded as a broad description of hearing levels. The hearing levels associated with the degrees of hearing loss are as indicated below:

Within the range of normal limits	−10 to 15 dB HL
Minimal hearing loss	16 to 25 dB HL
Mild hearing loss	26 to 40 dB HL
Moderate hearing loss	41 to 55 dB HL
Moderately severe hearing loss	56 to 70 dB HL
Severe hearing loss	71 to 90 dB HL
Profound hearing loss	91+ dB HL

Although −10 to 25 dB was generally considered the range of normal hearing for adults, children require more audibility in order to learn language. Research over the past 25 years has shown the impact of minimal hearing loss (16 to 25 dB) on children's auditory functioning (Crandell, 1993; Tharpe et al., 2009). Therefore, normal hearing for children is defined as −10 to 15 dB HL.

The range of frequencies represented in the speech spectrum is well beyond the PTA frequencies of 500, 1000, and 2000 Hz, as demonstrated in Killion and Mueller's Count the Dot audiogram shown in Figure 4–1. The one hundred dots represent frequencies and intensities of speech at normal conversational level. The greater the number of dots at a frequency, the more important it is for speech perception. Note that there are more audible dots above 4000 Hz in the speech spectrum than was previously thought, thus

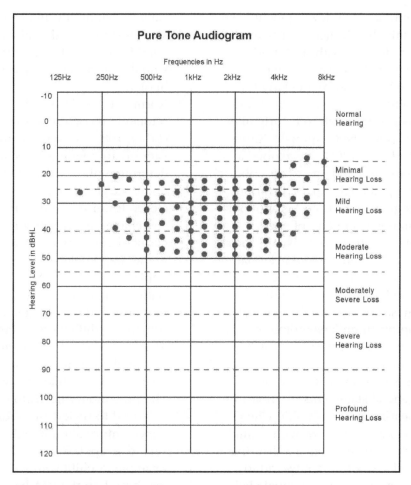

Figure 4-1. Pure tone audiogram–count the dot audiogram. Adapted from Killion and Mueller (2010).

increasing the demand for amplification at these higher frequencies. The greater the degree of hearing loss, the more likely the child will not be able to access the full frequency spectrum through conventional amplification.

Classification of degree of hearing loss does not take into account the *shape* of the hearing loss. High frequency hearing loss, low frequency hearing loss, precipitously sloping hearing loss, and "cookie bite" configurations where hearing loss occurs at only the mid frequencies create different acoustic challenges for a child, and speech testing is essential to assess the impact on understanding of spoken language.

Guidance for the Practitioner

■ Degree of hearing loss was first used as a guide to develop expectations for auditory skills by Winnifred Northcott (1972). Since then, technology and age of identification have advanced dramatically and expectations for auditory skill development have similarly advanced, particularly for children with profound hearing loss using cochlear implants, and particularly for children whose parents choose AVT as the preferred early intervention (see Chapter 1). Karen Anderson (2007) developed a series of handouts to describe the potential impact of various degrees of hearing loss not only on understanding of speech and language, but also on social development and educational accommodations and services. As illustrated in Appendix 4-A, these are very useful in developing an understanding of the impact of hearing loss for families.

- It is useful to consider the general statements of impact of hearing loss as a guide when beginning to work with a child who is deaf or hard of hearing and his or her family, and to be aware of the potential challenges of the particular degree of hearing loss. Think about what you might anticipate will be difficult for the child auditorily, socially, emotionally, educationally. As work with the child advances, the practitioner will delve more deeply into the child's individual auditory abilities.
- With varying slopes in hearing losses, it is critical to review the speech awareness and speech recognition testing to better understand the impact of hearing loss and the implications for AVT with the child, specifi-

cally the audibility and clarity of speech sounds with and without amplification and/or electrical stimulation provided by cochlear implants.

- Norman Erber's GASP 1 phoneme recognition test (Erber, 1982) is useful to administer on an ongoing basis, to determine phoneme audibility under varying conditions—close, distance, noise, with any change in amplification or earmold coupling or changes in the mapping of the cochlear implant (CI).
- With unusual audiometric configurations on the audiogram, it is sometimes difficult for a family to understand the discrepancies that might appear between test results and the child's responses. The practitioner needs to be prepared to review the audiological information in light of such discrepancies. Example: A child with a severe loss based on the PTA has excellent low frequency hearing and parents wonder why the child responds to his name when called without the hearing aids on. The practitioner can explain that the response to the name is due to the low frequency hearing thresholds.

Ear Differences

Hearing levels can vary between ears at some or all frequencies, which may also affect speech understanding. It is important to know whether the hearing difference between ears is minimized with the use of amplification or the CI, or if the child will continue to hear better with the right or left ear. If children have been fit sequentially rather than simultaneously with cochlear implants, they may develop a preference for the earlier fitted side.

Guidance for the Practitioner

▪ The practitioner and/or the parent (when coached by the practitioner during AVT sessions) may want to sit on the side of the ear with better auditory capacity.

▪ If child comes to the AVT session without amplification on their better ear due to repairs, or if he or she is unable to use amplification due to ongoing fluid drainage from the middle ear, the practitioner needs to adjust the expectations for the child's responsivity due to the reduced auditory capacity for that particular AVT session.

▪ Remind the parents to adjust their auditory expectations in similar situations at home and in the community.

Auditory Brainstem Response

ABR is an electrophysiological test that evaluates auditory function and is used when behavioral audiological procedures cannot be reliably obtained. In the pediatric world, this could occur with infants and very young children or children with behavioral or developmental challenges in addition to hearing loss.

Unlike pure tone testing in sound field or with insert phones where test-

ing can provide tonal information on octave or mid octave frequencies from 250 up to 8000, results of ABR testing reflect, primarily, responses to a few frequencies, clicks centered around the frequency region of 2000 to 4000 Hz, or brief frequency-specific tone bursts. The maximum intensity level used in ABR is typically less than the maximum level used in behavioral testing with insert phones. Finally, intervals are much more discrete in behavioral testing. Whereas pure tone thresholds are obtained in 5 dB intervals, ABR is usually obtained using 20 dB changes in presentation levels. Thus, the results of ABR testing provide degree of hearing loss at selected frequency regions but do not have the specificity of pure tone thresholds.

Guidance for the Practitioner

▪ ABR provides information on the degree of hearing loss in each ear and the presence or absence of a conductive component and does so without the active participation of the child.

▪ When reviewing the results of ABR testing with the family, remember that there is less specific information on frequency sensitivity and thresholds than behavioral testing and is not a substitute, but rather a first step toward behavioral testing. It will not be used for monitoring hearing levels unless behavioral testing is not possible.

▪ It is possible to have much better hearing at the low frequencies and still be reported as a severe loss due to responses at the higher frequencies.

- "No response" on ABR testing does not mean no measurable hearing. It simply means no response at the maximum intensity tested at that frequency region.
- If you or the family see discrepancies between the results reported on ABR testing and behavioral responses, this may reflect hearing at frequencies not tested.
- Observations of the child's auditory responsivity by yourself and the parents is extremely useful to the audiologist working with your child. Questionnaires such as the PEACH (Ching & Hill, 2007), LittlEARS (Weichbold et al., 2005), and ELF (Anderson, 2000) provide direction for observations in the home or the clinic.

Otoacoustic Emissions

Evoked otoacoustic emissions (EOAE) is another electrophysiologic measure of auditory function. The main types of EOAE are transient-evoked otoacoustic emissions (TEOAE) and distortion product otoacoustic emissions (DPOAE) and both can be used to evaluate the status of the cochlea. Like the ABR, TEOAE and DPOAE testing do not require the child's cooperation. In fact, because it is non-invasive, there is minimal preparation required of the child. However, middle ear function must be normal in order to obtain an accurate test. In addition, otoacoustic emissions (OAEs) are an essential part of the diagnostic battery to identify ANSD.

Guidance for the Practitioner

- EOAE testing is used as a hearing screening measure in newborn screening protocols and families may have some familiarity with this type of test.
- EOAE testing permits the audiologist to differentiate between sensory and neural hearing loss. Reduction in otoacoustic emissions reflects sensory loss due to damage to the cochlear, and abnormal evoked potentials on the ABR testing reflect neural loss due to damage to the auditory nerve and brainstem. Therefore, through the addition of these tests, the audiologist's ability to differentiate the nature of sensorineural hearing loss has improved significantly.

Speech Awareness Threshold

The speech awareness threshold (SAT), sometimes called the speech detection threshold, is an additional verification measure of the pure tone thresholds, using a speech stimulus. As with the pure tone thresholds, speech is presented at softer and softer levels to find the dB level at which the child detects speech 50% of the time. Young children may respond to speech at softer levels than pure tone stimuli so, at times, there may be a discrepancy between pure tone thresholds and the SAT that may be attributed to the greater familiarity of speech. In the case of sloping or rising hearing loss configurations, the SAT will agree with or be similar to the better hearing thresholds, since the child only needs to hear a portion of the speech spectrum in order to respond to the speech stimulus.

Guidance for the Practitioner

Here are suggested guidelines for interpretation of the SAT for training purposes:

- The softest level at which a child could detect some part of the speech spectrum would be as follows:
  Whispered speech level if the SAT = 30 dB
  Quiet conversational level if the SAT = 40 dB
  Average conversational level if the SAT = 50 dB
  Loud conversational level if the SAT = 60 to 65 dB
- The SAT reflects the optimal level for detection of speech in a quiet one-to-one environment. When a child is in noisier environments such as a preschool, a family gathering, or an outdoor setting, his or her response level will be necessarily reduced. Therefore, if a child obtains an SAT of 40 dB, the softest level of speech that he or she could detect in ideal listening conditions is quiet, normal, and loud conversational levels. If listening in less than optimal conditions, such as at a distance or in background noise, the child may only be able to detect normal or loud conversational levels. Use of remote microphone technology can enhance audibility for softer speech sounds. Note

that the SAT does not confirm audibility at all frequencies but simply provides evidence of the ability to detect speech of sufficient intensity at one or more frequencies.
- The range between the softest consonant and the loudest vowel is approximately 30 dB. Therefore, a child needs significantly greater loudness to identify speech than the SAT.

Speech Reception Threshold

For a child who identifies some simple words through hearing only, the speech reception threshold (SRT), sometimes called *spondee threshold*, is both a measure of reliability of pure tone thresholds and a guide for presentation levels of any further word recognition tests. The SRT is the softest level at which a child recognizes selected spondee words 50% of the time.

Guidance for the Practitioner

- The first audiological indication of the child's emerging ability to identify speech sounds and words on formal testing is the child's ability to establish an SRT. Therefore, it is an important step in auditory development.
- The ability to establish an SRT is primarily based on the child's ability to differentiate vowels. A child with poor consonant identification skills will often have little or no difficulty establishing an SRT.

■ Similar to the SAT, the SRT provides an indication of the optimal level for the identification of speech. Children require speech at approximately 30 dB higher than the SRT in order to achieve optimal speech recognition scores. For example, for a child with an SRT of 30 dB, an intensity level of 60 dB would be optimal for reception of the full speech spectrum.

■ Questions to explore with the clinical audiologist: Can we achieve an optimal level for speech reception with the child's current hearing technology? Can we enhance speech reception with the use of remote microphone technology?

Middle Ear Function

Middle ear function as measured by impedance audiometry is critical to monitor with children not just at the first assessment, but at each audiological visit. For children for whom permanent hearing loss is already present, the presence of middle ear dysfunction can cause anywhere from a 5 dB to 40 dB additional decrease in hearing levels at one or more frequencies. All children are at risk for developing middle ear dysfunction during preschool and school age years. The presence of middle ear dysfunction has significant implications for the child's capacity to learn through listening in AVT sessions and at home because of the impact on hearing levels and its transitory nature, which makes it more difficult to detect and address in the moment. The child's need to listen more intently due to temporary decrease

in hearing levels and resulting auditory fatigue are rarely discussed, and yet have a significant impact.

Nature of middle ear dysfunction can be typically categorized:

■ *Negative Middle Ear Pressure and Normal Tympanic Mobility* This condition reflects a retracted eardrum and yet normal mobility within the middle ear system and creates the least reduction in hearing thresholds. The physical sensation is similar to the pressure experienced during airplane takeoff and landing and is often seen when young children have upper respiratory congestion.

■ *Negative Middle Ear Pressure and Reduced Tympanic Mobility* This condition reflects a stiff middle ear system due to conditions commonly seen in young children including impacted wax, extreme negative middle ear pressure, or fluid buildup in the middle ear. There is a greater reduction in hearing thresholds than with negative middle ear pressure.

■ *Extremely High Tympanic Mobility* This reflects a highly mobile middle ear system due to conditions such as flaccid eardrum or ossicular discontinuity and is less frequently seen in children.

Guidance for the Practitioner

■ If there is any decrease in the child's auditory performance, it may be due to decreased middle ear function. Therefore, the first check is to obtain an impedance audiometry test to determine if there is any middle ear involvement.

▪ Find out from the family or the audiologist about any chronic middle ear history such as repeated middle ear dysfunction, date of the last episode, typical length of episodes, history of ventilating tubes, number of tube insertions, and if ventilating tubes are currently present.

▪ Do you and/or the parents notice a change in hearing levels when the child has middle ear dysfunction? If so, there is a need to be sensitive to the child's need for auditory rest during periods of middle ear dysfunction, and to put less auditory demands on the child. In addition, if the middle ear dysfunction is chronic, the audiologist may suggest increasing the volume of the child's hearing devices or using a different hearing program in response to decreased hearing levels. It is important to be aware that significant interruptions in auditory learning can occur during episodes of fluid buildup in the middle ear.

▪ The majority of episodes of middle ear dysfunction may be symptom free, other than a decrease in hearing levels. Therefore, it is important for the practitioner to be alert to any changes in hearing sensitivity.

▪ It is wise to schedule impedance audiometry every 3 months for children with chronic histories of middle ear dysfunction to monitor the status of middle ear until middle ear dysfunction clears.

ONGOING AUDIOLOGICAL ASSESSMENT

Listening Skills

Once hearing acuity has been established, the focus of ongoing audiological assessment is to determine any changes in hearing acuity, middle ear function and understanding of speech. The initial speech measures provide a baseline prior to beginning AVT, and ongoing assessment demonstrates the changes in speech recognition as a result of using hearing technology, intervention through AVT, and support from parents and teachers in home and educational settings. The rate of progress through various speech tasks is also a reflection of the child's overall development.

Children's listening skills change both quantitatively and qualitatively over time. Quantitatively the audiologist assesses the level at which children can detect various speech sounds, their ability to identify words, phrases, and sentences in quiet and in noise, and their ability to comprehend and track conversation. Equally important to listening skill development are the qualitative changes over time, including: their ability to maintain and sustain attention; their level of confidence in listening; their communicative engagement with others; their ability to recognize and clarify miscommunications; and their ability to advocate for themselves. It is important that the practitioner keep a careful systematic record about these qualitative changes as a significant measure of auditory skill development that is often unreported in formal testing.

Detection

There is a variety of auditory responses that the clinical audiologist is looking for in order to determine the infant's or toddler's ability to detect sound. The child's early responses in the clinical setting can include the following:

- searching for the sound
- turning of the eyes or head toward the sound
- cessation of activity
- quieting, startling, or vocalizing when a detectable sound occurs.

Early behavioral testing relies on these observations. When a child begins to demonstrate some spontaneous responses to sound, it is a good indication that the child has attached meaning to sound.

Audiological testing then proceeds to assess conditioned responses to sound using visual reinforcement audiometry (VRA), where the child is conditioned to turn to sounds presented through speakers or insert phones. By the age of 2 to 3 years of age, using conditioned play audiometry (CPA), the child is taught to perform a specific action when he or she hears a sound delivered through insert phones or speakers. VRA and CPA provide the most detailed and specific information on the child's auditory capacity and confirm the behavioral observations and electrophysiological results obtained earlier.

The SAT, previously mentioned, measures the child's ability to detect any speech stimuli. There are two additional formal tests that can be administered in the clinic and in the AVT session to provide more detailed information.

Ling's Six Sound Test (Ling, 2002) is a detection task of six speech sounds: /m/, /u/, /a/, /i/, /ʃ/, and /s/ presented at normal conversational level when the child is using hearing technology. Each of these sounds represents critical information in a different frequency range of the speech spectrum. This test can provide information for a variety of purposes:

- to predict the ability to recognize various speech features
- to measure effects of distance from the speaker on the audibility of various speech features if presented at distances from 6 inches to 10 feet away
- to observe increases in audibility when remote microphone technology is used
- to observe differences in audibility with different remote microphones from omnidirectional, directional, boom, and pass around microphones
- to monitor changes in hearing due to middle ear dysfunction or changes in aided performance when there are differences in response from day to day.

The Glendonald Auditory Screening Procedure (GASP) Test 1 (Erber, 1982) is an expansion of the Ling Six Sound Test and presents 10 vowels and 12 consonants (nasals, laterals, voiced and unvoiced fricatives) at normal conversational level. Erber described several additional purposes for this test, including:

▪ evaluation of audibility of the speech spectrum of the practitioner's voice and/or the parent's voice by having either present the speech sound to the child

▪ evaluation of any strategies to enhance audibility of the phoneme tested, such as talking closer to the microphone of the child's amplification, using remote microphone technology, or intentionally distorting the speech sound by directing the breath stream across the microphone opening.

Note that the Six Sound Test and the GASP 1 can also be used as identification tasks if the child's auditory skills are more advanced. For an identification task, the child is asked to repeat the specific sound heard.

The practitioner and parents need to assist by teaching the child a conditioned play response in preparation for audiological testing. This serves two purposes: to consolidate the child's conditioned response to sound and to have a tool to detect changes in hearing levels due to middle ear dysfunction, overall decrease in hearing levels, and/or malfunctions in hearing technology. *Note: the sounds used in training need to be presented at random intervals without visual clues to ensure that the child does not develop a timed response to the task.*

Guidance for the Practitioner

▪ Detection of the three vowels /u/, /a/, /i/, and /m/ suggests potential for audibility of the speech spectrum from 250 to 1000 Hz.

▪ Detection of the three vowels /u/, /a/, /i/, and/m/ and /ʃ/ suggests potential for audibility of the speech spectrum from 250 to 2000 Hz.

▪ Detection of the three vowels /u/, /a/, /i/, and/m/, /ʃ/ and /s/ suggests potential for audibility of the speech spectrum from 250 to 4000 Hz or higher.

▪ Although it is important to experiment with detection of a variety of sounds, children need not be frustrated by perseverance with listening activities that continue to focus on sounds they are unable to detect.

Observational Tools

There is a variety of parent observational questionnaires for detection of sound that the audiologist or the practitioner may give to the parents to fill out as they observe their child in everyday environments that can provide more ongoing information about the child's responses to sound. LittlEars is a parent questionnaire designed for young children between birth and 2 years of age (Weichbold, Tsiakpini, Coninx, & D'Haese, 2005). The first half of the 35 question survey relate to many different aspects of detection. The Early Listening Function (ELF), designed for children between 5 months and 3 years, teaches families how to observe children's responses in 12 listening situations at different distances and then suggests activities to stimulate alerting responses in the young child (Anderson, 2002). The Infant Toddler Meaningful Auditory Integration Scale (IT-MAIS) provides 10 questions that evaluate the child's meaningful use of sound in daily living, from vocal behavior, to use of hearing instruments, to the ability to alert to sound, to the ability to attach meaning to sound (Zimmerman-Phillips, Osberger, & Robbins, 1997).

Guidance for the Practitioner

- Use of any of the parent observational tools provides a much broader perspective on the child's emerging detection skills in the everyday environment and supplements the information gleaned from single session audiological testing and the weekly AVT session (see Chapter 17).
- It is sometimes a lengthy journey in auditory development from detection to recognition of sound for a child with hearing loss, and families can get discouraged by the wait. Giving families detailed observational frameworks that show the variety of responses for detection of sound can provide considerable encouragement in this initial stage of development.

Discrimination

Discrimination is the ability to perceive similarities and differences between two or more sounds. This skill precedes the ability to identify specific sounds and demands that the child attend to differences between sounds or respond differently to different sounds. This is not tested in the audiological evaluation but is a highly useful assessment tool for the practitioner in ongoing AVT, to determine if the child has difficulty

discerning differences between two auditory stimuli. It is typically not used as an instructional step in therapy but rather for clarification and further training when the child makes identification or comprehension errors.

At the suprasegmental level, the practitioner can present sound pairs that vary in duration, loudness, or pitch and ask the child to indicate if the pairs are the same or different. Alternately one can present a series of sounds—where only one variation occurs and ask the child to indicate when the sound changes. At the segmental level, if the practitioner is unsure if the child is detecting /s/ in a word, he or she could present pairs such as cat-cat and cat-cats and ask the child to tell whether the words in each pair are the same or different, or say cat-cat-cats-cat-cat and ask when the sound changed.

Guidance for the Practitioner

- When a child has difficulty identifying a particular speech sound or characteristic, there are a number of strategies that can be used for this skill, including use of a same/different discrimination task to determine if the child can detect the auditory difference. If the child cannot, then the auditory tasks need to focus on that differentiation before moving on to a recognition task.

Identification or Recognition

Identification or recognition is the ability to reproduce a speech stimulus or environmental sound by labeling it through pointing to the object or picture, by repeating the word or sound heard, or by writing it. (Note that audiologists refer to these word or sentence tests as "discrimination" tests. This is a different meaning for the word *discrimination* than is used in listening skills training.)

There is a wide variety of identification tasks within the audiological test battery ranging from identification of single phonemes through to words and sentence materials and ranging in difficulty from closed set to open set formats. They can also be administered through listening only, through listening with speechreading, and in both quiet and noise conditions. The child's age, language level, speech intelligibility, and degree of hearing loss will determine which tests can be administered at a particular time.

Word discrimination tests measure the child's ability to recognize monosyllabic words under ideal and typical listening conditions. Ideal listening conditions include listening at 30 dB above the SRT without background noise. Typical conditions may include presenting speech at quiet or normal conversational levels with and without background noise. The child is asked to repeat 25 or 50 words and the word discrimination score (WDS) is calculated as a percentage reflecting the number of words repeated correctly (Example: 15/25 = 60%). The score can also be expressed as a phoneme score where one point per phoneme is given so that each word is scored as three points for the three sounds in the word. This provides a better estimate of the child's degree of difficulty with specific speech sounds, especially for children with high frequency hearing losses. Word lists such as the PBK and NU-6

are used with older children where speech is fully intelligible and vocabulary is well developed.

For children in the early stages of vocabulary development when speech may not be easily understood, a closed set or multiple-choice picture word discrimination task is more appropriate. The NU-CHIPS or WIPI was designed for children 3 years and above; four or six words are pictured on each page of a 25- or 50-page booklet and the child is asked to point to one of the pictures on each page.

There are varying interpretations for the percentage score obtained on word discrimination testing. Ninety to 100% may be described as excellent, 75 to 89% as slight difficulty, 60 to 74% as moderate difficulty, 50 to 59% as poor, and below 50% as very poor word discrimination ability. In order to understand the interpretation, one must remember the specific conditions of the test—single words with no context is the most difficult recognition task possible. This does not reflect the typical listening conditions in which children find themselves. However, the score allows a comparison on a standardized test and reflects their phoneme skills; it is not a generalized statement of the child's ability to understand speech. Children will always perform better in everyday situations when they have support of contextual and syntactic clues inherent in sentence and connected conversation.

Guidance for the Practitioner

▪ When reviewing a child's word discrimination scores, consider whether an open set or closed set test was used. Closed set tasks are easier than open set tasks so scores cannot be directly compared. A high score on a closed set task does not necessarily reflect the same auditory capacity as a high score on an open set task.

- The child's ability to move from a closed set discrimination test to an open set test is a measure of his or her progress in auditory development.
- For children with high frequency precipitous or steeply sloping hearing loss, word discrimination scores will not represent their actual auditory functioning; scores will underestimate their auditory ability. When given the context of sentence material, children with high frequency hearing losses do considerably better; therefore testing with sentence material is essential.
- Speech production skills are integrally linked to speech discrimination skills; it is important to find out the nature of the child's errors on word discrimination testing in order to include further practice in the AVT session and at home and to determine any auditory limitations in phoneme recognition.
- Ask the audiologist for the differences in scores between audition and audition and speechreading to determine the support offered by speechreading cues.
- Ask the audiologist for score differences between speech presented in quiet versus background noise, in order to

determine if more practice is needed in background noise.

Sentence repetition tests are used to assess the child's ability to use contextual clues for identification of speech. Although single word repetition is the most commonly used speech recognition task, it does not reflect the auditory challenges presented in the child's everyday environment, which requires recognition and comprehension of sentence material.

A wide variety of sentence tests is available in the literature. The child's task is to repeat the entire sentence, as in the BKB Sentences (Bench, Kowal, & Bamford, 1979) or the HINT test (Nisson, Soli, & Sullivan, 1994), or the last word in the sentence as in the Speech Perception in Noise (SPIN) test (Kalikow, Stevens, & Elliott, 1977). The SPIN test adds an additional testing feature by creating sentences with high predictability (where other words in the sentence provide additional clues to the content) versus low predictability (where no other clues are provided to the content) in order to assess the child's ability to use context.

Guidance for the Practitioner

- The child's performance on sentence testing provides a measure of typical functioning at home or in the classroom; the word discrimination test results provide the direction for specific phoneme training.
- Results of sentence testing in background noise also indicate areas for further listening skills development.

▪ Results of sentence testing with added speechreading cues may indicate where visual clues will be supportive.

Comprehension

Comprehension is the ability to understand the meaning of speech by a variety of responses such as answering questions, following instructions, paraphrasing, and participating in conversation. By definition, the child's response must be qualitatively different from the stimulus presented (Erber, 1982).

There are, unfortunately, very few formal audiological tests at the comprehension level currently in use. It falls to the practitioner to develop and assess the child's ability to follow single or multi-step directions, sequence directions, or track a story and answer questions about it with or without context. Paraphrasing, a higher-level comprehension skill that blends cognitive, linguistic, and auditory skills, is also an essential skill when the child is learning clarification strategies. These higher order skills of listening and responding are substantive long-term goals in AVT.

Descriptive measures often give the most instructive indicators of comprehension through qualitative questionnaires completed by the parent in the preschool years or the teacher and the child in the elementary and secondary years. The Children's Home Inventory for Listening Difficulties (CHILD) (Anderson & Smaldino, 2000) is designed for children between the ages of 3 and 12 years. It is completed by the parent and at later ages by the parent and the child, in which the parents assess their child's abilities in 15 different listening situations in everyday living. The Listening Inventory for Education–Revised (LIFE-R) (Anderson, Smaldino, & Spangler, 2011) is designed for teachers and children from 6 years and older and looks at challenging listening situations in the classroom. This inventory and additional self-assessment tools for the adolescent who is deaf or hard or hearing are outside the scope of this chapter. Readers are referred to the Self-Assessment of Communication (SAC-A) and the Significant Other Assessment of Communication (SOAC-A) (Crowell, English, McCarthy, & Elkayam, 2005) for unique questionnaires to evaluate teenagers and their friends' perceptions of their communication difficulties, offering a rare opportunity for discussion of different perspectives with the student who is deaf or hard of hearing.

Guidance for the Practitioner

▪ Qualitative data are equally useful in determining the current impact of hearing loss on a child's communication experiences and can provide additional directions for AVT.

▪ Feedback from the family and/ or the child's teacher is useful to determine the amount of integration of therapy goals that occurs in the child's everyday environment.

▪ Feedback from the various questionnaires can provide a basis for discussion of difficult listening situations with the child and/or the family and lead to introduction of additional listening strategies to support the child in the everyday world.

Overhearing

Overhearing is an essential skill in the development of spoken language; in fact, research clearly indicates that language learning often occurs incidentally through overhearing other children's conversations (Moeller, 2007). In the past, the focus on listening skill training was only to help children attend to the primary signal, but now practitioners and parents, particularly in AVT, include a focus on overhearing as a vital auditory skill. This begins at the detection level and continues throughout children's listening skill development.

Guidance for the Practitioner

- Attending to all sounds in the child's learning environment is an important first step in auditory development; in other words, the practitioner needs to shift the auditory figure-ground frequently for the child in order to bring attention to the *figure* of interest and then back to the *ground* where overhearing occurs.
- In later stages of AVT the practitioner and parents will help the children to learn how to *listen in* on the conversations of others in order to increase their vocabulary, language, and knowledge of the world around them.
- There is a need to create assessment tools to evaluate how well

children extract information from overhearing.

ONGOING MONITORING

Electroacoustical Evaluation

Children's hearing technology needs to be evaluated regularly to ensure satisfactory functioning. The clinical audiologist assesses a variety of electroacoustic characteristics:

- gain (intensity across various frequencies)
- frequency response (bass, mid and treble response)
- saturation sound pressure level (maximum intensity produced at various frequencies)
- equivalent input noise level (internal noise produced by the hearing aid)
- distortion levels (clarity of the sound)

For very young children who do not have the communication skills to report issues with their hearing technology, it is desirable to obtain an electroacoustical evaluation every three to six months, *or any time there is a decrease in the child's auditory responsiveness or clarity of speech*.

Example: Parents of a young preschooler who had a sloping severe to borderline profound sensorineural hearing loss tracked their child's auditory and speech development carefully over the past year in AVT. The child was able to identify all the vowel sounds and produce them accurately in everyday speech. One day the parents noticed that the child was unable to recognize the difference between /u/ and /i/ ("oo" and "ee"). After the child's sound confusion persisted for several days, they called the audiologist. Electroacoustical and real-ear measurement of aided function showed that the bore on the child's new earmolds was narrower than previously and was reducing the amount of high frequency amplification. So, the child was unable to hear the second formant of /i/ and consequently discrimination between /u/ and /i/ was impossible. Modifications to the new earmold restored the child's high frequency perception, and speech production returned to previous levels.

When a child is using remote microphone technology in combination with personal hearing technology, the electroacoustical response of the combined system also needs to be evaluated to ensure compatibility and optimal response.

Guidance for the Practitioner

▪ Optimal functioning of the child's hearing technology is the first determinant of his or her auditory performance. Therefore, any time there is a drop in auditory performance, it is important to have hearing technology evaluated.

▪ When the child is having difficulty detecting or identifying specific speech sounds, ask the clinical audiologist if there are any modifications to the hearing device or earmold coupling that would enhance audibility and/or perception.

▪ Ask the clinical audiologist if there are any accessories that would enhance audibility of speech in various listening environments with remote microphone technology such as the use of a boom microphone, a pass around microphone, or patch cords to audio or audiovisual equipment.

Real-Ear or Simulated Real-Ear Measurement

For hearing aids, the acoustic performance of the hearing aid fitting can be measured in the child's ear canal using real-ear measurement or for infants and very young children using a simulated real-ear or coupler approach to verification of amplification. Real-ear or simulated real-ear measurement is used to determine:

▪ audibility of various speech features with the child's amplification, specifically the gain, frequency response, and saturation sound pressure level of the device in the child's ear
▪ effects of altering amplification settings
▪ effect of the shape and size of the child's ear canal on the acoustic response of the child's amplification
▪ effects of various earmold modifications on the amplification response

Hearing aid fitting protocols using real-ear or simulated real-ear measurement provide a means of selecting and fitting hearing aids for children that is more reliable, provides more comprehensive and reliable data across frequencies, and requires less cooperation from the child than traditional aided sound-field testing. This is of great benefit for very young children who were previously dependent on behavioral testing for hearing aid fitting.

Table 4–1 summarizes predictions for the audible frequencies needed for recognition of various speech features as measured through real-ear and simulated real-ear testing. The goal of fitting hearing devices is for the child to have sufficient audibility at each frequency to detect and identify speech features. A detailed discussion of the principles of speech science and the development of speech applicable to AVT can be found in Chapter 11 and includes reference to the work of Daniel Ling (1976, 1989). Without audibility, the child cannot perceive spectral differences. Only through ongoing assessment of auditory perceptual skills will the practitioner determine the capacity to utilize acoustic cues at various frequencies.

Guidance for the Practitioner

- Discuss the implications of the child's real-ear or simulated real-ear measurements for perception of speech with the clinical audiologist to determine which frequencies are audible for the child with hearing technology and if there is any enhancement possible with the additional use of remote microphone technology.
- Determine what speech features are inaccessible, if any, and

add visual, motor, or other prompting strategies for those specific speech features.

COUNSELING OVER TIME

A child's sense of self develops over time and in response to his or her changing environment. Much of the audiological data is focused on content: What did the child hear? What were the optimal thresholds for audibility? What were the scores under a variety of conditions? But equally important is how the child approached the task. We need to ask other questions as well, such as:

- Was the child encouraged or discouraged by the listening tasks?
- Was the child anxious as greater listening demands occurred in the testing?
- Was the child curious about ways to enhance his or her listening?
- Was the child creative in finding new strategies to cope with difficult listening situations?
- How did the child engage with others in communication—tentatively, in an exploratory way, or confidently?
- How does the child express his or her concerns or challenges to others?

The answers to these questions will determine the directions for discussion, coaching, and counseling. For example, if the child appears discouraged or anxious, other strategies may need to be incorporated in AVT to ease the stress

Table 4–1. Frequency Spectrum Required for Audibility of Various Speech Features

Auditory Potential for:	Audibility @250 Hz	Audibility @500 Hz	Audibility @1000 Hz	Audibility @2000 Hz	Audibility @3000 Hz	Audibility @4000 Hz
Detection of suprasegmentals (duration, loudness, and pitch)	■	■				
Identification of suprasegmental features		■				
Detection of all vowels		■	■			
Identification of back and mid vowels		■	■			
Identification of front vowels			■	■	■	
Detection of voiced consonants		■	■			
Detection of voiceless consonants			■	■	■	■
Recognition of consonant voicing characteristics		■				
Recognition of consonant manner characteristics		■	■	■		
Recognition of consonant place characteristics			■	■	■	■
Identification of voiced consonants		■	■	■		
Identification of voiceless consonants		■	■			■

of communication. If the child looks tentative in communication with others, we need to determine where the challenges lie and support the child there. That is a primary role of the practitioner in diagnostic therapy. Use of questionnaires such as the LIFE(R) can provide information on the child's perspective and experience that can form the basis for further discussion and directions in AVT. *Growing Up with Hearing Loss*, created by the Ida Institute (2017), provides an excellent tool for supporting children and families through transitions from infancy, to toddler, early childhood, teenage, and the adult years.

The question that must be asked is, how best can audiologists and practitioners empower the child and family so that they can communicate more effectively and with more confidence over time? As practitioners, we need to continue to expand our repertoire of skills in co-empowerment to support and enhance the child's and family's journey throughout the AVT journey and well beyond.

SUMMARY

The journey for a child and family in Auditory-Verbal Therapy begins with a comprehensive audiological assessment. The clinical audiologist and the practitioner become professional partners with the child and family, to provide support for the development and enhancement of the child's communication and to assist the child to become a fully interactive member of a chosen community (see Chapter 1). Ongoing dialogue among members of the child's team—the child, the family, the practitioner, the audiologist, and ultimately the school personnel—will ensure that auditory issues are addressed as they arise. The child's auditory potential and current capacity, listening skill development, response to listening experiences, and hearing technology needs are the subject of exploration for the hearing professional team at time of initial assessment and throughout the work of Auditory-Verbal Therapy.

REFERENCES

Anderson, K. L. (2000). *Early Listening Function (ELF)*. User's manual. Available at: http://successforkidswithhearingloss.com/uploads/ELF_Questionnaire.pdf

Anderson, K. (2007). *Relationship of hearing loss to listening and learning needs*. Retrieved from Supporting Success for Children with Hearing Loss at http://successforkidswithhearingloss.com

Anderson, K. L., & Smaldino, J. J. (2000). *Children's Home Inventory of Listening Difficulties (CHILD)*. Tampa, FL: Educational Audiology Association.

Anderson, K., Smaldino, J., & Spangler, C. (2011). *Listening Inventory for Education-Revised (LIFE-R)*. Retrieved from Supporting Success for Children with Hearing Loss at http://successforkidswithhearingloss.com

Bench, J., Kowal, A., & Bamford, J. (1979). The BKB (Bamford-Kowal-Bench) sentence lists for partially-hearing children. *British Journal of Audiology, 13*, 108–112.

Ching, T., & Hill, M. (2007). The Parents/Evaluation of Aural/Oral Performance of Children (PEACH) scale: Normative data. *Journal of the American Academy of Audiology, 18*, 220–235.

Crandell, C. (1993). Speech reception in noise by children with minimal degrees of hearing loss. *Ear and Hearing, 14*(3), 210–216.

Crowell, R., English, K., McCarthy, P., & Elkayam, J. (2005). Use of a self-assessment technique in counseling adolescents with hearing loss. *Journal of Educational Audiology, 12*, 86–99.

Erber, N. (1982). *Auditory training.* Washington, DC: A. G. Bell Association for the Deaf and Hard of Hearing.

Ida Institute (2017). *Growing up with hearing loss.* Available under Tools at https://idainstitute.com

Kalikow, D., Stevens, K., & Elliott, L. (1977). Development of a test of speech intelligibility in noise with sentence materials using controlled word predictability. *Journal of the Acoustical Society of America, 61*, 1337–1351.

Killion, M., & Mueller, H. (2010). Twenty years later: A new count the dot method. *Hearing Journal, 63*(1), 10.

Ling, D. (1976). *Speech and the hearing-impaired child.* Washington, DC: A. G. Bell Association for the Deaf and Hard of Hearing.

Ling, D. (1989). *Foundations of spoken language for hearing-impaired children.* Washington, DC: A. G. Bell Association for the Deaf and Hard of Hearing.

Ling, D. (2002). *Speech and the hearing-impaired child* (2nd ed.). Washington, DC: A. G. Bell Association for the Deaf and Hard of Hearing.

Moeller, M. P. (2007). What's in a word? In R. Seewald & J. Bamford (Eds.), *A sound foundation through early amplification 2007: Proceedings of the Fourth International Conference* (pp. 19–31). Staefa, Switzerland: Phonak AG.

Nisson, M., Soli, S., & Sullivan, J. (1994). Development of the Hearing in Noise Test for the measurement of speech reception thresholds in quiet and in noise. *Journal of the Acoustical Society of America, 95*, 1085–1099.

Northcott, W. (1972). *Curriculum guide: Hearing impaired children: Birth to three years and their parents.* Washington, DC: A. G. Bell Association for the Deaf.

Tharpe, A. M., Dodd-Murphy, J., Sladen, D., & Boney, S. (2009). Minimal hearing loss in children: Minimal but not inconsequential. *Seminars in Hearing 30*(2), 80–93.

Weichbold, V., Tsiakpini, L., Coninx, F., & D'Haese, P. (2005). Development of a parent questionnaire for assessment of auditory behavior of infants up to two years of age. *Laryngorhinootologie, 84*, 328–334.

Zimmerman-Phillips, S., Osberger, M. F., & Robbins, A. M. (1997). *Infant-Toddler: Meaningful Auditory Integration Scale (IT-MAIS).* Sylmar, CA: Advanced Bionics Corp.

Appendix 4-A

RELATIONSHIP OF HEARING LOSS TO LISTENING AND LEARNING NEEDS

16–25 dB HEARING LOSS

Possible Impact on the Understanding of Language and Speech	Possible Social Impact	Potential Educational Accommodations and Services
Impact of a hearing loss that is approximately 20 dB can be compared to ability to hear when index fingers are placed in your ears. Child may have difficulty hearing faint or distant speech. At 16 dB student can miss up to 10% of speech signal when teacher is at a distance greater than 3 feet. A 20 dB or greater hearing loss in the better ear can result in absent, inconsistent or distorted parts of speech, especially word endings (s, ed) and unemphasized sounds. Percent of speech signal missed will be greater whenever there is background noise in the classroom, especially in the elementary grades when instruction is primarily verbal and younger children have greater difficulty listening in noise. Young children have the tendency to watch and copy the movements of other students rather than attending to auditorily fragmented teacher directions.	May be unaware of subtle conversational cues that could cause child to be viewed as inappropriate or awkward. May miss portions of fast-paced peer interactions that could begin to have an impact on socialization and self-concept. Behavior may be confused for immaturity or inattention. May be more fatigued due to extra effort needed for understanding speech.	Noise in typical classroom environments impede child from having full access to teacher instruction. Will benefit from improved acoustic treatment of classroom and sound-field amplification. Favorable seating necessary. May often have difficulty with sound/letter associations and subtle auditory discrimination skills necessary for reading. May need attention to vocabulary or speech, especially when there has been a long history of middle ear fluid. Depending on loss configuration, may benefit from low power hearing aid with personal FM system. Appropriate medical management necessary for conductive losses. In-service on impact of "minimal" 15–25 dB hearing loss on language development, listening in noise and learning, required for teacher.

Possible Impact on the Understanding of Language and Speech	Possible Social Impact	Potential Educational Accommodations and Services
Effect of a hearing loss of approximately 20 dB can be compared to ability to hear when index fingers are placed in ears therefore a 26–40 dB hearing loss causes greater listening difficulties than a "plugged ear" loss. Child can "hear" but misses fragments of speech leading to misunderstanding. Degree of difficulty experienced in school will depend upon noise level in the classroom, distance from the teacher, and configuration of the hearing loss, even with hearing aids. At 30 dB can miss 25–40% of the speech signal; at 40 dB may miss 50% of class discussions, especially when voices are faint or speaker is not in line of vision. Will miss unemphasized words and consonants, especially when a high frequency hearing loss is present. Often experiences difficulty learning early reading skills such as letter/sound associations. Child's ability to understand and succeed in the classroom will be substantially diminished by speaker distance and background noise, especially in the elementary grades.	Barriers begin to build with negative impact on self-esteem as child is accused of "hearing when he/she wants to," "daydreaming," or "not paying attention." May believe he/she is less capable due to difficulties understanding in class. Child begins to lose ability for selective listening, and has increasing difficulty suppressing background noise causing the learning environment to be more stressful. Child is more fatigued due to effort needed to listen.	Noise in typical class will impede child from full access to teacher instruction. Will benefit from hearing aid(s) and use of a desk top or ear level FM system in the classroom. Needs favorable acoustics, seating and lighting. May need attention to auditory skills, speech, language development, speechreading and/or support in reading and self-esteem. Amount of attention needed typically related to the degree of success of intervention prior to 6 months of age to prevent language and early learning delays. Teacher in-service on impact of so called "mild" hearing loss on listening and learning to convey that it is often greater than expected.

Please Consider Indicated Items in the Child's Educational Program:

____ Teacher inservice and seating close to teacher
____ Contact your school district's audiologist
____ Screening/evaluation of speech and language
____ Educational consultation/ program supervision by specialist(s) in hearing loss
____ Periodic educational monitoring such as October and April teacher/student completion of SIFTER, LIFE

____ Hearing monitoring at school every _____ mos.
____ Protect ears from noise to prevent more loss
____ Note-taking, closed captioned films, visuals
____ Regular contact with other children who are deaf or hard of hearing

____ Amplification monitoring
____ Educational support services/evaluation
____ FM system trial period

NOTE: All children require full access to teacher instruction and educationally relevant peer communication to receive an appropriate education.
Distance, noise in classroom and fragmentation caused by hearing loss prevent full access to spoken instruction. Appropriate acoustics, use of visuals, FM amplification, sign language, notetakers, communication partners, etc. increase access to instruction. Needs periodic hearing evaluation, rigorous amplification checks, and regular monitoring of access to instruction and classroom function (monitoring tools at www.hear2learn.com or www.SIFTERanderson.com).

41–55 dB HEARING LOSS

Possible Impact on the Understanding of Language and Speech	Possible Social Impact	Potential Educational Accommodations and Services
Consistent use of amplification and language intervention prior to age 6 months increases the probability that the child's speech, language and learning will develop at a normal rate. Without amplification, understands conversation at a distance of 3–5 feet, if sentence structure and vocabulary are known. The amount of speech signal missed can be 50% or more with 40 dB loss and 80% or more with 50 dB loss. Without early amplification the child is likely to have delayed or disordered syntax, limited vocabulary, imperfect speech production and flat voice quality. Addition of a visual communication system to supplement audition may be indicated, especially if language delays and/or additional disabilities are present. Even with hearing aids, child can "hear" but may miss much of what is said if classroom is noisy or reverberant. With personal hearing aids alone, ability to perceive speech and learn effectively in the classroom is at high risk. A personal FM system to overcome classroom noise and distance is typically necessary.	Barriers build with negative impact on self-esteem as child is accused of "hearing when he/she wants to," "daydreaming," or "not paying attention." Communication will be significantly compromised with this degree of hearing loss if hearing aids nor worn. Socialization with peers can be difficult, especially in noisy settings such as cooperative learning situations, lunch or recess. May be more fatigued than classmates due to effort needed to listen.	Consistent use of amplification (hearing aids + FM) is essential. Needs favorable classroom acoustics, seating and lighting. Consultation/program supervision by a specialist in childhood hearing impairment to coordinate services is important. Depending on intervention success in preventing language delays, special academic support necessary if language and academic delays are present. Attention to growth of oral communication, reading, written language skills, auditory skill development, speech therapy, self-esteem likely. Teacher in-service required with attention to communication access and peer acceptance.

56–70 dB HEARING LOSS

Possible Impact on the Understanding of Language and Speech	Possible Social Impact	Potential Educational Accommodations and Services
Even with hearing aids, child will typically be aware of people talking around him/her, but will miss parts of words said resulting in difficulty in situations requiring verbal communication (both one-to-one and in groups). Without amplification, conversation must be very loud to be understood; a 55 dB loss can cause a child to miss up to 100% of speech information without functioning amplification. If hearing loss is not identified before age one year and appropriately managed, delayed spoken language, syntax, reduced speech intelligibility and flat voice quality is likely. Age when first amplified, consistency of hearing aid use and success of early language intervention strongly tied to speech, language and learning development. Addition of visual communication system often indicated if language delays and/or additional disabilities are present. Use of a personal FM system will reduce the effects of noise and distance and allow increased auditory access to verbal instruction. With hearing aids alone, ability to understand in the classroom is greatly reduced by distance and noise.	If hearing loss was late-identified and language delay was not prevented, communication interaction with peers will be significantly affected. Children will have greater difficulty socializing, especially in noisy settings such as lunch cooperative learning situations, or recess. Tendency for poorer self-concept and social immaturity may contribute to a sense of rejection; peer in-service helpful.	Full time, consistent use of amplification (hearing aids + FM system) essential. May benefit from frequency transposition (frequency compression) hearing aids depending upon loss configuration. May require intense support in development of auditory, language, speech, reading and writing skills. Consultation/supervision by a specialist in childhood hearing impairment to coordinate services is important. Use of sign language or a visual communication system by children with substantial language delays or additional learning needs, may be useful to access linguistically complex instruction. Note-taking, captioned films, etc. accommodations often needed. Requires teacher in-service.

Please Consider Indicated Items in the Child's Educational Program:

___ Teacher inservice and seating close to teacher	___ Hearing monitoring at school every ___ mos.	___ Amplification monitoring
___ Contact your school district's audiologist	___ Protect ears from noise to prevent more loss	___ Educational support services/evaluation
___ Screening/evaluation of speech and language	___ Note-taking, closed captioned films, visuals	___ FM system trial period
___ Educational consultation/ program supervision by specialist(s) in hearing loss	___ Regular contact with other children who are deaf or hard of hearing	
___ Periodic educational monitoring such as October and April teacher/student completion of SIFTER, LIFE		

NOTE: All children require full access to teacher instruction and educationally relevant peer communication to receive an appropriate education.
Distance, noise in classroom and fragmentation caused by hearing loss prevent full access to spoken instruction. Appropriate acoustics, use of visuals, FM amplification, sign language, notetakers, communication partners, etc. increase access to instruction. Needs periodic hearing evaluation, rigorous amplification checks, and regular monitoring of access to instruction and classroom function (monitoring tools at www.hear2learn.com or www.SIFTERanderson.com).

© 1991. Relationship of Degree of Longterm Hearing Loss to Psychosocial Impact and Educational Needs. Karen Anderson & Noel Matkin, revised 2007 (thanks to input from the Educational Audiology Association listserv.

	71–90 dB and 91+ dB	
Possible Impact on the Understanding of Language and Speech	**Possible Social Impact**	**Potential Educational Accommodations and Services**
The earlier the child wears amplification consistently with concentrated efforts by parents and caregivers to provide rich language opportunities throughout everyday activities and/or provision of intensive language intervention (sign or verbal), the greater the probability that speech, language and learning will develop at a relatively normal rate. Without amplification, children with 71–90 dB hearing loss may only hear loud noises about one foot from ear. When amplified optimally, children with hearing ability of 90 dB or better should detect many sounds of speech if presented from close distance or via FM. Individual ability and intensive intervention prior to 6 months of age will determine the degree that sounds detected will be discriminated and understood by the brain into meaningful input. Even with hearing aids children	Depending on success of intervention in infancy to address language development, the child's communication may be minimally or significantly affected. Socialization with hearing peers may be difficult. Children in general education classrooms may develop greater dependence on adults due to difficulty perceiving or comprehending oral communication. Children may be more comfortable interacting with peers who are deaf or hard of hearing due to ease of communication. Relationships with peers and adults who have hearing loss can make positive contributions toward the development of a healthy self-concept and a sense of cultural identity.	There is no one communication system that is right for all hard of hearing or deaf children and their families. Whether a visual communication approach or auditory/oral approach is used, extensive language intervention, full-time consistent amplification use and constant integration of the communication practices into the family by 6 months of age will highly increase the probability that the child will become a successful learner. Children with late-identified hearing loss (i.e., after 6 months of age) will have delayed language. This language gap is difficult to overcome and the educational program of a child with hearing loss, especially those with language and learning delays secondary to hearing loss, requires the involvement of a consultant or teacher with expertise in teaching children with hearing loss. Depending on the configuration of the hearing loss and individual speech perception ability, frequency transposition (frequency

with 71–90 dB loss are typically unable to perceive all high pitch speech sounds sufficiently to discriminate them or benefit from incidental listening, especially without the use of FM. The child with hearing loss greater than 70 dB may be a candidate for cochlear implant(s) and the child with hearing loss greater than 90 dB will not be able to perceive most speech sounds with traditional hearing aids. For full access to language to be available visually through sign language or cued speech, family members must be involved in child's communication mode from a very young age.

compression) aids or cochlear implantation may be options for better access to speech. If an auditory/oral approach is used, early training is needed on auditory skills, spoken language, concept development and speech. If culturally deaf emphasis is selected, frequent exposure to Deaf, ASL users is important. Educational placement with other signing deaf or hard of hearing students (special school or classes) may be a more appropriate option to access a language-rich environment and free-flowing communication. Support services and continual appraisal of access to communication and verbal instruction is required. Note-taking, captioning, captioned films and other visual enhancement strategies necessary. Training in pragmatic language use and communication repair strategies helpful. In-service of general education teachers is essential.

Please Consider Indicated Items in the Child's Educational Program:

___ Teacher inservice and seating close to teacher
___ Contact your school district's audiologist
___ Screening/evaluation of speech and language
___ Educational consultation/ program supervision by specialist(s) in hearing loss
___ Periodic educational monitoring such as October and April teacher/student completion of SIFTER, LIFE

___ Hearing monitoring at school every ___ mos.
___ Protect ears from noise to prevent more loss
___ Note-taking, closed captioned films, visuals
___ Regular contact with other children who are deaf or hard of hearing

___ Amplification monitoring
___ Educational support services/evaluation
___ FM system trial period

NOTE: All children require full access to teacher instruction and educationally relevant peer communication to receive an appropriate education.

Distance, noise in classroom and fragmentation caused by hearing loss prevent full access to spoken instruction. Appropriate acoustics, use of visuals, FM amplification, sign language, notetakers, communication partners, etc. increase access to instruction. Needs periodic hearing evaluation, rigorous amplification checks, and regular monitoring of access to instruction and classroom function (monitoring tools at www.hear2learn.com or www.SIFTERanderson.com).

UNILATERAL HEARING LOSS

Possible Impact on the Understanding of Language and Speech	Possible Social Impact	Potential Educational Accommodations and Services
Child can "hear" but can have difficulty understanding in certain situations, such as hearing faint or distant speech, especially if poor ear is aimed toward the person speaking. Will typically have difficulty localizing sounds and voices using hearing alone. The unilateral listener will have greater difficulty understanding speech when environment is noisy and/or reverberant, especially when normal ear towards the overhead projector or other competing sound source and poor hearing ear towards the teacher. Exhibits difficulty detecting or understanding soft speech from the side of the poor hearing ear, especially in a group discussion.	Child may be accused of selective hearing due to discrepancies in speech understanding in quiet versus noise. Social problems may arise as child experiences difficulty understanding in noisy cooperative learning, or recess situations. May misconstrue peer conversations and feel rejected or ridiculed. Child may be more fatigued in classroom due to greater effort needed to listen, if class is noisy or has poor acoustics. May appear inattentive, distractible or frustrated, with behavior or social problems sometimes evident.	Allow child to change seat locations to direct the normal hearing ear toward the primary speaker. Student is at 10 times the risk for educational difficulties as children with 2 normal hearing ears and 1/3 to 1/2 of students with unilateral hearing loss experience significant learning problems. Children often have difficulty learning sound/letter associations in typically noisy kindergarten and grade 1 settings. Educational and audiological monitoring is warranted. Teacher in-service is beneficial. Typically will benefit from a personal FM system with low gain/power or a sound-field FM system in the classroom, especially in the lower grades. Depending on the hearing loss, may benefit from a hearing aid in the impaired ear.

MID-FREQUENCY HEARING LOSS or REVERSE SLOPE HEARING LOSS

MID-FREQUENCY HEARING LOSS or REVERSE SLOPE

Possible Impact on the Understanding of Language and Speech	Possible Social Impact	Potential Educational Accommodations and Services
Child can "hear" whenever speech is present but will have difficulty understanding in certain situations. May have difficulty understanding faint or distant speech, such as a student with a quiet voice speaking from across the classroom. The "cookie bite" or reverse slope listener will have greater difficulty understanding speech when environment is noisy and/or reverberant, such as a typical classroom setting. A 25–40 dB degree of loss in the low to mid-frequency range may cause the child to miss approximately 30% of speech information, if unamplified; some consonant and vowel sounds may be heard inconsistently, especially when background noise is present. Speech production of these sounds may be affected.	Child may be accused of selective hearing or "hearing when he wants to" due to discrepancies in speech understanding in quiet versus noise. Social problems may arise as child experiences difficulty understanding in noisy cooperative learning situations, lunch or recess. May misconstrue peer conversations, believing that other children are talking about him or her. Child may be more fatigued in classroom setting due to greater effort needed to listen. May appear inattentive, distractible or frustrated.	Personal hearing aids important but must be precisely fit to hearing loss. Child likely to benefit from a sound-field FM system, a personal FM system or assistive listening device in the classroom. Student is at risk for educational difficulties. Can experience some difficulty learning sound/letter associations in kindergarten and 1st grade classes. Depending upon degree and configuration of loss, child may experience delayed language development and articulation problems. Educational monitoring and teacher in-service warranted. Annual hearing evaluation to monitor for hearing loss progression is important.

Please Consider Indicated Items in the Child's Educational Program:

____ Teacher inservice and seating close to teacher
____ Contact your school district's audiologist
____ Screening/evaluation of speech and language
____ Educational consultation/ program supervision by specialist(s) in hearing loss
____ Periodic educational monitoring such as October and April teacher/student completion of SIFTER, LIFE

____ Hearing monitoring at school every ____ mos.
____ Protect ears from noise to prevent more loss
____ Note-taking, closed captioned films, visuals
____ Regular contact with other children who are deaf or hard of hearing

____ Amplification monitoring
____ Educational support services/evaluation
____ FM system trial period

NOTE: All children require full access to teacher instruction and educationally relevant peer communication to receive an appropriate education.
Distance, noise in classroom and fragmentation caused by hearing loss prevent full access to spoken instruction. Appropriate acoustics, use of visuals, FM amplification, sign language, notetakers, communication partners, etc. increase access to instruction. Needs periodic hearing evaluation, rigorous amplification checks, and regular monitoring of access to instruction and classroom function (monitoring tools at www.hear2learn.com or www.SIFTERanderson.com).

© 1991. Relationship of Degree of Longterm Hearing Loss to Psychosocial Impact and Educational Needs. Karen Anderson & Noel Matkin, revised 2007 thanks to input from the Educational Audiology Association listserv.

HIGH FREQUENCY HEARING LOSS

Possible Impact on the Understanding of Language and Speech	Possible Social Impact	Potential Educational Accommodations and Services
Child can "hear" but can miss important fragments of speech. Even a 25–40 dB loss in high frequency hearing may cause the child to miss 20%–30% of vital speech information if unamplified. Consonant sounds t, s, f, th, k, sh, ch likely heard inconsistently, especially in noise. May have difficulty understanding faint or distant speech, such as a student with a quiet voice speaking from across the classroom and will have much greater difficulty understanding speech when in low background noise and/or reverberation is present. Many of the critical sounds for understanding speech are high pitched, quiet sounds, making them difficult to perceive; the words: cat, cap, calf, cast could be perceived as "ca," word endings, possessives, plurals and unstressed brief words are difficult to perceive and understand. Speech production may be affected. Use of amplification often indicated to learn language at a typical rate and ease learning.	May be accused of selective hearing due to discrepancies in speech understanding in quiet versus noise. Social problems may arise as child experiences difficulty understanding in noisy cooperative learning situations, lunch or recess. May misinterpret peer conversations. Child may be fatigued in classroom due to greater listening effort. May appear inattentive, distractible or frustrated. Could affect self-concept.	Student is at risk for educational difficulties. Depending upon onset, degree and configuration of loss, child may experience delayed language and syntax development and articulation problems. Possible difficulty learning some sound/letter associations in kindergarten and 1st grade classes. Early evaluation of speech and language skills is suggested. Educational monitoring and teacher in-service is warranted. Will typically benefit from personal hearing aids and use of a sound-field or a personal FM system in the classroom. Use of ear protection in noisy situations is imperative to prevent damage to inner ear structures and resulting progression of the hearing loss.

FLUCTUATING HEARING LOSS

Possible Impact on the Understanding of Language and Speech	Possible Social Impact	Potential Educational Accommodations and Services
Of greatest concern are children who have experienced hearing fluctuations over many months in early childhood (multiple episodes with fluid lasting three months or longer). Listening with a hearing loss that is approximately 20 dB can be compared to hearing when index fingers are placed in ears. This loss or worse is typical of listening with fluid or infection behind the eardrums. Child can "hear" but misses fragments of what is said. Degree of difficulty experienced in school will depend upon the classroom noise level, the distance from the teacher and the current degree of hearing loss. At 30 dB can miss 25–40% of the speech signal; child with a 40 dB loss associated with "glue ear" may miss 50% of class discussions, especially when voices are faint or speaker is not in line of vision. Will frequently miss unstressed words, consonants and word endings.	Barriers begin to build with negative impact on self-esteem as the child is accused of "hearing when he/she wants to," "daydreaming," or "not paying attention." Child may believe he/she is less capable due to understanding difficulties in class. Typically poor at identifying changes in own hearing ability. With inconsistent hearing, the child learns to "tune out" the speech signal. Children are judged to have greater attention problems, insecurity, distractibility and lack self-esteem. Tend to be non-participative and distract themselves from classroom tasks; often socially immature.	Impact is primarily on acquisition of early reading skills and attention in class. Screening for language delays is suggested from a young age. Ongoing monitoring for hearing loss in school, communication between parent and teacher about listening difficulties and aggressive medical management is needed. Will benefit from sound-field FM or an assistive listening device in class. May need attention to development of speech, reading, self-esteem, or listening skills. Teacher in-service is beneficial.

Source: Karen L. Anderson, PhD., Supporting Success for Children with Hearing Loss. Download single page versions from http://successforkidswithhearingloss.com/for-professionals/relationship-of-hearing-loss-to-listening-and-learning

Please Consider Indicated Items in the Child's Educational Program:

___ Teacher inservice and seating close to teacher	___ Hearing monitoring at school every ___ mos.	___ Amplification monitoring
___ Contact your school district's audiologist	___ Protect ears from noise to prevent more loss	___ Educational support services/evaluation
___ Screening/evaluation of speech and language	___ Note-taking, closed captioned films, visuals	___ FM system trial period
___ Educational consultation/ program supervision by specialist(s) in hearing loss	___ Regular contact with other children who are deaf or hard of hearing	
___ Periodic educational monitoring such as October and April teacher/student completion of SIFTER, LIFE		

NOTE: All children require full access to teacher instruction and educationally relevant peer communication to receive an appropriate education. Distance, noise in classroom and fragmentation caused by hearing loss prevent full access to spoken instruction. Appropriate acoustics, use of visuals, FM amplification, sign language, notetakers, communication partners, etc. increase access to instruction. Needs periodic hearing evaluation, rigorous amplification checks, and regular monitoring of access to instruction and classroom function (monitoring tools at www.hear2learn.com or www.SIFTERanderson.com).

© 1991, Relationship of Degree of Longterm Hearing Loss to Psychosocial Impact and Educational Needs. Karen Anderson & Noel Matkin, revised 2007 thanks to input from the Educational Audiology Association listserv.

5

HEARING AIDS AND AUDITORY-VERBAL THERAPY

Ryan W. McCreery and Elizabeth A. Walker

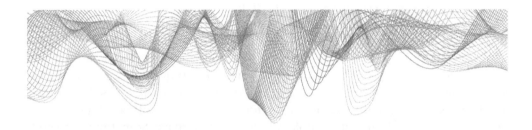

INTRODUCTION

Hearing aids are the most frequently used technology to help improve auditory access for children who have hearing loss. Without amplification, children who are deaf or hard of hearing will experience reduced access to sound, including acoustic cues that are needed to develop spoken language. As a result, optimizing speech audibility with amplification and promoting consistent hearing aid use are essential for promoting listening and spoken language skills. Parents, audiologists, and Auditory-Verbal practitioners (AV practitioners) all play important roles in maximizing auditory access for children who wear hearing aids. Knowledge of the benefits of hearing aids for supporting Auditory-Verbal Therapy (AVT), therefore, is critical for parents and practitioners.

In this chapter, the authors provide a detailed overview of how hearing aids support listening and spoken language in children who are deaf or hard of hearing and demonstrate in detail how hearing is fundamental in the planning, evaluating, and delivery of AVT for most such children (see Chapter 17). Because speech and spoken language are among the most important sounds that children can hear, the importance of making those sounds audible is a key theme. The basic function of hearing aids will be discussed, including the latest advances in how hearing aids process sound. Since hearing aids are not beneficial if they are not worn, strategies for promoting consistent hearing aid use across a wide range of listening situations are presented. Children with mild bilateral hearing loss, children with unilateral hearing loss, and children with auditory neuropathy spectrum disorder are three unique groups for whom amplification benefits have been debated and are included at the end of the chapter.

HOW DO HEARING AIDS SUPPORT THE GOALS OF AUDITORY-VERBAL THERAPY?

One key feature of AVT is the emphasis on using the child's listening and auditory skills as the foundation for promoting the development of spoken language in conversations and literacy (see Chapters 10, 11, and 14). The emphasis on listening and development of auditory skills means that hearing aids and cochlear implants (see Chapter 6) are fundamental to AVT. Hearing aids enhance the child's access to sound by increasing its intensity and by processing the sound to enhance audibility of speech in specific ways that are discussed in detail here. We will focus broadly on how hearing aids support the short-term and long-term goals of AVT.

Maximizing Residual Hearing

The use of auditory skills for processing spoken language effectively requires the maximization of the child's remaining auditory abilities. Children who are born with profound or complete hearing losses that eliminate the child's access to sound may only be able to receive usable auditory access through cochlear implants. However, most children with hearing loss have some amount of hearing and can access some sound, even without amplification. The remaining hearing in children with hearing loss is known as *residual hearing*. Hearing aids amplify sounds to maximize the child's ability to use this residual hearing. The range of residual hearing is often referred to as the *dynamic range of hearing*. The dynamic range is the difference between the softest sounds we can hear (hearing thresholds) and the loudest sounds we can tolerate without experiencing discomfort. Hearing thresholds increase with hearing loss, but the listener's ability to tolerate loud sounds does not increase. Sometimes, the ability to tolerate loud sounds decreases with hearing loss. As a result, residual hearing decreases as degree of hearing loss gets worse, as illustrated by the different panels in Figure 5–1.

Amplified sound that is above threshold and within the child's dynamic range is considered to be audible to the child. The dynamic range of hearing may be large for children with mild and moderate hearing losses, which makes amplification of speech sounds relatively easy to accomplish. In contrast, the dynamic range becomes narrow for children with severe or profound hearing losses. Hearing aids make speech and other sounds audible to maximize the residual hearing of each child and increase the dynamic range. The amount of amplification, also known as *gain*, provided by a hearing aid is cus-

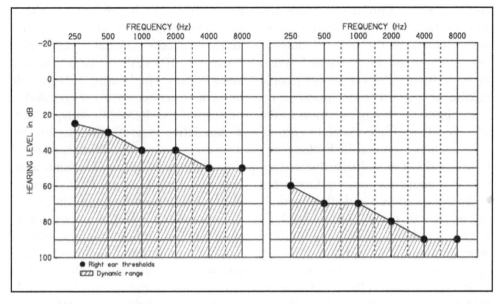

Figure 5-1. Audiograms demonstrating the dynamic range for two different degrees of hearing loss. Actual dynamic ranges for two individuals with these audiograms may vary.

tomized based on the child's residual hearing. The gain of a hearing aid is simply the difference between the level of the input and level of the output. The individual prescription of the amount of gain is crucial to providing auditory access and maximizing audibility across the speech frequency range.

Making Speech and Other Environmental Sounds Audible

Children are exposed to a wide range of sounds in their everyday listening environments, and in AVT, parents and the practitioner will focus on increasing the child's access to and subsequent awareness and understanding of such sounds. The amount of access that a child has to sound with his or her residual hearing is known as *audibility*. Audibility is

often defined in reference to how well a listener can hear the sounds that make up speech. The audibility for speech can be quantified using metrics like the Speech Intelligibility Index (SII; ANSI S3.5:1997 R2007), which utilizes a number between 0 and 1 that describes the amount of the speech spectrum that is audible. Higher numbers mean that more of the speech spectrum is audible to the listener. However, identification and comprehension of environmental sounds also serve important purposes for extensive learning and for safety. Children often encounter listening situations with multiple talkers and different sources of background noise where these sound sources can change in terms of location or intensity. For example, in daycares and pre-school classrooms, a child may need to attend to the teacher and other children during a discussion while also hearing steady background noise from the air-conditioner and intermittent noise from children in the hallway outside. In social settings, children may listen to multiple friends with different people talking at once. These situations require the child to pay attention to the specific talker of interest and to ignore talkers who are part of the background. Hearing aids can help in these complex listening situations by increasing audibility for speech and all the sounds of everyday living. In places with high levels of background noise, additional hearing assistance technology, such as remote-microphone frequency or digital-modulation (FM or DM, respectively) systems may be used to enhance the child's access to a specific talker of interest (see Chapter 7).

Increasing Auditory Stimulation to Promote Linguistic and Cognitive Development

For a child with hearing loss, hearing aids provide access to the acoustic cues needed to support learning to listen and listening to learn. More recently, the positive impact of auditory stimulation on brain development in children who are deaf or hard of hearing has been reported in the literature. Limited auditory exposure has been linked to lack of development of the auditory areas of the brain (Sharma, Dorman, & Spahr, 2002), but auditory stimulation from hearing aids and cochlear implants is likely to promote development of these areas (Sharma, Dorman, & Kral, 2005). Research suggests that there are two mechanisms by which auditory stimula-

tion provided by hearing aids can support development. Children with better auditory access will have higher performance on a wide range of auditory tasks because the hearing aids provide immediate access to the cues needed to perform the task. Additionally, there is a cumulative impact of increasing auditory access on the development of linguistic, cognitive, and academic abilities over time (Pisoni, 2000; Tomblin et al., 2015; Tomblin et al., in press). The cumulative effect of auditory stimulation is that children with greater auditory experience will develop stronger cognitive and linguistic skills that will enhance their ability to listen, speak, and learn over time, and in AVT that is a highly desired outcome.

Consider two hypothetical children who wear hearing aids and are entering school. Jimmy has good audibility for speech through his hearing aids and has worn his hearing aids during all waking hours since he was diagnosed with hearing loss in early childhood. Brian has good audibility for speech through his hearing aids but has experienced long periods of time without amplification during infancy and early childhood because of frequent hearing aid repairs and ear infections. Both Jimmy and Brian have the same immediate auditory access to the speech of the teacher and children in the preschool, but Jimmy is more likely to have acquired the cumulative benefits of auditory experience because of greater hearing aid use over time. When access to the acoustic cues needed to understand speech is reduced, listeners must rely on top-down processing to help them understand the message. Top-down processing skills are cognitive and linguistic skills that enable a listener to understand and process incoming information. As a result of enhanced cumulative auditory experience, Jimmy may have better cognitive and linguistic skills to support speech recognition when audibility is reduced by background noise. Brian may lag behind due to limited device use. This comparison of two children highlights the importance of promoting consistent early auditory experience, not only for immediate access to sounds in the environment, but also for increasing the cumulative auditory stimulation needed to support the development of auditory, linguistic, and cognitive abilities that enhance listening in everyday life.

AN INTRODUCTION TO HEARING AIDS

A deep understanding of how hearing aids work is essential to practitioners and parents. Examples of two types of behind-the-ear hearing aids are displayed in Figure 5–2.

Hearing aids receive sounds from the environment through a microphone. Sound from the environment is converted to an electrical signal. In most modern hearing aids, the electrical signal from the microphone is converted to a digital signal. Digital hearing aids contain a small computer that modifies the digital signal based on the listener's hearing needs. After processing, the digital signal is converted back to an electrical signal and sent to a speaker, known as the receiver. The receiver changes the electrical signal back into amplified sound that is sent to the ear. The entire amplification process must happen in less than ten-thousandths of a second or the listener may notice that the amplified sound is delayed compared with the visual cues in the environment. For most children who are deaf or hard of hearing, the hearing aid produces sound that is routed into the ear canal using air conduction. In some cases, children may be born without an ear canal or with physical differences that prevent sound from being routed through the ear canal with air conduction. Using bone

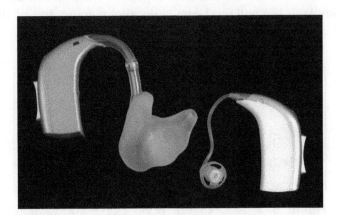

Figure 5-2. A behind-the-ear hearing aid coupled to an earmold (left) and a behind-the-ear hearing aid coupled to a receiver-in-the-ear with a comfort dome.

conduction, amplified sound can also be converted to mechanical vibrations by the hearing aid, which can be transmitted to the skull using a hard or soft headband or surgical implant. Different bone conduction hearing aid devices are shown in Figure 5–3.

Who Should Wear Hearing Aids?

Generally, hearing loss of any degree can have a negative impact on a child's development of spoken language. Therefore, organizations such as the American Academy of Audiology (2013) and Australian Hearing (King, 2010) recommend that every child who is deaf or hard of hearing be considered a candidate for hearing aids. Figure 5–4 shows the range of hearing thresholds that are usually recommended for hearing aids in children.

Hearing aids are typically recommended for children with mild to severe hearing losses. Children in the severe or profound hearing loss range are often considered to be candidates for cochlear implants but will use hearing aids prior to cochlear implantation to provide auditory stimulation and, hopefully, at least awareness of sound.

When Should Hearing Aids Be Fit?

Although babies often do not say their first words until around 12 months of age, auditory experience during infancy is crucial for promoting the development of spoken language (Kuhl, Conboy, Padden, Nelson, & Pruitt, 2005). For example, an infant's ability to hear the difference between two vowel sounds at 6 months of age is a strong predictor of his or her spoken language development up to 2 years of age (Tsao, Liu, & Kuhl, 2004). Therefore, early provision of amplification for children who are deaf or hard of hearing can ensure that the process of neural maturation and awareness of speech sounds begins as soon as possible. A shift toward early identification of hearing loss and fitting of amplification has occurred rapidly over the past two decades. In a paper by Moeller in 2000, for example, the average age of diagnosis for

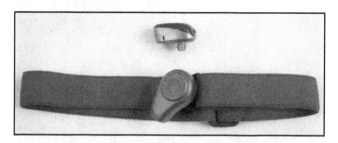

Figure 5-3. A Cochlear Baha bone conduction sound processor (top) and an Oticon Ponto bone conduction sound processor coupled to a soft headband. Both devices take incoming acoustic energy and convert it to vibrations for conduction to the inner ear.

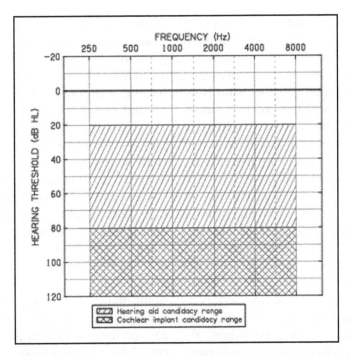

Figure 5–4. The typical candidacy range for hearing aids (hatched area) and for cochlear implants (cross-hatched area). Other factors beyond the audiogram are also important for determining cochlear implant candidacy, including the child's development, aided audibility, and speech recognition ability in older children.

children with hearing loss was around 2½ years of age. More recently, studies have shown that the median age of diagnosis is around 3 to 4 months, with a median age of hearing aid fitting around 6 to 7 months of age (Holte et al., 2012). Generally, children who are deaf or hard of hearing should be fitted with amplification as soon as possible after hearing loss has been diagnosed to minimize the amount of time that auditory stimulation is limited, consistent with the core tenets of AVT. The timing of amplification may be affected by a wide range of factors, including inconclusive diagnostic results, waiting time for audiology appointments, the pres-

ence of middle ear fluid or other general health concerns, and not returning for care after the diagnosis (Walker et al., 2014). Many of these factors are preventable, and audiologists and others who serve children with hearing loss strive to support children and their caregivers to minimize delays in fitting amplification.

THE HEARING AID FITTING PROCESS

Fitting children with hearing aids is not a one-time event. Rather, it is an ongoing process that occurs regularly throughout the child's development and ideally involves the audiologist, parents, practitioners, and others. The hearing aid fitting process is initiated with the confirmation of permanent hearing loss with a diagnostic hearing evaluation by an audiologist. Based on the results and input from parents, the audiologist selects the most appropriate hearing aids and signal processing technologies for the child. The hearing aids are then programmed and fitted on the child, and the audibility provided by the hearing aids is verified. Parents and other professionals involved in the use of hearing aids are oriented as to the care, maintenance, and function of the devices by the audiologist. Finally, the benefits of hearing aids must be assessed by parents, practitioners, and/or audiologists during the outcome validation phase of the process. Each of these steps is repeated as necessary based on the child's progress and development.

Diagnostic Assessment

To know whether or not a hearing aid is needed and how much amplification should be provided, a diagnostic assessment of hearing (discussed more specifically in Chapter 4) is an important first step in the process of providing hearing aids to infants and young children. If hearing loss is suspected from newborn hearing screening or other assessments, hearing thresholds in each ear are measured using either behavioral audiometry or estimates of behavioral hearing based on electrophysiological measures, such as the auditory brainstem response (ABR) or

auditory steady-state response (ASSR). Unlike adults, where the entire audiogram may be measured in both ears in a single test, children may provide less information in both electrophysiological and behavioral tests. Electrophysiological measures of hearing can often only be completed while an infant or child sleeps, so the amount of information that can be obtained may be limited because the child may wake up at any time. Behavioral hearing assessment is contingent on the child's cooperation and can be limited if the child loses interest during the test. Other tests, such as tympanometry and otoacoustic emissions, may provide supplemental information about the status of the middle ear and inner ear organ of hearing (cochlea) but do not measure frequency-specific hearing thresholds that are needed to fit hearing aids. After a diagnosis of hearing loss is made based on the diagnostic hearing evaluation, the audiologist will refer the family to an ear, nose, and throat (ENT or otolaryngologist) physician for medical evaluation and clearance for hearing aids. This process helps to ensure that any underlying medical concerns related to the hearing loss are identified. Additionally, referrals to ophthalmology and medical genetics may be recommended to assess the child's vision and potential genetic causes of hearing loss, respectively.

Earmolds

Earmolds are molds of the child's ear that are used to connect a behind-the-ear hearing aid to the child's ear canal for air-conduction hearing aids. Impressions of the ear for earmolds are often taken at the diagnostic evaluation and confirmation of permanent hearing. Taking ear impressions early in the process allows time for fabrication prior to the fitting and avoids delays in the amplification fitting. The earmold is not simply a conduit for sound to reach the child's ear canal from the hearing aid but can be manufactured to alter the sound that passes through it. Dampers or filters can be used to enhance or minimize specific frequencies. Increasing or decreasing the diameter of the tubing can affect the amount of amplification at specific frequencies. Even with digital hearing aid signal processing that allows precise manipulation of the amount of gain provided by the hearing aid, selecting earmolds with specific characteristics to enhance the acoustic frequency response of the hearing aid can be useful. The audiologist will select the earmold characteristics that are appropriate for the child's ear and degree of hearing loss. For young children, audiologists are likely to select a soft earmold material that is easy to modify, such as silicone or vinyl. Older children may transition to harder acrylic material depending on their preference and skin texture. Parents and children can select from a wide range of earmold colors from clear or skin color to bright neon or mixtures of colors.

Earmolds have a limited life span and need to be regularly replaced to ensure consistent coupling with the ear canal. An earmold that provides a good connection with the ear canal ensures that the amount of gain provided by the hearing aid is consistent as the child's ear canal grows. The length of time that each earmold lasts depends on the age of the child, the earmold material, and the care and maintenance of the earmold. Infants and younger children usually experience significant ear canal growth, particularly during the first year of life, which means that a new earmold may be needed as often as every 3 months. As children get older, their ear canals continue to grow, but the rate of growth is much slower, and earmolds can provide a good fit of the ear canal, in some cases, for over a year. Hard earmold materials, such as vinyl and acrylic, tend to last longer than softer materials, such as silicone.

Selection of Amplification

After the diagnostic assessment indicates the presence of permanent hearing loss, the audiologist, in consultation with the family, needs to select the hearing aid and signal processing characteristics that will provide the child with the best auditory access. The audiologist may select a hearing aid for an infant, but the device needs to adapt to the child's needs over a period as long as 5 years. Although the child's earmold will be replaced numerous times as the child's ear grows, replacement of hearing aids is cost prohibitive. As a result, behind-the-ear (BTE) hearing aids are most frequently recommended for use with infants and young children. Another consideration when selecting a BTE hearing aid is the color of the case, which can be selected by the child or family. Bright colors are easier to find if the hearing aid is misplaced compared with beige or other neutral colors. Additional advantages of BTE hearing aids over other styles of hearing aids for children are summarized in Table 5–1.

Levels of Technology

Most hearing aid manufacturers offer at least three different levels or tiers of technology. The cost of the hearing aid increases as the level of technology increases. Higher cost often leads to the perception that higher (and more expensive) levels of technology might lead to better hearing and developmental outcomes. There is little evidence to suggest, however, that higher levels of technology create better outcomes in speech recognition or language development. If an audiologist recommends a higher level of technology, the parents need to ask for research to support the recommendation. Parents and practitioners also can ask the dispensing audiologist for hearing aid specifications for the specific makes and models of hearing aids recommended. Fortunately, audibility for speech can be achieved using hearing aids at all levels of technology. Selecting a less expensive hearing aid may allow the family to purchase additional hearing assistance technology or other devices that support connectivity. So, more expensive hearing aids do not necessarily yield "better outcomes."

Selection of Hearing Aid Signal Processing

As part of the selection process, the dispensing audiologist determines what specific signal processing features in the hearing aid will be activated for the child. Nearly all modern digital hearing aids include a wide range of signal processing features that can be activated using a computer programming interface. The audiologist needs to use a pediatric, evidence-based rationale for activating specific features. Preferably, the research used to justify the activation of specific signal processing features needs to be based on data obtained from children who wear hearing aids. The research evidence to support specific signal processing features for children is increasing but remains extremely limited. Following is a brief review of the major types of hearing aid signal processing and considerations of common features for parents and practitioners. A more complete review of hearing aid signal processing considerations for children and evidence-based systematic reviews are available on the topics of amplitude compression (McCreery et al., 2012a), digital noise reduction and direction microphones (McCreery et al., 2012b), and frequency lowering (McCreery et al., 2012c).

Amplitude Compression

As mentioned earlier, the sounds comprised by speech need to be made audible with amplification without making those sounds uncomfortably loud. In order to provide audibility across a wide range of different sound intensities, nearly all hearing aids use a feature called *amplitude compression*, to adjust the amount of amplification or gain that sounds receive. Soft sounds receive the most gain, average sounds receive slightly less gain, and loud sounds receive little or no gain. In other words, as the input level of sound to the hearing aid increases, the amount of amplification provided by the hearing aid decreases. Amplitude compression provides enough amplification to make soft

Table 5–1. Advantages of Behind-the-Ear (BTE) Hearing Aids for Children

1. **Durability**: BTE hearing aids are more resistant to moisture and debris than smaller in-the-ear (ITE) hearing aids. On average, the increased durability means that BTE hearing aids need fewer repairs and last 2–3 years longer than ITE hearing aids.
2. **Growth**: As the child's ear grows, the earmold used with a BTE hearing aid can be replaced to improve the fit of the device. Replacing the shell on an ITE means that the entire device must be sent to the manufacturer to make a new shell. Time without amplification reduces auditory experience and access for children who are deaf or hard of hearing and should be minimized.
3. **Adaptability**: If the child experiences a change in hearing, the amount of amplification provided by a BTE hearing aid can be adjusted over a much larger range than with an ITE hearing aid. The ability to change the amount of gain provided by the hearing aid decreases the potential that new hearing aids will be needed if the child's hearing changes.
4. **Real-ear-to-coupler difference**: The acoustics of the child's earmold can be estimated using a RECD measurement with a BTE hearing aid. Verification for ITE hearing aids must occur with all of the measurements in the child's ear canal, which may not be possible for many children.
5. **Connectivity**: BTE hearing aids are more likely to connect hearing aids to accessories via hard-wired, wireless, or Bluetooth connections compared with ITE hearing aids. The connectivity of BTE hearing aids can increase access to different listening environments and devices like computers and tablets that can be important educationally and socially.

sounds audible without making loud sounds uncomfortable. The amount of amplitude compression prescribed will depend on the child's degree of hearing loss. Different amounts of amplitude compression can be used to accommodate children with different amounts of residual hearing.

Guidance for the Practitioner

If the parent or practitioner notices that a child is having difficulty hearing soft sounds or is experiencing loudness discomfort, the audiologist needs to adjust the amplitude compression pa-

rameters of the hearing aid. Conversely, too much amplitude compression can reduce the intensity contrasts between speech sounds and make speech understanding more difficult. Providing specific information for the audiologist about the types of speech sounds that are inaudible or uncomfortable can help him or her to pinpoint the specific areas of difficulty without compromising audibility for other speech sounds. *The practitioner may ask the child's audiologist*: How is the amount of amplitude compression in the hearing aid fitting determined? How audible are soft sounds with and without the hearing aid? How does the hearing aid make the sounds of conversational speech more audible? How does the hearing aid process louder speech compared with average or soft speech? Following a discussion about questions such as these, the practitioner can refer to the literature provided by various hearing aid manufacturers.

Feedback Suppression

The whistling sound that is produced by a hearing aid when it is held in the hand or not fully inserted is known as *acoustic feedback*. Acoustic feedback most commonly occurs when amplified sound from the hearing aid reaches the microphone and is amplified over and over again in a feedback loop. Children who wear hearing aids may not even hear feedback, but parents and practitioners may when inserting the hearing aids or holding them in their hands. Most hearing aids contain some type of signal processing to minimize the likelihood of feedback. Feedback suppression systems in hearing aids may limit the gain of the hearing aid at high frequencies in an attempt to limit feedback. In some cases, it may be possible to preserve gain for high-frequency sounds by addressing feedback through new earmolds that provide a better seal to the child's ear canal. Feedback suppression needs to be activated for children at all ages, as long as it does not impose significant limitations on amplification for high-frequency sounds.

Guidance for the Practitioner

Practitioners or parents may be the first to notice that the fit of the ear-

mold is insufficient. Signs to watch for include difficulty with keeping the earmold in the ear or excessive feedback. Gaps around the earmold may become larger as children's ears grow. Large gaps in the earmold might indicate that new earmolds may be needed. Feedback suppression makes changes to the sound coming out of the hearing aid that can lead to the distortion of sounds, particularly for children with severe or profound hearing loss. Prompt replacement of earmolds can help to minimize the unnecessary application of feedback suppression and distortion of speech. *The practitioner may ask the child's audiologist*: Does the feedback management system in this hearing aid limit the amount of high-frequency amplification? If so, is it possible to provide more amplification and better audibility with a new earmold? Does feedback suppression, when activated, change the quality of speech?

Frequency Lowering

High-frequency speech sounds such as /s/ and mid-high frequency sound such as /sh/ serve important functions for communication. The /s/ sound, for example, is the third most frequently occurring phoneme in English. Recent research suggests that even well-fit hearing aids may not provide enough amplification in the high frequencies to make /s/ audible (Kimlinger et al., 2015), and this, of course, will negatively affect speech and language development (Koehlinger et al., 2015; Moeller et al., 2007). An alternative to amplifying high-frequency sounds is to process those sounds at lower frequencies, where the child's degree of hearing loss might be less and the amount of amplification provided by the hearing aid could be greater. Different hearing aid manufacturers use different approaches to frequency lowering, but most are in two categories. Frequency compression lowers high-frequency sounds by moving them to lower frequencies and compacting those sounds into a smaller range. Frequency transposition moves high-frequency information to lower frequencies using a "cut-and-paste" approach that places those sounds on top of speech sounds at lower frequencies. The type of frequency lowering used for any child may depend on the child's degree and configuration of hearing loss and the specific type of frequency lowering available in the child's hearing aids, but the overall goal is to make high-frequency sounds more audible and more intelligible.

Guidance for the Practitioner

Practitioners need to be aware that without frequency lowering, many children will not be able to discriminate between /s/ and /sh/ easily, because those sounds are not sufficiently amplified. Limited high-frequency amplification can be related to the child's degree of hearing loss, limited high-frequency gain in hearing aids, or a combination of these factors. Frequency lowering can increase audibility for high-frequency sounds for children with mild to moderate hearing losses (McCreery et al., 2014; Wolfe et al., 2011) and those with severe to profound hearing loss (Glista et al., 2009). Audiologists may not always communicate that frequency lowering has been activated. In some cases, the initial setting for frequency lowering may not optimize

audibility. Therefore, practitioners may need to inquire about the activation of frequency lowering, particularly when children are not perceiving or producing high-frequency speech sounds.

The practitioner may want to ask the child's audiologist: Is frequency lowering activated in the hearing aid? What type of frequency lowering is used? What speech sounds are likely to be lowered? How does frequency lowering affect vowel and consonant discrimination when appropriately used? What types of errors would be expected if frequency lowering settings need to be adjusted? If the speaker moves closer to the microphone of the hearing aid, will this affect frequency lowering?

Directional Microphones

Background noise is a persistent problem in most everyday listening environments, where children need to learn, socialize, and communicate. Although hearing assistance technologies, such as remote-microphone (RM) systems, can be used in nursery and preschool classrooms, these options may not be optimal for listening situations with more than one talker. Hearing aids often have multiple microphones that can be used to determine the location of sound relative to the listener and reduce the amount of gain provided to sounds that originate from the side or behind the listener. Omnidirectional microphones are equally sensitive to sounds from all directions. Directional microphones are more sensitive to sounds that arrive from a specific direction, usually in front of the listener, while providing less amplification for sounds that arrive from the sides and behind the listener. Intuitively, reducing sound from the sides and behind the listener will enhance listening for sounds in front of the listener. However, children are not always facing the people with whom they are communicating. If the parent or other important speaker is to the side or behind the child, audibility for those listeners may be reduced, although typically the amount of reduction is very small (1 to 3 dB; Ching et al., 2009). Overhearing is also an important mechanism to support vocabulary and subsequent language development in children (Akhtar, 2005). Opportunities for overhearing language may be reduced if children are using directional microphones. Consequently, directional microphones need to be used selectively in children who can orient toward the talker of interest. In some hearing aids, directionality can be activated automatically when the hearing aid detects that the listener is in a noisy environment. An automatic directional microphone may be preferable in cases where the child is unable to switch the hearing aid to a directional mode him/herself.

Guidance for the Practitioner

Practitioners need to know whether or not a child's hearing aid has directional microphones. If so, he or she can help the audiologist, child, and parents to determine the listening environments where directional microphones will be most beneficial (when the child is facing the talker of interest with noise sources behind) and situations where the benefit of directional microphones may be limited (the speaker of interest may move around the child and/or where sources of noise come from in front of the child).

The practitioner may ask the child's audiologist: Does the hearing aid have directional microphones? How are the directional microphones activated (automatically or manually)? Who is responsible for switching the hearing aid to directional mode? If the directional microphone is used in therapy sessions, how can I help my child or client to listen if I need to sit facing him or her? Is there a way that the hearing aid can tell automatically whether omnidirectional or directional microphones should be activated?

Noise Reduction

In addition to directional microphones, many hearing aids include additional signal processing that reduces the amount of gain provided by the hearing aid when the hearing aid detects background noise. Noise reduction reduces the amount of gain provided by the hearing aid, and, in some cases, can also reduce audibility for speech sounds. Many hearing aids avoid this by reducing input only when steady-state noises, such as noise from ventilation systems or a computer fan, are detected by the hearing aid. The frequencies where gain is reduced can depend on the type of noise reduction system. In some devices, gain is reduced only in the low frequencies, and in other systems gain may be reduced across the entire speech frequency range. The reduction in gain also means that current noise reduction systems cannot improve speech understanding in noise. However, research suggests that noise reduction may improve the comfort of listening situations for children without negatively affecting speech understanding (Stelmachowicz et al., 2010).

Because most digital noise reduction systems would be unlikely to have a negative or positive effect on speech understanding, noise reduction should be considered as a feature that can be activated to maximize listening comfort in noise.

Guidance for the Practitioner

For children who experience loudness discomfort in background noise, *the practitioner may ask the audiologist: Is noise reduction activated in the hearing aid?* If so, how much reduction in gain or audibility occurs when the noise reduction is activated? What signs will be present if there is too much or not enough noise reduction? What methods do you use to determine the benefits of noise reduction? *Would you recommend that noise reduction be activated, or the amount of noise reduction increased?*

Hearing Aid Fitting and Verification

Following the selection of the device and the features to be activated, the child can be fitted with the hearing aid. The primary goals at the hearing aid fitting are to verify that the hearing aid provides audibility for speech sounds and to orient the caregivers and the child to the device. Verification is crucial to determine that the hearing aid is making speech audible without exceeding predicted levels of loudness discomfort. A hearing aid orientation increases the comfort level of caregivers and children with managing amplification on a day-to-day basis, including insertion and removal of earmolds,

care and maintenance of the hearing aids and earmolds, and establishing a schedule for hearing aid use.

Verification

Ear canal size varies across children and over time as they grow. Hearing aids deliver sound to the ear canal, but the amount of sound in the ear canal depends on its size. A hearing aid set to provide a specific amount of gain in an adult ear canal produces a much louder sound level than in a child's smaller ear canal, since sound pressure increases in smaller spaces. Since there are differences in ear canal size among children of the same age, accurate measurements are required to ensure the levels of sound are safe and that sounds are audible. Changes in ear canal size over time affect the sound level delivered by the hearing aid. Therefore, hearing aid verification needs to be repeated periodically as the child grows.

Hearing aid verification is completed using a probe microphone system. A small, flexible tube, known as a probe tube, is placed into the child's ear canal. This is connected to a microphone that typically hangs over the child's ear. It compares the sound delivered outside the ear with the sound level inside the ear canal to estimate the output of the hearing aid. There are two types of probe microphone measures that can be completed, depending on the age of the child. For older children, the output of the hearing aid in the ear canal is measured using recordings of speech at soft, average, and loud levels to ensure that the intensity range of speech is audible. For infants and younger children who may not have the attention and patience to cooperate with multiple measurements in each ear canal, the audiologist can measure the acoustics of the child's ear canal with the earmold. This is called the real-ear-to-coupler difference (RECD). The RECD is actually a comparison of a soft sound presented through the child's earmold to the same sound measured in a coupler that is designed to mimic the volume of an adult ear canal. By taking an RECD measurement in the child's ear, the child's individual ear canal acoustics can be incorporated into hearing aid measurements completed in the coupler. This requires only a single measurement in the child's ear. Age-related average RECD values are available but are not as accurate as RECD values from individual children.

Once the aided levels of speech have been measured as presented above, the audibility of each level can be calculated. The aided level of speech measured in the child's ear canal is compared with the child's hearing thresholds to determine how much of the aided speech

energy is above the child's threshold. Most verification equipment provides an estimate of the aided audibility as the SII. Research has demonstrated that children who wear hearing aids who have better aided audibility have higher language abilities (Tomblin et al., 2015) and better speech recognition (McCreery et al., 2015) than children with poorer audibility. The audiologist may also measure a loud sound through the hearing aid in order to ensure that the hearing aid does not exceed a level that is uncomfortably loud. The audiologist is encouraged to report the level of aided audibility in each ear to the parents and the practitioner so they can monitor the audibility provided by hearing aids over time. Figure 5–5 includes two examples of children with different amounts of audibility provided by their hearing aid fittings. Verification needs to be repeated at the initial hearing aid fitting as well as at any time that there is a change in the audiogram, earmold, or hearing aid. Typically, hearing aid

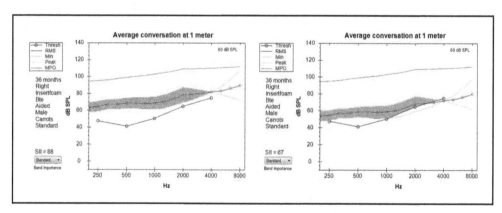

Figure 5–5. Audibility for the long-term average speech spectrum for a hearing aid fitted to optimize audibility (left panel) and fitted at less than optimal audibility (right panel). Note the lower Speech Intelligibility Index (SII) for the right panel, even though the audiogram is the same.

verification is repeated every 3 months for children under 1 year of age, every 6 months for children under 3 years of age, and annually for children over 3 years of age.

Guidance for the Practitioner

Verification measures can help the practitioner to set realistic goals and expectations for sound detection and speech recognition. For example, if probe microphone verification indicates that high-frequency (4000 Hz and above) audibility is limited, the child may not be able to discriminate between fricative speech sounds like /s/ and /sh/ without frequency lowering (see Chapter 8). Results from verification can also help the practitioner to visualize the relative amounts of amplification for soft, average, and loud speech signals to determine if the speech spectrum is audible and how much amplitude compression is present. *The practitioner may ask the child's audiologist: How audible are soft speech sounds with and without the hearing aid? Is the amount of audibility within the expected range for this child's degree of hearing loss? Does the verification suggest that the speech spectrum is receiving too much or too little amplitude compression? How audible are high-frequency sounds?*

Hearing Aid Validation

Verification ensures that the hearing aids provide audibility for speech and thus for successful listening and language development in AVT. Therefore, the child's progress needs to be docu-

mented through validation and through other formal developmental assessments. Two types of validation are commonly recommended for children: parental questionnaires and aided speech perception assessment. McCreery and colleagues (2015) have cited outcomes on parent questionnaires and aided speech recognition measures for a large group of children who use hearing aids. Both types of assessments, however, provide important information about the child's auditory development (see Chapters 4 and 9).

Parent Questionnaires

Questionnaires about the child's progress in audition and spoken communication provide valuable information about the parents' perspectives on their child's development. A large number of these are available that cover age ranges from infancy through adolescence. Most questionnaires can be completed by parents independently or by an interview. Many provide an age-equivalent score and give parents and the practitioner a perspective on the child's development of auditory skills. Questionnaires need to be appropriate for a child's developmental age, rather than chronological age, as parents may become frustrated if the questions refer to developmental milestones that the child has yet to achieve or if the child has advanced beyond skills assessed by the questionnaire. Comparing questionnaire scores with normative data for children with typical hearing and repeated administrations of parent questionnaires can provide some evidence of progress, but can only really be substantiated by standardized speech, language, and hearing assessments (see Chapter 19).

Aided Speech Perception Assessment

Unaided speech recognition assessment was discussed in Chapter 4. Similarly, aided speech recognition assessment provides valuable information about how the child uses audibility provided by hearing aids to support listening and spoken language. Awareness of speech can be assessed during infancy. Starting at the developmental age of 18 to 24 months, most children can participate in some form of generative speech recognition assessment. Some tasks, such as the Ling Six Sound Test (Ling, 1978), are used to assess a child's detection or discrimination of isolated speech sounds. The ability to recognize familiar words or sentences can also be assessed using speech materials that are appropriate. If children have limited expressive speech or language skills, speech recognition can be assessed using toys or pictures to which the child can point. Once a child has achieved high levels of word or sentence recognition in quiet, speech recognition in the presence of background noise can be tested. This approximates conditions in everyday listening situations.

Since children who wear hearing aids have a wide range of auditory skills and abilities, it can be difficult to determine whether or not they are achieving an appropriate level of aided speech recognition. Even on the few speech recognition tests with normative data for children with hearing aids, the range of performance can be variable. Poor speech recognition abilities in such children may be due to a number of factors. If a child with hearing aids has poorer speech recognition than expected, the audibility of the hearing aid can be verified to ensure the speech signal is audible. Speech recognition is dependent on language and cognitive abilities, so children with deficits in these areas may have lower speech recognition than children with hearing loss who have stronger skills in these areas. Repeated speech recognition assessment over time can provide evidence in development of auditory skills.

Aided Pure Tone Thresholds or Functional Gain

Prior to the development of probe microphone systems used for verification of audibility, audiologists would often measure a listener's audiometric thresholds through a loudspeaker to provide evidence that amplification was improving the detection of pure tones compared with their unaided thresholds. Although the approach of measuring the same pure tones used to assess unaided hearing with amplification may seem intuitive, the limitations of this approach are numerous. Pure tones used for hearing assessment are affected by signal processing in hearing aids, leading to responses that are not reflective of audibility of speech. Even if a child can detect pure tones at very soft levels in a sound booth, aided pure tone thresholds provide limited information about how well the child can understand speech in real life situations. In a study by Davidson and Skinner (2006), the range of open-set speech recognition scores for children with normal aided detection thresholds for pure tones was 0% to 68% for soft speech. Aided pure tone thresholds need to be completed only when other measures of audibility are not possible (when children use bone-conduction devices or cochlear implants). Aided speech recognition assessment has greater validity for predicting speech recognition in everyday listening situations, because the stimulus is speech.

HEARING AID USE

The principles of AVT are closely aligned to maximizing audibility, but the benefits of audibility are commensurate with the amount of time hearing aids are worn throughout the day. As previously stated, even the most optimally fit hearing aids cannot help in AVT or in life if the child does not wear them. Anyone with a toddler or preschooler knows how challenging it can be to even get the child to wear socks some days, let alone a device that goes in his or her ears and can be easily removed. The following section describes strategies for maximizing hearing aid use, and ways that parents and practitioners can track this.

How to Measure Hearing Aid Use?

The target for daily hearing aid use in infants and children is for all waking hours (with the exception of bath time and other water activities). Parents and practitioners have several tools to determine how often hearing aids are being worn throughout the day. When parents estimate the average number of hours the child wears hearing aids, it is difficult to determine what an "average" day

is. Walker et al. (2013) found that parents' self-report of consistency of their child's hearing aid use often depended on the situation; for example, infants and toddlers were less likely to wear hearing aids in unsupervised settings such as in the car or playtime in the daycare. Parents also noted that it is difficult to keep hearing aids on during activities such as nursing, in the presence of loud background noise, or when the child is tired, ill, or having a tantrum (Moeller, Hoover, Peterson, & Stelmachowicz, 2009). The amount of time a child wears his or her hearing aids is likely to highly depend on the situation. For example, if the child is in the car seat as the parents run errands, the hearing aids may not be worn because of concerns about losing them. Busy, fluctuating schedules of typical families may make it difficult to estimate daily use time, even for the most attentive parents. Therefore, we may need to use other, more objective tools for determining daily hearing aid use.

One technology available in most modern hearing aids is data logging (Gustafson, Ricketts, & Tharpe, 2017). Data logging is an automatic feature that reports on how often hearing aids are turned on (more specifically, how often the battery door is closed, and the battery is activated). Audiologists can use the data logging function by connecting hearing aids to the programming software for that particular hearing aid manufacturer. It records the average amount of time a child is wearing each hearing aid per day, based on the most recent date that the hearing aid was hooked up to the software.

Investigators have used data logging to find out how often children are wearing hearing aids. Jones and Feilner

(2013) examined a national database with anonymous data logging results from 6696 children who are deaf or hard of hearing, ranging in age from infancy to 18 years. Children wore hearing aids an average of 6.1 hours per day, based on data logging. Infants and toddlers averaged less, around 5.5 hours per day. For the whole sample of children, data logging showed that only 33% wore hearing aids more than 8 hours a day, considered a low estimate for use time during all waking hours. Walker et al. (2015a) looked at data logging results from a longitudinal sample of 290 children between the ages of 5 months and 9 years. Their findings indicated that all the children in the group were wearing hearing aids around 8.5 hours per day. Infants had an average use time of 4.5 hours per day, while preschoolers increased their usage to around 7.5 hours. Gustafson et al. (2017) followed 13 school-age children between 7 and 10 years of age. Data logging results collected over a median of 283 days indicated that children were wearing hearing aids 6 hours per day, on average. Together, this research indicates that some children are wearing hearing aids at less-than-optimal amounts, particularly at younger ages. Given the importance of early, consistent auditory exposure for later cognitive and language skills, practitioners and audiologists need to guide parents in helping their children achieve full-time use of their hearing aids (Eyes open, Ears on!).

How Does Hearing Aid Use Affect Outcomes?

It may seem sensible that children who wear hearing aids more hours will have better outcomes than children who wear them less often. Greater daily use of hearing aids provides better access to speech sounds, and subsequently more progress will happen in listening and spoken language. One of the principles of AVT concerning the recommendation of the use of amplification to obtain benefits of auditory stimulation is based on this notion. Until recently, however, there was not much evidence to support it. Tomblin and colleagues (2015) followed 317 preschool-age children with mild to severe hearing loss over a period of up to 4 years. They looked at performance on different outcome measures (articulation, vocabulary, grammar, social use of language). They were particularly interested in whether amount of hearing aid use made a difference in the outcomes of these children. In support of the principles of AVT, results from this study showed that amount of hearing aid use does matter. Average daily hearing aid use was a significant predictor of better language outcomes, regardless of the degree of hearing loss of the children. In other words, children with milder hearing loss benefited from more daily hearing aid use as well as children with moderate or severe hearing losses.

The same research group also looked at how daily hearing aid use affected growth of language skills. One expects a child who is typically developing to show steady growth in language skills over time, making 1 year of language growth over 12 months. Young children who are deaf or hard of hearing may start off with delays compared with peers with typical hearing, so they need to make even greater gains over time. Closing the gap can only be done with consistent all-day use of amplification and it is critical for success in the aca-

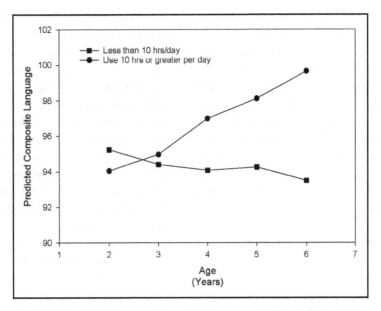

Figure 5-6. Longitudinal patterns in language growth for children who wore hearing aids more than 10 hr per week (black circles) and less than 10 hr per week (black squares). Modified from a figure in Tomblin et al. (2015).

demic setting (Tomblin et al., in press). Therefore, research results that show a steeper growth trajectory are positive findings. As Figure 5–6 shows, amount of hearing aid use influenced the language growth trajectory; children who wore hearing aids more often throughout the day displayed steeper change in language skills over time, while children who wore hearing aids less showed a flat trajectory (Tomblin et al., 2015).

More specifically, children who wore their hearing aids for less than 10 hours a day showed no change in their rate of language growth between 2 and 6 years of age (i.e., the gap between their language skills compared with average performance for same-age children with typical hearing remained the same over time). In contrast, children who wore hearing aids more than 10 hours a day made more than a year's language gains in 12 months' time, ef-

fectively closing the language gap between themselves and children with typical hearing. These results provide strong evidence for the importance of consistent amplification use for achieving maximum benefits from auditory stimulation, particularly during important periods of early brain development.

Situational Assessment of Hearing Aid Use

What can be done to improve the amount of time a child wears amplification, particularly in the case of noncompliant toddlers? Consistent with the AVT principle of *administering formal and informal assessments for the purpose of developing treatment plans, monitoring progress, and evaluating the effectiveness of them*, practitioners and audiologists encourage parents and service providers to regularly monitor hearing aid use as part of treatment plans, and they work together: to identify situations of successful hearing aid use; to encourage families to be aware of situations that pose problems; and to take proactive steps to limit challenges. In doing so, the child's entire management team can implement the principles of AVT to *create environments that support listening for the acquisition of spoken language throughout the child's daily activities.*

An informal tool to monitor situational assessment of hearing aid use can be found in articles by Moeller et al. (2009) and Walker et al. (2013). Both studies used a parent-report measure in which families rated consistency of pediatric hearing aid use in specific situations, based on a 5-point scale of always, often, sometimes, rarely, and never. The situations included (a) riding in the car, (b) daycare, (c) mealtimes, (d) playing with parents, (e) playing alone, (f) book sharing, (g) playing outside, and (h) in public (e.g., zoo, restaurant). Moeller and her colleagues completed telephone interviews using the rating scale with seven mothers of infants who were deaf or hard of hearing, starting when their children were around 10 months old. The mothers reported that certain situations were more challenging in achieving consistent hearing aid use than others, particularly riding in the car, outdoor play, and going out in public. This was primarily due to concerns about safety or losing the hearing aids. There were also situations that were easier for achieving consistent hearing aid use, including mealtimes, one-on-one playing time with parents, and especially book sharing opportunities (essentially, all times

when the mothers were able to monitor their children closely). Walker et al. (2013) used a similar questionnaire with a wider age range (6 months to 6 years). As children grew older, situations such as riding in the car became less of an issue, while child-specific factors such as degree of hearing loss were more significant. For both going out in public and school, parents of children with milder hearing losses reported less consistent hearing aid use than children with more severe hearing losses.

The take-home message from these studies is that consistency of hearing aid use differs among children, across families, and across developmental periods. The process of achieving consistent hearing aid use is multifaceted and is affected by child-specific issues, parent-child issues, situational issues, and parental adjustment issues (Moeller et al., 2009). By working with the practitioner and using a rating scale for determining consistency of use in different contexts (see Table 5–2), parents can formulate plans for creating positive listening environments and monitoring progress related to hearing aid use. Parents who make an informed choice of AVT usually *buy into* the notion of consistent hearing aid use during all waking hours from the very beginning.

Strategies for Enhancing Hearing Aid Use

Once parents have begun to identify challenging situations, there are direct and indirect strategies that can be implemented to overcome barriers and integrate hearing aid use. Given the fact that many challenging situations seem to be related to parental safety

Table 5–2. Example of Parent Rating Questionnaire for Situational Hearing Aid Use

Situation	Never (0)	Rare (1)	Sometimes (2)	Often (3)	Always (4)	N/A
1. Car						
2. PreSchool/school						
3. Daycare						
4. Mealtime						
5. Playing alone						
6. Book sharing						
7. Playground						
8. Public (store, zoo, restaurant)						

concerns, hearing aid retention devices may be a feasible option for reducing the risk of losing the hearing aids. Retention devices include bonnets, Oto or Critter Clips, toupee tape, EarGear, and Hearing Aid Headbands, to name a few options (see Figure 5–7).

Infants, toddlers, and preschoolers are persistent, however, and will likely find many innovative ways to remove their hearing aids even while wearing retention devices. For example, some young children remove the hearing aids to get attention or during tantrums. Parents need to learn to respond neutrally to behaviors such as throwing hearing aids and reinsert the hearing aids after a few minutes when the child has had time to regulate himself or herself (Moeller et al., 2009). In difficult situations such as in the car or going to the park or zoo, using a remote microphone system, such as personal FM, may address some of the challenges by improving communication related

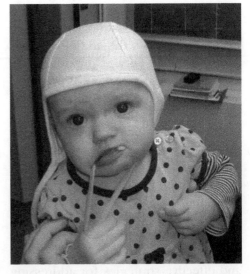

Figure 5-7. Caps and bonnets are one option for keeping hearing aids secure on infants and toddlers.

to distance and background noise between the parent and an active child (Thibodeau & Schafer, 2002) (see Chapter 7). The website Supporting Success for Children with Hearing Loss (http://

successforkidswithhearingloss.com/ hearing-aids-on) lists additional recommendations for supporting full-time hearing aid use and includes survey results that describe options preferred by parents and audiologists.

Audiologists are becoming increasingly aware that communication about data logging may also be useful in trying to increase hearing aid use (McCreery, 2013; Munoz, Preston, & Hicken, 2014). The term *data logging* may make parents feel slightly apprehensive about privacy, because it is not clear what data are being collected. Parents need to be assured that the information collected via hearing aid data logging is related to the number of hours the battery is activated, and no conversations are recorded. Data logging needs to be considered as a strategy to monitor the function of the hearing aids, in collaboration with the audiologist and AV practitioner. Service providers may also encounter defensiveness from parents when discussing data logging and addressing hearing aid use (Meibos et al., 2016). Occasionally parents' estimations of hours of daily hearing aid use do not correspond with the reported average number of hours obtained through data logging. Parents, practitioners, and audiologists can view this as an opportunity to discuss the situations that pose challenges to hearing aid use and effective strategies for addressing these challenges.

AVT purports that parents become the primary facilitators of their child's listening and spoken language development (see Chapter 1). Research shows that parents who feel more engaged in early intervention tend to have children who wear amplification more often (Desjardin, 2003, 2005). This is particularly true of mothers who are confident in their abilities to troubleshoot and maintain their child's sensory devices (hearing aids and/or cochlear implants). Desjardin proposed that this relationship is the result of personal beliefs of self-efficacy and that these beliefs lead to more persistence in the challenge of achieving consistent hearing aid use. Parents who perceive that they have the knowledge and competence to manage their child's amplification are more likely to persist with meeting specific goals related to AVT. Although this is not a direct strategy for keeping hearing aids on a child, parents who take an active role in hearing aid management, including performing daily listening checks and troubleshooting the equipment, feel more empowered (Desjardin, 2005). Families can embrace hearing aids as something that makes their child unique (see Figure 5–8). For younger children, this can include customizing their devices by choosing colorful earmolds. Older children can add removable tube decorations such as TubeRiders that can be selected to fit children's personalities and hobbies.

SPECIAL CASES: MILD BILATERAL OR UNILATERAL HEARING LOSS

Children with mild bilateral or unilateral hearing loss have significant amounts of residual hearing and often appear to be able to *get by* without hearing aids during conversation. At the same time, there are a number of studies that indicate that this population of children is at risk of experiencing difficulties in language,

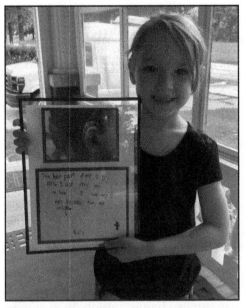 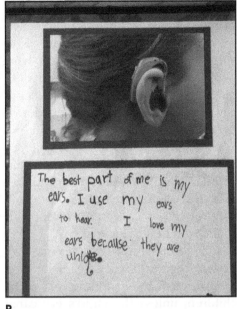

The best part of me is my ears. I use my ears to hear. I love my ears because they are unique.

A   **B**

Figure 5-8. We encourage families and children to talk to classmates about hearing aids and how they work. Children who are comfortable with talking about their hearing aids are more likely to wear them on a regular basis.

academic, and psychosocial outcomes (Bess, Dodd-Murphy, & Parker, 1998; Đoković et al., 2014; Griffin, Poissant, & Freyman, in press; Porter, Sladen, Ampah, Rothpletz, & Bess, 2013; Walker et al., in press). There is evidence that children with mild bilateral or unilateral hearing loss are less likely to wear their hearing aids on a consistent basis (Fitzpatrick, Durieux-Smith, & Whittingham, 2010; Walker et al., 2013).

The Outcomes of Children with Hearing Loss (OCHL) project is a longitudinal, multicenter study that followed a large group of children with bilateral mild to severe hearing loss. The OCHL team looked specifically at the question of hearing aid use and language outcomes in a subset of 38 children with mild hearing loss (Walker et al., 2015b). The children were divided into three groups based on the amount of daily hearing aid use. The researchers determined amount of daily hearing aid use by a combination of parent-report measures and hearing aid data logging. Group 1 consisted of children with mild hearing loss who had never worn hearing aids, Group 2 consisted of children who wore hearing aids part time (on average, 5.5 hours per day), and Group 3 consisted of children who wore hearing aids full time (on average, 11 hours per day). The full-time users had significantly higher scores on grammar and vocabulary measures, compared with children who did not wear hearing aids. Children with mild bilateral hearing loss who wore hearing aids part time had average language scores between the non-users and the full-time users. These findings are powerful examples of how consistent hearing aid use can benefit language development, even for children who have some access to speech sounds. These findings also have implications for practitioners and audiologists. Practitioners coach parents in ways that can facilitate consistent device use and help optimize listening and spoken language development in children with all degrees of hearing loss who are following AVT. Cumulative auditory experience influences outcomes of all children in AVT, even children with slight or mild hearing loss.

The behavioral audiogram may underestimate the degree of hearing loss, particularly in infants or young children, unless the child's ear canal acoustics are taken into consideration. Insert earphones often used to assess hearing in this population are acoustically calibrated using a coupler that is designed to reflect an average adult ear canal, as previously indicated. When the insert earphones are placed in the child's ear canal, the residual volume is much smaller. Just like a hearing aid programmed for an adult can have a higher output in a child's ear canal than an adult ear canal, the sound level from the insert earphone can be higher in the child's ear canal. This enhancement leads to the impression that the child's hearing thresholds are better than they really are. One recent study examined an approach to using the child's ear canal acoustics to assess unaided audibility for speech, which is simply the amount that the hearing loss negatively impacts audibility (McCreery et al., in press). When ear canal acoustics were considered, children with an unaided SII that was 80 or lower were at higher risk for language problems compared with chil-

dren with typical hearing than peers with unaided SII greater than 80. The audiologist can calculate the unaided SII based on the hearing assessment results to determine whether a child with mild hearing loss would be considered a candidate for hearing aids.

When working with children with mild hearing loss who receive hearing aids, it is critical that audiologists follow best-practice guidelines when fitting and verifying hearing aids. Earlier, the authors described the real-ear-to-coupler difference (RECD) as a tool for measuring a child's individual ear canal acoustics during hearing aid verification. As noted above, children's ear canals change rapidly in size over time, and this change affects the loudness of sounds as they are presented through the hearing aid. The size of the child's ear canal can also affect the loudness of sounds used to test hearing, but also the output of hearing aids in the ear canal. The equipment used to test hearing is calibrated on a coupler that is designed to mimic the volume of an adult ear canal. Another potential application of the RECD beyond hearing aid verification is to estimate the child's hearing thresholds, while taking into account the effect of his or her ear canal acoustics on the level of sound in the ear. In many cases, hearing loss that appears to be in the mild range for infants and young children can be more significant because the actual sound level used during the hearing test is much higher in the ear canal. When ear canal acoustics are taken into account using the RECD, the impact of the child's hearing loss and ear canal acoustics on audibility for speech can be more accurately determined. As with any degree of hearing loss, obtaining regular audiograms and individually measured RECDs ensures that the audiologist is providing adequate gain at soft and average conversational speech levels, as the child gets older and the acoustic properties of the ear canals change (Bagatto & Tharpe, 2013).

Similar to children with mild bilateral hearing loss, children with unilateral hearing loss present a unique challenge for practitioners and audiologists. Unilateral hearing loss negatively affects the ability to use information from both ears to listen, also known as binaural hearing. Even when a child has normal hearing in one ear, deficits in binaural hearing can create particular difficulties listening in background noise or identifying the location of sound sources. While some children with unilateral hearing loss will not experience noticeable difficulties during development, the current evidence does suggest that they are at risk for language and educational delays (Lieu, Tye-Murray, Karzon, & Piccirillo, 2010). Children with unilateral hearing loss are as likely as children with bilateral hearing loss to experience listening-related fatigue throughout the day (Bess et al., in press) and may also show differences in brain connectivity structures compared with children with typical hearing (Jung et al., 2017). The challenge for service providers, then, is whether to recommend hearing aids or other hearing assistance technologies and if so, what type (Bagatto, 2019).

For children with unilateral hearing loss who have usable residual hearing (i.e., in the mild to severe range), early fitting of BTE air-conduction hearing aids for the affected side can help to improve sound localization and enhance quality of life (Briggs et al., 2011; Johnstone, Náblek, & Robertson, 2010). Hearing aid fitting and verification procedures need to be consistent with the procedures described earlier in this chapter for children with bilateral hearing loss. Because the amplified sound in the affected ear may not approximate the same loudness or sound quality, adjustments may be needed to balance the inputs between ears if hearing aids are selected. More research is needed to determine whether loudness balancing between the aided and normal hearing ear is helpful for improving sound quality for children with unilateral hearing loss who use hearing aids on their affected ear (Bagatto, 2019).

Children with unilateral hearing loss in the severe to profound range (i.e., limited usable hearing) are less likely to benefit from traditional hearing aids due to their reduced dynamic range of hearing and potential crossover of amplified sound through bone conduction to the normal-hearing ear. Some families of these children may elect to pursue surgical options such as a cochlear implant or an osseointegrated bone conduction hearing aid. For children who are not surgical candidates or decide to pursue non-surgical options, current guidelines recommend remote microphone systems (in the classroom) (American Academy of Audiology, 2013). Contralateral routing of signal (CROS) hearing aids may also be recommended for children who are mature enough to orient themselves to the sound source of interest (Picou, Davis, & Tharpe, in press). Regardless of the recommended treatment approach, children with unilateral hearing loss benefit from early intervention services (Wininger, Alexander, & Diefendorf, 2016).

SPECIAL CASES: AUDITORY NEUROPATHY SPECTRUM DISORDER (ANSD), HEARING AIDS, AND AVT

ANSD is a relatively rare subtype of sensorineural hearing loss in which the auditory nerve or auditory brainstem is functioning abnormally, but the outer hair cells in the cochlea are working appropriately. For infants with ANSD, it is critical to identify this type of hearing loss as early as possible, because methods for clinical management are less straightforward than other types of sensorineural hearing loss. The reason for this lies in the measures used to determine the severity of the hearing loss in infants who cannot participate in behavioral audiometry. In children with ANSD, ABRs are absent or abnormal and may not correspond with auditory thresholds that are documented on an audiogram, making it more of a challenge to accurately determine how much residual hearing the child has.

Clinical management for ANSD is further complicated by the fact that individuals who have ANSD with similar amounts of residual hearing can have very different abilities in terms of how they understand speech. Speech recognition abilities in ANSD may be better or poorer than expected, based on their audibility levels (Rance, 2005). This feature of ANSD is different from having a sensorineural hearing loss, in which level of audibility corresponds with the ability to understand speech (in other words, people with better audibility with sensorineural hearing loss tend to have higher speech recognition scores; people with poorer audibility tend to have lower speech recognition scores). In addition, understanding speech in noise is particularly difficult for people with ANSD, even more so than for people with sensorineural or conductive hearing losses (Kraus et al., 2000; Rance & Barker, 2008). It is not entirely clear why speech recognition skills vary so much in individuals with ANSD. Researchers suspect that it may be related to the degree to which ANSD affects the ability of the auditory system to process timing differences in speech (Rance, McKay, & Grayden, 2004). Currently, an important area of research involves developing appropriate evidence-based clinical interventions for this population, given the challenges in diagnosing and providing clinical management with ANSD (Roush, Frymark, Venediktov, & Wang, 2011).

Children with ANSD may be candidates for three different types of hearing technology: cochlear implants, hearing aids, or remote microphone technology. Even if children with ANSD eventually receive a cochlear implant, the American Academy of Audiology (AAA) recommends that they receive hearing aids as soon as it is determined that their hearing loss limits their ability to understand speech. In general, children with ANSD who have thresholds in the severe-to-profound range show only minimal benefit from hearing aids, and therefore are candidates for cochlear implants (Rance, Cone-Wesson, Wunderlich, & Dowell, 2002). Evidence for appropriate intervention for children with significant residual hearing is mixed. Some children with ANSD may have the potential to benefit greatly from the audibility provided by hearing aids (Ching et al., 2013; Rance, Barker, Sarant, & Ching, 2007). At the same time, some children with ANSD who have residual hearing have difficulty understanding speech, even when wearing hearing aids (Rance et al., 2002). The practitioner has an important role in carefully monitoring children with ANSD, to establish if they are receiving benefit from hearing aids, if cochlear implantation is warranted, and if a suitable trajectory of listening, spoken language acquisition, and cognition is being achieved.

Earlier, we described how audiologists may use electrophysiological measures of hearing to determine how much amplification needs to be provided via hearing aids. Unfortunately, electrophysiological measures such as ABR cannot provide valid estimates of behavioral thresholds for children with ANSD, in contrast to children with sensorineural hearing loss. The AAA Pediatric Amplification guidelines suggest that hearing aids may initially be fit based on careful behavioral observations to sound, by the clinician and/or the parent until a reliable behavioral audiogram can be obtained. Because of the difficulty in obtaining reliable behavioral audiometry, children with ANSD who wear hearing aids may need to see their audiologist a minimum of every 3 months until the child is 6 years old.

Once the audiologist is able to obtain behavioral responses to sound, the child needs to be fitted with behind-the-ear hearing aids using prescriptive targets that optimize the audibility of speech (Bagatto et al., 2005). As for children with sensorineural hearing loss, the output of the hearing aids needs to be verified using probe microphone measures, at soft, average, and loud conversational levels of speech. These measures may be obtained in the child's ear canal or via simulated measurements of the hearing aid output in a coupler with a real-ear-to-coupler-difference measure (AAA, 2013; Bagatto, Scollie, Hyde, & Seewald, 2010; King, 2010).

Since ANSD was first identified in children and adults who are deaf or hard of hearing, researchers and practitioners have debated about the best approach for providing hearing aids to children with ANSD. Some have argued for a conservative approach—providing low-gain hearing aids, similar to how a hearing aid would be fit for someone with mild hearing loss. There is no empirical evidence, however, to support this conservative approach for children who have ANSD with mild-severe behavioral thresholds. Using this approach could limit the ability to acquire listening and spoken language, because it underamplifies sounds and reduces the child's access to the speech spectrum and sounds of the environment. The major differences in hearing aid fitting and verification for children with ANSD, compared with children with sensorineural hearing loss, are that audiologists cannot use ABR results to help estimate auditory thresholds and fitting amplification, and this population needs to be monitored more closely, both before and after the hearing aid fitting. This close monitoring allows the audiologist to determine that behavioral thresholds are stable and that progress is appropriate.

One of the hallmark features of ANSD is poor performance in background noise (Rance, 2005; Starr et al., 1998). Therefore, another important recommendation for this population is the use of remote microphone systems to improve the ability to listen in noise (Kraus et al., 2000; Rance, 2005). This is particularly important for children with ANSD who have significant residual hearing. Just like children with typical hearing and children with sensorineural hearing loss, children with ANSD are expected to learn academic material while listening in noisy and reverberant acoustic conditions in regular classrooms (Crandell & Smaldino, 2000). Remote microphone technology will help with understanding speech in these adverse listening conditions.

Guidance for the Practitioner

Practitioners need to be aware that children with ANSD may or may not demonstrate improvements in speech understanding once they have been fit with hearing aids. Questionnaires such as the LittlEARS (Coninx et al., 2009) and the Parents' Evaluation of Aural/Oral Performance of Children (PEACH; Ching & Hill, 2007) may help in counseling, in that they will provide information about functional auditory skills and developmental progress. *The practitioner may ask the child's audiologist*: Is the child showing any improvement with or without the hearing aids using speech perception measures? What type of remote microphone technology should be used in combination with the hearing aids?

CONCLUSION

This chapter provided an overview of the importance of hearing aids in children with hearing loss whose families have chosen to follow AVT. Hearing aids are an essential component to providing auditory access for listening and the development of spoken language. Hearing aids maximize residual hearing and make speech and other environmental sounds audible to give each child the greatest opportunity to develop the skills needed for listening, spoken language, and cognitive development. A wide range of advanced signal processing features in hearing aids can benefit children and increase auditory access, if appropriately prescribed. Consistent audibility and use of hearing aids provide children with the essential opportunities to learn to listen and talk as their parents chart a course toward the expected outcomes in AVT.

REFERENCES

Akhtar, N. (2005). The robustness of learning through overhearing. *Developmental Science, 8*(2), 199–209.

American Academy of Audiology. (2013). *Clinical practice guidelines: Pediatric amplification*. Reston, VA.

American National Standards Institute. (1997). *American national standard: Methods for calculation of the speech intelligibility index*. Melville, NY: Acoustical Society of America.

Bagatto, M. (2019). Audiological considerations for managing mild bilateral or unilateral hearing loss in infants and young children. *Language, Speech, and Hearing Services in Schools*.

Bagatto, M., Moodie, S., Scollie, S., Seewald, R., Moodie, S., Pumford, J., & Liu, K. R. (2005). Clinical protocols for hearing instrument fitting in the Desired Sensation Level method. *Trends in Amplification, 9*(4), 199–226.

Bagatto, M., Scollie, S. D., Hyde, M., & Seewald, R. (2010). Protocol for the provision of amplification within the Ontario infant hearing program. *International Journal of Audiology, 49*(suppl. 1), S70–S79.

Bagatto, M. P., & Tharpe, A. M. (2013). Decision support guide for hearing aid use in infants and children with minimal/mild bilateral hearing loss. *Proceedings from a Sound Foundation in Amplification.* Stafa, Switzerland: Phonak, AG.

Bess, F., Davis, H., Camarata, S., & Hornsby, B. (In press). Listening-related fatigue in children with unilateral hearing loss. *Language, Speech, and Hearing Services in Schools.*

Bess, F. H., Dodd-Murphy, J., & Parker, R. A. (1998). Children with minimal sensorineural hearing loss: Prevalence, educational performance, and functional status. *Ear and Hearing, 19*(5), 339–354.

Briggs, L., Davidson, L., & Lieu, J. E. (2011). Outcomes of conventional amplification for pediatric unilateral hearing loss. *Annals of Otology, Rhinology & Laryngology, 120*(7), 448–454.

Ching, T. Y., Day, J., Dillon, H., Gardner-Berry, K., Hou, S., Seeto, M., . . . Zhang, V. (2013). Impact of the presence of auditory neuropathy spectrum disorder (ANSD) on outcomes of children at three years of age. *International Journal of Audiology, 52*(S2), S55–S64.

Ching, T. Y., & Hill, M. (2007). The parents' evaluation of aural/oral performance of children (PEACH) scale: Normative data. *Journal of the American Academy of Audiology, 18*(3), 220–235.

Ching, T. Y., O'Brien, A., Dillon, H., Chalupper, J., Hartley, L., Hartley, D., . . . Hain, J. (2009). Directional effects on infants and young children in real life: Implications for amplification. *Journal of Speech, Language, and Hearing Research, 52*(5), 1241–1254.

Coninx, F., Weichbold, V., Tsiakpini, L., Autrique, E., Bescond, G., Tamas, L., . . . Le Maner-Idrissi, G. (2009). Validation of the LittlEARS® auditory questionnaire in children with normal hearing. *International Journal of Pediatric Otorhinolaryngology, 73*(12), 1761–1768.

Crandell, C. C., & Smaldino, J. J. (2000). Classroom acoustics for children with normal hearing and with hearing impairment. *Language, Speech, and Hearing Services in Schools, 31*(4), 362–370.

Davidson, L. S., & Skinner, M. W. (2006). Audibility and speech perception of children using wide dynamic range compression hearing aids. *American Journal of Audiology, 15*, 141–153.

Desjardin, J. L. (2003). Assessing parental perceptions of self-efficacy and involvement in families of young children with hearing loss. *Volta Review, 103*(4), 391–409.

Desjardin, J. L. (2005). Maternal perceptions of self-efficacy and involvement in the auditory development of young children with prelingual deafness. *Journal of Early Intervention, 27*(3), 193–209.

Đoković, S., Gligorović, M., Ostojić, S., Dimić, N., Radić-Šestić, M., & Slavnić, S. (2014). Can mild bilateral sensorineural hearing loss affect developmental abilities in younger school-age children? *Journal of Deaf Studies and Deaf Education, 19*, 484–495.

Fitzpatrick, E. M., Durieux-Smith, A., & Whittingham, J. (2010). Clinical practice for children with mild bilateral and unilateral hearing loss. *Ear and Hearing, 31*(3), 392–400.

Glista, D., Scollie, S., Bagatto, M., Seewald, R., Parsa, V., & Johnson, A. (2009). Evaluation of nonlinear frequency compression: Clinical outcomes. *International Journal of Audiology, 48*(9), 632–644.

Griffin, A., Poissant, S., & Freyman, R. (In press). Auditory comprehension in school-aged children with normal hearing and with unilateral hearing loss. *Language, Speech, and Hearing Services in Schools.*

Gustafson, S. J., Ricketts, T. A., & Tharpe, A. M. (2017). Hearing technology use and management in school-age children: Reports from data logs, parents, and teachers. *Journal of the American Academy of Audiology, 28*(10), 883–892.

Holte, L., Walker, E., Oleson, J., Spratford, M., Moeller, M. P., Roush, P., . . . Tomblin, J. B. (2012). Factors influencing follow-up to newborn hearing screening for infants who are hard of hearing. *American Journal of Audiology, 21*(2), 163–174.

Johnstone, P. M., Náblek, A. K., & Robertson, V. S. (2010). Sound localization acuity in children with unilateral hearing loss who wear a hearing aid in the impaired ear. *Journal of the American Academy of Audiology, 21*(8), 522–534.

Jones, C., & Feilner, M. (2013). What do we know about the fitting and daily life usage of hearing instruments in pediatrics? In *A sound foundation through early amplification: Proceedings of the 2013 international conference* (pp. 97–103). Chicago, IL: Phonak AG.

Jung, M. E., Colletta, M., Coalson, R., Schlaggar, B. L., & Lieu, J. E. (2017). Differences in interregional brain connectivity in children with unilateral hearing loss. *The Laryngoscope, 127*(11), 2636–2645.

Kimlinger, C., McCreery, R., & Lewis, D. (2015). High-frequency audibility: The effects of audiometric configuration, stimulus type, and device. *Journal of the American Academy of Audiology, 26*(2), 128–137.

King, A. M. (2010). The national protocol for paediatric amplification in Australia. *International Journal of Audiology, 49*(suppl. 1), S64–S69.

Koehlinger, K., Van Horne, A. O., Oleson, J., McCreery, R., & Moeller, M. P. (2015). The role of sentence position, allomorph, and morpheme type on accurate use of s-related morphemes by children who are hard of hearing. *Journal of Speech, Language, and Hearing Research, 58*(2), 396–409.

Kraus, N., Bradlow, A., Cheatham, M., Cunningham, J., King, C., Koch, D., . . . Wright, B. (2000). Consequences of neural asynchrony: A case of auditory neuropathy. *Journal of the Association for Research in Otolaryngology, 1*(1), 33–45.

Kuhl, P. K., Conboy, B. T., Padden, D., Nelson, T., & Pruitt, J. (2005). Early speech perception and later language development: Implications for the "critical period." *Language Learning and Development, 1*(3–4), 237–264.

Lieu, J. E., Tye-Murray, N., Karzon, R. K., & Piccirillo, J. F. (2010). Unilateral hearing loss is associated with worse speech-language scores in children. *Pediatrics, 125*(6), e1348–e1355.

Ling, D. (1978). Speech development in hearing-impaired children. *Journal of Communication Disorders, 11*(2), 119–124.

McCreery, R. (2013). Data logging and hearing aid use: Focus on the forest, not the trees. *Hearing Journal, 66*(12), 18–19.

McCreery, R. W., Alexander, J., Brennan, M. A., Hoover, B., Kopun, J., & Stelmachowicz, P. G. (2014). The influence of audibility on speech recognition with nonlinear frequency compression for children and adults with hearing loss. *Ear and Hearing, 35*(4), 440–447.

McCreery, R. W., Venediktov, R. A., Coleman, J. J., & Leech, H. M. (2012a). An evidence-based systematic review of amplitude compression in hearing aids for school-age children with hearing loss. *American Journal of Audiology, 21*(2), 269–294.

McCreery, R. W., Venediktov, R. A., Coleman, J. J., & Leech, H. M. (2012b). An evidence-based systematic review of directional microphones and digital noise reduction hearing aids in school-age children with hearing loss. *American Journal of Audiology, 21*(2), 295–312.

McCreery, R. W., Venediktov, R. A., Coleman, J. J., & Leech, H. M. (2012c). An evidence-based systematic review of frequency lowering in hearing aids for school-age children with hearing loss. *American Journal of Audiology, 21*(2), 313–328.

McCreery, R. W., Walker, E. A., Spratford, M., Oleson, J., Bentler, R., Holte, L., & Roush, P.

(2015). Speech recognition and parent ratings from auditory development questionnaires in children who are hard of hearing. *Ear and Hearing, 36*, 60S–75S.

McCreery, R. W., Walker, E. A., Stiles, D., Spratford, M., Oleson, J., & Lewis, D. (In press). Audibility-based hearing aid fitting criteria for children with mild bilateral hearing loss. *Language, Speech, and Hearing Services in Schools.*

Meibos, A., Munoz, K., White, K., Preston, E., Pitt, C., & Twohig, M. (2016). Audiologist practices: Parent hearing aid education and support. *Journal of the American Academy of Audiology, 27*(4), 324–332.

Moeller, M. P. (2000). Early intervention and language development in children who are deaf and hard of hearing. *Pediatrics, 106*(3), e43.

Moeller, M. P., Hoover, B., Peterson, B., & Stelmachowicz, P. (2009). Consistency of hearing aid use in infants with early-identified hearing loss. *American Journal of Audiology, 18*(1), 14–23.

Moeller, M. P., Hoover, B., Putman, C., Arbataitis, K., Bohnenkamp, G., Peterson, B., . . . & Stelmachowicz, P. (2007). Vocalizations of infants with hearing loss compared with infants with normal hearing: Part I—phonetic development. *Ear and Hearing, 28*(5), 605–627.

Mueller, H. G. (2007). Data logging: It's popular, but how can this feature be used to help patients? *Hearing Journal, 60*(10), 19–26.

Munoz, K., Preston, E., & Hicken, S. (2014). Pediatric hearing aid use: How can audiologists support parents to increase consistency? *Journal of the American Academy of Audiology, 25*(4), 380–387.

Picou, E., Davis, H., & Tharpe, A. M. (In press). Considerations for choosing microphone technologies for students with limited useable hearing unilaterally. *Language, Speech, and Hearing Services in Schools.*

Pisoni, D. B. (2000). Cognitive factors and cochlear implants: Some thoughts on perception, learning, and memory in speech perception. *Ear and Hearing, 21*(1), 70–78.

Porter, H., Sladen, D. P., Ampah, S. B., Rothpletz, A., & Bess, F. H. (2013). Developmental outcomes in early school-age children with minimal hearing loss. *American Journal of Audiology, 22*(2), 263–270.

Rance, G. (2005). Auditory neuropathy/dys-synchrony and its perceptual consequences. *Trends in Amplification, 9*(1), 1–43.

Rance, G., & Barker, E. J. (2008). Speech perception in children with auditory neuropathy/dyssynchrony managed with either hearing aids or cochlear implants. *Otology and Neurotology, 29*(2), 179–182.

Rance, G., Barker, E. J., Sarant, J. Z., & Ching, T. Y. (2007). Receptive language and speech production in children with auditory neuropathy/dyssynchrony type hearing loss. *Ear and Hearing, 28*(5), 694–702.

Rance, G., Cone-Wesson, B., Wunderlich, J., & Dowell, R. (2002). Speech perception and cortical event related potentials in children with auditory neuropathy. *Ear and Hearing, 23*(3), 239–253.

Rance, G., McKay, C., & Grayden, D. (2004). Perceptual characterization of children with auditory neuropathy. *Ear and Hearing, 25*(1), 34–46.

Roush, P., Frymark, T., Venediktov, R., & Wang, B. (2011). Audiologic management of auditory neuropathy spectrum disorder in children: A systematic review of the literature. *American Journal of Audiology, 20*(2), 159–170.

Sharma, A., Dorman, M. F., & Kral, A. (2005). The influence of a sensitive period on central auditory development in children with unilateral and bilateral cochlear implants. *Hearing Research, 203*(1), 134–143.

Sharma, A., Dorman, M. F., & Spahr, A. J. (2002). A sensitive period for the development of the central auditory system in children with cochlear implants: Implications for age of implantation. *Ear and Hearing, 23*(6), 532–539.

Starr, A., Sininger, Y., Winter, M., Derebery, M., Oba, S., & Michalewski, H. (1998). Transient deafness due to temperature-sensitive auditory neuropathy. *Ear and Hearing, 19*(3), 169–179.

Stelmachowicz, P., Lewis, D., Hoover, B., Nishi, K., McCreery, R., & Woods, W. (2010). Effects of digital noise reduction on speech perception for children with hearing loss. *Ear and Hearing, 31*(3), 345.

Thibodeau, L. M., & Schafer, E. (2002). Issues to consider regarding use of FM systems with infants with hearing loss. *SIG 9 Perspectives on Hearing and Hearing Disorders in Childhood, 12*(1), 18–21.

Tomblin, J. B., Harrison, M., Ambrose, S. E., Walker, E. A., & Moeller, M. P. (2015). Language outcomes in young children with mild to severe hearing loss. *Ear and Hearing, 36,* 76S–91S.

Tomblin, J. B., Oleson, J., Ambrose, S. E., Walker, E. A., McCreery, R. W., & Moeller, M. P. (in press). Aided hearing moderates the academic outcomes of children with mild to severe hearing loss. *Ear and Hearing.*

Tsao, F.-M., Liu, H.-M., & Kuhl, P. K. (2004). Speech perception in infancy predicts language development in the second year of life: A longitudinal study. *Child Development*, 1067–1084.

Walker, E. A., Holte, L., McCreery, R. W., Spratford, M., Page, T., & Moeller, M. P. (2015b). The effects of hearing aid use on outcomes of children with mild hearing loss. *Journal of Speech, Language, and Hearing Research, 58,* 1611–1625.

Walker, E. A., Holte, L., Spratford, M., Oleson, J., Welhaven, A., & Harrison, M. (2014). Timeliness of service delivery for children with later-identified mild-to-severe hearing loss. *American Journal of Audiology, 23*(1), 116–128.

Walker, E. A., McCreery, R. W., Spratford, M., Oleson, J. J., Van Buren, J., Bentler, R. A., Roush, P., & Moeller, M. P. (2015a). Trends and predictors of longitudinal hearing aid use for children who are hard of hearing. *Ear and Hearing, 36,* 38S–47S.

Walker, E. A., Sapp, C., Dallapiazza, M., Spratford, M., & McCreery, R. W. (In press). Language and reading outcomes in fourth-grade children with mild hearing loss compared to age-matched hearing peers. *Language, Speech, and Hearing Services in Schools.*

Walker, E. A., Spratford, M., Moeller, M. P., Oleson, J., Ou, H., Roush, P., & Jacobs, S. (2013). Predictors of hearing aid use time in children with mild-to-severe hearing loss. *Language, Speech, and Hearing Services in Schools, 44*(1), 73–88.

Winiger, A. M., Alexander, J. M., & Diefendorf, A. O. (2016). Minimal hearing loss: From a failure-based approach to evidence-based practice. *American Journal of Audiology, 25*(3), 232–245.

Wolfe, J., John, A., Schafer, E., Nyffeler, M., Boretzki, M., Caraway, T., & Hudson, M. (2011). Long-term effects of non-linear frequency compression for children with moderate hearing loss. *International Journal of Audiology, 50*(6), 396–404.

6

IMPLANTABLE HEARING TECHNOLOGIES AND AUDITORY-VERBAL THERAPY

Sara Neumann and Jace Wolfe

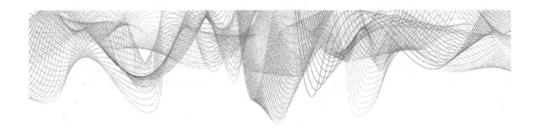

INTRODUCTION

Implantable hearing technologies include a wide range of cochlear implants, auditory brainstem implants, bone conduction, and middle ear devices. The availability of modern implantable hearing technologies has created opportunities for children with all degrees, types, and configurations of hearing loss to develop age-appropriate listening and spoken language abilities that are commensurate with those of their peers with typical hearing. The majority of this chapter focuses on cochlear implants (CIs) and bone conduction hearing devices, the implantable hearing technologies most commonly used by children with severe to profound hearing loss as well as the implications of such technologies for Auditory-Verbal Therapy (AVT).

COCHLEAR IMPLANTS

Cochlear implants are the most successful sensory prosthetic devices in medicine. Cochlear implants deliver electrical stimulation to the cochlear nerve in an effort to restore access to a wide range of acoustic input levels throughout the speech frequency range. Cochlear implant systems comprise two main components, an external sound processor and the cochlear implant (see Figure 6–1). The external sound processor contains microphones that capture sound and deliver it to a digital signal processor for analysis and processing. The digital signal processor determines how much electrical stimulation the CI recipient should receive in response to the given input acoustic signal. The digitally processed signal is converted to an electrical signal and delivered from the processor to an external transmitting coil that converts the electrical current into an electromagnetic signal. The electromagnetic signal is delivered from the external transmitting coil across the skin to the internal receiving coil of the CI by way of electromagnetic induction (i.e., nearfield magnetic induction/radio frequency transmission). The internal coil converts the electromagnetic signal to an electrical current that is delivered to the digital signal processor within

the CI. After processing, current generators deliver electrical pulses to electrode leads, which then deliver the electrical pulses to intracochlear electrode contacts. Of note, high-frequency information is delivered to intracochlear electrode contacts located at the base of the cochlea, whereas low-frequency information is delivered to intracochlear electrode contacts located at the apical end of the cochlea. The electrical pulses are then delivered from the intracochlear electrode contacts to the cochlear nerve to elicit an auditory response.

Cochlear implantation is generally considered to be the standard of care for children and adults with severe to profound sensory hearing loss. Many children with auditory neuropathy spectrum disorder (ANSD) also receive substantial benefit from cochlear implantation. Research has shown that most children who receive CIs prior to 12 months achieve age-appropriate listening and spoken language outcomes (Ching, Dillon, Leigh, & Cupples, 2018; Dettman et al.,

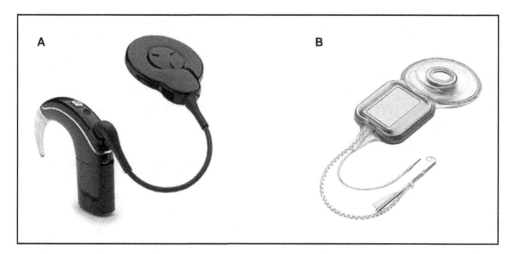

Figure 6-1. An example of a cochlear implant external sound processor (**A**) and a cochlear implant (**B**). Courtesy of Cochlear Americas.

2016; Hoff et al., 2019; Leigh, Dettman, & Dowell, 2016).

Assessment of Cochlear Implant Candidacy for Children

The decision to pursue cochlear implantation for a child should be based on two questions. First, will the provision of a CI (or CIs) most likely improve a child's quality of life? Second, will the provision of a CI (or CIs) most likely optimize a child's listening and spoken language abilities? If the answer to one or both of those questions is yes, then cochlear implantation should be considered. These two questions should be answered by an interdisciplinary team of hearing health care practitioners who are experienced in providing care for children who are deaf or hard of hearing.

Regulatory bodies, such as the United States Food and Drug Administration (FDA), approve indications for use of CIs in children and adults (also known as guidelines for cochlear implantation). Pediatric CI guidelines vary by manufacturer and global region. Indications for use of CIs in children vary by age of implantation, degree of hearing loss, aided auditory performance, etc. For example, indications for use in some countries state that children should be at least 12 months old, whereas other countries have approved cochlear implantation for children under 1 year of age.

In general, current indications for use suggest that infants with severe to profound sensorineural hearing loss should be considered for cochlear implantation when the child receives limited to no benefit from appropriately fitted hearing aids. A discussion of the selection, fitting, verification, and validation of hearing aids for children is beyond the scope of this chapter. The reader is referred to Chapter 5 for additional information on matters pertaining to hearing aids for children. Infants and toddlers typically are unable to complete aided speech recognition assessment. As a result, the decision to recommend cochlear implantation for infants and young children is typically based on the child's degree of hearing loss, functional auditory performance, and spoken language development.

Cochlear Implant Candidacy and Degree of Hearing Loss

In recognition of the fact that degree of hearing loss is a central factor determining CI candidacy in infants and young children, Leigh and colleagues (2016) sought to identify an audiometric criterion that identifies children who are likely to understand speech better with a cochlear implant relative to use of a hearing aid. Leigh et al. reported that almost 75% of children with CIs achieved word recognition that was as good or better than the average score of children who used hearing aids and had a 60 dB HL pure tone average. Of note, 95% of children with CIs in the Leigh et al. study scored as well or better than children who used hearing aids and had a pure tone average of 80 dB HL. Similarly, Ching and colleagues (2013) reported that spoken language outcomes of children with CIs were as good as the outcomes of children who used hearing aids and had a four-frequency pure tone average (500, 1000, 2000, and 4000 Hz) of 66 dB HL. In short, recent research suggests that many children with severe to profound hearing loss will achieve better speech recognition with a CI relative to use of hearing aids (Ching et al., 2013; Leigh et al., 2016).

Cochlear Implant Candidacy and Aided Speech Recognition Assessment

Aided speech recognition should also be measured from children who are old enough to participate in speech recognition assessment. A comprehensive discussion of speech recognition assessment of children who are deaf or hard of hearing exceeds the boundaries of this chapter. However, the interested reader should review the Pediatric Minimum Speech Test Battery (PMSTB) for information pertaining to the assessment of speech recognition abilities of pediatric CI candidates and recipients (Uhler & Gifford, 2014; Uhler, Warner-Czyz, Gifford, & Working Group, 2017). The PMSTB provides a recommendation for a number of different tests and tools that may be used to evaluate children's speech recognition across the age range (e.g., visual reinforcement infant speech discrimination, Lexical Neighborhood Test, Consonant-Nucleus-Consonant monosyllabic word recognition test, Baby Bio sentence recognition test). Additionally, the PMSTB provides a recommendation for how the clinician should select the test that is most appropriate for evaluating the speech recognition of a given child. Moreover, the PMSTB recommends the use of several testing parameters, including recorded materials rather than monitored live voice, assessment of speech recognition in quiet at 50 and 60 dBA, assessment of speech recognition in noise at a +5 dB signal-to-noise ratio (SNR), etc. Of note, aided speech recognition assessment should ideally be completed in at least three conditions: the right ear, left ear, and binaurally aided conditions.

The US FDA guidelines for cochlear implantation in children also include aided speech recognition criteria. For instance, the FDA-approved indications for use of the Cochlear Ltd. cochlear implant suggest an aided word recognition score of no greater than 30% correct. The Leigh et al. (2016) study found that 75% of children who received a CI prior to 3 years of age scored over 40% correct on word recognition assessment with use of a CI. Moreover, Dettman et al. (2016) reported a mean word recognition score of 84% correct for school-age children who received their CIs prior to 12 months of age. When the results of the Leigh et al. and Dettman et al. studies are viewed collectively, it is fair to suggest that current US FDA guidelines for cochlear implantation for children are too conservative. Indeed, Carlson and colleagues (2015) reported on CI outcomes for a group of 51 children who underwent off-label cochlear implantation (e.g., users who receive a CI even though they did not meet the criteria specified in the manufacturer's indications for use). A mean improvement of 63 percentage points was found for speech recognition of the implanted ear and of 40 percentage points in the bimodal condition. Furthermore, all 51 subjects experienced significant improvement in speech recognition after cochlear implantation and there was significant improvement in speech and language development. FDA indications for CI in children are made infrequently, and as a result, the indications of use do not always match the evidence-based, best practice standard of care.

Cochlear Implant Candidacy and Assessment of Functional Auditory Performance

Determination of pediatric CI candidacy should also include an assessment of the child's functional auditory performance and spoken language development that is provided by the AV practitioner and the child's parents. Bagatto (2012) has suggested a protocol for evaluating the functional auditory development of children using hearing technology. These measures may be administered by asking the family to complete norm-referenced, standardized questionnaires that are designed to evaluate auditory and spoken language development and performance in the child's day-to-day life. Specifically, Bagatto recommended the use of the LittlEARS questionnaire (Tsiakpini et al., 2004) for children birth to 24 months of age. Once the child reaches 24 months of age or attains a score of at least 27 (out of a total of 35) on the LittlEARS questionnaire, Bagatto recommends use of the Parents' Evaluation of Aural/Oral Performance of Children (PEACH) (Ching & Hill, 2005) to evaluate the functional auditory development of children who are deaf or hard of hearing. Based on the normative data available for the LittlEARS and PEACH questionnaires, Bagatto recommended the use of scoring sheets to plot the child's score relative to the normative range for a child of the same age with typical hearing abilities. Plotting the score in this manner allows the child's practitioners and family to simply determine whether

the child is making satisfactory progress relative to her/his peers with typical hearing abilities. The Auditory Skills Checklist (Meinzen-Darr, Wiley, Creighton, & Choo, 2007) is an additional criterion-referenced evaluation tool that follows Erber's Auditory Hierarchy and can be administered in interview format or by having the practitioner complete it prior to the audiology appointment so the audiologist can see the child's progress or lack thereof with his/her auditory skills development. Cochlear implantation may be considered when a child who has severe to profound hearing loss and appropriately fitted hearing aids demonstrates a delay in functional auditory performance. The reader is referred to the work of Bagatto and colleagues (2011) for more information on the use of standardized, norm-referenced questionnaires to evaluate auditory skill development in children who are deaf or hard of hearing.

Cochlear Implant Candidacy and Assessment of Spoken Language Development

An audiologist cannot be certain of the efficacy of her/his services for a child who is deaf or hard of hearing without knowledge of that child's listening and spoken language development. A child's listening and spoken language aptitude is another key determinant of CI candidacy. If a child is making insufficient progress with optimally selected and fitted hearing aids, then the child's hearing health care team should consider whether a CI would allow the child to make better progress in the development of her/his spoken language skills. Ideally, the listening and spoken language development of children who are deaf or hard of hearing should be on par with their peers with typical hearing. Additionally, in one calendar year, children who are deaf or hard of hearing should make one year of progress in their language development as evaluated via standardized speech and language measures. At the very least, a child's standard scores attained on standardized listening and spoken language measures should be commensurate with their nonverbal IQ.

In summary, the decision to move forward with cochlear implantation for a child should be made by a team of professionals who are experienced in the evaluation of auditory, speech, and language development of children who are deaf or hard of hearing. A CI needs to be considered for a child when it is likely that implantation will improve the child's quality of life and the child's auditory, speech, and language abilities. The CI team should consider a cochlear implant for young children with severe to profound hearing loss when standard, norm-referenced measures (e.g., LittlEARS, PEACH) indicate that the child is not making satisfactory progress. Additionally, cochlear implantation can be considered when the practitioner reports speech and language progress that does not meet age-appropriate norms or when the child does not achieve one year of development in speech and language over the time of one year. Finally, limited speech understanding on a linguistically appropriate measure of speech recognition is an indicator for cochlear implantation. Ideally, children should score at least 80% correct in the best aided condition. Otherwise, they will be inclined to experience considerable difficulty in real-world situations. Certainly, cochlear implantation should be strongly considered for children who cannot achieve this criterion with the use of well-fitted current hearing aid technology.

Factors that Complicate the Cochlear Implant Candidacy Process

A number of factors can complicate the decision to move forward with cochlear implantation. First, 35% to 40% of children who are deaf or hard of hearing have additional disabilities, many of which affect cognitive/neurological status (Ching et al., 2018; Gallaudet Research Institute, 2008). Cognitive challenges obviously present the potential to delay speech and language progress. In the case of children who have cognitive disabilities and profound hearing loss, cochlear implantation will likely optimize the child's potential to communicate by using spoken language, particularly when provided at an early age (e.g., less than 12 months old) (Ching et al., 2018; Cupples et al., 2018). Once again, the CI team relies on the practitioner and a multidisciplinary team of professionals to evaluate the needs of a child who has hearing loss and additional disabilities in order to holistically consider the needs of the child and identify the optimal interventions to meet those needs.

Children may also make poor progress with hearing aids when they do not receive optimal support at home (Tomblin et al., 2015). It is critical for hearing health care practitioners, including AV practitioners, to provide all families with the necessary supports required to optimize each child's individual potential to listen and talk. The pediatric hearing health care team should include a social worker who can assist the family in locating the resources required for the needs of the child.

Audiologic Management of Children with Cochlear Implants

To optimize the outcome a child achieves with her/his CIs, clinicians must set the stage for success. Prior to activation of the CI, the audiologist and AV practitioner must establish the importance of full-time use of the cochlear implants. Use of the adage "eyes open, ears on" is a great way to succinctly remind families that when the child's is awake, she/he should be using her/his CIs. In order to optimize auditory brain development and listening and spoken language, a child with hearing loss must have consistent audibility of speech throughout her/his day. The only way to provide consistent audibility is through consistent use of the cochlear implants.

Prior to activation of the CI, the practitioners also inform the family of what they should expect in the early stages following cochlear implantation. Infants and young children typically exhibit three types of responses during the initial activation of their cochlear implant. Some children show clear responses to sound and are happy with the new auditory signal provided from the CI. Other children may become upset when they first respond to their CI because it is the first time they have received auditory stimulation. However, it should be noted that stimulation from the CI should not be uncomfortable if the audiologist programs the implant and introduces auditory stimulation appro-

priately. Finally, some children produce little to no overt response to the initial stimulation even though certain measures, such as the electrically evoked compound action potential (e.g., neural response telemetry [NRT]) or the electrically evoked stapedial reflex threshold, indicate that the CI is providing audibility across the speech frequency range. It is important for the family to be prepared for each of these different types of reactions, so they are prepared to respond and support their child accordingly.

Cochlear Implant Activation

Physical and Audiologic Examination

The audiologist must select the appropriate magnet strength for the child's transmitting coil so that it is strong enough to allow for consistent adherence of the coil to the head but not so strong that it compromises blood flow to the implant site and/or causes discomfort. The implant site should be monitored at each implant checkup to ensure satisfactory health of the soft tissue at the implant site. Ideally, the practitioner should also routinely inspect the child's implant site and refer the child to the audiologist if there are any signs of inflammation, irritation, or swelling. The audiologist should also complete otoscopy and tympanometry to evaluate the status of the external and middle ears.

For children who have a considerable amount of acoustic hearing prior to implantation (70 dB HL or better), it is prudent to complete an audiometric assessment prior to CI activation to determine whether it may be preferable to provide acoustic stimulation in the low-frequency range rather than electrical stimulation. Low-frequency acoustic stimulation needs to be considered for all frequencies (125 to 1000 Hz) at which the air conduction threshold is 75 dB HL or better.

Cochlear Implant Programming

CI programming, which is also often referred to as cochlear implant mapping, is a term that describes the process in which an audiologist selects and determines the electrical stimulation parameters that seek to optimize the cochlear implant recipient's hearing performance and listening experience. An almost limitless combination of parameters may be adjusted in the CI programming process, including but not limited to the signal coding strategy, electrical stimulation levels, stimulation rate, input dynamic range, mixing ratio, microphone mode, etc. Of note, there are numerous differences in the signal coding strategies, input processing schemes, programming parameters, and programming methods found in the different commercially available cochlear implant systems. A full discussion of these parameters is beyond the scope of this chapter. The interested reader is referred to Wolfe (2020) and Wolfe and Schafer (2015) for a comprehensive discussion of CI programming.

In most cases, children will perform well with their cochlear implants when the audiologist selects the programming parameters recommended by the implant manufacturer (e.g., signal coding strategy, input dynamic range). The most important parameter the audiologist must adjust to optimize an individual child's hearing performance and listening experience is the electrical stimulation levels provided by the CI. In general, there are two types of electrical stimulation levels an audiologist sets for a CI recipient. The minimum amount of electrical stimulation the recipient can detect is typically referred to as the T level (e.g., the threshold for detection of electrical stimulation). The audiologist must also set the upper stimulation level, which refers to the maximum amount of electrical stimulation the recipient will receive. The upper stimulation level typically refers to the amount of electrical stimulation that is most comfortable to the recipient or loud but not uncomfortable.

Figure 6–2 provides an example of T levels and upper stimulation levels (i.e., C levels) set for a 3-year-old child. As shown, the electrical threshold (T level) and upper stimulation level (C level) have been set for each of the 22 channels of the child's CI. Each channel corresponds to a specific frequency analysis band (e.g., sounds ranging from 188 to 313 Hz are delivered to Channel 22) and to an electrode contact located within the cochlea. Electrical stimulation arising from the low-frequency channels is delivered to electrode contacts located in the apex of the cochlea, whereas stimulation from the high-frequency channels is sent to electrode contacts located in the base of the cochlea. Within each channel, low-level sounds elicit electrical stimulation that is near T level, whereas high-level sounds elicit stimulation that is near upper stimulation level.

Of note, not all cochlear implant manufacturers recommend routine measurement of electrical threshold levels. Instead, electrical threshold levels are set to zero or some percentage of the

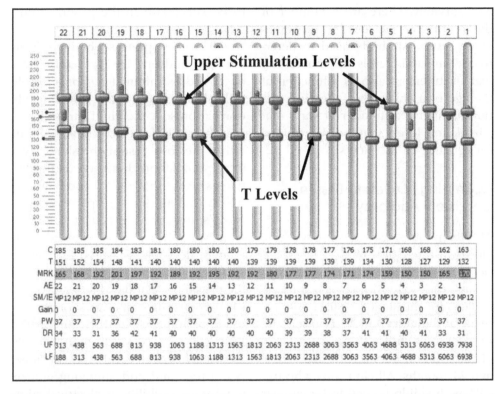

Figure 6-2. An example of cochlear implant stimulation levels. Courtesy of Cochlear Americas.

upper stimulation levels (e.g., 10% of upper stimulation levels). Some research has suggested that cochlear implant recipients receive adequate access to low-level sounds with the use of estimated T levels (Spahr & Dorman, 2005), whereas other studies have shown better audibility and speech recognition with the use of measured T levels (Holden, Reeder, Firszt, & Finley, 2011). The definition of upper stimulation level (e.g., most comfortable, loud but comfortable, maximally loud without discomfort) and the method of determining upper stimulation level vary by cochlear implant manufacturer. The audiologist must have a good understanding of the CI programming process and how it varies by manufacturer.

A number of research studies have shown that the outcomes that CI recipients achieve are influenced by the stimulation levels they receive from their cochlear implant (Busby & Arora, 2016; Geers, Brenner, & Davidson, 2003; Holden et al., 2011, 2013; Wolfe & Kasulis, 2008). The use of insufficient stimulation levels can result in compromised audibility, poor sound quality, and reduced speech recognition, whereas the use of excessive stimulation levels can result in reduced speech recognition, distortion and poor sound quality, discomfort, and in extreme and rare cases, possible damage to the auditory system. To optimize a child's auditory performance with a CI, it is imperative that stimulation levels are set appropriately. There are a number of different techniques used to set stimulation levels. Methods used to determine stimulation levels vary not just by manufacturer but also as a function of the age of a child. The following section highlights a number of ways that stimulation levels may be determined for pediatric CI recipients.

Optimizing T Levels to Ensure Consistent Audibility

The techniques used to measure the electrical thresholds (e.g., T levels) of pediatric implant users are similar to techniques used to measure behavioral audiometric thresholds. Visual reinforcement audiometry (VRA) is often the procedure of choice to measure T levels in children between the ages of 8 and 24 months. All clinicians who use VRA with children need to be familiar with excellent resources that address this topic (Diefendorf & Tharpe, 2017; Gravel, 2000; Gravel & Hood, 1999; Widen, 1993).

Conditioned play audiometry (CPA) is excellent for measuring T levels. CPA involves setting up a game in which the child performs an action every time he or she hears a sound. A conditioned play response needs to be developed as early as possible, because young children often become disinterested in the VRA tasks after multiple programming sessions. The child's practitioner may strive to establish a CPA response in weekly therapy sessions. With focused practice, it is possible for children who are deaf or hard of hearing to develop CPA as young as 18 months of age, although expected to perform these consistently at 24 months. As with VRA, an assistant is often necessary for CPA

to be successful in the programming session.

T level responses obtained from young children are probably best described as minimal response levels (MRLs). In other words, the T levels don't represent the child's true detection threshold for electrical stimuli but rather the lowest suprathreshold level (e.g., stimulation that exceeds the listener's true threshold of audibility) at which the child will respond to electrical stimulation. In fact, it has been suggested that audiologists need to globally decrease measured T levels for small children in order to account for the possibility that the child's responses to programming stimuli are suprathreshold in nature (Zwolan & Griffin, 2005). Provision of excessively high T levels may result in low-level ambient noise being too loud and annoying and/or persistent audibility of electrical stimulation from the implant. Ultimately, ideal sound-field detection thresholds are obtained at 20 to 25 dB HL. If sound-field detection thresholds are elevated, then the audiologist may need to increase T levels to improve audibility of low-level sounds. Again, some CI manufacturers recommend alternative programming adjustments to optimize audibility of low-level sounds (e.g., increase input dynamic range, increase Maplaw).

Optimizing Upper Stimulation Levels to Ensure Comfort, Sound Quality, and Speech Recognition

Determining optimal sufficient upper stimulation levels can be particularly challenging, especially for infants and young children. Audiologists must rely on their knowledge of typical electrical dynamic range and upper stimulation levels for particular cochlear implant systems as well as their observations of the child's behavior and responsiveness to sound as upper stimulation levels are increased. As the upper stimulation levels are slowly increased, the audiologist and assistant observe the child's behavior for signs that the stimulation from the implant is too loud. It may be helpful to use noisemakers, such as a xylophone, a drum, a tambourine, electronic toys, etc., that may be used to produce moderate to high-level noise while upper stimulation levels are being increased in live speech mode. The child's caregiver may also speak to the child while upper stimulation levels are being increased.

The child's responses to increasing upper stimulation levels may be subtle and may occur in many forms. If the child is playing with the noisemakers, then he or she may stop playing with the toy, push it away, and/or decrease the intensity with which he or she is playing with it (e.g., banging on a drum may change to tapping). Also, as upper stimulation levels are increased to a point that may be too loud, the child may change facial expression and/or his or her breathing pattern (e.g., stop smiling, hold breath), reach for a caregiver for affirmation, throw a toy from the highchair tray, attempt to remove the sound processor, etc. The practitioners observe these behaviors closely in an effort to avoid increasing upper stimulation levels that are too loud. If they feel the child is exhibiting behaviors suggesting that the stimulation may be approaching the child's upper loudness limits, then upper stimulation levels will be decreased slightly, until they may confirm that the stimulation is com-

fortable. If the child appears to be fine, then upper stimulation levels may be increased in small steps again, while the practitioners continue to observe the child's responses. These steps continue until the desired upper stimulation levels are reached or until the child exhibits behavior suggesting the stimulation is approaching a level that may be too loud.

Some children may show signs of discomfort prior to reaching the aforementioned upper stimulation levels, particularly during the early stages of implant use. In these cases, the practitioners refrain from aggressively pursuing the typical upper stimulation levels previously mentioned. Instead, upper stimulation levels are set to provide audibility and avoid any discomfort. Subsequently, the audiologist may seek to increase upper stimulation levels at future appointments.

Getting Objective: The Use of Objective Measures in Cochlear Implant Programming and Management

The audiologist may also use objective measures of auditory responsiveness to electrical stimulation as a guide to create programs, evaluate function, and manage the needs of children with cochlear implants. A number of different objective measures have been used to evaluate a child's response to a CI, with the most common being the electrically evoked compound action potential (eCAP) (e.g., NRT) and the electrically evoked stapedial reflex threshold (eSRT). A comprehensive discussion of the eCAP and eSRT are beyond the scope of this chapter. However, the eCAP can be used to determine a level of stimulation that is audible to the recipient, but it is not a satisfactory predictor of T levels or upper stimulation levels (Gordon, Papsin, & Harrison, 2004). The eCAP may be used in conjunction with behavioral measures to aid in the determination of stimulation levels for children who cannot provide verbal feedback about the auditory stimulation they receive from their CI. In contrast, the eSRT has been shown to be an excellent predictor of upper stimulation level and needs to be used routinely as a guide to determine upper stimulation levels in children (Gordon et al., 2004). Wolfe and Schafer (2015) and Wolfe (2020) provide more information regarding the use of the eCAP and eSRT for CI programming in children.

Follow-Up: Touching Base to Ensure Optimal Performance for the Long Run

Children with CIs need to be scheduled for frequent audiology appointments to evaluate post-activation outcomes, ensure that the CI system is functioning appropriately, and ensure that the CI program/MAP is set to optimize recipient performance. The family needs to be encouraged to contact the audiologist to report any concerns that arise regarding the child's performance and/or progress with the CI. Also, the child's AV practitioner and audiologist need to maintain a continual dialogue, and an unscheduled appointment may be set if the practitioner believes the child's progress is being impeded by his or her inability to hear optimally with the CI. At follow-up audiology appointments, attempts are made to measure aided sound-field thresholds to ensure that

the child has good access to low-level sounds (as indicated by sound-field thresholds of 20 to 25 dB HL). Also, speech recognition in quiet (at a presentation level consistent with average and soft level speech) and in noise need to be evaluated. Finally, standardized questionnaires are recommended to assess the child's functional auditory development.

Factors Influencing Cochlear Implant Outcomes

Several factors influence the outcomes children achieve with CIs. For instance, the etiology of the hearing loss can impact the outcome a child receives from CIs. Children with etiologies such as connexin 26, enlarged vestibular aqueduct, Usher syndrome, otoferlin mutation, and non-syndromic hearing loss without additional disability often achieve excellent listening and spoken language outcomes after cochlear implantation (Bauer, Geers, Brenner, Moog, & Smith, 2003; Miyamoto, Bichey, Wynne, & Kirk, 2002; Rouillon et al., 2010; Wu, Liu, Wang, Hsu, & Wu, 2011). In contrast, children with cochlear nerve deficiency often experience poorer listening and spoken language outcomes after cochlear implantation (Govaerts et al., 2003; Teagle et al., 2010; Wu et al., 2015; Young, Kim, Ryan, Tournis, & Yaras, 2012).

Some etiologies are associated with varied results. For example, a number of studies suggest that children with a wide range of temporal bone abnormalities (e.g., Mondini's dysplasia) frequently receive considerable benefit from cochlear implantation, whereas children with more severe cochlear anatomical abnormalities may experience limited outcomes (Buchman et al., 2004; Papsin, 2005). Likewise, some children with profound hearing loss secondary to bacterial meningitis develop age-appropriate listening and spoken language skills, whereas children who have severe cochlear ossification and/or neurological injury after bacterial meningitis are likely to experience delays in spoken language development. Similarly, children who suffer neurological insults after cytomegalovirus (CMV) are more likely to experience delays in listening and spoken language development. Research has also suggested variable outcomes after cochlear implantation for children with ANSD. Some researchers have reported reduced auditory and spoken language skills for children who have ANSD and receive CIs (Buchman et al., 2006; Teagle et al., 2010). More recently, the Longitudinal Outcomes of Children with Hearing Impairment (LOCHI) study found similar spoken language outcomes for children with ANSD compared with children with sensorineural hearing loss (Ching et al., 2013, 2018). The LOCHI researchers have suggested that the relatively favorable outcomes for the children with ANSD can be attributed to the fact that they received their cochlear implants at an early age. Of note, the site-of-lesion of the ANSD is likely to influence the outcomes achieved after cochlear implantation. If the ANSD is caused by a disorder in the cochlea or at the synapse between the cochlea and the cochlear nerve, outcomes are likely to be satisfactory. If the site-of-lesion exists at the cochlear nerve and/or

central auditory nervous system, then outcomes after implantation are likely to be poorer (Rapin & Gravel, 2006).

Several other factors have been shown to influence outcomes after cochlear implantation. As previously discussed, better spoken language outcomes are generally observed in children who receive their CIs prior to 12 months of age (Ching et al., 2018; Dettman et al., 2016; Hoff et al., 2019; Leigh et al., 2016). Also, better listening and spoken language outcomes are typically observed in children whose primary mode of communication is spoken language (i.e., children who communicate via spoken language achieve better listening, spoken language, and literacy outcomes than children who communicate via sign language and spoken language) (Ching et al., 2018; Chu et al., 2016; Dettman et al., 2013; Geers et al., 2003, 2011). In contrast, children whose families have lower income and educational levels are more likely to achieve lower listening and spoken language outcomes (Ching et al., 2018; Niparko et al., 2010). Also, children who have additional disabilities other than hearing loss are more likely to experience poorer outcomes after cochlear implantation, particularly when the disability involves cognitive deficits (Ching et al., 2018; Cupples et al., 2018). However, children with additional disabilities achieve better outcomes when they receive their CIs at an earlier age (Cupples et al., 2018). Additionally, children with additional disabilities are able to achieve listening and spoken language skills that are commensurate with their cognitive abilities, and their listening and spoken abilities can develop into one of their strengths.

Additional Considerations Pertaining to Pediatric Cochlear Implantation

Bilateral Cochlear Implantation

A wealth of research suggests that children with bilateral severe to profound hearing loss are typically best served through the use of bilateral cochlear implantation (Litovsky, Johnstone, & Godar, 2006; Schafer, Amlani, Paiva, Nozari, & Verret, 2011). Namely, speech recognition in quiet and in noise as well as localization are typically better with use of two cochlear implants relative to the unilateral condition (Litovsky et al., 2006). It has also been suggested that better language outcomes are prevalent among children who use bilateral CIs. But, in order to obtain maximum benefit from bilateral cochlear implantation, research has suggested that implantation needs to occur at an early age with a relatively short delay in implantation between ears (Gordon, Jiwani, & Papsin, 2011, 2013; Peters, Litovsky, Parkinson, & Lake, 2007; Wolfe et al., 2007).

Bimodal

The bimodal condition (use of a CI on one ear and a hearing aid on the other ear) generally provides better hearing performance than that obtained with use of a CI alone (Ching et al., 2014; Ching, van WanRooy, & Dillon, 2007; Litovsky et al., 2006). Specifically, children understand speech better in noise with bimodal use compared with performance with the implant alone (Ching et al., 2007, 2014; Litovsky et al., 2006). Bimodal use typically provides a limited improvement in localization, because

electrical stimulation does not adequately preserve low-frequency timing cues necessary for localization via interaural time differences, while the hearing aid typically provides poor audibility of high-frequency sounds necessary for localization via interaural level differences. Bimodal use can be considered essential for children with bilateral hearing loss who are not deemed to be good candidates for bilateral cochlear implantations. A recent study outlined the effects of early acoustic hearing on suprasegmental and segmental perception (Davidson, Geers, Uchanski, & Firszt, 2019) and seeks to help clinicians make a decision regarding bimodal or bilateral CI use. Suprasegmental information can convey prosodic information that is useful in sentence comprehension at lexical and syntactic levels. These suprasegmental cues are conveyed acoustically and cannot be easily transmitted by a CI, so in some cases, a child with some amount of residual hearing may benefit from the acoustic information through a bimodal fitting rather than using bilateral CIs. The authors of this study suggested an increased benefit of extended bimodal use to support language development and suprasegmental and segmental perception. They found optimal benefit with bimodal use of 3.6 years or longer in children with severe hearing loss (pure tone average, ~73 dB HL in the non-implanted ear) provided the child demonstrated bimodal benefit, rather than detriment). Children with severe to profound loss (~92 dB HL) had benefit in suprasegmental perception without observed effect on segmental perception with bimodal use of up to approximately 3.6 years, and children in the profound range (~111 dB) did not receive any benefit; the authors recommended bilateral CIs either simultaneously or with short duration between ears.

Additional research is needed to set best practice guidelines for provision of bimodal or bilateral CI use. In the absence of evidence-based guidelines, the authors of this chapter suggest the following criteria for selection of technology for children with bilateral hearing loss:

- When better ear thresholds are flat and better than 75 dB HL, try bimodal.
- When low-frequency thresholds are better than 70 dB HL with severe to profound high-frequency hearing loss, consider hybrid cochlear implantation and/or use of an acoustic component on the sound processor for preserved residual hearing with longer electrode arrays.
- When hearing loss is flat and in the 75 to 85 dB HL range, lean toward bimodal until evidence of bilateral disruption or poor progress exists.
- When hearing loss exceeds 85 to 90 dB HL for both ears, consider bilateral implantation.

(Note: low-frequency = 125 to 750 Hz; high-frequency = 1500 Hz and up)

Single-Sided Deafness

An emerging trend in pediatric cochlear implantation is the consideration of a CI for children with single-sided deafness (SSD) (e.g., severe to profound hearing loss in one ear and normal hearing sensitivity in the poorer ear). Historically, children with SSD have been considered as candidates for contralateral-routing-of-signal (CROS) hearing aids, implantable bone conduction hearing devices, and/or remote microphone technology. However, none of these technologies are able to effectively stimulate the impaired ear, and as a result, binaural processing cannot be restored. Also, the continuation of auditory deprivation for the impaired ear may result in irreversible changes in the auditory cortex opposite the impaired ear (Gordon, Henkin, & Kral, 2015; Kral, Heid, Hubka, & Tillein, 2013; Kral, Hubka, Heid, & Tillein, 2013). Consequently, pediatric hearing health care professionals have begun to consider cochlear implantation for children with SSD. Indeed, if an MRI indicates that the child has an intact cochlear nerve for the impaired ear, then cochlear implantation is the only hearing technology that allows for auditory stimulation to the poorer ear. Early cochlear implantation may prevent negative effects associated with auditory deprivation and may serve to partially restore interaural auditory cues, and subsequently may improve localization and speech recognition in noise. Indeed, researchers have shown that children with congenital SSD routinely use their CIs, a finding that would suggest that the children find the implant to be beneficial (Polenko, Papsin, & Gordon, 2017). Additional research is needed to further clarify the advantages and limitations of cochlear implantation for children with SSD. In particular, research is needed to determine the relationship between age at implantation and benefit from cochlear implantation for children with congenital SSD. The US FDA recently approved cochlear implantation for individuals who are at least 5 years old and who have profound hearing loss in one ear with normal hearing in the opposite ear or profound hearing loss in one ear and mild to moderately severe hearing loss in the opposite ear.

AUDITORY BRAINSTEM IMPLANTS

The overwhelming majority of those who have severe to profound hearing loss and are candidates for an implantable hearing device will receive and benefit from a cochlear implant. However, a small number will be unresponsive to or unsuitable for one. Some may be candidates, therefore, for an *auditory brainstem implant.*

An auditory brainstem implant is similar to a CI, but the electrode array is typically inserted on the cochlear nucleus at the inferior, dorsolateral area of the pons. Figure 6–3 provides an example of an auditory brainstem implant system.

Auditory brainstem implants function in a similar manner to CIs, but instead of providing stimulation to the auditory nerve, the cochlea is bypassed and electrical stimulation is delivered via a paddle electrode array to the auditory brainstem. A neurotologist places the paddle electrode in the lateral recess of the fourth ventricle over the cochlear nucleus.

Typical Outcomes with Auditory Brainstem Implants

Auditory brainstem implants were originally developed for persons with neurofibromatosis type 2 (NF2), a condition that causes tumors to proliferate along the central nervous system. In some patients with NF2, the cochlear nerve is severed during the process of tumor removal, and as a result, a CI is unsuccessful. The auditory brainstem implant bypasses the damaged cochlear nerve and stimulates the auditory areas of the lower brainstem directly. Unfortunately, many persons with NF2 experience a substantial amount of degeneration of the neurons in the cochlear

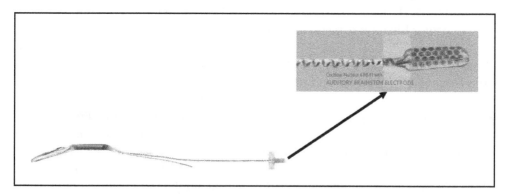

Figure 6–3. An example of an auditory brainstem implant. Courtesy of Cochlear Americas.

nerve as well as in the auditory centers of the brainstem. As such, the auditory brainstem may not produce a favorable outcome for many persons with NF2 (Colletti & Shannon, 2005; Colletti, Shannon, Carner, Veronese, Colletti, 2009).

Outcomes appear to be more favorable in studies examining performance of persons with auditory brainstem implants and etiologies other than NF2 (Colletti & Shannon, 2005; Colletti et al., 2009; Noij et al., 2015). For example, Colletti et al. (2009) reported on the open-set speech recognition of 48 auditory brainstem implant users who did not have NF2. These participants achieved a mean score of 59% correct, with performance ranging from 10% to 100% correct. Of note, participants with cochlear nerve deficiency and cochlear nerve injury typically performed quite well with their auditory brainstem implants. In short, auditory brainstem implants are a worthy consideration for children who have cochlear nerve deficiency or cochlear ossification.

IMPLANTABLE BONE CONDUCTION HEARING DEVICES

Implantable bone conduction hearing devices (IBCHDs), also commonly referred to as osseointegrated auditory devices, bone anchored hearing aids, or BAHAs, were created as an option to treat conductive or mixed types of hearing losses as well as single-sided deafness. IBCHDs aim to transmit acoustic information to the cochlea via vibratory transmission through the skull. IBCHDs essentially operate on the same physiologic bases as what is found in bone conduction hearing assessment. All IBCHD devices possess an external sound processor and a titanium implanted component. In short, sound is received at the microphone of the external sound processor and converted from acoustic to mechanical energy. Then, the mechanical, vibratory signal is transmitted to the implanted component either across the skin or via direct connection. The vibratory oscillations are then delivered from the implanted component through the bones of the skull to vibrate the structures of the cochlea. Some IBCHD devices require osseointegration between the skull and the implantable component called a fixture, whereas others do not require osseointegration. Osseointegration describes the process in which a functional connection is established between the bone and implant. Specifically, the osteoblasts and connective tissue of the bone migrate into small pores in the titanium of the implant.

IBCHDs are typically classified into three broad categories, *percutaneous, transcutaneous,* and *active* systems. Percutaneous devices contain an implantable fixture that is surgically inserted into the mastoid bone of the skull. An abutment, which is connected to the fixture, protrudes through the skin so that the surface resides just over the skin. The IBCHD external sound processor is connected to the abutment so that the mechanical oscillations of the sound processor may be delivered directly to the skull via the implanted fixture/abutment. See Figure 6–4A for an example of percutaneous IBCHDs.

Transcutaneous IBCHDs feature an implantable titanium component that is surgically fixed to the mastoid bone of the skull by biocompatible titanium screws. The implanted component also possesses a magnet or magnets. The external sound processor is connected to a magnetic plate that adheres to the magnet(s) of the implanted component residing under the skin. As such, the external sound processor sits on the skin above the mastoid bone by way of magnetic attraction to the implanted component. The vibratory oscillations of the external sound processor are delivered across the skin to the implanted component and then to the cochleae via bone conduction through the skull. See Figure 6–4B for examples of transcutaneous IBCHDs.

Active IBCHDs contain a vibratory (typically piezoelectric transducer) device that is implanted in the skull with a titanium fixture (see Figure 6–5). This IBCHD also contains an electromagnetic receiving coil that is used to receive an electromagnetic radio frequency signal from the external sound processor. A magnet resides in the center of the internal receiving coil and the external sound processor to allow for adherence of the external sound processor to the internal device. Acoustic inputs are captured by the microphone of the external sound processor, processed by the digital signal processor within the external sound processors, and delivered to the internal receiving coil by way of a short-range electromagnetic induction link. Then, the signal is sent to the internal oscillator, which creates vibratory oscillations that are delivered to the skull.

Percutaneous and transcutaneous IBCHDs are approved for use in children 5 years of age and older. Younger children typically do not receive IBCHDs, because their skull thickness is insufficient to accommodate the implant-

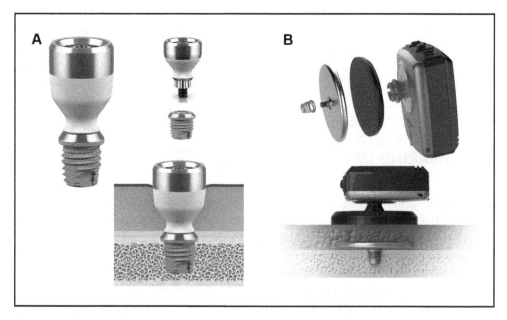

Figure 6–4. An example of a percutaneous implantable bone conduction hearing device (**A**) and a transcutaneous implantable bone conduction hearing device (**B**). Courtesy of Cochlear Americas.

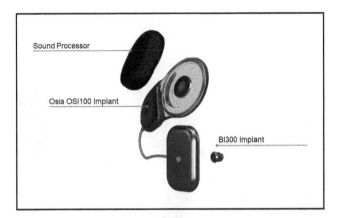

Figure 6-5. An example of an active implantable bone conduction hearing device. Courtesy of Cochlear Americas.

able fixture. Also, active IBCHDs are approved for children 12 years of age and older, because additional skull thickness is required to accommodate the presence of the internal oscillator. However, infants and young children may also use modern bone conduction technologies. The external sound processor of an IBCHD may be connected to a "softband" or a "sound arc" so that the processor resides on the head similar to a conventional non-implantable bone conduction device (see Figures 6–6 and 6–7). Moreover, an alternative option is to use a bone conduction sound processor that connects to the head via an adhesive pad. For all non-implantable wearing configurations, however, the signal is attenuated in a frequency-specific manner as it crosses the skin to be delivered to the skull.

Assessment of IBCHD Candidacy with Various Indications for Use

IBCHDs are considered to be the standard of care for treating children with permanent conductive hearing loss (CHL) or mixed hearing loss (MHL) that may not be ameliorated through surgical intervention. In particular, children diagnosed with congenital aural atresia and/or microtia or other outer and middle ear hearing losses are excellent candidates for an IBCHD. These hearing losses can occur in one or both ears, but more commonly occur unilaterally. Other common causes of CHL and MHL include chronic otitis media and chronic otitis externa (middle and outer ear infections) with resulting hearing loss, cholesteatoma, and ossicular chain abnormalities such as congenital stapes fixation. Specific examples of children who commonly benefit from an IBCHD include those who have congenital syndromes such as Goldenhar, Treacher-Collins, and Down syndrome. Individuals with single-sided deafness (severe to profound hearing loss in one ear) are also common candidates for an IBCHD.

Bone conduction hearing devices are recommended over conventional air conduction hearing aids for those with CHL or MHL with an air–bone gap

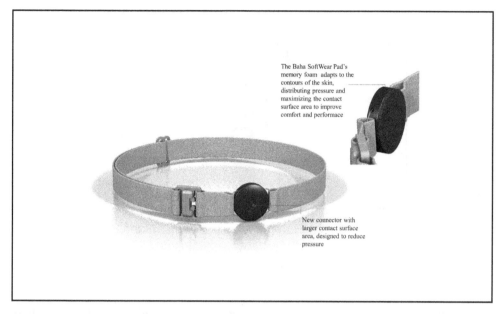

Figure 6–6. An example of a bone conduction processor worn on a softband. Courtesy of Cochlear Americas.

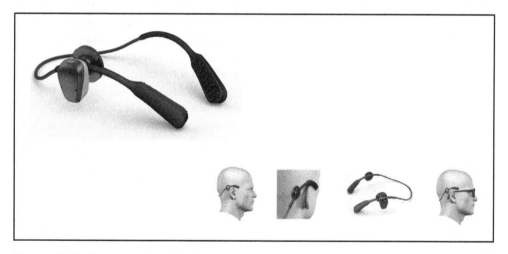

Figure 6–7. An example of a bone conduction processor worn on a sound arc. Courtesy of Cochlear Americas.

exceeding 30 dB and normal to near-normal bone conduction hearing sensitivity (Hol, Bosman, Snik, Mylanus, & Cremers, 2005; Hol, Snik, Mylanus, & Cremers, 2005). IBCHDs can bypass the affected middle ear and directly stimu-late the intact inner ear(s). As a result, a higher fidelity signal with lower distortion can be provided.

IBCHDs may also be considered for children with SSD. In such cases, an IBCHD may be used to send the signal captured at the side of the poorer ear to the better ear via bone conduction. In essence, the IBCHD works like a CROS hearing instrument by delivering the signal of interest from the poor ear to the better ear by way of bone conduction, which assists in overcoming the head shadow effect. However, the impaired ear is not being stimulated in this situation. Also, use of an IBCHD for children with SSD will not improve localization, and speech recognition in quiet and in noise will not improve unless the signal of interest arrives on the side of the impaired ear.

Audiologic Criteria for Candidacy for IBCHD

From an audiologic perspective, children must have a conductive or mixed hearing loss with an average air–bone gap (average bone conduction thresholds at 500, 1000, and 2000 Hz) of at least 30 dB to benefit from an IBCHD. The FDA guidelines state that the bone conduction pure tone average (an average of bone conduction thresholds at 500, 1000, and 2000 Hz) has to be less than or equal to 55 to 65 dB HL. Ideally, however, bone conduction thresholds should be in the normal to near-normal range. IBCHD sound processor selection is an important consideration when the sensorineural component is more severe (e.g., bone conduction 25 dB HL or poorer), because those individuals may do best with a more powerful external sound processor. The manufacturers of IBCHD have delineated the selection of external sound processors on the basis of bone conduction pure tone average criteria. For example, "standard" sound processors are recommended for persons with

bone conduction pure tone averages of 45 dB HL or better, while "power" processors are suggested for persons with poorer bone conduction hearing thresholds (45 to 65 dB HL).

Assessment of Auditory Outcomes of Children with IBCHD/Expectations

Beyond the provision of an IBCHD, verification and validation are necessary to ensure ongoing benefit. For children using IBCHDs, the expectations and outcomes need to be similar to those of children who wear traditional hearing aids or to cochlear implants. Aided sound-field warble tone thresholds need to be ideally no less than 30 dB HL. Additionally, percutaneous IBCHDs may now be evaluated with the use of real ear verification measures with the IBCHD output level matched to evidence-based prescriptive targets (Hodgetts & Scollie, 2017).

Speech recognition assessments need to be completed at normal (60 dBA/45 dB HL) and soft (50 dBA/35 dB HL) conversational levels in quiet and in noise. Given the normal to near-normal cochlear status for children with IBCHD, substantial open-set speech recognition capacity can be expected with device use.

The youngest children fit with IB-CHDs may be at a disadvantage because practitioners are not always able to assess benefit objectively through audiologic measures, at least not at first. Instead, subjective measures can be administered. Questionnaires can be an effective way to validate the IBCHD fitting. Also, the child's practitioner can provide valuable information regarding auditory and spoken language development. At least one year of growth in auditory and spoken language development needs to occur for each chronological year.

IMPLICATIONS OF IMPLANTABLE HEARING TECHNOLOGIES FOR THE AV PRACTITIONER

Many children with severe to profound hearing loss, auditory neuropathy spectrum disorder, or significant, permanent conductive hearing loss may receive limited benefit from hearing aids. In such cases, the practitioner needs to consult with the child's hearing health care team (e.g., audiologist, otologist) to determine whether the child's needs may be met more effectively with implantable hearing technology. Implantable hearing technologies are continuously evolving, and practitioners who coach and guide parents need to have current knowledge of the changes in these technologies in order to optimize the child's listening and spoken language development.

Determination of a child's candidacy for implantable hearing technology is a multifaceted process that involves audiological, otological, and speech and language assessments. The practitioner plays a critical role in the CI candidacy process. The status of a child's auditory skills and spoken language development is one of the primary and most instrumental factors governing the CI candidacy decision-making process. With modern hearing technology and AVT, many children who are deaf or hard of hearing can achieve age-appropriate auditory and spoken language abilities and make at least one year of progress in spoken language development for every chronological year. Thus, sessions with the practitioner are critical both pre and post cochlear implantation.

The practitioner is required to have a thorough understanding of a child's unaided and aided auditory function, including the degree, type, and configuration of the hearing loss, aided thresholds, and aided speech recognition in quiet (at an average and soft conversational level) as well as in noise. With this knowledge and ongoing diagnostic sessions in AVT, the practitioner can move forward or consider modifying the child's services (e.g., hearing technology) when aided performance is inadequate.

Audiologists and practitioners work in partnership to effectively optimize the progress and performance of the child (Estabrooks, MacIver-Lux & Houston, 2014; MacIver-Lux et al., 2016). This partnership takes place throughout the assessment and management processes. Management of implantable hearing technologies (e.g., device programming, troubleshooting, evaluation of aided performance) is a complex process that is best navigated when the audiologist and practitioner work in tandem. Ideally, the practitioner needs to be an intimate part of managing the child's implantable hearing technology, including the provision of assistance in device programming, assessment, and troubleshooting. The audiologist and practitioner can work collaboratively to improve hearing performance when aided assessment of auditory function, or the practitioner's assessment of auditory and spoken language development, indicates insufficient performance and/or progress.

CONCLUSION

Implantable hearing technology makes age-appropriate spoken language a possibility for the vast majority of children with hearing loss, regardless of their degree, configuration, or type of hearing loss. Pediatric hearing health care providers need to be vigilant about the advances in implantable hearing technology to ensure that children with hearing loss are able to reach their full potential in the development of listening and spoken language abilities. Audiologists, AV practitioners, otologists, and families work together in order to optimize the benefit children receive from implantable hearing devices.

REFERENCES

Bagatto, M. (2012). 20Q: Baby steps following verification—outcome evaluation in pediatric hearing aid fitting. *Audiology-Online*. Retrieved on August 28, 2015 from http://www.audiologyonline.com /articles/20q-baby-steps-following-verification-783

Bagatto, M. P., Moodie, S. T., Malandrino, A. C., Richert, F. M., Clench, D. A., & Scollie, S. D. (2011). The University of Western Ontario audiological monitoring protocol (UWO PedAMP). *Trends in Amplification, 15*(1), 57–76.

Bauer, P. W., Geers, A. E., Brenner, C., Moog, J. S., & Smith, R. J. (2003). The effect of GJB2 allele variants on performance after cochlear implantation. *Laryngoscope, 113*(12), 2135–2140.

Buchman, C. A., Copeland, B. J., Yu, K. K., Brown, C. J., Carrasco, V. N., & Pillsbury, H. C. (2004). Cochlear implantation in children with congenital inner ear malformations. *Laryngoscope, 114*(2), 309–316.

Buchman, C. A., Roush, P. A., Teagle, H. F., Brown, C. J., Zdanski, C. J., & Grose, J. H. (2006). Auditory neuropathy characteristics in children with cochlear nerve deficiency. *Ear and Hearing, 27*(4), 399–408.

Busby, P. A., & Arora, K. (2016). Effects of threshold adjustment on speech perception in nucleus cochlear implant recipients. *Ear and Hearing, 37*(3), 303–311.

Carlson, M. L., Sladen, D. P., Haynes, D. S., Driscoll, C. L., DeJong, M. D., Erickson, H. C., . . . Gifford, R. H. (2015). Evidence for the expansion of pediatric cochlear implant candidacy. *Otology and Neurotology, 36*(1), 43–50.

Ching, T. Y. C., Day, J., Van Buynder, P., Hou, S., Zhang, V., Seeto, M., . . . Flynn, C. (2014). Language and speech perception of young children with bimodal fitting or bilateral cochlear implants. *Cochlear Implants International, 15*(suppl. 1), S43–S46.

Ching, T. Y., Dillon, H., Leigh, G., & Cupples, L. (2018). Learning from the longitudinal outcomes of children with hearing impairment (LOCHI) study: Summary of 5-year findings and implications. *International Journal of Audiology, 57*(2), S105–S111.

Ching, T. Y., Dillon, H., Marnane, V., Hou, S., Day, J., Seeto, M., . . . Yeh, A. (2013). Outcomes of early- and late-identified children at 3 years of age: Findings from a prospective population-based study. *Ear and Hearing, 34*(5), 535–552.

Ching, T. Y., & Hill, M. (2005). *The Parents' Evaluation of Aural/Oral Performance of Children (PEACH) Rating Scale*. Chatswood, New South Wales, Australia: Australian Hearing. Retrieved from http://www.outcomes.nal.gov.au /LOCHI%20 assessments.html

Ching T. Y., & Hill, M. (2007). The parents' evaluation of aural/oral performance of children (PEACH) scale: Normative data. *Journal of American Academy of Audiology, 18*(3), 220–235. Retrieved from http://www.audiology.org/resources/journal/Pages/default.aspx

Ching, T. Y. C., van Wanrooy, E., & Dillon, H. (2007). Binaural-bimodal fitting or bilateral implantation for managing severe to profound deafness: A review. *Trends in Hearing, 11*(3), 161–192.

Chu, C., Choo, D., Dettman, S., Leigh, J., Traeger, G., Lettieri, S., Courtenay, D., & Dowell, D. (2016). *Early intervention and communication development in children using cochlear implants: The impact of service delivery practices and family factors*. Podium presentation at the Audiology Australia National Conference 2016, May 22–25, Melbourne, Australia.

Colletti, V., & Shannon, R. V. (2005). Open set speech perception with auditory brainstem implant? *Laryngoscope, 115*(11), 1974–1978.

Colletti, V., Shannon, R., Carner, M., Veronese, S., & Colletti, L. (2009). Outcomes in nontumor adults fitted with the auditory brainstem implant: 10 years' experience. *Otology and Neurotology, 30*(5), 614–618.

Cupples, L., Ching, T. Y. C., Button, L., Leigh, G., Marnane, M., Whitfield, J., Gunnourie, M., & Martin, L. (2018). Language and speech outcomes of children with hearing loss and additional disabilities: Identifying the variables that influence performance at five years of age. *International Journal of Audiology, 57*(S2): S93–S104.

Davidson, L. S., Geers, A. E., Uchanski, R. M., & Firszt, J. B. (2019). Effects of early acoustic hearing on speech perception and language for pediatric cochlear implant recipients. *Journal of Speech, Language, and Hearing Research, 62*, 3620–3637.

Dettman, S. J., Dowell, R. C., Choo, D., Arnott, W., Abrahams, Y., Davis, A., . . . Briggs, R. J. (2016). Long-term communi-

cation outcomes for children receiving cochlear implants younger than 12 months: A multicenter study. *Otology and Neurotology, 37*(2), e82–e95.

Dettman, S., Wall, E., Constantinescu, G., & Dowell, R. (2013). Communication outcomes for groups of children using cochlear implants enrolled in auditory-verbal therapy, aural-oral, and bilingual-bicultural early intervention programs. *Otology and Neurotology, 34*, 451–459.

Diefendorf, A. O. (1988). Behavioral evaluation of hearing-impaired children. In F. Bess (Ed.), *Hearing impairment in children* (pp. 133–151). Parkton, MD: York Press.

Diefendorf, A. O., & Tharpe, A. M. (2017). Behavioral audiometry in infants and children. In A. M. Tharpe & R. Seewald (Eds.), *Comprehensive handbook of pediatric audiology* (2nd ed.; pp. 591–607). San Diego, CA: Plural Publishing.

Estabrooks, W., MacIver-Lux, K., & Houston, K. T. (2014). Therapeutic approaches following cochlear implantation in cochlear implants. In S. Waltzman & T. Roland (Eds.), *Cochlear implants* (3rd ed.). New York, NY: Thieme.

Gallaudet Research Institute (2008). *Regional and national summary report of data from the 2007–08 annual survey of deaf and hard of hearing children and youth*. Retrieved August 28, 2015 at http://research.gallaudet.edu/Demographics/2008_National_Summary.pdf

Geers, A., Brenner, C., & Davidson, L. (2003). Factors associated with development of speech perception skills in children implanted by age five. *Ear and Hearing, 24*(S1), 24S–35S.

Geers, A. E., Strube, M. J., Tobey, E. A., & Moog, J. S., (2011). Epilogue: Factors contributing to long-term outcomes of cochlear implantation in early childhood. *Ear and Hearing, 32*(1, suppl.), 84S–92S.

Gordon, K., Henkin, Y., & Kral, A. (2015). Asymmetric hearing during development: The aural preference syndrome and treatment options. *Pediatrics, 136*(1), 141–153.

Gordon, K. A., Jiwani, S., & Papsin, B. C. (2011). What is the optimal timing for bilateral cochlear implantation in children? *Cochlear Implants International, 12*(2):8–14.

Gordon, K. A., Jiwani, S., & Papsin, B. C. (2013). Benefits and detriments of unilateral cochlear implant use on bilateral auditory development in children who are deaf. *Frontiers in Psychology, 4*(719), 1–14.

Gordon, K. A., Papsin, B. C., & Harrison, R. V. (2004). Toward a battery of behavioral and objective measures to achieve optimal cochlear implant stimulation levels in children. *Ear and Hearing, 25*(5), 447–463.

Govaerts, P. J., Casselman, J., Daemers, K., De Beukelaer, C., Yperman, M., & De Ceulaer, G. (2003). Cochlear implants in aplasia and hypoplasia of the cochleovestibular nerve. *Otology and Neurotology, 24*(6), 887–891.

Gravel, J. S. (2000). Audiologic assessment for the fitting of hearing instruments: Big challenges from tiny ears. In R. C. Seewald (Ed.), *A sound foundation through early amplification: Proceedings of an international conference* (pp. 33–46). Stafa, Switzerland: Phonak AG.

Gravel, J. S., & Hood, L. J. (1999). Pediatric audiologic assessment. In F. E. Musiek & W. F. Rintelmann (Eds.), *Contemporary perspectives in hearing assessment* (pp. 305–326). Needham Heights, MA: Allyn and Bacon.

Hodgetts, W. E., & Scollie, S. D. (2017). DSL prescriptive targets for bone conduction devices: Adaptation and comparison to clinical fittings. *International Journal of Audiology, 56*(7), 521–530.

Hoff, S., Ryan, M., Thomas, D., Tournis, E., Kenny, H., Hajduk, J., & Young, N. M. (2019). Safety and effectiveness of cochlear implantation of young children, including those with complicating conditions. *Otology and Neurotology, 40,* 454–463.

Hol, M. K. S., Bosman, A. J., Snik, A. F., Mylanus, E. A. M., & Cremers, C. W. R. J. (2005). Bone-anchored hearing aids in unilateral inner ear deafness: An evaluation of audiometric and patient outcome measurements. *Otology and Neurotology, 26*(5), 999–1006.

Hol, M. K., Snik, A. F., Mylanus, E. A., & Cremers, C. W. (2005). Long-term results of bone-anchored hearing aid recipients who had previously used air-conduction hearing aids. *Archives of Otolaryngology–Head and Neck Surgery, 131*(4) 321–325.

Holden, L. K., Finley, C. C., Firszt, J. B., Holden, T. A., Brenner, C., Potts, L. G., & Skinner, M. W. (2013). Factors affecting open-set word recognition in adults with cochlear implants. *Ear and Hearing, 34*(3), 342–360.

Holden, L. K., Reeder, R. M., Firszt, J. B., & Finley, C. C. (2011). Optimizing the perception of soft speech and speech in noise with the Advanced Bionics cochlear implant system. *International Journal of Audiology, 50*(4), 255–269.

Kral, A., Heid, S., Hubka, P., & Tillein, J. (2013). Unilateral hearing during development: hemispheric specificity in plastic reorganizations. *Frontiers in Systems Neuroscience, 7,* 93.

Kral, A., Hubka, P., Heid, S., & Tillein, J. (2013). Single-sided deafness leads to unilateral aural preference within an early sensitive period. *Brain, a Journal of Neurology, 136*(pt. 1), 180–193.

Leigh, J. R., Dettman, S. J., & Dowell, R. C. (2016). Evidence-based guidelines for recommending cochlear implantation for young children: Audiological criteria and optimizing age at implantation. *International Journal of Audiology, 55,* S9–S18.

Litovsky, R. Y., Johnstone, P. M., & Godar, S. P. (2006). Benefits of bilateral cochlear implants and/or hearing aids in children. *International Journal of Audiology, 45*(suppl. 1), S78–S91.

MacIver-Lux, K., Estabrooks, W., Lim, S. R., Siomra, R. A., Visser, W., Sansom, J. K., . . . Atkins, D. (2016). Professional partnerships and auditory-verbal therapy. In W. Estabrooks, K. MacIver-Lux, & E. Rhoades (Eds.), *Auditory-verbal therapy: For young children with hearing loss and their families, and the practitioners who guide them* (pp. 507–543. San Diego, CA: Plural Publishing.

Meinzen-Derr, J., Wiley, S., Creighton, J., & Choo, D. (2007). Auditory skills checklist: Clinical tool for monitoring functional auditory skill development in young children with cochlear implants. *Annals of Otology, Rhinology & Laryngology, 116*(11), 812–818.

Miyamoto, R. T., Bichey, B. G., Wynne, M. K., & Kirk, K. I. (2002). Cochlear implantation with large vestibular aqueduct syndrome. *Laryngoscope, 112*(7, Pt. 1), 1178–1182.

Niparko, J. K., Tobey, E. A., Thal, D. J., Eisenberg, L. S., Wang, N. Y., Quittner, A. L., & Fink, N. E. (2010). Spoken language development in children following cochlear implantation. *Journal of the American Medical Association, 303*(15), 1498–1506.

Noij, K. S., Kozin, E. D., Sethi, R., Shah, P. V., Kaplan, A. B., Herrmann, B., & Lee, D. J. (2015). Systematic review of nontumor pediatric auditory brainstem implant outcomes. *Otolaryngology Head and Neck Surgery, 153*(5), 739–750.

Papsin, B. C. (2005). Cochlear implantation in children with anomalous cochleovestibular anatomy. *Laryngoscope, 115*(suppl. 1), S1–S25.

Peters, B., Litovsky, R., Parkinson, A., & Lake, J. (2007). Importance of age and post-implantation experience on speech perception measures in children with sequential bilateral cochlear implants. *Otology and Neurotology, 28*(5), 649–657.

Polenko, M., Papsin, B. C., & Gordon, K. (2017). Children with single-sided deafness use their cochlear implant. *Ear and Hearing, 38*(6), 681–689.

Rapin, I., & Gravel, J. S. (2006). Auditory neuropathy: A biologically inappropriate label unless acoustic nerve involvement is documented. *Journal of the American Academy of Audiology, 17*(2), 147–150.

Rouillon, I., Marcolla, A., Roux, I., Marlin, S., Feldmann, D, Couderc, R. . . . Loundon, N. (2006). Results of cochlear implantation in two children with mutations on the OTOF gene. *International Journal of Pediatric Otorhinolaryngology, 70*(4), 689–696.

Schafer, E. C., Amlani, A. M., Paiva, D., Nozari, L., & Verret, S. (2011). A meta-analysis to compare speech recognition in noise with bilateral cochlear implants and bimodal stimulation. *International Journal of Audiology, 50*(12), 871–880.

Spahr, A. J., & Dorman, M. F. (2005). Effects of minimum stimulation settings for the Med-El Tempo+ speech processor on speech understanding. *Ear and Hearing, 26*(suppl. 4), 2S–6S.

Teagle, H. F. B., Roush, P. A., Woodard, J. S., Hatch, D. R., Buss, E., Zdanski, C. J., & Buchman, C. A. (2010). Cochlear implantation in children with auditory neuropathy spectrum disorder. *Ear and Hearing, 31*(3), 325–335.

Tomblin, J. B., Harrison, M., Ambrose, S. E., Walker, E. A., Oleson, J. J., & Moeller, M. P. (2015). Language outcomes in young children with mild to severe hearing loss. *Ear and Hearing, 36*(suppl. 1), 76S–91S.

Tsiakpini, L., Weichbold, V., Kuehn-Inacker, H., Coninx, F., D'Haese, P., & Almadin, S. (2004). *LittlEARS auditory questionnaire.* Innsbruck, Austria: MED-EL.

Uhler, K., & Gifford, R. H. (2014). Current trends in pediatric cochlear implant candidate selection and postoperative follow-up. *American Journal of Audiology, 23*, 309–325.

Uhler, K., Warner-Czyz, A., Gifford, R., & Working Group, P. (2017). Pediatric Minimum Speech Test Battery. *Journal of the American Academy of Audiology, 28*(3), 232–247.

Widen, J. E. (1993). Adding objectivity to infant behavioral audiometry. *Ear and Hearing, 14*(1), 49–57.

Wolfe, J. (2020). *Cochlear implants: Audiologic management and considerations for implantable hearing devices*. San Diego, CA: Plural Publishing.

Wolfe, J., Baker, S., Caraway, T., Kasulis, H., Mears, A., Smith, J., & Wood, M. (2007). 1-Year postactivation results for sequentially implanted bilateral cochlear implant users. *Otology and Neurotology, 28*(5), 589–596.

Wolfe, J., & Kasulis, H. (2008). Relationships among objective measures and speech perception in adult users of the HiResolution Bionic Ear. *Cochlear Implants International, 9*(2),70–81.

Wolfe, J., & Schafer, E. C. (2015). *Programming cochlear implants* (2nd ed.). San Diego, CA: Plural Publishing.

Wu, C. C., Liu, T. C., Wang, S. H., Hsu, C. J., & Wu, C. M. (2011). Genetic characteristics in children with cochlear implants and the corresponding auditory performance. *Laryngoscope, 121*(6), 1287–1293.

Wu, C. M., Lee, L. A., Chen, C. K., Chan, K. C., Tsou, Y. T., & Ng, S. H. (2015). Impact of cochlear nerve deficiency determined using 3-dimensional magnetic resonance imaging on hearing outcome in children with cochlear implants. *Otology and Neurotology, 36*(1), 41–21.

Young, N. M., Kim, F. M., Ryan, M. E., Tournis, E., & Yaras, S. (2012). Pediatric cochlear implantation of children with eighth nerve deficiency. *International Journal of Pediatric Otorhinolaryngology, 76*(10), 1442–1448.

Zwolan, T. A., & Griffin, B. L. (2005). How we do it: Tips for programming the speech processor of an 18-month-old. *Cochlear Implants International, 6*(4), 169–177.

7

HEARING ASSISTANCE TECHNOLOGIES AND AUDITORY-VERBAL THERAPY

Sarah E. Warren, Tina Childress, and Olivia G. Naegle

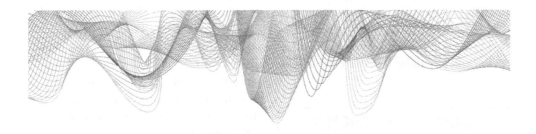

INTRODUCTION

In Auditory-Verbal Therapy (AVT), parents work collaboratively with AV practitioners (practitioners) and audiologists to ensure that their children who are deaf or hard of hearing can obtain maximum benefits of auditory stimulation by using appropriately fit hearing aids (Chapter 5) and implantable technologies (Chapter 6) so that hearing can be used as the primary sensory modality in developing listening and spoken language. While practitioners guide parents to use strategies that support listening for the acquisition of spoken language throughout the child's daily activities, they also realize that the majority of children's daily activities take place in complex listening environments. For example, 80% of a young child's time in preschool daycare is estimated to be in competing noise (Cruckly, Scollie, & Parsa, 2011) where the ambient noise levels range 60 to 70 dBA (Cruckley et al., 2011; Maisse & Dillon, 2006). The American National

Standards Institute (ANSI) recommends that maximum background noise level in unoccupied classrooms should not exceed 35 dBA (ANSI, 2010).

The first course of action is to decrease the noise; however, implementing steps to decrease sound levels is not always feasible, or may still not be sufficient for optimal listening. When decreasing the impact of complex listening environments is not an option, improving children's access to the signal is recommended with the use of hearing assistance technology (HAT). Practitioners provide valuable feedback to audiologists in their recommendations and verification of HAT with information about the listening demands of the child's daily environment and the child's auditory functioning with/without HAT. They also guide parent(s) in the use of HAT (when and where) and how to maintain equipment. A list of terminology can be found in Table 7–1.

COMPLEX LISTENING ENVIRONMENTS

Three primary variables make a listening environment complex: noise, listener distance from the speaker, and reverberation. An infant and/or young child's environment is full of sounds that do not directly contribute to a child's language learning, and these sounds are typically referred to as noise. *Noise* can interfere with the signal of interest, typically speech, and unintentionally mask the signal. The relationship of the level of the signal compared with the level of the noise, both at the level of the listener's ear, is referred to as the *signal-to-noise ratio* (SNR). Also, the perception of speech can be affected by the distance from the speaker. Sound pressure is subject to the inverse square law that states there is a decrease of 6 dB for each doubling of distance between the sound source and listener. Another way to think of this is that children hear optimally if the signal is within their "listening bubble" (Cole & Flexer, 2011). As a general rule of thumb: if the signal is more than about an adult's arm's length away, the child may have poor perception because it is beyond the "bubble." In addition to noise, reverberation creates perceptual disadvantages. *Reverberation* is defined as the prolongation of sound as sound waves reflect off hard surfaces. Examples of highly reverberant rooms include places such as a cafeteria, gym, and a classroom if it contains hard surfaces and/or high ceilings. Each of these variables compromises infants' and young children's ability to understand speech in complex environments, even in children with normal hearing (Boothroyd, 1997; Wolfe et al., 2013).

COMPLEX LISTENING ENVIRONMENTS AND CHILDREN WHO ARE DEAF OR HARD OF HEARING

Even though all infants and young children face difficulties in understanding speech in complex listening environments (Crandall & Smaldino, 2000), children who are deaf or hard of hearing are at a particular disadvantage (Crandall & Smaldino, 2000; Wolfe et al., 2013). Although hearing aids and implantable devices help children who are deaf or hard of hearing to achieve satisfactory speech understanding abilities in quiet, performance is still negatively impacted to a higher degree compared with normal-hearing peers (Boothroyd & Medwetsky, 1992; Crandell & Smadino, 2000; Glista et al., 2009; Schafer & Thibodeau, 2006a; Wolfe et al., 2013). In noise, speech understanding abilities decrease by up to 30 to 60 percentage points among children with cochlear implant(s) (Schafer & Thibodeau, 2003, 2004; Spahr, Dorman, & Loiselle, 2007; Wolfe et al., 2013), hearing aids, or both (are bimodal) (Ching et al., 2007, 2014; Litovsky et al., 2006; Wolfe, Morais, & Schafer, 2016). The extreme reductions in performance in complex listening environments warrant the use of HAT in order to overcome the adverse effects of noise, reverberation, and distance in children who are deaf or hard of hearing, as these allow children with bilateral cochlear implants to achieve similar levels of speech understanding in noise as in quiet (Schafer & Kleineck, 2009; Wolfe & Schafer, 2008). The use of HAT in children with hearing aids has been shown to provide a 15 to 20 dB increase in SNR compared with listening without HAT (Hawkins, 1984; Schafer & Thibodeau, 2006a). Thus, while the use of appropriately fit hearing aids and implantable devices is the first intervention recommended for implementing the principles of AVT, additional technology and accessories may be required to maximize speech audibility and intelligibility in specific situations, including complex listening environments, as well as to provide alternate access to other signals for communication.

HEARING ASSISTANCE TECHNOLOGY

HAT can be defined as a device or system that directly delivers sound to the listener in an effort to minimize the barriers of hearing loss. The sound may be amplified or even converted to light, vibration, or text. Other terms used, often interchangeably, include hearing assistive technology (HAT), hearing assistance technology system (HATS), assistive listening device (ALD) or assistive listening system (ALS), access technology, remote microphone (RM) technology or remote microphone hearing assistance technology (RMHAT), and wireless accessories.

Hearing deficits in noise have the most significant impact in the early stages of life, particularly when the child is developing foundational speech and language skills (Ambrose, VanDam, & Moeller, 2014; Christakis et al., 2009; Flexer, 2016). HAT for infants and toddlers will most likely be used in places like the home, car, playground, parent/child programs, daycares, and preschools. As children enter preschool and become more mobile and independent, families may identify more advantages of HAT. Preschoolers often use portable touch technology such as cellphones and tablets for entertainment or in the school setting. Connectivity options for their hearing aids and/or implantable devices ensure they are getting the best possible signal at all times no matter where they are. While the purpose of this chapter is to address HAT in relation to children ages 0 to 6 years old in AVT, much of the information on HAT here can apply to individuals

Table 7-1. Terminology

Transmitter	This is worn by the talker. A transmitter sends the signal (e.g., speech, music, other desired sound) to another component called a receiver, which is coupled with the hearing aid or implantable device. The terms "transmitter" and "microphone" or "mic" are often used interchangeably.
Receiver	This is worn by the listener. The receiver accepts the signal from the transmitter and delivers it to the hearing aid or implantable device. RMHAT systems only work when both transmitter and receiver components communicate with each other.
Coupling	Coupling refers to how the technology connects the receiver component to the hearing aid or an implantable device. Coupling may be wireless or wired. As technology miniaturization continues to evolve, more wireless options will become available. Technology that connects two devices with a physical auxiliary cable (and sometimes uses an adapter) may be described as wired or direct audio input (DAI).
Compatibility	Compatibility is the ability for different devices or technologies to work with one another. Some hearing assistive technologies are designed to be universally compatible across devices from different manufacturers, whereas others are proprietary and only work with specific brands and models.
Mixing ratio	The relationship between the external and enhanced sound input relative to the signal received at the environmental microphone on a hearing aid or implantable device is known as the mixing ratio.

throughout their life span. This information is included to allow the reader to imagine future possibilities even if a particular technology is not appropriate in the early stages of life.

REMOTE MICROPHONE HEARING ASSISTANCE TECHNOLOGY

RMHAT is used in situations where distance, reverberation, and competing noise are negatively affecting the ability of a child to attend to and/or understand one talker individually or within a group of talkers. These situations might include AVT sessions where providing optimal auditory input is necessary, in a noisy restaurant with family, or sitting on the couch at home and watching a movie on a mobile device. There are various technologies used by RMHAT that connect an audio signal with hearing aids and implantable devices: frequency modulation (FM), digital modulation (DM), Bluetooth®, intermediary devices (sometimes known as "wireless accessories" or "streamers"), induction, infrared (IR), and direct audio input (DAI). While FM and DM systems are most commonly used in young children, Bluetooth and intermediary devices/streamers offer additional options as the child becomes older. With RMHAT, the microphone is typically worn 4 to 6 inches away from the talker's mouth. This is comparable to a talker speaking 4 to 6 inches away from the child's hearing aid or implantable device, which means the talker's voice will be more robust, clearer, and louder than the competing background noise. Because the microphone travels with the parents and/or daycare teacher and the distance from the talker's mouth to the microphone does not change, the effects of distance are also ameliorated.

One disadvantage to RMHAT is that listeners cannot hear people as well if they are not speaking into the microphone, or when they are "off mic," even if the environmental microphone on the hearing aid or implantable device is active. For this reason, it is important for speakers to repeat questions.

Table 7–2 is a reference for the many connectivity options for hearing aids and implantable devices using a remote microphone, phone and cellphone, media device, television, and sound systems.

Frequency Modulation and Digital Modulation

FM and DM systems are forms of RMHAT and both consist of two components: a transmitter (or microphone) and a receiver. They are the most popular types of RM technology used with young children as these technologies

have the ability to improve the audio signal over the barriers of distance, noise, and reverberation. These systems can broadcast a signal over a long range (generally 50 to 70 feet) and to numerous receivers if they are on the same channel (FM) or network (DM).

FM and DM systems have similar functions but differ in the technology used to transmit the signal. *FM systems* are considered older technology, having been used for decades, and use analog transmission, similar to the technology used in a car radio. Like a car radio that needs to be set to a certain station with the tuning knob, FM transmitters and receivers need to be on the same channel or frequency. If the channel/frequency is too close or if there are multiple transmitters in the room, channel interaction can occur and listeners might hear someone else's transmitter nearby or electrical interference. *DM systems* are newer technology, developed in the past 10 years, and use digital transmission that allows for simultaneous processing and calculations of additional information compared with FM. "Frequency hopping" is a method in DM systems that eliminates the chances of channel interaction because it uses the versatility and speed of digital processing to constantly switch frequency channels in a predetermined pattern while keeping the transmitter and receiver in communication with each other. In today's world with various electronic sound sources, children need a variety of options for connectivity.

FM and DM systems improve the SNR by systematically scanning the listening environment and providing an amplified signal through the transmitter with respect to the varying levels of background noise. Some systems use a

Table 7–2. Hearing Assistive Technology Listening and Connectivity Options

	Source of the Audio Signal				
	Remote Microphone	(Cell) Phone	Media Player (e.g., tablet, game console, laptop)	TV	Sound System (e.g., movie, live theater)
Original audio signal					
Direct to environmental Microphone on HA/CI/BAHS		•	•	•	
To headphones (wired or Bluetooth) then env mic		•	•	•	
To external speaker (wired or Bluetooth) then env mic	•	•	•	•	•
Induction					
Direct to T-coil setting on HA/CI/BAHS		•	•	•	
Bluetooth to amplified neckloop to T-coil		•	•	•	
Bluetooth to induction earhooks/HATIS to T-coil		•	•	•	
Room loop (large area) to T-coil	•		•	•	•
Personal loop (small area) to T-coil			•	•	
FM or DM to neckloop receiver to T-coil	•		•	•	•
Infrared to neckloop receiver to T-coil	•			•	•
Intermediary device/streamer					
FM or DM to int device to HA/CI/BAHS	•		•	•	•
Bluetooth to int device to HA/CI/BAHS	•	•	•	•	
Direct audio input					
Aux cable plugged into source and HA/CI/BAHS		•	•	•	
Aux cable plugged into source and FM or DM transmitter to FM or DM receiver	•	•	•	•	•

fixed-gain approach, where the loudness level of the signal is a constant set amount above the background noise (e.g., the FM system will ensure that the signal has a +10 SNR). Other systems use an adaptive-gain approach, where there is a set SNR for lower level noise, but once noise reaches a certain loudness level (also known as a "kneepoint"), the SNR increases to a higher level (e.g., +15 SNR) to help the listener hear better in louder background noise. A child may do well in situations where there is moderate background noise (e.g., 55 dBA) but may really struggle in environments where the noise is louder, like in a cafeteria—an adaptive-gain system is advantageous in this environment. Studies have compared cochlear implant users' speech understanding in noise with adaptive and fixed-gain remote microphone systems. Wolfe et al. (2009) discovered that cochlear implant users experienced improvements up to 50 percentage points when using adaptive remote microphone technology in moderate-to-high levels of noise compared with fixed-gain devices. Thibodeau (2010) confirmed these findings, and through subjective report, found that most users preferred the adaptive systems over the fixed-gain devices.

Some FM and DM systems also have data-logging capabilities. If enabled by the programming audiologist, information such as how and when the transmitter is being used, overall ambient noise levels present when the microphone is active, as well as providing a record of monitoring activities, are able to be analyzed. This information can be invaluable to determine if, for example, there are certain times of the day when the microphone is not being used appropriately, or if there is a malfunction. It can help not only the audiologists and practitioner to gain information about the consistency of HAT use and the listening environment where the child spends most of his/her time, but will also give parents a better understanding of how to use RM technologies most advantageously. For example, if the child tends to act out during a certain time of day, data-logging might point out that there is excessive noise at that time. It is an opportunity for parents and AV practitioners to discuss appropriate expectations and strategies to cope in those situations as well as have a discussion with the audiologist about perhaps changing the child's hearing aid settings to compensate for this excessive noise.

Transmitters/Microphones

Microphones can detect sound in a variety of patterns. **Omnidirectional** microphones pick up sound from all directions. **Directional** microphones focus on a fixed point and have a narrower focus. **Adaptive directional** microphones can be arranged in a cluster, straight line, or circular array of multiple microphones which automatically or manually detect a primary signal/voice and adjusts the beam-forming capabilities of the microphones to focus on that signal. There are also transmitters that contain accelerometers that can automatically switch to a directional mode when pointed at or worn by a talker, and then switch to an omnidirectional or adaptive directional mode when placed on a flat surface.

There are different wearing styles for microphones. **Lavalier** microphones are secured on a special lanyard and worn around the neck. **Lapel** microphones can be clipped onto clothing.

For these first two styles, it is important that the microphone is located at the midline of the body, about 4 to 6 inches away from the speaker's mouth and not in contact with items like jewelry or other lanyards that can strike the microphone by accident (Leavitt & Flexer, 1991). Unless an adaptive directional system or boom microphone is being used, the microphone signal will be less robust if the speaker turns his/her head, since that person would not be speaking directly into the microphone anymore. Lavalier and lapel microphones are the most common styles worn both in home and school settings due to ease of use. **Boom** microphones look like what singers use on stage and are worn along the side of the cheek and are plugged into the transmitter. This style of microphone does not have the problem of a degraded signal with head turns because the mic moves with the entire head and is always in front of the speaker's mouth. While this style of microphone is recommended for the best possible signal, it should be noted that the boom style can be uncomfortable because there is a headband, and teachers, for example, are more resistant to using this style. **Wand** microphones can point at what the speaker or listener wants to be heard but may be more appropriate for older children who are more independent with their equipment and have sufficient self-advocacy skills to control their listening environment. With this style, it is possible that the child may be pointing the mic at a talker but then another talker starts talking with the child unaware. In this situation, educating the talkers to raise their hand or wave to show that they are talking would be necessary. **Pass-around** microphones are hand-held and used as an additional mic for situations such as group activities where there is a main talker using a primary transmitter/microphone and peers or perhaps another teacher speaking at select times. One advantage to this style is that the child knows who is talking because the talker is holding the microphone. Lastly, some microphones are multi-functional and can be used in more than one style. For example, a microphone worn on a teacher's lapel during direct instruction can be removed and put in the middle of the table to function as a table mic during snack time.

Receivers

Just as there are different styles of transmitters/microphones, there are different styles of receivers. **Universal receivers** are external and plug into an adapter that is coupled to a hearing aid or implantable device. They can also be directly plugged into an intermediary device that sends the signal wirelessly to a child's hearing aid or implantable device. This added weight and length may not be appropriate for young children with smaller ears, since it may cause the hearing aid or implantable device to fall off. Some universal receivers have LEDs to indicate function (e.g., not connected/connected). They also can be easily transferred from one personal device to another as long as an appropriate adapter is available. This is helpful if the child has to upgrade the hearing aid or transition using a cochlear implant because the same universal receiver can be used. **Dedicated receivers** do not require any kind of adapter, are integrated into the battery compartment, and are smaller and lighter in size than universal receivers. They are designed to only work with specific brands and models of hearing aid or cochlear implant, meaning they are proprietary. This is an extra financial burden for preschools if the child leaves and that receiver does not fit anyone else's hearing aid or implantable device. An ***integrated receiver*** is built directly into the circuitry of a hearing aid or implantable device, transferring the functionality of a universal receiver to an internal receiver on the hearing aid computer chip via an external interface, or to an "installer" and firmware upgrade. Because there is no external receiver to add to the size and weight of a hearing aid or implantable device, this smaller size option can be an excellent option for very young children. One disadvantage is that if either the hearing aid or integrated receiver stops working, the whole device needs to go in for repair, which could leave the child without amplification unless a loaner hearing aid or implantable device is available (Eiten, 2010).

Induction

Induction is a method of transmission where sound that has been converted into an electromagnetic signal is picked up by the ***telecoil*** (also known as ***T-coil***) on a hearing aid or implantable device. When the telecoil is activated, transmission of the signal can happen ***directly***, as in the case of holding a phone up to the hearing aid or implantable device. It can also occur ***indirectly***, where the audio signal first communicates with an intermediary device such as a neckloop (worn around the neck), induction earhooks (hooks that sit on the ear next to the hearing aid or implantable device), or induction loop system (physical loop of copper wire installed around the perimeter of an area), and

then the telecoil program picks up the electromagnetic signal. Intermediary devices are often used to interface with sound sources such as computers, tablets, and mobile devices. Induction loop systems can be installed in a small area (e.g., a favorite chair, part of a living room near a television, taxi cab, a customer service counter) or a large area (e.g., library conference room, sports arena, theater). Induction loop systems are prevalent in Europe but there is a movement in the US promoting the use of this system as well.

For younger children, there is a variety of listening situations where using induction is an option. In a public setting like a room at the local library where a mother/child activity is being held, if there is a hearing loop installed, merely switching to the telecoil setting means that the child will have improved auditory access to the signal without any extra equipment. Using the telecoil setting on a hearing aid or implanted device when using the phone can overcome the problem of feedback because the child is not using/covering his/her environmental microphone. It is also possible to use the telecoil setting with a cochlear implant if the child wants to hear the phone signal only and block out competing environmental sounds.

When in the telecoil setting, it should be noted that hearing aids and implantable devices can be more susceptible to electromagnetic interference so children might report hearing a buzzing sound if they are in a room with an abundance of overhead fluorescent lights, nearby power lines, or electrical equipment like computers.

Conducting a listening check for telecoil function can be complicated. It is possible to listen for telecoil function with a hearing aid; with cochlear implants, however, depending on the make and model of the device, this is not always possible. If considering using the telecoil function, it is important that the AV practitioner and parents ensure that the child learns to be a good reporter of functionality because it may not always be possible to do a traditional listening check.

Lastly, the orientation of a telecoil varies from device to device, meaning that while one child can hear well using his/her telecoil setting in one situation, another child with a different hearing aid or implantable device may not hear as well. This is most evident in situations with room loops or while using neckloop receivers. Children may need to use an external telecoil accessory and tilt their head or move the neckloop to hear the signal better, and that is not ideal. It is important to have a discussion with the child's audiologist to confirm telecoil orientation so that the family and the AV practitioner know which situations work best with any particular child's telecoil orientation.

Neckloop receivers send the FM or DM signal from the transmitter to hearing aids and implantable devices via the telecoil setting. An advantage is that one neckloop receiver can reach both ears, whether bilateral or bimodal, as long as both devices have a telecoil setting. Because it is worn around the neck, this option may not be ideal for very young children who are prone to fidgeting or have sensory issues.

Though not considered personal FM or DM and not easily portable, *classroom audio distribution systems (CADS)* consist of remote microphone(s) and a single or multiple soundfield speakers that are placed strategically in a room. They can be considered receivers, since they take the transmitted FM or DM signal and amplify it for a small or large area to hear. CADS are often used with children who have fluctuating hearing levels or unilateral hearing loss or cannot use ear-level receivers coupled to their hearing aid or implantable device because they are not good reporters if their equipment is connected and functioning. Since the whole classroom would be able to hear if CADS is working or not, it is easier for the teacher to know if the transmitter is communicating appropriately with the receiver/speaker.

Infrared System

An *IR system* picks up sounds from a transmitter and converts the sound from an electric signal to invisible light waves. The light waves are sent from a transmitter (sometimes called an emitter) to a receiver which converts the signal back into acoustic sound which is heard by the listener. The energy conversion is the same technology used in a television's remote control, and similarly, the receiver must be in the line of sight of the transmitter due to the signal's transference by light waves. This means the transmitter will not send signals to a receiver in another room, nor is it sensitive to electrical noise or other transmitting systems. This is an advantage over FM systems because the person wearing the infrared transmitter does not have to be concerned with "bleed over" from room to room and the user does not have to turn the transmitter off when leaving the room—the signal stops at the walls. Infrared transmission also has disadvantages, such as the inability to work around corners or when the pathway between the transmitter and receiver may be blocked. Additionally, these systems cannot be used outside because sunlight interferes with the signal transmission.

Infrared systems are not integrated into hearing aids and implantable devices and thus require an external receiver. These systems are often used with neckloops or headphones in settings that plug into this receiver like a movie or live theater, or with mounted speakers on walls or ceilings in a classroom. Additional disadvantages of infrared systems include difficulty in installment and maintenance, and generally higher costs than other available options.

Bluetooth Technology

Bluetooth is a specific standard used for short-range, low power, wireless connectivity that can be used by a wide variety of devices. For children with hearing loss, this technology can provide access to everyday sound sources such as remote microphones, tablets, cellphones, computers, and game consoles. It is also possible to connect via Bluetooth with a smartphone to access features on a proprietary app such as checking battery life, changing programs or settings, and using geolocation to find a lost hearing aid or implantable device.

Compatible hearing aids and implantable devices which are Made for iPhone (MFi) or Made for Android/ Made for All (MFA) can directly connect to these portable devices via Bluetooth. If the devices are not MFi or MFA, the sound source will take an indirect route. First, it will need to connect with an intermediary device such as a streamer

or amplified neckloop via Bluetooth. Second, the signal is accessed by the hearing aid or implantable device via the telecoil setting (used with an amplified neckloop) or streamer setting. Bluetooth protocol is typically one-to-one, which means that the hearing aid or implantable device can only connect to one Bluetooth-compatible sound source at a time. Occasionally, the user will have to unpair from one device to pair with another device or will have to re-pair devices due to losing a connection, which can result in loss of auditory access due to the time needed to switch devices. A contingency plan and awareness of this situation is necessary in the school setting so that the child does not miss critical auditory information. There are newer Bluetooth protocols and technologies that allow for connectivity to more than one device but require the user to manually switch to this other device. Parents are cautioned to check Bluetooth pairing when sharing a Smart Device with a child, as they would want to deactivate this function before resuming personal use.

Direct Audio Input

Direct Audio Input (*DAI*) involves using an auxiliary cable to directly connect a hearing aid or implantable device with a sound source. If children do not have access to RMHAT, they can still connect to sound sources like computers, tablets, and mobile devices with a headphone jack via DAI. An advantage to DAI is that there is almost no possibility for interference (with the most common source of interference being a short in the wire). One disadvantage is that the user is tethered to the device and most people opt for wireless options when available. For hearing aids, a special battery door or adapter is necessary to accept one end of the auxiliary cable. This male end of this auxiliary cable is three-pronged so you also need a three-pronged female part (commonly known as an "audio-shoe") to accept this connection. The other male end plugs into the 3.5-mm headphone jack of the audio source. For older models of cochlear implant processors, each implant company has proprietary cables that are used with its device. One end of these proprietary cables plugs into a port or receptacle accessory on the implant and the other end plugs into the headphone jack of the audio source. With the advent of more wireless accessories, DAI is not as frequently used.

A message of caution is necessary with cochlear implants and DAI connections because of the special transmission across the scalp from the external implant device to the internal receiver stimulator inside the child's head. Cochlear implants should not be directly connected via DAI to any device that is plugged into the wall. In the event of a power surge, the extra current could enter the building, travel through the hard-wired electrical circuitry, through the DAI cable, and damage a child's external cochlear implant processor and, on rare occasions, traverse the scalp and damage the cochlear implant's internal device and perhaps cause a serious injury. It is highly recommended that an auxiliary cable with surge protection be used if the cochlear implant is going to be plugged directly into a device such as a desktop computer that also plugs into a wall outlet.

Similarly, DAI should not be used with portable devices (e.g., cellphone, tablet, laptop) without surge protection while these devices are plugged into the wall.

Integration of HAT with Hearing Aids and Implantable Devices

Access to RM systems should always be a consideration when hearing technology is recommended and fit. Current ear-level technology includes a wide variety of options, including hearing aids or implantable devices (including implantable bone-anchored hearing systems, or BAHS), and contralateral-routing-of-the-signal (CROS) devices. A child may have the same devices on each ear (referred to as "bilateral") or a combination of implantable devices and a hearing aid or CROS receiver on the contralateral ear (referred to as "bimodal"). Both hearing aids and cochlear implants will facilitate improved hearing performance across many environments compared with residual hearing alone (Tharpe & Seewald, 2016); however, as stated previously, reverberation, competing noise, and increasing distance between sound source and listener will reduce the child's access to speech sounds even with the use of these interventions (Anderson & Goldstein, 2004; Anderson, Goldstein, Colodzin, & Iglehart, 2005). Not only do the effects of noise and poorly managed classroom acoustics affect speech perception, but evidence suggests that these potential deficits can affect a child's psychoeducational and psychosocial outcomes (Crandell & Smaldino, 2000). Thus, the importance of hearing assistance technology in the child's holistic success is emphasized.

A consideration with bimodal technology and HAT connectivity is that the cochlear implant and hearing aid must both be compatible with the wireless accessory it may be sharing. At the time of writing this chapter, Cochlear has a collaboration with ReSound, and Advanced Bionics and Phonak are owned by the same parent company, so they are able to share a common streaming device. While MED-EL does not currently have a hearing aid partner, the devices have connectivity options if using an FM or DM system which can reach both the cochlear implant and hearing aid.

For individuals with modern cochlear implant devices from Cochlear, a compatible contralateral ReSound hearing aid can benefit from binaural streaming of the signal through a hearing assistance device. Both devices are compatible with Cochlear's Mini Microphone 2+, universal receiver when paired with Cochlear's Mini Microphone 2+, and Cochlear's Personal Neckloop System. Additionally, with the newest technology, users will be able to access all compatible accessories available from ReSound. All modern Cochlear sound processors have an ear-level FM and DM system option from Phonak available, depending on the sound processor model. Cochlear and ReSound devices are also capable of direct streaming to both Android and Apple devices (Cochlear Limited, 2018).

Children with a modern Advanced Bionics (AB) sound processor and a compatible Phonak hearing aid are able to achieve binaural streaming as well. The hearing aid and cochlear implant sound processor can take advantage of the same HAT and automatic features in dynamic listening environments. Devices from both manufacturers are compatible with the Phonak Roger™ System, Phonak ComPilot accessories, and phone accessories. The Phonak Roger System accessories can provide binaural streaming through on-ear receivers and clip-on or remote microphones. A wireless remote microphone or a neckloop version of Phonak's ComPilot may also be selected to achieve binaural streaming for the child. If needed, both hearing aid and sound processor may receive binaural streaming from any smartphone device via Phonak's EasyCall accessory (Advanced Bionics, 2004, 2016, n.d.).

Modern MED-EL cochlear implants are compatible with Phonak's Roger system. The Roger 21 dedicated receiver slips over the processor's battery compartment and is compatible with the various Roger transmitter options. The latest MED-EL sound processors are also compatible with the AudioLink, a remote microphone with universal connectivity. Earlier sound processors, however, must be coupled with the FM battery pack available from MED-EL to be compatible with the Roger platform. It should also be noted that sound processors without a behind-the-ear component must connect a wireless receiver, such as the Roger X, to the Mini Battery Pack provided by MED-EL to be compatible with the Roger accessories (MED-EL, n.d.).

Through bone conduction, BAHS achieve the transmission of sound from the external environment to the inner ear through vibrations of the bones of the skull. Like other device users, individuals with BAHS report difficulty when listening in noise and on the phone (Stephens, Board, & Cooper, 1996). Minimal research is available describing the benefits of HAT with this population. BAHS available from Cochlear, called bone-anchored hearing aids (BAHAs), are compatible with the Mini Microphone 2+, universal receiver when paired with the Mini Microphone 2+, and Cochlear's Personal Neckloop System (Cochlear Limited, 2018). MED-EL's Samba processor has the option of the miniTek, a device that can stream audio to the device through Bluetooth. The miniTek can wirelessly transmit the signal from a remote microphone to the child's device. However, other MED-EL BAHS can only be connected to FM systems via MED-EL's audio cable (MED-EL, n.d.). Lastly, modern Oticon Medical BAHS are also compatible with assistive devices and wireless technology. The Oticon Medical Streamer is an assistive device that is designed with a built-in telecoil and can act as a remote microphone or FM system for most sound processors. The latest sound processors from Oticon Medical are fully wireless and can seamlessly connect with the user's internet-enabled devices when using the Oticon phone application. Therefore, these users will not require the Oticon Medical Streamer (Oticon, 2015, 2019).

Hearing assistance technology will continue to evolve with advancements in hearing instrument technology. It is critical that practitioners understand current device options and be aware of future advances as they become available. Parents and practitioners may contact the child's audiologist or reference manufacturer publications to stay up-to-date with new technology options and to confirm that technologies are compatible with each other.

ASSISTANCE DEVICES

Assistance devices refers to any device, system, or technical service that provides access to an individual who is deaf or hard of hearing. This technology does not enhance direct communication between a child and the speaker in the same way as a remote microphone, but can still contribute value to a family's ability to communicate with their child (in the case of alerting or warning devices) or facilitate the development of spoken language skills (in the case of Smart Device applications). Additionally, these technologies can provide opportunities for the child to develop independence.

Alerting and Warning Devices

There are times when hearing aids or implantable devices are being repaired or when they are not being worn (e.g., sleeping, taking a bath). With or without amplification or electrical stimulation via implantation, it is vitally important to be aware of safety alerts. As young children who are deaf or hard of hearing grow and mature, the use of alerting or warning devices not only provide improved safety, they promote environmental awareness and independence. Devices can be simple and single function such as an alarm clock with a very loud audible signal, or they may have multiple functions such as very loud alarms with built-in flashing lights or bed shaker attachments when the doorbell rings or there is a baby crying. Other systems have remote receivers so one can keep the main system at the bedside with the bed shaker and have a remote system in the living room connected to a lamp that flashes or a body-worn pager that vibrates. There are also stand-alone fire/smoke or carbon monoxide detector systems that have a strobe light or a bed shaker attachment, or a special low-pitched and very loud tone. Some local fire departments may distribute these free of charge. Otherwise, there are online vendors that have these specialized products.

Regardless of alerting devices present in the home, *a family emergency plan is necessary* when someone in the family has a hearing loss. In an emergency, there may not be time to grab hearing aids or implantable devices. The child will have great difficulty without his or her hearing technologies, especially if the emergency is at night. A serious discussion of the emergency plan is imperative ahead of time so that everyone knows what to do and the child understands all the instructions. The practitioner can help families develop emergency plans and perhaps help determine appropriate and accessible alerting devices.

Smart Device Applications

Greater opportunities for access, independence, and mobile learning have come with *Smart Devices* like cell phones, tablets, and their accompanying apps. Their portability, easy manipulations with swipes, taps, and pinches make them very appealing due to their multi-modal capabilities. In addition, using Smart Devices can be instantly stimulating with games, movies, and engaging colors and displays. There are many apps specifically designed to foster learning. Couple these advantages with the fact that they are widely adopted in today's society, and it is evident they are powerful tools.

Conversely, there are concerns about using Smart Devices with young children, and their effect on cognitive, language, and emotional development. However, "research regarding the impact of this portable and instantly accessible source of screen time on learning, behavior, and family dynamics has lagged considerably behind its rate of adoption" (Ambrose et al., 2014; Radesky et al., 2015). General guidelines based on age can be found in the "Family Media Plan" tool, developed by the American Academy of Pediatrics (https://www.healthychildren.org/En glish/media/Pages/default.aspx). Especially for children under age 2, these devices should not become electronic parents, babysitters, or teachers or used by the child in isolation. Parents should limit the time that children above the age of 2 use this technology sparingly.

There are several features on Smart Devices that make them accessible to children who are deaf or hard of hearing. Front-facing cameras can provide more opportunities for lipreading for those children who need a visual reinforcer when communicating with relatives and friends through videochat apps, such as making a Sunday "phone" call to grandparents. Although the sound quality of a Smart Device may not be optimal (e.g., not loud enough, playing in a complex listening environment), the practitioner and parent can use their own voices to repeat what was misheard or to provide the linguistic support for what is happening on the screen.

Most television and movie streaming apps now have the ability to display closed captions or subtitles. Studies have shown that reading captions while watching/listening to digital media, especially if it is a topic that is interesting to the reader, can improve literacy (Lindenbarger, 2001).

Selecting Apps for Learning Experiences

When determining whether an app is appropriate for a child, the practitioner and parent should consider features and questions such as: Does it fulfill a therapy goal such as expanding vocabulary, a higher-level auditory task, or self-advocacy? Does it have features that are accessible for the child, like being able to turn text on/off for working on reading? Does it have record keeping options so that one can track progress and data? Will it engage my child? How can I best use this app interactively with my child?

Buying apps can be cost prohibitive, but there are opportunities to get apps free or at reduced prices. Anecdotally, popular times for app sales seem to be April/May and September/October/November, which surround events that promote speech, language, and hearing awareness. Social media and developer websites also provide information about sales, and parents can sign up for developer e-newsletters. Social media can also be used to preview apps in action and view online tutorials. There are also sites that categorize apps by Individualized Education Plan (IEP) goals and video channels that demonstrate the app. AV practitioners and parents can check with regional special education departments to see if there are any opportunities to buy apps in bulk, which can also reduce the price.

At http://bit.ly/Apps4HL-iOS and http://bit.ly/Apps4HL-Android, one can find lists entitled "Apps for Kids (and Adults) with Hearing Loss" for iOS and Android platforms, respectively, which are updated several times per year. The apps are grouped into categories including: Accessibility, Advocacy, Audiology, Classroom Tools, Hearing Test, Listening Therapy, Media Player, Personal Amplifier, Sound Level Meter, Speech/Language, and Telecommunication. The most popular and populated category is Listening Therapy. Here, parents and therapists can find ideas for engaging apps for working on specific auditory skills.

As children become older, they may be able to take advantage of apps to become more independent. Coupling their Smart Devices, apps, and HAT, they might work on listening to audiobooks or watching videos online (with and without captions). There are apps that connect via Bluetooth to portable bed shakers so they can work on waking themselves up without parent intervention. Speech-to-text apps can help during communication breakdowns (a list of recommended speech-to-text apps can be found at http://bit.ly/SpeechToTextOptions). New apps are being developed every day, so the possibilities are vast.

Selecting a Phone

Parents often have questions about which phones work best with hearing aids and implantable devices. Currently, all wireline and a percentage of wireless phones are required by the Federal Communications Commission (FCC) in the USA to be "hearing aid compatible (HAC)." HAC phones have strong induction signals and are less likely to have microphone interference when used in hearing aids and implantable devices. All wireline phones (sometimes known as "land line" phones) are required to be HAC and in 2020, phones that use Voice Over Internet Protocol (VOIP) will be required to be HAC as well. In order to hear best on a cellular phone, families will want to look for an HAC rating of M3 or M4 (indicates microphone strength) and T3 or T4 (indicates telecoil strength). If the child's environmental microphone is worn higher above the ear, they may benefit from a longer phone so they do not have to move the earpiece up to the environmental microphone and then back down to speak into the mouthpiece. Younger children also benefit from M3/M4 phones when used in speakerphone mode, since the signal is louder and parents and AV practitioners can listen in on the conversation to check for comprehension.

SELECTION, USE, AND VERIFICATION OF HAT IN CHILDREN

In order for children who are deaf or hard of hearing to receive optimal benefit from HAT, consistent collaboration among the parent(s) and the adults who provide intervention or care for their child needs to take place. In most cases, it's usually the AV practitioner who makes the determination if HAT could be beneficial for the child based on hearing the parents' weekly reports of the child's auditory functioning

within the family's daily environment. This determination is on an individual and situational basis. The clinical audiologist then discusses choices for HAT with hearing aid or implantable devices with the family. After a determination of which HAT device is most appropriate, the audiologist proceeds to dispense and/or fit the HAT. It is usually the audiologist who explains to parents how the HAT works, how it can be maintained, and how to troubleshoot. The practitioner and parent(s) usually educate the child's other family members, teachers, and/or those of the multidisciplinary intervention team on the appropriate usage of HATs. Audiologists, parents, AV practitioners, and/or teachers usually connect or "pair" the HAT with the child's hearing aid or implantable device at home, in AVT sessions, or daycare or preschool and troubleshoot the HAT whenever necessary. Instructions for connecting the device to the HAT vary, based on manufacturer. It is incumbent on the audiologist and practitioner to remain knowledgeable about device connectivity options. Finally, most pediatric audiologists will disable program controls due to the possibility of children unintentionally changing settings, meaning these changes may have to be done by an adult with a remote control.

HAT Selection

Considerations in device selection include children's age and developmental skills, technology and connectivity options available on their hearing aid or implantable device, the setting where access is needed, possible sensory issues, and the parents' technological savvy.

Determining which style of receiver to use with a child depends on several other factors, such as: compatibility with the child's hearing aid or implantable device, added size, monaural or binaural transmission, need for LED indicators, and portability.

Deciding between a personal remote microphone and CADS can be a challenge, particularly when the decision is being funded by the educational system. Although a costly option, studies have indicated that personal remote microphones yield the greatest increase in SNR compared with personal desktop systems and soundfield systems (Anderson & Goldstein, 2004; Anderson, Goldstein, Colodzin, & Iglehart, 2005; Wolfe et al., 2013). Logically, this makes sense as the signal will directly be delivered to the listener, not traveling through the air as with speaker systems. To confirm this idea, a meta-analysis conducted by Schafer and Kleineck (2009) compared the performance of each of these systems: personal, personal desktop, and soundfield systems. Across the studies included, soundfield systems produced insignificant improvements in speech understanding compared with conditions with cochlear implants alone. However, speech recognition improved by about 17% when using personal desktop systems and by about 38% when using the personal system, both compared with cochlear implants alone. This information can be particularly useful when determining devices that may be best suited for this population on an individual basis.

It should be noted that simultaneous delivery of the signal from the HAT to both worn devices will achieve optimum benefit, as described earlier in research describing speech understanding in noise. Children with hearing loss will have improved speech recognition in noise with the signal routed to both devices compared with conditions with no assistance technology or with monaural signal delivery (e.g., Schafer & Thibodeau, 2006).

Before purchasing any kind of equipment, one should see if there are opportunities to "try it before you buy it." Local clinics or hospitals, university-based audiology programs, vendors with demonstration rooms, centers for independent living, and consumer event exhibit halls are all places where one could touch and play with a piece of technology before purchasing it. Many HATs have a return policy that should be considered prior to purchase.

In addition to the options described in this chapter, parents and practitioners need to be aware that using no HAT is acceptable, and sometimes preferred, in certain situations. For example, HAT may not be appropriate in a classroom during independent play or center-based activities when the child is interacting with peers. Young children should also work on spontaneous listening skills such as hearing their parent's voice in quiet, in noise, at a distance, listening to music coming through the car speakers, having a conversation in a noisy restaurant—all by hearing sounds that enter the environmental microphone on their hearing aid or implantable device. Use of ear-level HAT could also be contraindicated if children have not yet bonded to their primary hearing aid or implantable device, since they will not likely be good reporters if their equipment is working or not. If RM systems are added to this scenario, chances are the child will reject the equipment. Therefore, decisions to use or not use HAT can vary depending on the situation.

Due to inherent differences between acoustic stimulation with hearing aids and electric stimulation of cochlear implants, the default gain of assistive listening devices may be inappropriate for cochlear implant users (Tharpe & Seewald, 2016). Most remote microphone manufacturers offer instructions to adjust receiver settings in order to provide adequate gain and enhance patient performance. Additionally, enabling of certain advanced features in cochlear implant programming may positively influence individuals' speech understanding when using assistive listening devices (Wolfe et al., 2009, 2015). These considerations should be discussed with the child's audiologist.

Educating Parents, Teachers, and Other Professionals

Just as a team of individuals play a role in maximizing access of spoken language for children who are deaf or hard of hearing, these individuals are responsible for appropriate usage of HAT. Not only AV practitioners and clinical and educational audiologists, but parents, educators, daycare workers, coaches and instructors, and other individuals contributing to a child's language development need to be educated on when and how to use HAT. For very young children, adults have exclusive control of the microphone. Adults involved with the care of children who are deaf or hard of hearing should be educated that the use of HAT would be appropriate any time a child would benefit from improved SNR, particularly during AVT

sessions, at school, at home, in the community, during outdoor activities, in the car, or when listening to a sound source such as a computer or tablet. Another potential use of RM systems is to have children talk into the microphone themselves during an AVT session or in the classroom to help them monitor or detect their own produced speech sounds. As children become more independent, they may choose to change styles of microphones to something like a multi-function or table mic so they can hear their peers better in small group work. They may also develop the ability to switch programs in different listening environments. Over time, adults should encourage children to develop self-advocacy skills regarding their devices and HAT. Table 7–3 lists some tips for teachers who are using RMHAT for the first time or need a refresher. Table 7–4 lists some red flags to consider if concerned about a student's hearing.

For young children, the default mixing ratio set by the audiologist is to be equal (i.e., the input level from a DM system would be the same as the sound received at the hearing aid environmental microphone) so that they have access to environmental sounds, hearing their own voice and opportunities for incidental learning when overhearing others. Under age 2, it is possible that adding an FM or DM receiver will make their hearing aid or implantable device difficult to wear due to size and weight. For the most part, children of this age only need RM systems in "listening environments in which communication would be difficult or impossible without a remote microphone" (Eiten, 2010). These situations include when the child needs to be listening to environmental sounds (such as playing with peers on the playground or during independent play), when the child is communicating with peers for learning (such as center-based play), and when the person with the remote microphone is not intending to speak directly to the child (having a personal conversation or leaving the classroom). Adults using microphone technology should be aware that their voice is being transmitted to the child at all times and should take caution in sensitive conversations or situations while wearing the remote microphone.

Verification of HAT

The goal of fitting and validating HAT is to mitigate the negative effects of noise, distance, and reverberation and provide the child with optimal audibility. When verifying HAT with a hearing aid, it is assumed that the aid is already optimized to meet the audibility needs of the child. To ensure these goals are being met, it is essential that the device function be verified, particularly when

Table 7-3. Tips for Teachers

When to use the microphone:

- when the student needs to hear you or peer(s) or needs to hear an audio signal from a sound source like a computer
- for younger students, it is recommended that an adult facilitates passing a microphone around until the students are able to do it independently.

When *not* to use the microphone (put it on mute):

- when the student does not need to be included in the conversation (e.g., talking to another adult, having a private discussion with another student) or hear environmental sounds (e.g., talker going to the bathroom, going into a different noisy environment)

At the start of every day:

- make sure the equipment is working by:
  - asking the student random questions (e.g., What did you have for breakfast? What color are your shoes? What color is your friend's shirt?) from a distance in auditory-only condition.
  - checking that student is able to detect and discriminate the Ling Six Sounds from a distance in auditory-only condition.

Ensure that:

- there is a designated contact person who will be responsible for the equipment and contact the (educational) audiologist for troubleshooting help.
- there is a designated place for your student to pick up, take off and plug in their equipment. Younger students will need help with this task.

Table 7-3. *continued*

- there is nothing hitting the microphone (e.g., lanyard, jewelry) and that it is being worn in the correct location about 4 to 6 inches from your mouth, toward the center of your body. If worn on the lapel, make sure that the lapel doesn't fold back on itself, since the mic will be pointing at your body instead of your mouth.
- during class discussions, your hand is used to point to who is talking and repeat their name, question or comment. This helps the student to follow the discussion or conversation.
- there is a way to connect the transmitter to a sound source (e.g., computer, tablet) (the (educational) audiologist or teacher of the deaf/hard of hearing can provide guidance).

Caution:

- If you need to raise your voice, understand that the remote microphone system as well as the student's hearing aid or implanted device have a "ceiling," so sounds should never become uncomfortably loud.
- The student will hear the microphone strike a table or desk so please lay it down gently.
- Please turn your head or cover your mouth for any coughs or sneezes.

Table 7-4. Red Flags: When the Child Needs to See an (Educational) Audiologist

Transmitter and receiver are not maintaining a consistent or clear connection
   . . . as reported by the child
   . . . as seen on the transmitter monitoring feature
   . . . as determined by a listening check of the equipment

Changes in baseline or characteristic responses such as:
   Responding to quiet sounds
   Responding to sounds at a distance
   Responding in competing background noise
   Not responding to sounds that they typically have in the past
   Responses to Ling sounds
   Providing answers unrelated to questions asked
   Asking for more repetition

Changes in speech production such as:
   Mixing up, substituting, or omitting sounds (especially at the beginning or end of words)
   Different tonality in their voice
   Louder or softer voice than is typical

working with infants and young children who will not have the skills to report poor functionality. This is when the practitioner's report on the child's auditory functioning with the HAT (and without) is essential for the audiologist to have to support objective verification measures.

SUMMARY

Hearing assistance technology and assistance devices are often necessary to fulfill the principles of AVT, particularly when access to speech cannot be optimized with hearing aids or implantable devices alone. AV practitioners are often the first to evaluate the need for HAT and work collaboratively with audiologists to help parents identify when HAT should be used, how they should be used, and how they can be maintained. The purpose of HAT is to increase the SNR and provide the listener with greater access to speech in a time when these skills are rapidly developing. To do this effectively, practitioners, parents, and educators must understand how HAT can be used and when it is most beneficial. Additionally, practitioners who provide AVT must be knowledgeable about the access technology available to educate parents on maximizing communication and awareness of their listening environment within their family. Using these technologies will not only allow better access to language in a critical period of auditory development, it will allow for opportunities to teach advocacy to families and even children who are deaf or hard of hearing as they gain independence.

REFERENCES

Advanced Bionics (2004). *Hearing with two ears: Technical advances for bilateral cochlear implantation*. White paper.

Advanced Bionics. (2016). *Adaptive Phonak digital bimodal fitting formula: optimizing hearing for listeners with a cochlear implant and contralateral hearing aid*. White paper.

Advanced Bionics. (n.d.). *Connect like never before*. Retrieved from https://advancedbionics.com/us/en/home/products/naida-ci-connect.html

AG Bell Academy for Listening and Spoken Language (2019). *Principles of LSLS certified auditory-verbal therapists*. Retrieved September 16, 2019, from https://agbellacademy.org/certification/principles-of-lsl-specialists/

American Academy of Audiology. (2013). *Pediatric amplification practice guidelines*. Retrieved from https://www.audiology.org/publications-resources/document-library/pediatric-rehabilitation-hearing-aids

American Academy of Pediatrics. (n.d.). *Family media plan*. Retrieved from https://www.healthychildren.org/English/media/Pages/default.aspx

American National Standards Institute/Acoustical Society of America. (2010). *Acoustical performance criteria, design requirements, and guidelines for schools (ANSI/ASA S12.60-2010)*. Melville, NY: Acoustical Society of America.

Ambrose, S. E., VanDam, M., & Moeller, M.P. (2014). Linguistic input, electronic media, and communication outcomes of toddlers with hearing loss. *Ear and Hearing, 35*(2), 139–147. doi: 10.1097/AUD.0b013e3182a76768

Anderson, K. L., & Goldstein, H. (2004). Speech perception benefits of FM and infrared devices to children with hearing aids in a typical classroom. *Language, Speech, and Hearing Services in Schools, 35*(2), 169–184.

Anderson, K., Goldstein, H., Colodzin, L., & Iglehart, F. (2005). Benefit of S/N enhancing devices to speech perception of children listening in a typical classroom with hearing aids or a cochlear implant. *Journal of Educational Audiology, 12*, 14–28.

Bess, F., Tharpe, A., & Gibler, A. (1986). Auditory performance of children with unilateral sensorineural hearing loss. *Ear and Hearing, 7*(1), 20–26.

Boothroyd, A. (1997). Auditory development of the hearing child. *Scandinavian Audiology Supplement, 46*, 9–16.

Boothroyd, A., & Medwetsky, L. (1992). Spectral distribution of /s/ and the frequency response of hearing aids. *Ear and Hearing, 13*(3), 150–157.

Caldwell, A., & Nittrouer, S. (2013). Speech perception in noise by children with cochlear implants. *Journal of Speech, Language, and Hearing Research, 56*(1), 13–30.

Ching, T. Y. C., Day, J., Van Buynder, P., Hou, S., Zhang, V., Seeto, M. . . . Flynn, C. (2014). Language and speech perception of young children with bimodal fitting or bilateral cochlear implants. *Cochlear Implants International, 15*(suppl. 1), S43–S46.

Ching, T. Y. C., Psarros, C., Hill, M., Dillon, H., & Incerti, P. (2001). Should children who use cochlear implants wear hearing aids in the opposite ear? *Ear and Hearing, 22*(5), 365–380.

Ching, T. Y. C., van Wanrooy, E., & Dillon, H. (2007). Binaural-bimodal fitting or bilateral 1 implantation for managing severe to profound deafness: A review. *Trends in Hearing, 11*(3), 161–192.

Christakis, D., Gilkerson, J., Richards, J., Zimmerman, F., Garrison, M., Xu, D., . . . Yapanel, U. (2009). Audible television and decreased adult words, infant vocalizations, and conversational turns: A population based study. *Archives of Pediatric and Adolescent Medicine, 163*(6), 554–558.

Cochlear Limited. (2018). *Wireless technology in the classroom: For Nucleus and BAHA recipients*. Retrieved from https://cochlearlimited.showpad.com/share/RYlZxQYAQFky9iYGro5dX

Cole, E. B., & Flexer, C. A. (2011). *Children with hearing loss: Developing listening and talking, birth to six* (2nd ed.). San Diego, CA: Plural Publishing. Retrieved from http://search.ebscohost.com/login.aspx?direct=true&db=nlebk&AN=675771&site=eds-live&scope=site

Cox, R. M., DeChicchis, A. R., & Wark, D. J. (1981). Demonstration of binaural advantage in audiometric test rooms. *Ear and Hearing, 2*(5), 194–201. doi: 10.1097/00003446-198109000-00003

Crandell, C. (1993). Speech recognition in noise by children with minimal degrees of sensorineural hearing loss. *Ear and Hearing, 14*(3), 210–216.

Crandell, C. C., & Smaldino, J. J. (2000). Classroom acoustics for children with normal hearing and with hearing impairment. *Language, Speech, and Hearing Services in Schools, 31*(4), 362–370. doi: 10.1044/0161-1461.3104.362

Cruckley, J., Scollie, S., & Parsa, V. (2011). An exploration of nonquiet listening at school. *Journal of Educational Audiology, 17*, 23–35.

Cui, T. (2013, July 22). What are the advantages and disadvantages of using induction loops? Retrieved from https://www.audiologyonline.com/ask-the-experts/what-advantages-and-disadvantages-using-11957

Eiten, L. (2010). New developments in FM systems in infants and children. In *International pediatric audiology conference*, [online] pp. 167–177. Available at: https://www.phonakpro.com/com/en/training-events/events/past-events/2010/pediatric-conference-chicago.html [Accessed 3 Sep. 2019]

Fetterman, B. L., & Domico, E. H. (2002). Speech recognition in background noise of cochlear implant patients. *Otolaryngology–Head & Neck Surgery, 126*(3), 257–263.

Flexer, C. (2016). Maximizing outcomes for children with auditory disorders: Auditory brain development—listening for learning. *AudiologyOnline*, 1–8. Retrieved from: http://search.ebscohost.com.ez proxy.memphis.edu/login/aspx?direct =true&db=ccm&AN=124306818&site =eds-live&scope=site

Finitzo-Hieber, T., & Tillman, T. W. (1978). Room acoustics effects on monosyllabic word discrimination ability for normal and hearing-impaired children. *Journal of Speech, Language, and Hearing Research, 21*(3), 440–458.

Firszt, J., Holden, L., Skinner, M., Tobey, E., Peterson, A., Gaggl, W., & Ringe-Samuelson, C. (2004). Recognition of speech presented at soft to loud levels by adult cochlear implant recipients of three cochlear implant systems. *Ear and Hearing, 25*(4), 375–387.

Glista, D., Scollie, S., Bagatto, M., Seewald, R., Parsa, V., & Johnson, A. (2009). Evaluation of linear frequency compression: Clinical outcomes. *International Journal of Audiology, 48*(9), 632–644.

Hansen, M. R., Gantz, B. J., & Dunn, C. (2013). Outcomes after cochlear implantation for patients with single-sided deafness, including those with recalcitrant Ménière's disease. *Otology & Neurotology, 34*(9), 1681–1687. doi: 10.1097/MAO .0000000000000102

Hawkins, D. B. (1984). Comparisons of speech recognition in noise by mildly-to-moderately hearing-impaired children using hearing aids and FM systems. *Journal of Speech and Hearing Disorders, 49*, 409–418.

Hearing Aid Compatibility for Wireline and Wireless Telephones (2019). *Federal Communications Commission.* Retrieved from https://www.fcc.gov/sites/default /files/hearing_aid_compatibility_for_wire line_and_wireless_telephones.pdf

Hicks, C. B., & Tharpe, A. M. (2002). Listening effort and fatigue in school-age children with and without hearing loss. *Journal of Speech, Language, and Hearing Research, 45*(3), 573–584.

Kenworthy, O., Klee, T., & Tharpe, A. (1990). Speech recognition ability of children with unilateral sensorineural hearing loss as a function of amplification, speech stimuli, and listening condition. *Ear and Hearing, 11*(4), 264–270.

Leavitt, R., & Flexer, C. (1991). Speech degradation as measured by the Rapid Speech Transmission Index (RASTI). *Ear and Hearing, 12*, 115–118.

Lewis, M. S., Crandell, C. C., Valente, M., & Horn, J. E. (2004). Speech perception in noise: Directional microphones versus frequency modulation (FM) systems. *Journal of the American Academy of Audiology, 15*(6), 426–439.

Lindenbarger, D. L. (2001). Learning to read from television: The effects of using captions and narration. *Journal of Educational Psychology, 93*(2), 288–298.

Litovsky, R. Y., Johnstone, P. M., & Godar, S. P. (2006). Benefits of bilateral cochlear implants and/or hearing aids in children. *International Journal of Audiology, 45*(suppl. 1), S78–S91.

Maisse, R., & Dillon, H. (2006) The impact of sound-field amplification in mainstream cross-cultural classrooms: Part 1 Educational outcomes. *Australian Journal of Education, 50*(1), 62–77.

MED-EL. (n.d.). *Connectivity.* Retrieved from https://www.medel.com/hearing -solutions/accessories/connectivity.

Nabelek, A. K., & Pickett, J. M. (1974). Monaural and binaural speech perception through hearing aids under noise and reverberation with normal and hearing-impaired listeners. *Journal of Speech and Hearing Research, 17*(4), 724–739. doi: 10.1044/jshr.1704.724

Oticon Medical (2019). Get the Oticon Medical Streamer and connect. Retrieved from https://www.oticonmedical.com /bone-conduction/solutions/accessories /streamer.

Oticon Medical. (2015). Oticon Medical Streamer: Product Information. Retrieved from https://wdh01.azureedge.net/-/media /medical/main/files/bahs/products/om -streamer/pi/eng/product-information

-oticon-medical-streamer---english---15 3634.pdf?la=en-us&rev=5F84.

Phonak Communications AG. (2014). Phonak Roger inspiro: User guide. Retrieved https://www.phonak.com/content/phonak/us/en/support/product-support/accessories/roger-inspiro/_jcr_content/par/downloads_0/productdownloadspar/download/file.res/User_Guide_roger_inspiro_029-0264.pdf

Phonak Communications AG. (2017). Phonak Roger Touchscreen Mic: User guide. Retrieved from https://www.phonak.com/content/dam/phonak/gc_se/en/solution/accessories/roger_technology/documents/User_Guide_Roger_Touchscreen_Mic_GB_V1%2000_029-3222-02.pdf

Radesky, J., Miller, A. L., Rosenblum, K. L., Appugliese, D., & Kaciroti, N. (2015) Maternal mobile device use during a structured parent-child interaction task. *Academic Pediatrics, 15*(2), 238–244.

Schafer, E. C., & Kleineck, M. P. (2009). Improvements in speech-recognition performance using cochlear implants and three types of FM systems: A meta-analytic approach. *Journal of Educational Audiology, 15*, 4–14.

Schafer, E. C., & Thibodeau, L. M. (2003). Speech recognition performance of children using cochlear implants and FM systems. *Journal of Educational Audiology, 11*, 15–26.

Schafer, E. C., & Thibodeau, L. M. (2004). Speech recognition abilities of adults using cochlear implants interfaced with FM systems. *Journal of the American Academy of Audiology, 15*(10), 678–691.

Schafer, E. C. & Thibodeau, L. (2006a). Improving speech recognition in noise of children with cochlear implants; Contributions of binaural input and FM systems. *American Journal of Audiology, 15*(2), 114–126.

Schafer, E. C., & Thibodeau, L. M. (2006b). Speech recognition in noise in children with cochlear implants while listening in bilateral, bimodal, and FM-system arrangements. *American Journal of Audiology, 15*(2), 114–126.

Spahr, A. J., Dorman, M. F., & Loiselle, L. H. (2007). Performance of patients using different cochlear implant systems: Effects of input dynamic range. *Ear and Hearing, 28*, 260–275.

Stelmachowicz, P. G., Pittman, A. L., Hoover, B. M., Lewis, D. L., & Moeller, M. P. (2004). The importance of high-frequency audibility in the speech and language development of children with hearing loss. *Archives of Otolaryngology, 130*, 556–562. doi: 10.1001/archotol.130.5.556

Stephens D., Board T., Hobson J., & Cooper H. (1996). Reported benefits and problems experienced with bone-anchored hearing aids. *British Journal of Audiology, 30*(3), 215–220.

Tharpe, A. M., & Seewald, R. (2016). *Comprehensive handbook of pediatric audiology* (2nd ed.). San Diego, CA: Plural Publishing. Retrieved from http://search.ebscohost.com/login.aspx?direct=true&db=nlebk&AN=1283874&site=eds-live&scope=site

Thibodeau, L. (2010). Benefits of adaptive FM systems on speech recognition in noise for listeners who use hearing aids. *American Journal of Audiology, 19*, 1–10.

van Zon, A., Peters, J., Stegeman, I., Smit, A. L., & Grolman, W. (2015). Cochlear implantation for patients with single-sided deafness or asymmetrical hearing loss: A systematic review of the evidence. *Otology and Neurotology, 36*(2), 209–219.

Wolfe, J., Morais, M., Schafer, E., Agrawal, S., & Koch, D. (2015). Evaluation of speech recognition of cochlear implant recipients using adaptive, digital remote microphone technology and speech enhancement sound processing algorithm. *Journal of the American Academy of Audiology, 26*(5), 502–508.

Wolfe, J., Morais, M., & Schafer, E. (2016). Speech recognition of bimodal cochlear implant recipients using a wireless audio streaming accessory for the telephone.

Otology & Neurotology, 37(2). doi: 10.1097 /mao.0000000000000903

Wolfe, J., Morais, M., Neumann, S., Schafer E., Mülder, H. E., Wells, N., . . . Hudson, M. (2013). Evaluation of speech recognition with personal FM and classroom audio distribution systems. *Journal of Educational Audiology, 19,* 65–79.

Wolfe, J., Morais, M., Schafer, E., Mills, E., Mülder, H. E., Goldbeck, F., . . . Lianos, L. (2013). Evaluation speech recognition of cochlear implant recipients using personal digital adaptive radio frequency system. *Journal of the American Academy of Audiology, 24*(8), 714–724.

Wolfe, J., & Schafer, E. C. (2008). Optimizing the benefits of AuriaH sound processors coupled to personal FM systems with iConnectTM adaptors. *Journal of the American Academy of Audiology, 19*(8), 585–594.

Wolfe, J., Shafer, E. C., Heldner, B., Mülder, H., Ward, E., & Vincent, B. (2009). Evaluation of speech recognition in noise with cochlear implants and dynamic FM. *Journal of the American Academy of Audiology, 20*(7), 409–421.

Wolfe, J., Schafer, E. C., Mills, E., John, A. B., & Hudson, M. (2015). Evaluation of the benefits of binaural hearing on the telephone for children with hearing loss. *Journal of the American Academy of Audiology, 26,* 93–100.

8

SPEECH ACOUSTICS AND AUDITORY-VERBAL THERAPY

Helen McCaffrey Morrison

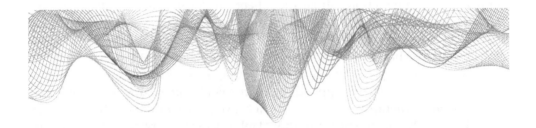

Auditory-Verbal practitioners and families apply speech acoustics to help children learn to comprehend and produce spoken language in a variety of ways. Consider the following scenarios:

- *A child misunderstands what his parents say—Why? Is the topic unfamiliar? Is the vocabulary in the message new or unknown? Is the language too complex? Or are aspects of the message inaudible or not discriminable?*
- *An Auditory-Verbal practitioner is helping a family prepare their child for a birthday party. Together they consider phrases and words the child might need to understand and use in con-*

versation at the celebration. Based on the child's acoustic access with hearing technology, are certain words and phrases going to be easier for a child to learn than others? Will others require more auditory practice?
- *A child produces speech errors— Why? Is he attempting to use language that is above his level in complexity? Is he using unfamiliar vocabulary? Are the errors consistent with developmental expectations for speech production? Does the child have motor difficulties or habits that impact production? Or are the errors a consequence of an inability to hear the speech sound clearly?*

Families and Auditory-Verbal practitioners apply their knowledge about speech acoustics every day to help children comprehend spoken language, to plan experiences for auditory-based language learning, and to help children develop appropriate speech production. Daily application of speech acoustics is second nature to Auditory-Verbal practitioners. This application requires an understanding of speech as sound, general principles of resonance, and the links between the postures and movements of speech production to the resulting acoustic signal. If we know how to produce a speech sound, we can make some predictions about the acoustic characteristics of that sound. Case descriptions throughout this chapter will illustrate how this can be accomplished and how knowledge of speech acoustics might be applied in Auditory-Verbal Therapy.

In its most fundamental form, the speech that children learn to listen to, comprehend, and produce is *sound*. Sound can be described along three dimensions:

- frequency
- intensity
- time

Each of the three dimensions has correlates in human auditory perception. Put simply, we perceive frequency as pitch, intensity as loudness or volume, and time as the duration of a sound. Each dimension can be measured, enabling us to explore how each impacts a listener's acoustic access to speech. The units of measurement presented here are hertz (Hz) for frequency, forms of the decibel (dBSPL or dBHL) for intensity, and milliseconds (msec) for time.

Analyses of the long-term components of conversational speech and the short-term speech components each contribute to our understanding of speech acoustics. Long-term analysis measures the overall intensity and frequency range of connected speech. Short-term speech analysis drills down to the building blocks of speech production and speech acoustics—suprasegmentals, vowels, and consonants. The short-term speech components are described not just by frequency and intensity measures. Speech timing plays a role as well.

The acoustic measures reported here are located in various references (e.g., Kent, Read, & Kent, 1992; Ladefoged, 1996; Ling, 1976, 1988, 2002; Peterson & Barney, 1951; Pickett, 1999). Although these sources are in general agreement, some variation is present as a consequence of differences in the syllables, words, or phrases that are analyzed, speaker groups, and measurement techniques. Unless noted otherwise, this chapter uses values cited by Ling, who consolidated information from seminal sources in his many publications. The figures that appear were created by the author using Praat acoustic analysis software (Boersma & Weenink, 2019).

Readers versed in the speech and hearing sciences may find that some of the following explanations have been simplified and that some aspects of acoustic physics and the mechanisms of speech production are excluded. This is intentional in order to make the material as accessible as possible while remaining accurate so that Auditory-Verbal practitioners, aspiring practitioners, and parents become empowered to apply speech acoustics in everyday life as effectively and efficiently as possible.

THE LONG-TERM COMPONENTS OF SPEECH

Examination of the long-term components of speech focuses on conversational speech in its entirety. The long-term acoustic speech spectrum (LTASS), the speech banana, and the Speech Intelligibility Index (SII) are audiological applications derived from such analyses. The speech banana and SII arise from LTASS findings. Each has been addressed in previous chapters (see Chapters 4 and 5). These topics are reviewed with particular regard to speech acoustics and Auditory-Verbal Therapy.

The LTASS is a measurement of the frequency and intensity range of connected speech (e.g., sentences, paragraphs, conversations). Calculations of the LTASS have been derived from recordings of both male and female speakers, various types of spoken material, different presentation levels and microphone placements, and from a variety of languages (Byrne et al., 1994; Niemoller, McCormick, & Miller, 1974; Stevens, Egan, & Miller, 1947). The LTASS is fairly consistent across speakers, speech material, and language. On average, connected speech ranges in frequency from 100 Hz to 10,000 Hz, and ranges in average intensity from 45 dB SPL for soft speech, through 65 dB SPL for conversational-level speech, and up to 85 dB SPL for loud speech. The mid-frequency range is the strongest, or most intense, frequency area in conversational speech. The LTASS is used as a reference during probe microphone verification of hearing aid fitting to determine that the output of the hearing aid is sufficiently audible to the listener (see Chapter 5).

The speech banana is an LTASS that has been converted from dBSPL values to dBHL, the intensity scale found on the audiogram (Fant, 2004). Speech ranges in average intensity from 25 dB HL for soft speech through 45 dB HL for conversational-level speech, and up to 65 dB HL for loud speech. The mid-frequency range remains the speech region with the strongest intensity. The shape of the LTASS when plotted on the audiogram in dBHL resembles a banana, hence the commonly used term. When auditory thresholds are plotted on an audiogram form that includes the speech banana, one can make some predictions regarding the frequency ranges in speech that have greater audibility for the listener.

The SII (ANSI, 1997) maps the LTASS according to the extent to which frequency bands within the speech spectrum contribute to speech recognition. Not all frequency regions are equally important to speech recognition. Although the greatest intensity in the LTASS is in the mid-frequency region, the greatest contribution to speech intelligibility appears in the region from 1500 Hz through 6000 Hz. The SII is reported as a score that represents the proportion of information in connected speech that is audible to a listener. Frequencies that are more important to speech intelligibility have greater impact on the score. An SII of 0 (or sometimes seen as 0%) suggests that none of the information in the LTASS that contributes to speech recognition is audible. In contrast, an SII of 1.0 (or 100%) suggests that all speech information in the LTASS is audible. The SII can be calculated from the predicted audible portions of the LTASS in probe microphone measures of hearing aid output. Chapter 5 shows a graphic version of the SII for the dBHL audiogram commonly referred to as the "Count-the-dots-audiogram" (Killion & Mueller, 2010). When hearing threshold levels are plotted on the Killion–Mueller audiogram, one can estimate an SII by counting the number of dots that appear at levels above the listener's thresholds.

Although the SII is not a direct measure of speech perception, there is a positive relationship between the SII score and speech recognition. Children require a higher SII, or greater audibility of the LTASS, than adults to reach equivalent levels of speech recognition. Children have a need for greater audibility in the 2000 Hz through 6000 Hz region (McCreery & Stelmachowicz, 2011; Stelmachowicz, Hoover, Lewis, Kortekaas, & Pittman, 2000; Stelmachowicz, Pittman, Hoover, & Lewis 2001). Audibility of the full speech spectrum is essential for children to learn to listen to, comprehend, and produce intelligible spoken language.

The overall frequency and intensity ranges of the speech signal provide just a sketch of what the acoustic speech signal is all about. For a full understanding of speech acoustics for application to Auditory-Verbal Therapy we need to know more about the acoustic building blocks of spoken language, the short-term components of speech.

THE SHORT-TERM COMPONENTS OF SPEECH

The short-term components of speech are those basic elements comprised by connected speech: suprasegmentals, vowels, and consonants. Examination of the long-term components of speech analyzes two of the three dimensions of sound, revealing the overall frequency and intensity of connected speech. The third acoustic dimension—time—is necessary for a complete understanding of the acoustics of the short-term speech components. The temporal dimension of speech (time) is its defining characteristic. Speech is the most quickly changing signal we process to gain information about the world. Most people speak at a rate of 3 to 8 syllables per second (Rafael, 2008) and about 13 phonemes per second (Boothroyd, 2019). Both spectral (frequency) and temporal cues contribute to recognition of speech sounds.

This discussion about the short-term components of speech begins with a description of the types of complex sounds that make up the short-term speech components, followed by the anatomical landmarks in the speech mechanism that play a role in the link between speech production and speech acoustics. The speech sounds referred to here are from English phonology. The principles that link speech production to speech acoustics, however, pertain across languages.

Speech as Complex Sound

Sound is transmitted from the speaker to the listener in the form of a sound wave that propagates across the molecules that make up the atmosphere. The shape of that sound wave varies with the category of sound that is propagated. Sounds fall into two categories based on their frequency content—simple and complex. *Simple* sound, frequently referred to as a pure tone, comprises only one frequency. Simple sounds don't really exist in nature. Simple sounds are generated electronically (or to a limited extent with tuning forks) and are used for such purposes as assessing hearing or conducting auditory research.

The sounds that we encounter in everyday life, including the sounds of speech, are *complex*. Complex sounds consist of more than one frequency. No single speech sound or acoustic aspect of speech production is manifested as a single frequency. Individual speech sounds or other aspects of speech are represented by a range of frequencies, with some frequencies appearing at greater intensity than others, depending upon that particular speech sound.

Complex sound, including speech, can be further categorized as being either periodic or aperiodic. The waveform of a *periodic* sound repeats over the duration of the sound. This is illustrated in Figure 8–1a, which is a display of the waveform of the vowel [u]. There is a repetitive shape to the waveform.

The tonal sound created by musical instruments is periodic. The component frequencies in periodic complex sound are organized in mathematical relationship to one another, which will be discussed below. Vowels and the nasal and approximant consonants are periodic complex sounds.

Aperiodic sounds are of two types, turbulent and transient. Listeners perceive *turbulent* sounds as noisy, hissy, or buzzing sounds. The waveform of the fricative consonant /s/ in Figure 8–1b illustrates the lack of periodicity in turbulent aperiodic sounds. It's just not possible to see a true repetition of the waveform across the duration of /s/ in this figure. *Transient* sounds are very short in duration, like a click, a clap, or the explosion of air that occurs in the production of the plosive consonant /p/, illustrated in Figure 8–1c. The listener perceives transients as short, percussive, or explosive sounds. The range of frequencies found in turbulent and transient aperiodic sounds are fairly wide, meaning that there's a broad range from lower to higher frequencies.

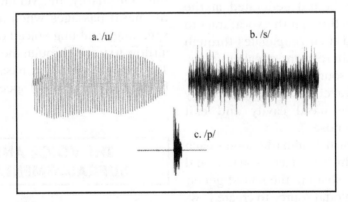

Figure 8-1. Waveforms of complex sound: **(a)** periodic /u/, **(b)** aperiodic turbulent /s/, **(c)** aperiodic transient /p/.

Speech Production as Sound Creation

Speech begins as airflow generated by the lungs and delivered to the larynx. The larynx houses the vocal folds, two membranes stretched across the larynx. The V-shaped opening between the vocal folds is called the glottis. Muscles within the larynx control the vocal folds to open or close the glottis and to thicken or thin the vocal folds by shortening or stretching.

When the vocal folds are almost completely closed, airflow from the lungs causes them to vibrate, which in turn traps and releases airflow from the lungs in puffs of air. Each puff of air is the initiation of a complex periodic sound wave that a listener will perceive as the speaker's voice and serves as the basis of the suprasegmental aspects of speech. The number of puffs generated per second determines the frequency of this periodic complex sound. Alternatively, when the vocal folds are open, airflow from the lungs is sent through the glottal opening as a voiceless, aperiodic complex sound. This serves as the source for voiceless consonants. Sound generated at the glottis flows through the vocal tract to the lips and then propagates through the atmosphere from speaker to listener. Nasal sounds (/m/, /n/, and /ŋ/), however, travel a different pathway through the nasal cavity and exit through the nose.

Anatomical landmarks along each of these pathways act as resonators and articulators, shaping the sound generated at the glottal source to create vowels and consonants. *Resonators* are the adjoining cavities proceeding from the larynx and include:

- the pharynx, the area in the throat that leads from the larynx to the mouth and the nasal cavity,
- the oral cavity, proceeding from the pharynx and leading to the lips, and
- the nasal cavity, also proceeding from the pharyngeal cavity.

Each resonator cavity "tunes" the sound generated at the glottis by permitting some frequencies to pass through the cavity more easily than others. This tuning creates a speech signal that is more intense at some frequency ranges than others. The volume and length of a cavity determine its resonance. Smaller volumes allow higher frequencies to pass through; larger volumes have lower resonant frequencies. Longer cavities pass lower frequencies through with greater strength; shorter cavities resonate to higher frequencies.

Articulators direct voice or airflow to the resonating cavities, change the shape and size of resonating cavities to vary cavity resonance, and constrict or block sound to create turbulent and transient consonants. Articulators include the jaw, tongue, lips, and velum. Ordinarily, the velum closes off the nasal passages when a person is speaking, enabling voiced or voiceless airflow to travel through the oral cavity. The velum opens the nasal passages for production of nasal speech sounds.

THE VOICE AND SUPRASEGMENTALS

Imagine what might be recorded if a microphone were placed at the glottis during voice production. Figure 8–2

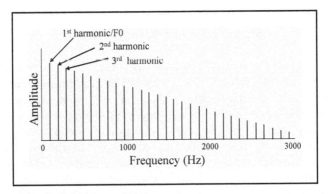

Figure 8-2. Amplitude spectrum of the periodic complex sound (voice) at the glottis showing the fundamental frequency (F0) and harmonics.

illustrates an acoustic analysis of such a recording, displaying the amplitude spectrum of the periodic signal generated at the glottis. Each of the vertical lines in this series of frequencies is called a harmonic. The harmonics are numbered—the first vertical line is the first harmonic, the second line is the second harmonic, etc. The first harmonic serves as the mathematical foundation for the others above it. The frequency of the second harmonic is two times the first harmonic, the frequency of the third harmonic is three times the first harmonic, and so forth. Accordingly, the first harmonic is also called the *fundamental frequency,* or *F0*, to designate it as the mathematical foundation for all the harmonics the lie above.

Average F0 varies with age and gender-related variations in vocal fold size and density that determine the natural frequency of vibration of the vocal folds. On average F0 is 125 Hz (± 1/2 octave) for adult males, 225 Hz (± 1/2 octave) for adult females, and 275 Hz (± 1/2 octave) for children (Ling, 1976, 2002). Adult females using infant-directed speech (aka motherese) and very young chil-

dren may produce F0s as high as 500 Hz. What do we mean by ± 1/2 octave? This is the range for these values, half an octave below the average frequency and half an octave above the average frequency. This range accommodates for the natural variation encountered across speakers due to their biology and the variation that speakers generate during conversational speech production. F0 is perceived by the listener as a speaker's voice. It is the basis for the suprasegmental aspects of spoken language.

Guidance for the Auditory-Verbal Practitioner

A child who can hear from 125 through 250 Hz will be able to detect and discriminate F0. This means that the child can detect the presence of speech or singing, the pauses at the ends of clauses/sentences, and voiced speech sounds (vowels, voiced consonants). He or she will be able to discriminate the following:

■ speaker gender
■ speaker emotion

Making Use of Valuable Time

The parents have arrived at an AVT session with 6-month-old Carlo as a new family. Carlo's audiological assessment indicates that he has a profound hearing loss. He has been fit with hearing aids binaurally. His parents' interpretation of the audiological assessment, probe microphone measures of hearing aid output, and behavioral observations of their baby in soundfield testing while wearing his hearing aids suggest to them that Carlo can hear their voices (F0), with his hearing aids but little more.

Carlo is scheduled to receive a cochlear implant at age 12 months. His parents wonder if there's any value at all to having their son wear his hearing aids prior to cochlear implant activation. The practitioner reassures Carlo's parents regarding the benefit of hearing aid use during this waiting period. The practitioner points out that when Carlo listens to auditory information in the F0 range he is developing his auditory cortex. Carlo's parents are encouraged to sing to him, talk to him using the natural variations in intonational contour that they would naturally use with babies, and provide the simple phrases and words that they might ordinarily use in daily routines. When the practitioner is able to help families take advantage of the available speech cues provided by F0, time waiting for the implant need not be time wasted.

- syllable number (up! *vs* bye-bye)
- duration of syllables or phrases (stop! *vs* gooooo!)
- syllable stress (con' tent *vs* con tent')
- melodies of simple songs

This low frequency information can help a child learn to use his voice to communicate and to control voice pitch, duration, and intensity of vocalizations, some of the earliest vocal behaviors.

VOWELS AND DIPHTHONGS

Vowel Production

English vowels are created by movements along two dimensions: tongue height and the position of the tongue on the front/back dimension in the oral track. Tongue height is controlled by movements of the jaw. When the jaw is lowered, the tongue is naturally in a lower position. Conversely, the tongue is in a higher position when the jaw is raised. The tongue also moves forward or backward like a piston and arches slightly during vowel production. The location of the tongue arch varies within the vocal tract with vowel place. Table 8–1 shows the *vowel quadrilateral*, a chart that displays the relative placement of English vowels on the height and place continua. Vowels are classified on the height dimension as high, mid, or low and as front, central, or back on the place dimension.

Vowel Acoustics

Vowels provide 90% of the intensity in the speech signal. The vowel /a/ (as

Table 8–1. The Articulatory and Acoustic Vowel Quadrilateral

		Back	Central	Front
	F2 in Hz	3000	1000	250
High	250	i (beet)		u (boot)
		ɪ (bit)		ʊ (but)
Mid	**F1 in Hz**	e (bait)		
		ɛ (bet)	ə, ʌ (about) ɔ (bought)	
		æ (bat)		
Low	1000		a (hot)	

277

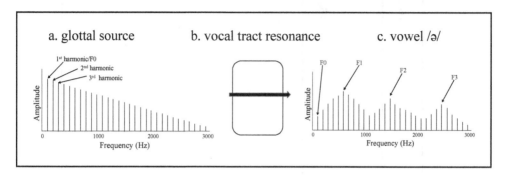

Figure 8–3. Transfer function of the vocal tract showing change in the amplitude spectrum of voice from the (**a**) glottal source, (**b**) shaped by resonant cavities to create (**c**) vowel /ə/ formants.

in "hot") is the most intense of all the English speech sounds. Vowels are longer in duration than consonants and are fairly steady state across the duration of production, meaning that there is little change in acoustics at the central portion of vowel production. Relative intensity, duration, and stability of sound all provide auditory perceptual cues that a speech segment is a vowel. These aspects are cued by the F0.

In order to fully identify a specific vowel, however, a listener must be able to hear the harmonics above F0. The harmonics at the glottis are changed by the time they emerge from the vocal tract, shaped by the pharyngeal and oral cavities, and even by the lips. Cavity resonances enhance some clusters of harmonics and diminish others. The enhanced harmonic clusters are *formants*, with the formant having the lowest frequency identified as F1, the next formant is F2, and so forth. This process, known as the *transfer function*, is illustrated in Figure 8–3. Figure 8–3a shows the amplitude spectrum of the vowel /ə/ (as in "about") at the glottis. Figure 8–3b represents cavity resonance along the vocal tract. Figure 8–3c shows the effects of trans-

mitting the glottal source through the vocal tract. The first 3 formants in the vowel are labeled F1, F2, and F3 in Figure 8–3c. A vowel can have as many as 10 measurable formants. F1 and F2 are the primary formants used by listeners to identify vowel height and place (see also McCaffrey & Sussman, 1994, for a discussion of the roles of F0 and F3 in vowel representation).

Let's take a closer look at the relationship between vocal tract resonances and vowel formants. F1 varies as a consequence of the impact on jaw movement on pharyngeal resonance and, accordingly, provides the acoustic cue for vowel height. F1 appears in the 250 through 1000 Hz range of the vowel spectrum. When the jaw is lowered for the production of low vowels it pushes the base of the tongue into the pharyngeal cavity, making it smaller, passing higher frequencies in the F1 range more effectively than low frequencies in the F1 range. In contrast, the pharyngeal cavity is larger for the production of high vowels (e.g., /u/ as in "who"), passing lower frequencies more effectively. *To summarize, F1 frequency is higher in low vowels and lower in high vowels.*

F2 varies as a consequence of the impact of tongue position in the oral tract and provides the acoustic cue for vowel place. F2 is observed in the 1000 Hz through 3000 Hz range of the vowel spectrum. The distance between the tongue arch and the front of the mouth during production of the front vowel /i/ (as in "ease") is shorter than that during production of the back vowel /u/ (as in "who"). The shorter distance from tongue arch to front of the mouth allows higher frequencies within the F2 range to be passed through more effectively. The longer distance from tongue arch to the front of the mouth for production of /u/ passes lower frequencies in the F2 range more effectively. The lips further enhance F2 as a differentiating cue for vowel place. The English back vowels /u, ʊ, o, ɔ/ are produced with rounded lips. This elongates the oral tract and drives F2 even lower in frequency. Conversely the front vowels /i/ and /ɪ/ are produced with the lips spread as if in a smile. This shortens the oral tract slightly and raises F2 frequency. *To summarize, F2 frequency is higher in front vowels and lower in back vowels.*

The F1 and F2 frequency ranges can be seen on the vowel quadrilateral in Table 8–1. By tracing the movement of F1 and F2 across vowels on the quadrilateral, one can see how F1 and F2 vary with vowel height and place. The speech spectrogram in Figure 8–4 provides further illustration of how formants vary depending on vowel height and place. A speech spectrogram displays all three dimensions of sound—frequency, time, and intensity—in a single picture. The vertical axis is frequency and the horizontal access is duration. Intensity is shown by the darkness of the tracing. Formants show up the darker horizontal or curved bands on the spectrogram because these are the frequency areas of greater intensity in the vowel. F1 and F2 are marked on the vowels in Figure 8–4.

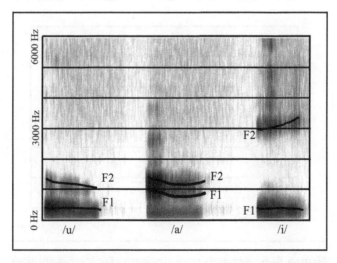

Figure 8-4. Speech spectrogram displaying F1 and F2 in the vowels /u, a, i/.

Figure 8–4 is a *speech spectrogram* of the high back vowel /u/, the low vowel /a/, and the high front vowel /i/. These 3 vowels represent the extremes of vowel height and place. F1 is higher in the low vowel /a/ compared with the high vowels /u/ and /i/. F2 is at the lowest frequency in the back vowel /u/, a bit higher in the central vowel /a/, and then at the highest frequency in the front vowel /i/. Absolute formant frequencies for each vowel vary with speaker age, gender, individual vocal tract characteristics, and the consonant context in which a vowel appears. What remains constant across speakers and contexts, however, is the relationship between F1 and F2. The relationship between *F1 and F2* provides an acoustic cue for *vowel identification*.

Diphthongs

Diphthongs are comprised of two vowels that are produced in succession and perceived as a single speech segment.

American English diphthongs are made up of vowels that *shift in height and place*, e.g., the mid-back to high-front /ɔɪ/ as in "boy," the low-central to high-back /aʊ/ as in "how," the low-central to high-front /aɪ/ as in "high." The acoustic result is a shift in F1 and in F2 over the duration of the diphthong, seen in Figure 8–5, a spectrogram of the diphthongs /aɪ/ (hi), /aʊ/ (how), /ɔɪ/ (hoy). Correct auditory identification of a diphthong requires audibility of F1 and F2 in *both* of the vowels that compose the diphthong and the recognition that these formants are *shifting* in frequency.

Guidance for the Auditory-Verbal Practitioner

A child who is able to access 250 Hz through 1000 Hz with hearing technology should be able to hear F0 and F1. This means that he should be able to (1) detect the presence of vowels, (2) dis-

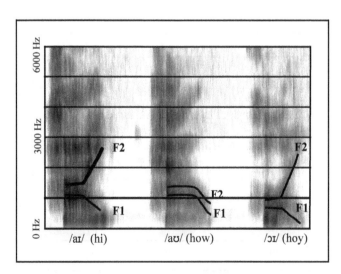

Figure 8-5. Speech spectrogram displaying shifting F1 and F2 in the diphthongs /aɪ/, /aʊ/, /ɔɪ/.

Vowel Sound-Alikes

Three-year-old Ariel and her family have been working with an Auditory-Verbal practitioner ever since she was fit binaurally with hearing aids at age 6 months. At the start of an AVT session, Ariel's parents voiced concerns about her hearing over the previous week. Ariel's practitioner listened to each of her hearing aids and did not find any apparent issues with them. The practitioner then conducted the Ling Six Sound Test. Ariel was not able to discriminate /u/ from /i/, nor could she detect /s/. This was a change from the previous session. The practitioner recommended that the par-

ents see the audiologist as soon as possible.

Audiological assessment indicated that Ariel had experienced a decrease in her hearing and no longer had auditory access to speech with her hearing aids at and above 2000 Hz. As a consequence, /u/ and /i/ sounded alike to Ariel because the F1 frequencies in /u/ and /i/ are almost identical, rendering F2 as an essential cue for discriminating the two vowels. F2 for /i/ was no longer available due to Ariel's decrease in hearing at 2000 Hz and above. Further testing of speech discrimination indicated confusions between /ʊ/ and /ɪ/ for the same reason.

---

criminate vowels that differ in height (e.g., "Pete" *vs* "pot"), and (3) identify some words based on the height of the vowel within the word. The child may be able to imitate or produce vowels along the height dimension, but might also be likely to make errors in vowel place without the added information that is provided by F2. A child who is able to access 250 Hz through 3000 Hz with hearing technology should be able to hear both F1 and F2, enabling discrimination and identification of *all* vowels.

CONSONANTS

Consonants contribute only 10% of the intensity in the speech signal but they make a much larger contribution to speech intelligibility. Consonants are categorized along three dimensions: *manner of articulation, place of articulation,* and *voicing,* as seen in Table 8–2. Con-

sonants are obstruents—airflow from the glottis is obstructed by an articulator. Consonant manner pertains to the way that articulators obstruct airflow, place pertains to the location in the oral tract where that obstruction occurs, and voicing indicates whether or not airflow is generated with vocal fold vibration (F0); *i.e.*, voiced *vs* voiceless consonants. The following descriptions of consonant acoustic characteristics are organized by consonant manner of production. Manner of production encompasses the acoustic signature of a consonant—whether turbulent or transient aperiodic sound is present, the overall frequency range, and the timing characteristics.

Nasals: /m/, /n/, and /ŋ/ (as in "ring")

Nasal consonants are voiced, periodic in sound type, and fairly steady state

Table 8–2. Consonants by Manner, Voicing, and Place

		Labials	Labiodental	Linguadental	Alveolar	Palatal	Velar/Glottal
Nasals	Voiced	m			n		ŋ (ri*ng*)
Approximants	Voiced	w			l, r		j (*yes*)
Plosives/stops	Voiced	b			d		g
	Voiceless	p			t		k
Fricatives	Voiced		v	ð (*th*at)	z	ʒ (measure)	
	Voiceless		f	θ (*th*ink)	s	ʃ (*sh*oe)	h
Affricatives	Voiced					dʒ (*j*u*dge*)	
	Voiceless					tʃ (*ch*air)	

282

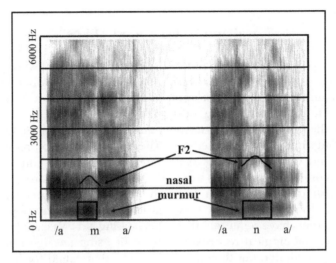

Figure 8-6. Speech spectrogram displaying nasal consonants /m and n/.

across duration of production. The pathway of sound for nasals proceeds from the glottis, through the velar opening into the nasal cavities, and exits through the nose. Sound is obstructed from exiting the mouth by the tongue or the lips at the place of articulation. Nasals consist of a series of harmonics that are enhanced by resonant cavities to create formants. The primary resonators for nasal consonants are the pharyngeal and nasal cavities. The oral tract serves as a secondary resonator that adds resonance to indicate the place of articulation.

F1 in nasals is low in frequency because the jaw is raised, increasing the size of the pharyngeal cavity. Nasal resonance adds even *more* low frequency energy around the F1 region. This resulting strong low frequency region that comprises both F1 and nasal resonance is known as the *nasal murmur*. The nasal murmur serves as a primary cue for identifying nasal consonant manner and ranges from approximately 125 Hz through 250 Hz. Nasal resonance also diminishes high frequency energy, enhancing the perception that nasals are predominantly low frequency speech sounds. Figure 8–6 shows the spectrograms of the nasal consonants /m/ and /n/. The nasal murmur is seen as a dark, thick band at the bottom of the speech spectrogram. The frequency region above the nasal murmur is less intense (lighter in shading) compared with the same frequency region in the consonants that precede and follow the nasal.

Place of articulation is signaled by F2. Nasal F2 tends to be centered around 1000 Hz (± 1/2 octave). The length of the oral cavity behind the place of obstruction for nasal production determines the frequency of F2. The oral cavity is longest when the lips are closed for production of /m/, a bit shorter with tongue obstruction at the alveolar ridge for /n/, and shortest with tongue placement for /ŋ/. As a consequence, F2 is lowest for /m/, a little higher for /n/, and highest for /ŋ/. This can be seen in Figure 8–6. Auditory access through

Nasal and Vowel Sound-Alikes

Vaseem is a 4-year-old boy with a moderately severe hearing loss who was fit with binaural hearing aids at age 18 months. He wears his hearing aids throughout the day, every day. Vaseem and his family have just relocated to a new city and started attending AVT sessions. His original hearing aids were replaced with new ones just a few months prior to moving to their new home. His parents have requested that copies of his audiological records be sent to the practitioner, but they have not yet arrived at the practitioner's office.

At his first AVT session, Vaseem quickly learned to exhibit a detection response to the Ling Six Sounds by placing a ring on a post for each of the six sounds /m, u, i, a, ʃ, s/. The practitioner then started to coach his parents to help him demonstrate an identification response to the Ling Sounds by picking up a toy or prop associated with the presented sound. He learned the task quickly and identified each of the sounds with the exception of /m/ and /u/, which he confused.

Upon further questioning from the practitioner, Vaseem's parents indicated that his current hearing aids were not fit by a pediatric audiologist,
but by a professional who typically fits adults. The practitioner encouraged the parents to find a pediatric audiologist in their new city to assess his auditory access with his hearing aids. The practitioner also provided a list of referrals they might consider.

Vaseem and his parents returned to the practitioner after seeing the pediatric audiologist, who re-programmed his hearing aids. Vaseem had originally been fit using an algorithm for adult listeners that called for less audibility in the low frequencies than recommended for children who are learning to listen and to talk (see Chapter 5). Consequently, the output of the hearing aids was inadequate below 250 Hz and it was difficult for him to hear the full range of the nasal murmur. Although Vaseem had adequate access to *detect* each of the sounds prior to re-programming, he was unable to *discriminate* /m/ from /u/ for two reasons: (1) the nasal murmur and the F1 for /u/ both appear at 250 Hz and (2) F2 for /m/ and /u/ both appear at 1000 Hz (± ½ octave). Re-programming the hearing aids to give audibility at and below 250 Hz provided the information Vaseem needed to recognize that /m/ and /u/ were two different sounds.

2000 Hz should be sufficient for identification of place of articulation for nasal consonants.

Approximants: /w/, /r/, /l/, /j/ (as in "yes")

Approximant consonants are seen on the spectrogram in Figure 8–7. Approximant
consonants are voiced, periodic in sound type, and produced like quickly changing diphthongs. The jaw and tongue both move, shifting F1 and F2 quickly, seen in Figure 8–7. Quickly changing F1 and F2 formant structure provides the acoustic cue for identification of approximant *manner of articulation*. F2 signals the *place of articulation*. F1 tends to center around 500 Hz (± 1/2 octave). F2 tends to

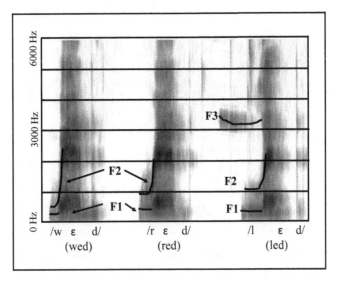

Figure 8-7. Speech spectrogram displaying approximant consonants /w, r, l/.

center around 1000 Hz (± 1/2 octave) and varies with *place of articulation*. The consonants /r/ and /l/ differ in the position and shape of the very tip of the tongue, which impacts oral tract resonance in the F3 region, illustrated in Figure 8–7. F3 for approximants ranges from 2000 through 3000 Hz (± 1/2 octave).

Plosives and stops: /p/, /b/, /t/, /d/, /k/, /g/

Plosives. Plosives appear at the beginning of syllables. Plosives are transient aperiodic sounds produced by a sequence of movements: (1) starting with occlusion of the oral tract that builds up airflow/pressure behind the occlusion, (2) followed by explosive release of the accumulated air pressure, and (3) terminating with movement, or transition, of the articulators into the vowel that follows the plosive. This is illustrated in Figure 8–8. During the occlusion phase there is a *silent gap*,

followed by a brief *noise burst*, seen as a narrow spike that extends vertically across a broad frequency range. Formants emerge after the noise burst, appearing as sloping bands leading from the burst to the vowel. These bands are *formant transitions* created by articulator movement from the consonant into the vowel. The brief amount of time between the noise burst and emergence of the formant transitions is known as the *voice onset time* (VOT), also seen in Figure 8–8.

Each of these acoustic markers for plosive production—the silent gap, noise burst, formant transitions, and VOT—supplies information for auditory identification of plosive consonants. *Manner of articulation* is signaled by (1) the silent gap created in the occlusion phase and (2) the noise burst. The noise burst in plosives ranges from 500 Hz through 4000 Hz (± 1/2 octave), depending upon the plosive. Listeners use either the absence of sound in the silent gap or detection of the transient

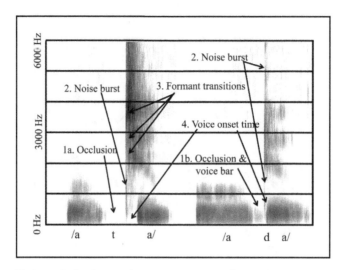

Figure 8–8. Speech spectrogram displaying plosive consonants /t and d/.

aperiodic sound in the noise burst, or both, to identify that a sound is plosive. Listeners whose auditory access to the speech spectrum is limited to 1000 Hz and below may be able to use the presence of silence within the stream of ongoing speech (occlusion phase) plus the low frequency end of the noise burst to identify plosive manner of articulation.

Place of articulation is cued by the noise burst and the F2 transitions from the plosive consonant to the succeeding vowel. The greatest concentration of energy in the noise burst appears around 2000 Hz (± 1/2 octave). The frequency of this energy concentration varies with place of articulation, or the location of plosive occlusion. The starting frequency of the F2 transition also averages around 2000 Hz (± 1/2 octave) and varies with place of articulation of both the plosive consonant *and* the succeeding vowel. Full identification of place of articulation of a plosive consonant requires auditory access to conversational speech through 3000 Hz.

The *voiced/voiceless contrast* in plosives is cued in two ways: (1) the presence of F0 during the occlusion phase of the voiced consonant and (2) the duration of VOT between the consonant and the succeeding vowel. This is illustrated in Figure 8–8. The presence of F0 during the occlusion phase in /ada/ can be seen as light gray shading (#1b in Figure 8–8). This is also known as the *voice bar*. VOT is shorter for voiced sounds than for voiceless sounds. The vowel following the /d/ in /ada/ emerges sooner than the vowel that follows the /t/ in /ata/ (seen as #4 in Figure 8–8). Listeners with auditory access limited to 500 Hz and below may be able to detect the earlier appearance of the vowel and the presence of F0 to discriminate voiced from voiceless plosives. These cues are so short in duration, however, that not all listeners with such limited auditory access will be able to achieve this discrimination when listening to quickly changing conversational speech.

Stops. Stops appear at the ends of syllables. Stops are also produced by an occlusion of the vocal tract, but the release is far less intense and generally not perceptible. The acoustic result is a quick termination of the vowel that precedes the stop consonant. Vowel formants shift as the jaw and tongue move from the position for vowel production into the stop consonant. This creates F1 and F2 formant transitions that are much shorter in duration than that seen in plosives. The F2 transition cues *place of articulation*, averages in the range of 2000 Hz (± 1/2 octave), and varies with the preceding vowel place and the place of articulation for the stop consonant. Auditory access through 3000 Hz is necessary to discriminate among all places of articulation for stop consonants.

The *voiced/voiceless contrast* is cued by the duration of the preceding vowel, longer in voiced stop consonants than in voiceless stops. If a listener has sufficient auditory access to detect vowels, it can be possible to discriminate syllables that terminate in voiced *vs* voiceless stop consonants (e.g., "bed" *vs* "bet").

Fricatives: /f/, /v/, /θ/ (as in "think"), /ð/ (as in "that"), /s/, /z/, /ʃ/ (as in "shine"), /ʒ/ (as in "azure"), /h/

Fricatives make up the largest manner class among the English consonants. The ability to identify /s/ is particularly important for auditory comprehension of English. The /s/ is one of the most commonly appearing consonants and performs several morphologic functions: plurals (cat**s**), possession (Mike'**s**), contraction for "is" (it'**s**), and third person singular verbs (he sit**s**).

Fricatives are turbulent aperiodic sounds that are fairly steady state across the duration of production. A fricative is created by constriction in airflow by an articulator that generates aperiodic noise, illustrated in Figure 8–9. The frequency range of fricative turbulence is

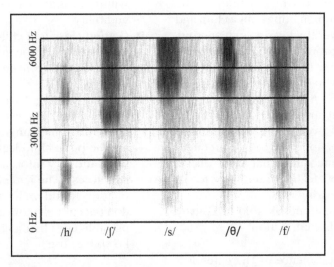

Figure 8-9. Speech spectrogram displaying fricative consonants /h, ʃ, s, θ, f/.

broad and can extend from 1000 Hz through 8000 Hz depending on the fricative consonant. Aperiodic turbulence provides the acoustic cue for identifying fricative *manner of articulation.*

Just as with the production of periodic speech sounds, oral tract resonance enables some frequencies within aperiodic fricative turbulence to pass through more effectively than others. The acoustic result is that some frequency regions within the turbulence for a particular fricative are more intense, while other regions have diminished intensity. The enhanced frequency regions are referred to as the primary frequency region. The range

and primary frequency region of aperiodic turbulence in fricatives are acoustic cues for *place of articulation.* The portion of the oral tract that is responsible for resonance in fricative production is the area in front of the place of constriction. Fricatives with the shortest tract length are those produced at the front—the interdentals /θ/ and /ð/ and the labials /f/ and /v/. Accordingly, these have the highest primary frequency at 6000 Hz (± 1/2 octave). The oral tract area in front of constriction for production of the glottal /h/ is the longest of the fricatives, and the primary resonance for this consonant is the lowest at 1000 Hz (± 1/2 octave).

Keeping High Expectations

Meahgan is a 2-year-old girl who has a severe high-frequency hearing loss and wears binaural hearing aids. She is playing with a little toy dog. Her practitioner leans close to her and starts to pant like a doggie, "hhh-hhh-hhh." Meahgan imitates the practitioner. The practitioner then brings out a cloth and places it over the toy dog, whispering, "Shhh, night-night doggie." Meaghan starts to pat the dog and whispers. Meahgan's parents are astounded. They had seen an audiogram with letters and pictures on it. The /h/ and a drawing of two people whispering to one another appeared to be at frequencies and intensities that were out of the range of Meahgan's auditory access with her hearing aids.

The practitioner is able to convey encouraging information:

■ The turbulence in /h/ extends into below 1000 Hz and has

a primary resonance around 1000 Hz (± 1/2 octave), within Meahgan's auditory access with her hearing aids.
■ Whispering is a form of /h/ and has sufficient turbulent energy within Meahgan's range of audibility.
■ Getting close to a child provides input that might be more difficult to hear at conversational distance.
■ Assume hearing. Give a child an opportunity to listen to speech in a meaningful context and help the child learn from what auditory information she *can* access. The letters and pictures found on an audiogram don't accurately convey all the possible cues that a child might be able to use.

The progression of primary resonances with place of production and oral tract length is seen in Figure 8–9. Identification of place of articulation for the full set of fricative consonants is achieved with auditory access through 6000 Hz.

The voiced fricatives /v/, /ð/, /z/, and /ʒ/ are produced with vocal fold vibration at the glottal source. Consequently, voiced fricatives have both periodic and aperiodic characteristics, with F0 as the periodic component and turbulence as the aperiodic component. The presence of F0 primarily cues the *voiced/voiceless* contrast in fricatives. In addition, the aperiodic turbulence in voiced fricatives is less intense than in voiceless fricatives.

Affricates: /dʒ/ (as in "judge"), /tʃ/ (as in "church")

Affricates are a combination of a plosive followed by a fricative. These are produced in such quick sequence to be perceived as a single consonant. There are two affricates in English, the voiced/voiceless pair /dʒ/ (as in "judge") and /tʃ/ (as in "church"), produced as an alveolar plosive followed by a palatal fricative. The sequence of motor acts for the two component consonants is as follows: (1) occlusion of the oral tract by the tongue at the alveolar ridge to build up airflow/pressure behind the occlusion, (2) explosive release of accumulated air pressure, and (3) constriction in airflow by the tongue in the palatal position to create aperiodic noise. The sound types produced by an affricate are aperiodic transient and turbulent, with periodic F0 generated by the voiced affricate /dʒ/. This is illustrated in Figure 8–10.

The acoustic markers for *manner of production* are from both the plosive and the fricative components: plosive silent gap and noise burst, followed by fricative steady state turbulence. This is seen in Figure 8–10. The noise burst

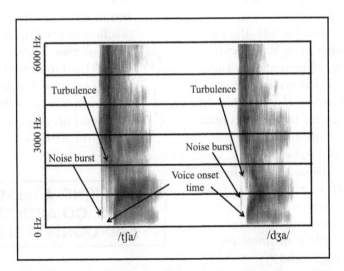

Figure 8-10. Speech spectrogram displaying affricate consonants /tʃa and dʒa/.

ranges from 2000 Hz to 4000 Hz; turbulence ranges from 2000 Hz to 8000 Hz. Identification of consonant manner is based on recognition of the noise burst and turbulence. Discrimination of the *voiced/voiceless contrast* is signaled by recognition of F0 during the turbulence phase of the affricate.

Summary

The postures and movements of consonant production create spectral and temporal acoustic cues for auditory recognition. Table 8–3 displays spectral cues for suprasegmentals, vowels, and consonants. Reading the table horizontally allows for a summary of the frequency regions for the acoustic characteristics of each speech sound type. Reading the table vertically makes it possible to consider what might be audible if hearing technology were to provide access through:

- *250 Hz:* suprasegmentals, consonant voicing with possible exception of plosives and affricates, the nasal murmur
- *500 Hz:* vowel height, the plosive noise burst in some contexts
- *1000 Hz:* all manners of consonant production with the exception of affricates, vowel height and place for back and central vowels, consonant place for nasals and some plosives, primary resonance for /h/
- *2000 Hz:* vowel place for front vowels; consonant place for nasals, approximants, and plosives; place distinctions between /h/ and /ʃ/
- *4000 Hz:* place distinctions among /h/, /ʃ/, and /s/

- *6000 Hz:* place distinctions among all fricatives.

Stability, rate of change, and duration are temporal cues that contribute to speech sound recognition.

- *Stability:* Vowel and nasal formants are fairly stable over the duration of production. In contrast, the formant frequencies in diphthongs and approximant consonants change over time.
- *Rate of formant change* is slower in diphthong production than in approximant consonant production.
- *Duration:* Vowels are longer in duration than consonants. Plosives have a sharp, fast noise burst. In contrast, the duration of turbulent aperiodic noise in fricatives is longer. Affricate timing is different from plosives and fricatives by shifting from a quick noise burst to turbulence of longer duration. Voice onset time is longer in voiced plosives and in affricates in the initial position of syllables compared with voiceless plosives and affricates. The duration of the preceding vowel is longer in voiced stops and affricates than vowel duration preceding voiceless stops and affricates.

MAKING A MESS OF THINGS: CO-ARTICULATION AND CONTEXT EFFECTS

The descriptions above are based on speech sounds produced in single syllables

Table 8–3. Spectral Cues for Short-Term Speech Components

	\multicolumn{9}{c}{**Frequency in Hz**}								
	125	**250**	**500**	**1000**	**2000**	**3000**	**4000**	**6000**	**8000**
Suprasegmentals	←— Voice & pitch								
	←— Intonational contour —→								
	←— Syllable duration & stress								
Vowels/ diphthongs		F1/u, i/	F1 others	F2 back vowels	F2 front vowels	F2 front vowels			
		↓ Voicing							
Consonants		↓ Voicing							
Nasals		↓ Nasal murmur		F2 transition					
Approximants	↓ Voicing		F1	F2	F3 /r, l/				
Plosives			←— Noise burst —→						
				←— F2 transition —→					
Fricatives				Turbulence ————————————————————→					
				Primary /h/	Primary /ʃ, ʒ/	Primary /ʃ, ʒ/	Primary /s, z/	Primary /θ, ð, f, v/	
Affricates					Noise burst ————→	Turbulence ————→			

291

using clearly articulated speech. The purpose of such highly controlled production is to obtain as clean a sample of the speech sound as possible for illustration and study. Conversational speech, however, is not that pristine. We don't produce one single sound at a time, but are constantly resolving from one movement to the next. We make a mess of things!

Speech sounds overlap. When we look at a spectrogram of a sentence, it can be difficult to separate out one sound from another, and one word from another. For example, the production of a nasal consonant in a word ("night") requires an open velum for passage of sound into the nasal cavity. The velum doesn't just immediately snap shut for production of the vowel that follows that nasal. The first few milliseconds of the vowel that follows a nasal carries nasal resonance and extended low frequency emphasis due to the fact that the velum is still partially open when the vowel begins.

Speakers also pre-program movement for upcoming productions. This means, for example, that if a speaker will be producing a word that contains a lip-rounded vowel such as /u/ ("sing a t*u*ne"), the muscles that round the lips for /u/ start to move into position prior to the appearance of the rounded vowel. As the lips start to round in preparation for vowel production, resonance in those preceding sounds is lowered.

This overlap from one speech sound to another is known as *co-articulation*. Co-articulation is present in the moments of transition from one speech sound to another. These transitions are "dually coded," containing acoustic information from both sounds. As a consequence, a speech sound varies a bit each time it

is produced in conversation depending upon the sound that precedes and follows it. This is called the *context effect*. Context effects pose one of the central questions in speech perception. Just how do we perceive these varied acoustic characteristics as a single speech sound? Speech perception theories offer several explanations (Kluender, Stilp, & Lucas, 2019).

- We perceive speech as words and phrases, rather than single sounds.
- Learning one's language enables the listener to ignore unimportant variability and focus on cues that differentiate sounds one from another.
- The auditory system processes speech differently from the way frequencies are laid out on the spectrogram, and stability can be seen in the firings in the neural pathways.

Guidance for the Auditory-Verbal practitioner

Practitioners translate theoretical explanations into action when they ensure that children with hearing loss are exposed to a wide range of consonant-vowel combinations for auditory learning. This is achieved when practitioners and parents have conversations with a child about what that child is experiencing and doing. The more words that a child listens to and is able to practice in conversation, the more likely it is that he will have exposure to the full range of context effects.

Practitioners can take advantage of context effects. For example, a practitioner can use the effect of lip rounding to lower resonance to help make surrounding speech sounds audible. A child who does not have good high frequency auditory access with hearing aids may have difficulty identifying the /s/ in the word "see," but not in the word "Sue."

THE LING SIX SOUND TEST

Audibility is key to the auditory recognition of speech cues. But how do we know what a child can hear? There is no single source that tells us definitively how a child makes use of acoustic cues. We rely upon multiple sources of information in collaboration with the child's audiologist and family. One quick approach that can be applied at the start of each AVT session and throughout the day is the Ling Six Sound Test, found in Appendix 8–A (Ling, 1988, 2013).

The Ling Six Sounds, /m/, /u/, /i/, /a/, /ʃ/, and /s/, encompass the frequency and intensity range of speech. A child's performance on the Ling Six Sound Test can help us understand what he/she is hearing within the speech spectrum. The ability to discriminate between the sounds can indicate a general ability to discriminate among the primary octaves within the speech spectrum. Parents conduct a Ling Six Sound Test at the start of each day and Auditory-Verbal practitioners start each therapy session with the Ling Six Sound Test. The test can help to quickly identify problems with a child's hearing technology or changes in hearing. The Ling Six Sound Test is the final verification that all is well following a listening and visual check of hearing technology.

Each sound is presented separately as a brief syllable, at about the same duration that syllables appear in spoken language. Some children may require longer syllable durations when they are first starting out. The Ling Six Sound Test is a check of audition so visual cues are not provided. The Ling Six Sound Test is conducted with the child wearing his or her hearing technology on one ear at a time. If the test were conducted with the child wearing hearing technology on both ears, it could be possible to miss discovering that one of the devices is not working.

Dr. Ling specified 1 meter, or about 3 feet, as the presentation distance between speaker and listener, since that is the distance at which conversation ordinarily occurs. One variation of the Ling Six Sound Test is to present the sounds at distances greater than 3 feet to know just how far away the speaker can be before any of the sounds become inaudible or confused. This information can be useful as a baseline measure because a reduction in distance hearing can often be the first sign that a child's technology is starting to have problems or that his hearing is changing.

The test should only take a few minutes. Very young children who are in the early weeks of intervention may require some time learning the expected response. The type of response that a child is instructed to give upon hearing a Ling sound depends upon his or her developmental and auditory skill level:

▪ *Detection*: A child drops a block, stacks rings on a stick, or performs some other simple action in response to hearing a Ling sound. This response demonstrates that a child can hear the syllable presented but fails to indicate whether auditory access is sufficient to make each sound distinct from one another.

■ *Discrimination* by imitation: A child imitates the phoneme that his parent or the Auditory-Verbal practitioner says to him or her. This requires that the child be able to produce the phonemes clearly enough that his parents or the Auditory-Verbal practitioner knows what he has perceived.

■ *Identification* from among the set of six sounds: A child picks up an object or points to a photo that represents the phoneme. This requires teaching the child to associate the sound with the object or picture.

The frequency information found in Table 8–3 can be used as a reference for interpreting a child's responses to the Ling Six Sound Test.

For example, if a child fails to *detect*:

■ /ʃ/ and /s/: There may be inadequate auditory access at 2000 Hz and above.
■ /s/: There may be inadequate auditory access at 4000 Hz and above.
■ any of the sounds except /a/: The child is hearing only the strongest phoneme in the set and auditory access is limited to the mid-frequency range of speech.

If a child fails to *discriminate*

■ /m/ from /u/: There may be inadequate auditory access below 250 Hz.

■ /u/ from /i/: There may be inadequate auditory access above 1000 Hz.
■ /ʃ/ from /s/: There may be inadequate auditory access above 2000 Hz.

The Ling Six Sound Test was developed for use with North American English but it is applied globally. Park and Kim (2016) confirmed via acoustic analysis that the Ling Six Sound Test is compatible with the Korean language. Adaptations of the Ling Six Sound Test have been developed and validated for Mandarin (Hung, Lee, & Tsai, 2018; Hung, Lin, Tsai, & Lee, 2016; Li, Zhang, & Sun, 2017). Agung, Purdy, and Kitamura (2005) suggested that the vowel /ɔ/ (as in "ought") be substituted for /u/ or added to the Ling Six Sound Test for administration in Australia to accommodate variations in how speakers of Australian English produce the vowel /u/.

CHAPTER SUMMARY

Daily application of speech acoustics in AVT requires understanding the links between the postures and movements of speech production and the resulting acoustic signal. The long-term components of effective conversational speech (overall intensity and frequency range) and the short-term components (suprasegmentals, vowels, and consonants) are described in this chapter, along with the spectral and temporal acoustic cues important to auditory speech recognition. Conversational speech is messy. Cues for speech sounds often overlap. The Ling Six Sound Test provides a check of the audibility of the Long-Term Speech Spectrum and a child's capacity to discriminate among frequency regions within the speech spectrum.

Speech ranges in frequency from 100 Hz through 10,000 Hz, with the greatest intensity appearing in the mid-frequency range. Full vowel recognition utilizes spectral information from 250 Hz through 3000 Hz, consonant recognition utilizes information through 125 Hz through 6000 Hz. The frequency range from 1500 Hz through 6000 Hz makes the greatest contribution to speech intelligibility.

The speech signal is complex. Some speech sounds are periodic in nature and others have aperiodic components, cuing consonants *vs* vowels and manner of production. Each speech sound comprises a range of frequencies. Particular frequencies within a speech sound appear at greater intensities than others, enhanced by vocal tract resonance created by production of that sound. Frequency, however, is not the only essential cue to speech recognition. Each speech sound also has a temporal signature. Temporal cues differentiate vowels from consonants, assist in identification of manner of consonant production and differentiate the voiced/voiceless pairs within plosive and affricate manners of production. Finally, the speech signal is not delivered as a series of separate individual speech sounds. Speech sounds overlap. A single vowel or consonant can vary depending upon the sound that precedes or follows it, particularly in the moments of transition from one sound to the next.

The Ling Six Sound Test is an essential event in a family's daily routine and in the practice of Auditory-Verbal Therapy. It helps families and Auditory-Verbal practitioners to confirm that all is well. Interpretation of the Ling Six Sound Test requires a basic understanding of the spectral cues in the speech signal. It helps families and Auditory-Verbal practitioners to confirm that all is well.

REFERENCES

Agung, K. B., Purdy, S. C., & Kitabura, C. (2005). The Ling Sound Test revisited. *Australian and New Zealand Journal of Audiology, 77*(1), 33–41.

ANSI. (1997). *American National Standard methods for calculation of the speech intelligibility index. ANSI S3.5–1997.* New York, NY: American National Standards Institute.

Boersma, P., & Weenink, D. (2019). Praat: Doing phonetics by computer. http://www.fon.hum.uva.nl/praat/

Boothroyd, A., (2019). The acoustic speech signal. In J. Madell, C. Flexer, J. Wolfe, & E. Schafer (Eds.), *Pediatric audiology: Diagnosis, technology, and management* (3rd ed., pp. 207–213). New York, NY: Thieme.

Byrne, D., Dillon, H., Tran, K., Arlinger, S., Wilbraham, K., Cox, R., . . . Kiessling, J. (1994). An international comparison of long-term average speech spectra. *Journal of the Acoustical Society of America, 96*(4), 2108–2120.

Fant, G. (2004). Speech related to pure tone audiograms. Speech acoustics and phonetics: Selected writings (pp. 216–223). Dordrecht, Netherlands: Kluwer.

Hung, Y. C., Lee, Y. J., & Tsai, L. C. (2018). Validation of the Chinese sound test: Auditory performance of hearing aid users. *American Journal of Audiology, 27,* 37–44.

Hung, Y. C., Lin, C. Y., Tsai, L. C., & Lee, Y. J. (2016). Multidimensional approach to the development of a Mandarin Chinese–oriented sound test. *Journal of Speech, Language, and Hearing Research, 59*(2), 349–358.

Kent, R. D., Read, C., & Kent, R. D. (1992). *The acoustic analysis of speech* (Vol. 58). San Diego, CA: Singular Publishing.

Killion, M. C., & Mueller, H. G. (2010). Twenty years later: A *NEW* Count-the-dots method. *The Hearing Journal, 63*(1), 10–17.

Kluender, K. R., Stilp, C. E., & Lucas, F. L. (2019). Long-standing problems in speech perception dissolve within an information-theoretic perspective. *Attention, Perception, & Psychophysics*, 1–23.

Ladefoged, P. (1996). *Elements of acoustic phonetics*. Chicago, IL: University of Chicago Press.

Li, A., Zhang, H., & Sun, W. (2017). The frequency range of "the Ling Six Sounds" in standard Chinese. *INTERSPEECH*, 1864–1868.

Ling, D. (1976, 2002). *Speech and the hearing-impaired child: Theory and practice*. Washington, DC: A. G. Bell.

Ling, D. (1988). *Foundations of spoken language for hearing-impaired children*. Washington, DC: A. G. Bell.

Ling, D. (2013). What is the Six Sound Test and why is it so important in auditory-verbal therapy and education? In W. Estabrooks (Ed.), *101 frequently asked questions about auditory-verbal practice* (pp. 58–62). Washington, DC: A. G. Bell.

McCaffrey, H. A., & Sussman, H. M. (1994). An investigation of vowel organization in speakers with severe and profound hearing impairment. *Journal of Speech and Hearing Research, 17*, 938–951.

McCreery, R. W., & Stelmachowicz, P. G. (2011). Audibility-based predictions of speech recognition for children and adults with normal hearing. *Journal of the Acoustical Society of America, 130*(6), 4070–4081.

Niemoller, A. F., McCormick, I., & Miller (1974). On the spectrum of spoken English. *Journal of the Acoustical Society of America, 55*, 461.

Park, H., & Kim, J. (2016). Comprehension and application of the Ling 6 sound test. *Audiology and Speech Research, 12*(4), 195–203.

Peterson, G. E., & Barney, H. L. (1951). Control methods used in a study of the vowels. *Journal of the Acoustical Society of America, 23*(1), 148–148.

Pickett, J. M. (1999). *The acoustics of speech communication: Fundamentals, speech, perception theory, and technology*. Boston, MA: Allyn and Bacon.

Raphael, L. J. (2008). Syllable production rate in conversational speech. *Journal of the Acoustical Society of America, 123*(5), 3074–3074.

Stelmachowicz, P. G., Hoover, B. M., Lewis, D. E., Kortekaas, R. W., & Pittman, A. L. (2000). The relation between stimulus context, speech audibility, and perception for normal-hearing and hearing-impaired children. *Journal of Speech, Language, and Hearing Research, 43*(4), 902–914.

Stelmachowicz, P. G., Pittman, A. L., Hoover, B. M., & Lewis, D. E. (2001). Effect of stimulus bandwidth on the perception of /s/ in normal- and hearing-impaired children and adults. *Journal of the Acoustical Society of America, 110*(4), 2183–2190.

Stevens, S. S., Egan, J. P., & Miller, G. A. (1947). Methods of measuring speech spectra. *Journal of the Acoustical Society of America, 19*, 771–781.

Appendix 8-A

THE SIX SOUND TEST*

Daniel Ling, PhD

The Six Sound Test, in which children learn to respond to the practitioner in less than 1 minute, enables parents and professionals to determine whether a child's audition is at least minimally adequate for hearing speech. Hearing aids and cochlear implants are designed to elevate the intensity levels of sounds across the complete frequency range of speech. They are constructed to provide comfortable and effective listening levels so that as many as possible (preferably, all) of the cues involved in speech perception and speech production are audible to most children who are deaf and hard of hearing. However, these conditions are not always met. Hearing aids frequently fail to provide optimal amplification, and cochlear implants are sometimes inappropriately mapped.

I devised the Six Sound Test to provide a speedy and face-valid check on a child's ability to detect sounds across the whole frequency range of speech. The practitioner can also use this test to check whether the child is able to identify each of the six sounds (/m/, /ah/, /oo/, /ee/, /sh/, and /s/). The test checks the integrity of all levels of the child's auditory system, beginning with the microphone of the hearing aid or cochlear implant and ending at the brain.

Both forms of the test involve a professional or a parent saying the six speech sounds, one at a time and in random order. The test can be administered by either a male or female professional. The child needs to be able to hear both professionals equally well. Although the pitch of voices may differ, the components of the sounds that permit the identification and comprehension of the sounds are sufficiently close for the purpose of this basic test. (If they were not closely similar, male and female professionals would not be able to understand one another's spoken language. Whatever difficulty men may have in understanding women or vice versa, it is unlikely to relate to the acoustics of speech.)

In the *detection* form of the test, the sounds are presented at a conversational level from different distances (as described later in this response). Young children can respond by playing a "go game"—placing an object in a box or putting a ring on a stick as soon as they detect the speech sound presented. In the detection form of the test, care needs to be taken to avoid presenting the sounds rhythmically because children are then likely to respond in time with the presentation and thus provide false positive responses. Older children can respond when they detect the sound presented by raising a hand or saying "yes." In the *identification* form of the test, children who have adequate speech simply imitate the sound presented when they hear it.

The focus of the test is on perception in the different regions of the speech frequency range from the lowest, voiced sounds to the highest, unvoiced sounds. The sounds selected, from low to high, are /m/ as in *me*, /oo/ as in *two*, /ah/ as in *aha!*, /ee/ as in *she*, /sh/ as in *fish*, and /s/ as in *us*. To control for duration, we use *continuant sounds*— those that can be made as long or as short as the tester finds necessary. To control for intensity, we administer the test in a typical conversation level from either 1 meter/3 feet (the average distance typically maintained between adult and child in one-on-one interaction) or 3 meters/ 10 feet (the average distance for interactions in a group). Sounds in an acoustically treated room vary in intensity by about 6 dB each time the distance between talker and listener is doubled (i.e., they are quieter) or halved (i.e., they are louder). Using the test at different distances is important because results obtained at 1 meter say nothing about what the child hears at greater distances, such as in a classroom. At no time should the six sounds be presented at levels that are louder or quieter than those the tester uses in real life during typical conversation. Doing so invalidates the test.

So, the Six Sound Test can be used to check a child's ability to detect and identify the basic speech patterns that occur over the frequency range of speech. Only when voice levels and distance are carefully controlled can the results of this test be valid.

WHY THESE SIX SOUNDS?

Low-Frequency Sounds

Our voices, as we speak and sing, are among the lowest sounds we produce.

So, too, are the resonances associated with the nasal sounds /m/, /n/, and /ng/, and the low vowels in words such as *shoe* and *toe*. If we cannot hear a sound such as /m/, then we are unlikely to be able to hear enough of the other low-frequency sounds to develop speech through hearing with typical prosody (tune) and without vowel errors.

So, we use the sound /m/ to check whether hearing for low frequencies is adequate. If /m/ cannot be heard at 3 meters or so, then poor prosody and nasalized speech are likely to develop.

Vowel Formant Range

Vowel sounds are very complex. They consist of *fundamental voice* (the sound made in the larynx when we vocalize) and some higher resonances (called *formants*) created in the mouth cavity that change in frequency as we move our tongues. Unless the first two of these formants are audible, a listener will not be able to identify the vowel with certainty. The two main formants of /oo/ are both in the low-frequency range. The two main formants of /ee/ are at very different frequencies—one is low, and the other is high. If the low one cannot be detected, then an atypical-sounding voice and an inability to hear tunes and sing songs will result.

So, we use the /oo/ vowel to check whether the low end of the vowel formant range can be detected. It also lets us ensure, in tests of identification, that sounds in the frequency range of /oo/ and /m/ are recognized and not confused. If they are confused, greater emphasis needs to be placed on listening skills.

Central Vowels

The formants in the vowel /ah/, as in the exclamation "Aha!," are at the center of the vowel range and, indeed, the center of the whole speech range. Central vowels are louder than others because the mouth is open wider during their production. If the /ah/ is inaudible or inadequately amplified, then unstressed words—particularly those that fall in the center of the speech range—are likely to be missing. Thus, instead of hearing all the words in a sentence such as "I went to the park," a child may hear only "I went park" and, as a result, may develop several grammatical problems. A child who uses hearing aids and who has substantial low-frequency hearing can usually detect the vowel /ah/. If this same child can detect the /ah/ but not the /m/ and /oo/ sounds, then other sounds in the low-frequency range are underamplified, or sounds in the mid-frequency range are overamplified. In either case, the hearing aids or cochlear implants require adjustment so that all vowels are equally detectable. Overamplification of the mid-frequency range is suggested when such a child can detect a stage-whispered /ah/ at 6 meters (20 feet) or so. For several reasons, the /ah/ is rarely confused with other vowels in tests involving identification.

So, we present /ah/ to check that the central vowels are audible and are neither underamplified nor overamplified.

The Vowel Sound /ee/

The vowel /ee/ may be detected through the audibility of either the low first formant or the high second formant, which is at the upper end of the frequency range of vowels. Thus, children may respond to /ee/ because they detect the low first formant, the high second formant, or both. Their response to the /ee/, therefore, needs to be interpreted by comparing it with other sounds in the test that have components in the same frequency range. The following deductions can be made relative to the /ee/:

1. No response indicates that neither formant can be detected.
2. A response indicates the detection of only the low-frequency formant if /oo/ and /m/ can be detected but /sh/ cannot be detected.
3. A response indicates the detection of only the high-frequency formant if /sh/ can be detected but /m/ and /oo/ cannot be detected.
4. A response indicates the detection of both formants if /sh/, /oo/, and /m/ can also be detected.
5. It is likely that the /ee/ and other vowels will be nasalized if /sh/ and /oo/ can be heard but /m/ cannot be detected.

So, we use the vowel sound /ee/ to check a range of possible problems.

High-Frequency and Unvoiced Sounds

The high and very high sounds in speech are mainly unvoiced plosives or stops such as /p/, /t/, and /k/ and unvoiced fricatives such as /sh/, /s/, /f/, and /th/. All of these are relatively quiet sounds. Also, the range of a child's hearing loss for high sounds is usually greater than for low sounds. For these reasons, high-frequency sounds are the most likely to be missed by children who have severe or profound hearing loss and whose hearing aids or cochlear implants are not well selected and adjusted (mapped). Remember: The test measures the effectiveness of the transmission of sounds from the microphone of the hearing aids or cochlear implant to the brain. The root of a problem in detecting or identifying sounds could, therefore, be with any link in the auditory chain, including a temporary middle-ear infection, a loss of fluid in the cochlea, or the auditory devices that are used. The reasons for any such failure require further audiological evaluation and, if the failure persists, perhaps modification of strategies used in teaching or therapy. Because the high sounds of speech carry most of the information required for the discrimination, identification, and comprehension of speech, the ability to detect them is of the utmost importance.

So, we use the sound /sh/ to check whether the moderately high sounds are audible, and we use the unvoiced sound /s/ to check whether the very high sounds can be detected.

OTHER APPLICATIONS

Although the Six Sound Test places a useful tool in the hands of parents and professionals, it has applications beyond those of detection or identification of speech sounds across the speech spectrum for those who wear hearing aids or cochlear implants. I also find it useful for checking the balance of my home entertainment system, the sound quality of amplifiers used in public address systems, and the quality of analog hearing aids that are suggested for a particular child. For this purpose, I have my own ear molds, and I listen to the aid as if it were prescribed for me. If I cannot hear all of the six sounds clearly, then others will not be able to either.

So, talkers who use the test can be more confident that they will, indeed, be heard. The Six Sound Test helps ensure that what parents and professionals are all working for truly comes about.

REFERENCE

*Adapted from Ling, D., in *Songs for learning! Songs for life!* By W. Estabrooks & L. Birkenshaw-Fleming (Eds.). Copyright © 2003 Plural Publishing, San Diego. Appendix 2: The six sound test, pp. 227–229.

Part III
DEVELOPMENTAL DOMAINS IN AUDITORY-VERBAL THERAPY

9

DEVELOPMENT OF LISTENING IN AUDITORY-VERBAL THERAPY

Helen McCaffrey Morrison

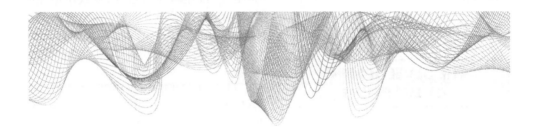

Listening enables a child to do many things—to acquire language, to develop speech production as a means to communicate, to comprehend conversations, and ultimately to keep the conversations going. Children listen to learn—from spoken language presented directly as well as from spoken language learned incidentally through "overhearing." One of the fundamental goals of Auditory-Verbal Therapy (AVT) is to help children who are deaf or hard of hearing learn to *listen*. Therefore, it is critically important for the Auditory-Verbal practitioner (practitioner) to have a comprehensive understanding of how listening develops in children with typical hearing and in children who are deaf or hard of hearing.

Hearing is automatic and proceeds along an open channel. We cannot close it off. The auditory pathways deliver acoustic information to the brain without conscious participation by the hearer. Electrophysiological evidence demonstrates that we hear even while sleeping (Gilley, Uhler, Watson, & Yoshinaga-Itano, 2017). Nevertheless, hearing does not achieve the same outcomes as *listening*. Listening involves attention. Listening, *the functional use of hearing*, is an active, cognitive process that takes place during interaction with others. This active process in AVT engages the child's attention and thinking during interactive play and conversation.

Today's children in AVT are likely to have been identified and fit with hearing technology at ages that enable them to pursue a typical developmental trajectory of *listening*. This chapter describes that trajectory, the processes that typically developing children use to listen to acquire language, how hearing loss impacts early listening development, and then shifts to the application of that information for assessing listening skills and planning opportunities for the child to learn to listen in daily life.

THE DEVELOPMENT OF LISTENING

The development of listening begins *in utero* during the third trimester of pregnancy when the human cochlea is fully formed and continues through adolescence with final maturation of the central auditory nervous system. Much happens along the way, as seen in evidence from investigations of auditory processing of acoustic signals and infant speech perception. By the end of their first year, infants have made great strides in extracting meaning from the perception of speech. They recognize words and phrases and are beginning to establish a language base for further development of receptive language and comprehension skills. Today's child in AVT is rarely presented with single words, since we know babies can ex-

tract meaningful information from sentence material.

Auditory Processes

Psychoacousticians (hearing scientists) and audiologists trace the processing of acoustic signals along the auditory pathway from the auditory periphery (cochlea and auditory nerve) to the cortex. Performance on tasks of auditory processing informs the researcher and audiologist about the status of neural waystations along this auditory pathway. Performance on four auditory processing tasks contributes to our understanding of auditory perceptual development—(1) auditory sensitivity (detection), (2) auditory specificity (discrimination), (3) auditory localization, and (4) signal perception in competing noise.

The basic auditory processes of detection and discrimination tend to be studied in infants using non-speech stimuli designed to isolate detection and discrimination of intensity, frequency, and duration. Experiments in *auditory detection* seek the lowest intensity that elicits a response. Infant detection of acoustic signals is poorer than adult detection, but this improves to adult levels throughout the first 2 years of life (Olsho, Koch, Carter, Halpin, & Spetner, 1988; Parry, Hacking, Bamford, Day, & Parry, 2003). Auditory detection by infants in the first 3 months of life is poorer for high frequency signals than for mid and low frequency signals (Tharpe & Ashmead, 2001).

Auditory discrimination is the detection of differences in sounds. Experiments in auditory discrimination seek to discover the smallest difference or change in sound that elicits an infant response. Auditory discrimination by infants is poorer than adults in the first few months of life, but improves during the first 6 months (Olsho, Koch, Halpin, & Carter, 1987; Schneider, Morrongiello, & Trehub, 1990; Werner, 2007), although there is also some evidence that children do not reach adult discrimination of differences in signal intensity until 12 years of age (Maxon & Hochberg, 1982).

The ability to *localize* sound improves over the first 10 months of life, as observed in experiments that elicit head turns toward the sound source. Infants are able to localize softer and softer sounds over the first year of life. The head-turn response becomes more complex during the first 10 months as well, proceeding from side to side at 3 months, a downward look at 8 months, and finally adding an upward look at 10 months (McConnell & Ward, 1967). This increased ability to search for sound is not only a product of improved sensitivity and auditory localization but also a consequence of increased trunk strength and neck control.

Among the various ways to investigate signal perception in competing noise, *speech understanding in noise* is the most relevant for AVT. Infants and young children have difficulty separating speech from noise compared with adults (Werner, 2007). This skill matures throughout childhood. Children's understanding of speech in competing noise greatly improves in adolescence (Eggermont & Moore, 2012). This is why the practitioner coaches parents of infants and young children to establish a listening environment that is as free of extraneous noise as possible. The real world is a noisy place, but children are

not miniature adults and do not have the ability or the experience to separate noise from speech signals as expertly as adults do. More on this can be found below under "Infant Speech Perception."

To summarize, infants improve their ability to localize sound over time, thus helping them to connect sounds in their environment to their meanings in daily life. Infants require greater signal intensity in order to demonstrate that they detect sound and this improves until age 2 years. It also appears that the ability to discern differences between sounds develops gradually and may require cumulative listening experience and practice. This is *not* observed, however, when the signal is speech, as described below. Infants and young children are particularly vulnerable while attempting to make sense of what they hear in noisy environments. Speech understanding in noise, however, improves into adolescence.

Information about basic auditory processes is the first step toward understanding listening development but it is limited. What is needed is a more direct approach that can illuminate *how* infants crack the speech code by listening. That information can be found in the study of infant speech perception.

Infant Speech Perception

Infants accomplish several tasks in order to decode the speech signal and acquire language. Newborns recognize speech as an interesting and important signal from among the many that they hear. They segment the steady stream of ongoing speech into chunks, extracting the recurrent phrases and words from which meaning is derived—the most salient acoustic information for them. They categorize the speech sounds they hear inside those phrases and words into the phonetic categories that are found in the language of the home. Infants have help to accomplish these tasks, gateways that guide the infant toward meaning-making (Kuhl, 2011). These gateways to *auditory learning* include the speech signal that is directed to the infant, daily interaction with parents and caregivers, and the infant's own perceptual and cognitive abilities. These are all clearly understood concepts in AVT.

Speech that is directed to infants is tailor-made for decoding and meaning. The acoustic features of infant-directed speech assist in the arousal of infant attention and segmentation of words and phrases (Thiessen, Hill, & Saffran, 2005; Werner, 2007). Infant-directed speech is higher and more variable in pitch than adult-directed speech, and is produced with exaggerated intonational contours that mark phrase boundaries. Key words appear at the ends of these clearly marked phrases and are further highlighted by changes in pitch (e.g., Here's your *nappy!*) (Fernald & Mazzie, 1991). Infant-directed speech helps infants discover the phonetic categories of their home language—speech rate is slower, vowels are longer in duration, consonants are more clearly articulated, and phonetic distinctions are exaggerated (Burnham, Kitamura, & Vollmer-Conner, 2002; Fernald & Simon, 1984). Infants whose mothers show greater exaggeration in speech tend to have better speech discrimination performance (Kuhl, Tsao, & Lui, 2003).

Infant-directed speech is easy to hear and is presented in routine interactive contexts that further support decoding and comprehension. The words and phrases parents repeat throughout routine daily events of caregiving, book sharing, and play give structure and predictability to the speech signal. Parents and infants maintain eye contact to establish a social bond that guides infants' auditory attention. Parents provide referential information that helps the infant make an association between speech sound patterns and meaning. They talk about the objects they are using or that the infant is playing with. They narrate the infant's actions. They use cues to lead the infant toward the object or event that is being referenced by pointing, shifting gaze, or leaning toward what they are talking about (Brooks & Meltzoff, 2002, 2005). Infants make use of these cues in auditory learning. In a study of the role of social cues and auditory learning, infants demonstrated short-term auditory memory for words and phrases embedded in an interactive book-sharing that included adult/infant eye contact, adult gestures toward the pictures, and joint attention toward the pages on the book. Infants who were read the same book without these interactive, social cues did not demonstrate auditory memory and learning (Kuhl, 2010, 2011. The role of infant-directed speech, interactive daily routines, and referential talk in child language acquisition is explored further in Chapter 10, with many examples of this provided throughout Chapters 12–15.

It is the *infant*, however, who does the real work of perceiving and decoding the speech signal for meaning. The cognitive processes of attention, memory, categorization, and statistical learning support speech perception to associate sound with meaning and acquire language (see Chapter 13). Infants detect patterns, regularities, and repeated events from their auditory experiences and use this information to make sense of what they hear. Infants also demonstrate a progression in the acoustic cues of the speech signal they use for speech perception, beginning with suprasegmental cues that are signaled by the fundamental frequency (F0). This is why, in AVT, the practitioner coaches the parents to use the Learning to Listen Sounds with their infants, to make the acoustic signal as meaningful as possible (see also Appendix 9–A).

Four levels of *auditory attention* support listening and language development (Gomes, Molholm, Christodoulou, Ritter, & Cowan, 2000). *Arousal* is the readiness to perceive and process auditory stimuli. Babies are born ready to listen. They are naturally motivated to explore their world and learn (Gopnik, Meltzoff, & Kuhl, 1999), and interaction with other people and the sounds of everyday life increase infant arousal (Kuhl, 2011). The next level of attention, *orienting*, is triggered by *auditory detection*. When an infant detects sound, he/she gathers attentional resources, becomes still, and seeks the source of the sound, recruiting the visual sense to support auditory information.

Auditory arousal and orientation prepare the infant for higher levels of auditory attention that facilitate learning. In order to learn from listening, the infant needs to engage *selective attention,* ignoring unimportant sensory input to focus on what he/she wants to hear. There's a lot going on in a baby's world—many new sounds and much to see. Yet, babies are able to focus on parent talk above all other interesting stimuli. This selective attention enables the infant to engage in *sustained atten-*

tion, listening for a sufficient duration so that the listening experience can be stored in memory. Selective and sustained attention work in tandem to support auditory learning.

Infants have *auditory preferences*, paying attention to the preferred sound for a longer time than to non-preferred sound. Auditory preferences develop from auditory experiences that occur frequently, become familiar, and are stored in the infant's auditory memory. Newborn auditory preferences are the product of *listening to the mother's voice while in the womb*. This experience leads to newborn recognition of *voice* and *stress patterns,* each signaled by the speaker's vocal fundamental frequency, or F0 (see Chapter 8).

Newborns prefer their mother's voice over the voices of other female speakers (DeCasper & Fifer 1980; Mehler, Bertoncini, & Barriere, 1978). They prefer to listen to human speech over synthesized speech or nonspeech signals (Jusczyk & Hohne, 1997; Vouloumanos & Werker 2007). They are able to discriminate speech that has stress patterns like the language that they heard in the womb from those with different kinds of stress patterns (Nazzi, Bertoncini, & Mehler, 1998; Ramus, Hauser, Miller, Morris, & Mehler, 2000). Newborn infants do not, however, demonstrate an auditory preference for infant-directed speech with its distinctive, spectrally varied intonational contours (Cooper, Abraham, Berman, & Staska, 1997). Nor do newborns discriminate languages with equivalent stress patterns but differing phonological content and organization (Nazzi et al., 1998).

This all changes once infants have had some time to listen to their parents while experiencing pleasurable, social, and interactive exchanges (see Chapters 10, 12–15). By age 3 months, infants demonstrate an auditory preference for infant-directed speech over an adult-directed speech style (Panneton, Abraham, Berman, & Staska, 1997). Sustained attention to infant-directed speech also helps the infant segment the continuous speech stream into meaningful units, beginning with *familiar phrases*. Phrases are subsumed within the exaggerated intonational contours that characterize infant-directed speech. Phrase recognition in infant-directed speech is accomplished by tracking the F0 variation that cues intonational contours. Infants are also able to discriminate the melodies in familiar songs by ages 2 to 3 months (Plantinga & Trainor, 2009), again showing the influence of experience tracking F0 and auditory memory.

Once an infant has segmented the speech stream into familiar phrases, he/she is able to listen *within* the phrase, to discover *familiar words*. By 3 months of age, infants pay attention for longer periods to sentences containing familiar words compared with ones with unfamiliar words (Seidl & Johnson, 2006). Infants are not yet demonstrating that they know the meaning of these words. Rather, they are engaging in *statistical learning*. They pay attention to the frequency of occurrence of an auditory event, in this case an often repeated word, and store it in memory. Attention to frequently occurring words leads to word comprehension at 8 months (Paul, 2007). There is also evidence that the infant is beginning to notice the *phonology*, or consonant and vowel organization, of words within phrases at 3 months as well, discriminating between languages that have the same stress patterns but different phonologies (Nazzi & Rasmus, 2003).

Paying attention to frequency of occurrence helps the infant categorize the many different vowel and consonant sounds he/she hears into the phoneme categories that make up the home language. In the first few weeks life, an infant is able to discriminate a wide variety of vowels (Swoboda, Kass, Morse, & Leavitt, 1976; Trehub 1976) and consonants (Lasky, Syrdal-Lasky, & Klein, 1975; Werker & Lalonde, 1988), including speech sounds not produced in the infant's home language. Accordingly, newborn speech perception abilities are said to be *language-general* (Jusczyk, 1993).

Auditory experience leads to a shift in perception from language-general to *language-specific* speech perception, coinciding with the emergence of infant word comprehension. From 6 to 8 months of age infants no longer discriminate vowels and consonants that are from outside their home language. The shift occurs at 6 months for vowels (Kuhl, Williams, Lacerda, Stevens, & Lindblom, 1992) and at 8 months for consonants (Werker, 1989; Werker & Tees, 1984). Here's an example. In English the consonants sounds of [r] and [l] are treated as separate phonemes that differentiate words such as "red" and "led." In Japanese, these consonants are not phonemes, but are considered to be *allophonic* variations within a single phoneme category that encompasses both [r] and [l]. Babies who live in homes where Japanese is spoken are able to discriminate [r] from [l] as newborns, but no longer perform that discrimination at age 8 months.

The shift toward language-specific speech perception is the product of infant statistical learning. Infants pay attention to the frequency of distribution of the speech sounds in their environment, note which sounds are used in words, and consolidate into single categories the allophonic variations of those sounds that don't differentiate words. It is not the case that babies have become poorer at auditory discrimination over the first 8 months of life. Rather, they are becoming *smarter listeners*. They have created phonemic categories for speech sounds to become more efficient at listening. It becomes easier to discover the acoustic patterns that signal a word when an infant must no longer treat each allophonic variation as a different sound, but as an unimportant variation within a larger phonemic category. Words that may have been perceived as different because the vowels and consonants each had a slightly different acoustic signature are now perceived as being the same words. This makes it much easier to recognize frequently heard words and store them into memory. The ability to engage in language-specific discrimination at 6 to 8 months is predictive of rate of language growth between 11 and 30 months (Kuhl, Conboy, Padden, Nelson, & Pruitt, 2005).

By the time infants reach their first birthday, they understand approximately 50 words, including nouns, verbs, and some attributes, and they respond to simple commands. The auditory preference for infant-directed speech shifts to a preference for an adult-directed speech style (Cooper & Aslin 1990; Fernald, 1985). Speech perception has shifted to *language comprehension*.

Summary

Table 9–1 summarizes milestones in infant speech perception, organized by age and the auditory skill the infant demonstrates by achieving this milestone. Learning to decode the speech signal and start on the path toward language acquisition is a more robust and complex process than simply detecting and discriminating the intensity, frequency, and duration of signals. Infants accomplish sophisticated perceptual and cognitive tasks over the first year of life. Facing an ongoing stream of sound, they pay attention to and scan for acoustic patterns that are repetitive and tied to meaningful experience. They recognize that the speech signal is important and engage in attention, memory, and statistical learning to recognize familiar words in ongoing speech and associate sound with meaning—leading to word comprehension. Infants categorize the vowels and consonants of their language into phonemic categories to further stimulate language acquisition. Parents help. They talk to their babies using infant-directed speech that is acoustically shaped to gain infants' attention and segment out meaningful phrases and words. Infant-directed speech that is delivered in daily routines that are repetitive and socially engaging arouses the infant's auditory attention and provides the auditory experience that is be stored in memory for learning.

Receptive Language and Language Comprehension in Early Childhood

Listening becomes intentional in early childhood. Toddlers listen to *act* upon what they hear. They begin to follow simple directions. They listen and *learn* new words at an increasing rate each year. Toddlers develop a *listening attitude* and *attend* to spoken language for longer periods of time. The more that young children are able to understand

Table 9–1. Milestones in Infant Speech Perception

Age	Behavior
Newborn	Pays more attention to speech over non-speech.
	Pays more attention to mother's voice over other female voices.
	Discriminates stress patterns in home language vs other languages.
	Discriminates vowels from numerous languages.
	Discriminates consonants from numerous languages.
3 months	Pays more attention to infant-directed speech over adult-directed speech style.
	Detects phrase boundaries at intonational contours in infant-directed speech.
	Detects familiar words in sentences.
	Discriminates familiar melodies.
	Discriminates languages that differ in phonology.
6 months	Discriminates only vowels from home language.
8 months	Discriminates only consonants from home language.
	Comprehends first words.
12 months	Shows enjoyment listening to rhymes, songs, stories. Dances to music.
	Pays more attention to adult-directed speech over infant-directed speech style.
	Comprehends approximately 50 words.
	Comprehends and responds to simple commands.

and use language, the greater the contribution of those language abilities in furthering intentional listening and language comprehension.

When children enter the preschool ages, listening becomes even more sophisticated. Preschoolers listen to gain information. They are better at deriving meaning from context and begin to understand conceptual vocabulary that relates to time, quantity, size, and relationships. Preschoolers answer questions of increasing complexity, comprehend more questions, and possess greater knowledge and a lexical base from which to retrieve answers. They follow increasingly complex commands. Receptive vocabulary explodes throughout early childhood and becomes more complex, more varied in use. Children learn to listen not just for content, but for the order of words and the morphemes that make up sentences.

Preschoolers can listen to and understand longer stories as time goes on. They remember stories they hear and even the sequence of events and they can remember messages to deliver from one person to another. They also display emerging phonological awareness that requires careful listening for words, rhymes, and sounds within words.

Table 9–2 lists milestones in receptive language and language comprehension from ages 1 through 6 years. These are organized first by the vocabulary types and language forms that children in early childhood learn to recognize by listening: general vocabulary, conceptual vocabulary, morphemes. This is followed by milestones for comprehension at the sentence level, such as following directions and responding to questions. The next grouping pertains to listening to and interacting with connected language: participation in conversations, and engaging with stories, rhymes, and other play with language. Finally, some specialized aspects of listening are included: phonological awareness and tasks of short-term memory. This list of milestones is not intended to encompass the full body of early childhood receptive language and language comprehension but is intended to help make evident the wide range of concepts and aspects of communication that young children develop. The milestones are drawn from information about the acquisition of

Table 9-2. Early Childhood Milestones in Receptive Language and Auditory Comprehension

Receptive Vocabulary	
6–12 months	Some 50+ words by 1 year Infant's own and names of family members Common items, action words, sound/object associations Action words/verbs: up, drink, go, come, give Recognizes words spoken at end and beginning of sentences
1–2 years	200–500 words by 2 years Recognizes words in the middle of sentences Capable of learning 1 new word per week
2–3 years	900–1500 words by 3 years (varies with reporting source) Capable of learning several new words each day
3–4 years	2,000 to 5,000 by 4 years (varies with reporting source)
4–5 years	3,000–6,000 words by 5 years (varies with reporting source)
5–6 years	13,000–20,000 words or more by 6 years (varies with reporting source)

continues

Table 9-2. *continued*

Conceptual Vocabulary (learned in phrases, not as single words)	
1–2 years	Develops category vocabulary
2–3 years	Quantity: one, two, all, many, a little bit, just one Spatial: in, off, on, under, out of, together, away from Size: big, little Time: soon, later, wait, yesterday and tomorrow Identifies familiar objects described by function: What do we use for eating?
3–4 years	Quantity: empty, full, a lot Equality: same/different, both Spatial: next to, beside, between, front/back Texture: hard/soft, rough/smooth Speed: fast/slow Weight: heavy Time: day, morning, afternoon, daytime *vs* nighttime activities Simple analogies (Daddy is a man, Mommy is a ____) Understands opposites
4–5 years	Quantity: whole Time: yesterday, today, tomorrow, days of the week, last week, next week Sequence: first, then, next, Spatial/positional: between, above, below, nearest, through, first, middle, last
5–6 years	More complex time phrases: for a long time, for years, a whole week, in the meantime
Morphology and Syntax	
6–12 months	Comprehends familiar phrases as an unanalyzed whole: go outside, wave bye-bye, let's get in the car
1–2 years	Comprehends simple sentences You, me, my, mine
2–3 years	Personal pronouns: he, she, we, they -est adjective marker: *e.g.,* biggest Irregular past tense: *e.g.,* ran, fell
3–4 years	/s/ morpheme: plurals *vs* singular noun (bear, bears) is *vs* is not not + adjective, noun: not hot, not mine Some comparatives: *e.g.,* I am faster Regular past tense: *e.g.,* walked Articles (a)

Table 9-2. *continued*

4–5 years	/s/ morphemes: Singular *vs* plural verbs: he walks/they Possessives Past, present, future verb tenses Comparative and superlative adjectives Understands sentences with dependent clauses: if, because, when, why
5–6 years	All pronouns Contractions: Jose's running, we're dancing Understands -er: skater, painter Irregular comparatives: good, better best
Following Directions	
6–12 months	Simple commands: sit down, no, hot, wave, bye-bye, give me Follows 1-step directions during play
1–2 years	1-step directions
2–3 years	2-step directions
3–4 years	3-step directions Follows 2 unrelated commands: Put down your cup and turn off the TV.
4–5 years	3 commands in 1 sentence
5–6 years	Follows classroom paper-and-pencil directions: On your paper, draw a circle around something that you eat.
Comprehending and Answering Questions	
6–12 months	Simple questions
1–2 years	Answers "What's this?" to familiar object Chooses object from choice of two: "Do you want milk or juice?" Finds object or person in response to "where" questions
2–3 years	Holds up fingers to tell age. Where . . . ?, What's that?, What's. . . . doing?, Who is . . . ?, Can you . . . ?
3–4 years	Questions about self: age, name, pets, etc. Rudimentary answers to why questions Quantity: How much? Time: How long?
4–5 years	How questions for quantity, distance: How many?, How far? Answers "What do you do when you're hungry/sleepy, etc.?" Begins to answer what if: "What would you do if . . . ?"

continues

Table 9–2. *continued*

Participating in Conversation	
6–12 months	Engages in joint attention, follows adult line of regard Takes part in interactive games: pat-a-cake, peek-a-boo Engages in vocal turn-taking
1–2 years	Engages in verbal turn-taking Overhears familiar words not directed to the child.
2–3 years	Takes turns in conversation Clarifies and requests clarification Overhears new words not directed to the child.
3–4 years	Carries on simple conversations Corrects others Requests and listens to explanations of why and how
4–5 years	Asks questions for information Understands most of what is said Follows discussion about past and present
5–6 years	Attends to peer conversation and takes turns
Stories, rhymes, songs, riddles, and jokes	
6–12 months	Joint attention: looks at pictures or objects with an adult Stops and pays attention to music
1–2 years	Listens as pictures are named Listens to simple stories Begins to join in with gestures to songs: *e.g.,* Itsy-bitsy spider Moves to music
2–3 years	Listens to longer stories Recognizes familiar sounds of TV commercials.
3–4 years	Listens to 20-minute story Requests favorite stories Protests when an adult changes the story Answers simple riddles
4–5 years	Understands story sequence Attends to a short story and answers simple questions Recalls 5 details from a story Memorizes lines of a song
5–6 years	Understands riddles and idioms: *e.g.,* hold your horses
Phonological Awareness	
3–4 years	Makes some letter/sound matches Participates in rhyming games
4–5 years	Discriminates rhyming vs non-rhyming word pairs
5–6 years	Recognizes letters and letter-sound matches

Table 9–2. *continued*

Short-term Auditory Memory	
3–4 years	Repeats a 6- to 7-word sentence
4–5 years	Repeats a 9-word sentence Repeats a 1-part message: "Go tell Mommy to . . ."
5–6 years	Repeats a 12-word sentence Repeats a 2-part message: "Go tell Mommy to . . ."

Sources: Estabrooks, Mac Iver-Lux, & Rhoades, 2016; Lanza & Flahive, 2009; Luinge, Post, Wit, & Goorhuis-Brouwer, 2006; Semel, Wiig, & Secord, 2004; Tuohy, Brown, & Mercer-Mosely, 2001; Wilkes, 1999; Zimmerman, Steiner, & Pond, 2011.

the English language, predominantly American English. Nevertheless, the overall perspective should be useful cross-linguistically.

These milestones can be thought of as the *content for listening practice in AVT*. The language that we direct to young children is what they are learning to comprehend. Listening goals need to be directly related to receptive language. It is common practice in AVT for these listening goals to be woven into each experience (see Chapters 12–16).

The Impact of Hearing Loss

Children who are deaf or hard of hearing are, for the most part, born with the same cognitive capacities as their typically developing peers. As explained in Chapter 2, hearing loss blocks the gateway of sound to the brain. When an infant or young child receives a hearing aid, that gateway is opened. The child's brain is ready and waiting to do its work. AVT is based in helping children engage their inherent cognitive abilities to use auditory information for learning. Practitioners and families help by making sure that sufficiently audible,

meaningful experiences are provided with care and intention so that children can make sense of what they hear.

Children who are deaf or hard of hearing start out with challenges even if they are optimally fitted with hearing technology in the earliest months of life. Practitioners and families are mindful of these challenges when they assess and plan for children's auditory learning. Typically developing newborns enter the world with several months of listening experience *in utero* that is unavailable to infants born with hearing loss. This adds a delay in auditory stimulation as a consequence of the time taken to fit the child optimally with hearing technology.

The difficulties that young typically developing children experience processing speech in competing noise is exacerbated by the attendant difficulties that listeners with hearing loss experience in noise (see Chapters 4 and 7). The challenging impact of listening at a distance can further reduce the amount of input an infant or young child might receive, even while using hearing technology. Reduced input, in turn, constrains the opportunities for infants and young children to use statistical learning to recognize and learn from regularities in language. Practitioners and families in AVT strive to create optimal acoustic environments with a variety of distances from the person talking, to ensure the child has many possible opportunities in each interaction to learn though listening.

The impact of hearing loss on the audibility and discriminability of speech sounds can impact a child's organization of speech input into the phonemic categories of his/her home language. This can create a need for the child to reorganize phonemic categories after fitting with hearing technology. It is possible that full discriminability of some speech sounds is not achieved after fitting with hearing technology. The practitioner and family, therefore, apply knowledge of speech acoustics to use words in input that provide discriminable contrasts between speech sounds to lead to the discovery of phonemic categories.

Perception of F0, or speaker voice, predominates the earliest listening milestones attained by typically developing infants, e.g., perception of voice, stress patterns, and intonational contours. Infants and young children with severe-to-profound loss who are candidates for cochlear implants are likely to be able to detect and make some use of F0 perception while wearing hearing aids prior to cochlear implantation. Auditory learning is possible for these aspects if F0 is audible, even while the infant is wearing hearing aids. This helps build neural pathways in the auditory system.

There is a growing body of evidence that indicates infants and young children who are deaf or hard of hearing attain listening milestones in a similar fashion as their typically developing peers. Early auditory preferences and abilities observed in typically developing children are also among the earliest milestones attained by children who are deaf or hard of hearing after receiving hearing technology. For example, within 1 to 2 months of listening with cochlear implants, infants and young children demonstrate that they can discriminate differences in syllable number and in duration (Houston, Pisoni, Kirk, Ying, Miyamoto, 2003; Kishon-Rabin, Harel, Hildesheimer & Segal, 2010). Infants and young children who receive cochlear implants prior to 2.5 years demonstrate auditory preferences within the first 6 months of listening for speech over non-speech signals (Segal & Kishon-Rabin, 2011) and for stress patterns in speech that are common to their home language (Segal, Houston, & Kishon-Rabin, 2016). They demonstrate a preference for infant-directed speech over an adult-directed speech style at hearing ages equivalent to the 3-month chronological age at which typically developing children demonstrate increased attention to infant-directed speech. Subsequently, children with cochlear implants and hearing aids switch to a preference for adult-directed speech at a hearing age of 12 months, equivalent to the chronological age at which typically developing children also make this attentional (Wang, Bergeson, & Houston, 2017, 2018).

The important evidence that infants and young children who are deaf or hard of hearing follow typical developmental milestones and sequences in auditory learning enables the practitioner to use typical developmental milestones as a foundation when assessing and supporting auditory development in AVT.

GUIDANCE FOR THE PRACTITIONER: SUPPORTING AUDITORY DEVELOPMENT AND LEARNING IN AVT

Models for Supporting Auditory Development and Learning

Today's children who are identified early and fit with hearing technology during the optimal language learning years are able to learn to listen in a similar manner to typically developing children. Practitioners in AVT use typical developmental milestones and the processes by which children reach these as the *foundational model* for assessing and supporting children's auditory development and learning. Learning through listening takes place in the same conversations and play that support young children's development. Listening skill development is not isolated from the global communication process. Children do not learn to listen in isolated auditory training exercises. Rather, listening, language, speech, and cognition are interacting, inseparable components. Learning to listen is essentially the process of acquiring the receptive language skills that lead to language comprehension.

Practitioners are mindful, however, of the particular challenges that children who are deaf or hard of hearing overcome in order to learn to listen and meet developmental milestones. Children in AVT are learning to listen after some delay in experience with auditory input, even when fit with hearing technology in the very early months of life. They are listening to a speech signal that is degraded to some extent by hearing technology, an atypical auditory system, and vulnerability to difficulty listening in the ordinary background noises of the everyday environments, even when optimally fit with hearing technology. Practitioners in AVT need to be able to identify when and how these challenges are impacting listening development so that they can be addressed. Accordingly, practitioners in AVT integrate a second model into developmental practice, an auditory processing model. The predominant auditory processing model that is integrated into developmental practice in AVT is the *Erber* (1982) model.

The hierarchy of auditory responses in the Erber model is familiar to many practitioners:

- *Detection*: response indicates an awareness that sound is present.
- *Discrimination*: response indicates awareness that one sound is different from another.
- *Identification*: response indicates that meaning is associated with sound.
- *Comprehension*: response indicates an understanding of connected language.

Erber introduced this hierarchy as the *response* component of what he called a *stimulus-response model*. In Erber's model, a child's response is understood fully only when the level of the *stimulus* that elicits that response is also considered. Erber's stimulus hierarchy, from the lowest to the highest stimulus level, includes:

- Phonemes
- Syllables
- Words

■ Phrases
■ Sentences

Erber did not intend his model to be applied in a rigidly prescribed manner. Rather, he proposed that it be used as an assessment tool and to guide *adaptive* conversational interactions that support auditory learning. In adaptive conversations, the practitioner and family use language that is natural and appropriate for a child. If a child fails to understand, the practitioner and family apply the stimulus-response model as a diagnostic tool to discover the source of breakdown, asking themselves questions such as:

■ Did the child hear what was said?
■ Were any words in the message unclear and might be confused?
■ Did the child know the language and make the appropriate identification?
■ Was the message too complex to enable the child to comprehend?

The answers to these questions can help practitioners respond to a child in a way that clarifies the message, helps the child to learn, and keeps the conversation going.

It can be tempting to position the Erber hierarchical model as the primary sequence of auditory skills that children need to learn because it is so clearly laid out. There are, however, aspects of a hierarchical model such as this that do not address the way that young children learn to listen. For example, the model can be interpreted that a child must discriminate syllables and speech features *before* understanding words. Developmentally, this is not exactly what happens. The reader is referred to Table 9–1, which displays the earliest speech perception milestones. Children are born able to discriminate syllables and learn to ignore unimportant discriminations in tandem with learning to understand words. Young children do not learn language from discrimination training such as drilling syllable imitations or pointing to pictures of words that differ in a single feature or speech sound.

Rather, practitioners and parents provide abundant examples of language in meaningful contexts. They anticipate that young children are likely to first recognize familiar words and phrases as an unanalyzed whole, encased in a recognizable intonational contour ("Uh oh! Fell down." "Night, night." "Kiss Mommy"). Eventually, when children understand words or sound-object associations, practitioners and parents give the child opportunities to listen and practice discrimination in appropriate social contexts such as putting away toys ("Hmmm, let's find the train that goes choooo-chooo. Oh, there it is! Now, have you seen the car that goes brrrrrrrr-beep-beep?").

Furthermore, a strict application of the Erber stimulus-response hierarchy might lead one to believe that children leap from identifying single words to understanding connected speech, and that, of course, is not the case. One approach to close the gap between identification and comprehension response levels is to add *auditory memory* and *auditory sequencing* between these levels. In this scenario, the practitioner might extend learning from single words to connected speech by setting auditory memory goals for the number of *critical units* in a sentence that a child processes and remembers. Critical units are the words in a sentence or phrase that a child needs to understand in order to comprehend that sentence. This enables practitioners and parents to target the child's ability to understand connected speech of increasing length and complexity. Table 9–3 lists examples of sentences and phrases with increasing numbers of critical units. Adding auditory memory does insert a more developmental aspect to the Erber response hierarchy, particularly with regard to increasing the syntactic complexity of what the child is expected to be able to comprehend. The practitioner needs to be mindful, however, of the many additional aspects of language and communication that a child learns to comprehend, as illustrated by Table 9–2.

Nevertheless, the Erber model is a powerful tool for understanding a child's early responses to sound and to ensure that a child is detecting sound and discriminating essential differences between the sounds that he/she is hearing. These developmental aspects occur so early in typical development that most milestones don't include this fundamental developmental aspect that is so important to children in AVT. It is recommended, therefore, that practitioners apply a developmental model founded in typical milestones as the primary model for assessing and supporting auditory development and use Erber's auditory processing model as a supplemental model that can promote attention to early skills. It is also a diagnostic tool that can address individual needs that a child might exhibit regarding how he/she accesses the speech signal, particularly for children who receive hearing technology later in childhood.

Supporting Auditory Development and Learning in AVT

Listening is not observable until the listener responds to what he/she hears. It can be tempting, therefore, for a practitioner to plan a session that is filled with tasks that elicit child responses to what adults say. In such a scenario the practitioner would present a stimulus and the child would respond. The practitioner would then deduce the child's listening ability from the adequacy of the response. However, a session that is filled with a child having to follow directions, pick up toys, or point to pictures is not only deadly boring, it is a *test*. First, a child needs to *learn*, and learning needs to be *fun*.

Think back to the description of how infants make sense of speech and acquire language. Auditory attention, or time spent *listening*, is the first step in learning. Children need time to listen to rich, learnable language in meaningful contexts. In AVT these contexts are play, conversations, language experiences, books and stories, and even songs. Quality input for auditory learning is that which follows the child's interest. The practitioner watches what happens when he/she brings out a toy, paying attention to what the child has noticed and how he/she plays. The strongest learning occurs when a child is listening to language that is aligned with that child's own play (Raab, Dunst, & Hamby, 2013). The following are ways that practitioners and parents provide quality learnable input and carry out AVT in the session and at home in a way that supports auditory development. (This is a segue into Chapters 12,

Table 9–3. Auditory Memory for Connected Language

A. Processing Single Words:

- Containing repetition of sound-word association in phrases: "The ball goes bounce, bounce, bounce."
- In single repetition of a sound-word association: "Where's the cat that goes meow?"
- In single objects varying in vowel content and syllables: "Where's the spoon?" *vs* "Where's the apple?" *vs* "Where's the ice cream cone?"
- In single objects representing nouns, verbs and adjectives with varied suprasegmentals and vowel content: "Pick the flower" *vs* "Wash, wash, wash your hands" *vs* "Mmm, that's good."
- With word presented at end of sentence: "Please get the bananas."

B. 2 Critical items:

- Two nouns: "Get your shoes and your hat."
- Noun and verb: "The baby is sleeping."
- Verb and object: "Wash the car."
- Two verbs: "Jump and sit down."
- Adjective and noun: "Go get your blue shirt."
- Number and noun: "I want three candies."
- Comprehension of prepositions in phrases: "in the closet" *vs* "under the bed"
- Pronoun development: "my book, your ball"
- Negatives, "no," "not the,"

C. 3 Critical items:

- Three nouns: "Don't forget your shoes, your coat and your books."
- Two nouns and a verb: "The boy and the dog are playing."
- Noun and two verbs: "Daddy is washing up and then having supper."
- Noun, preposition, and object: "Put your umbrella under your chair."
- Number, adjective, and noun: "I want two yellow balloons."
- Noun, conjunction, noun: "Put either the oranges or the bananas in the bowl."

D. 4 to 5 Critical items:

- Four nouns: "When we're shopping, we need bread, ice cream, fruit, and crackers."
- Nouns, preposition, and object: "Put your skateboard and your bike behind the house."
- Noun, conjunction, preposition, and object: "Get some popcorn or some chips and put them next to your backpack."
- Two noun-verb phrases: "The boy is swinging and the girls are sliding."
- Add a descriptive phrase: "See the girl wearing the blue hoodie in front of the store?"
- Add a time factor: "After you do your homework for one hour you can watch TV." "Before you wash your hands, you need to wipe your shoes."

15, and 17, where a discussion of these will be found in great detail.)

Starting Out

When an infant or young child first starts to use hearing technology, his/her auditory pathways automatically start sending acoustic information to the brain. The child is *hearing* but does not know *what* is heard or *how* to respond. Practitioners and parents help the child navigate this new soundscape. When a sound occurs, practitioners and parents delightedly point to their ears, verbalize their experience ("I hear that!"), and bring the child to the source so that an association can be made between the sound and its source. They repeat the sound whenever possible, e.g., making the microwave "ding" over and over, showing delight and pointing to their ears each time. Parents and practitioners give a name to this sound and imitate the sound so the child can have some fun imitating it as well, "I hear that! It's the microwave! Ding!"

It is a long-standing tradition in AVT to encourage new parents to take a "listening walk" with their child. Parents listen for all the sounds at home and throughout their community, and they point out each one to their child as it occurs (Pollack, 1970). This is not an "assignment" for parents to report back what sounds their child hears. It's an invitation for parents to share the exciting world of sound with their child. If parents believe that the assignment is to go for a walk to test their child's hearing, they will very likely become discouraged. A child who is just starting to listen does not yet know how to give a consistent and readily observable response to sound. By happily pointing

to their ears with delight, parents are teaching a valuable lesson about how to respond to sound.

Family members' voices are a very important part of an infant's or young child's soundscape. After listening to mother's voice for several months *in utero,* a typically developing infant is able to recognize and attend to mother's voice at birth, enabling the infant to start the process of language acquisition. Children who are deaf or hard of hearing who are just beginning to learn to listen benefit from experiences that help them learn to recognize their parents' voices and pay attention. For example, parents can play calling games with their child. A calling game can be as simple as Mom (for example) holding the child while Dad stands behind them, out of the child's sight. Dad calls the child and Mom turns around so they can all say "Hi!" Parents can take turns holding their child so there's an opportunity to listen to both parents, and of course the child gets a turn as well, playing with his/her voice and enjoying the power that comes with making Mom or Dad respond in delight.

Scaffolding Auditory Learning with Talk during Predictable Daily Routines and Play

Daily routines in the home—mealtime, dressing, toileting, going places in the car—provide a repeated sameness that is golden for learning. Children learn the phrases that accompany these daily actions by cumulative listening. They learn what parents say and what they are expected to say as well. When the practitioner and parents say many of the same things each time the child plays with a preferred toy, the language of play becomes predictable and learnable. For example, they say with play-doh: "open the can," "pull it out," "mmm. Smell it" or with wind-up toys: "turn, turn, turn," "wait," "1-2-3-go!" They take turns in the session so that the child has multiple opportunities to listen to each person in the setting. Practitioners and parents may even repeat favored activities from session to session. Sensitive practitioners and parents know when it's time to change things to prevent boredom.

Building a Phonology and Core Vocabulary with the Learning to Listen Sounds

The Learning to Listen Sounds (Estabrooks, 1994, 2006) (Appendix 9–1) focus on speech sounds in repeated, meaningful, play-based experiences. These are the fun sounds parents make for animals, vehicles, and toys that they can say again and again while playing (meow, woof-woof, ch-ch-ch-woo-woo, hop-hop-hop). By playing with a toy and hearing the Learning to Listen sound repeatedly, the child associates the repeated sound with the object. This is the basis for learning the sounds in his/her phonology and building vocabulary. Learning to Listen Sounds tend to be sounds that are easy for a young child to produce, enabling practitioners and families to target both listening and speech production in play. Each family will have particular sounds that they use for animals, vehicles, or toys and these become their child's Learning to Listen Sounds. Learning to Listen Sounds give a child experience listening to suprasegmentals, vowels, and consonants. The practitioner and parents pair the sound for a toy with its name so

that the child learns the name of the object as well as the sound association. They embed presentation of toys and the sound in language experiences that provide semantic and cognitive context. For example, while a child plays with farm animals he/she also rolls out a truck with grass from the garden for the animals to eat ("Eat, cow. Mooo! That's yummy grass"), puts together a fence for corralling the horses ("Jump, horse! Jump over the fence. Uh oh, don't fall down, Neigh!"), and walks the animals into a barn for bedtime ("Shhhh, night night, billy goat. Naaaaa!"). Learning to Listen Sounds can be found everywhere. They can be created for superheroes, Star Wars characters, or even mascots for sports teams.

Building Semantic Schemas with Themes

As children progress through the early childhood years, the practitioner sets up language experiences beyond daily routines or simple play with toys. Sessions might be organized around themes, perhaps in coordination with the themes in a child's early childhood classroom (see Chapter 20). Common early childhood themes include activities around holidays or the seasons, sports, taking a walk, and even dinosaurs. Thematic teaching can assist receptive language and comprehension development by helping a child develop a semantic schema for that theme or topic. A semantic schema is the map, or organization, we have in our minds about a topic that includes the words and phrases that are associated with that topic (Neuman, 2006). Schemas aid in the retrieval of information. When we know the topic of conversation, we can quickly go to that parcel of knowledge to access the relevant language. To put this in auditory learning terms, theme-based teaching and the formation of schemas help with:

- *Auditory Identification*: Themes and schema formation make new word learning more efficient because new words are associated with related ones that are already familiar.
- *Auditory memory and sequencing*: Asking a child to follow directions or retell a story when he or she knows the topic is aided by schematic-based retrieval.
- *Auditory closure*: When a child is listening in a noisy environment (which is any real-world environment), it is possible to miss words or phrases or confuse them. Schemas help a child narrow down the possibilities.

Analyzing Target Language Acoustically

The AVT session plan includes language that a child will be learning—phrases, words, perhaps even specific linguistic structures. The practitioner might build a language experience (scenario) around the language that a child needs at the moment. The language might be from a daily routine or playing with a favored toy or emerge from a planned theme. This becomes the *language for auditory skill building*. Prior to the AVT session, the practitioner needs to know how targeted language might be used to help a child practice auditory discrimination of speech sound contrasts, and can do that by:

- Listing key vocabulary for the activity or session.
- Grouping the vocabulary according to syllable number (e.g., 1 *vs* 2 *vs* multisyllabic words).
- Determining if the child's acoustic access with hearing technology is sufficient to hear the differences between words that differ in syllable number.
- Looking over the words within each group with the same number of syllables (e.g., look through all the one-syllable words). Within each syllable group, looking for pairs that might be easy or difficult to discriminate based on the child's acoustic access with hearing technology. Table 9–4 can assist the practitioner with this task. It lists speech sound contrasts that are likely to be found among the words that a child is learning during an AVT session. The table provides an example of each contrast along with a description of the acoustic cues that a listener should be able to use in order to make a successful discrimination.

Sharing Books and Telling Stories

Sharing books can reinforce everyday experience and language or take the child and parents to worlds far beyond the home. Book sharing can lead to conversations beyond the here-and-now, expanding a child's language and cognitive function. The language and pictures in children's texts provide a rich supply of new vocabulary and

Table 9-4. Speech Feature Discrimination Hierarchy

Stimulus	Examples	Auditory Task
Duration	Wheeee! *vs* Up!	F0 discrimination
Intonational contour	What's your name? *vs* That's my game!	F0 discrimination
Words differing in syllable number	shoe *vs* butterfly	F0 discrimination
Words with same syllable number that differ in consonant and vowel	card *vs* shoe	Multiple sources of differences between words: vowel formants and consonant features
Words with same syllable number and different vowels	bat *vs* boat	Discrimination based on F1 and/or F2 differences
Words with same syllable number and different initial consonant manner	bat *vs* mat	Manner differences tend to lie in the frequency range at 1000 Hz & below. In addition, manner differences incorporate differences in duration (*e.g.* nasals are longer than plosives).
Words with same syllable number and different final consonant manner	can *vs* catch	Low frequency manner differences. Final consonants appear after initial consonants in the hierarchy because they have fewer acoustic cues than initial consonants. Final consonants are softer in intensity and lack transitions into the following vowel.
Words with same syllable number and different final consonant voicing	bad *vs* bat	The duration of vowels preceding voiced consonants is longer than vowels preceding voiceless consonants.
Words with same syllable number and different initial consonant voicing Voice differences in initial continuants will be easier to perceive than plosives	Sue *vs* zoo is easier than dot *vs* tot	F0 signals the Sue *vs* zoo difference. Voice onset time is shorter for initial voiced consonants than voiceless.

Table 9-4. *continued*

Stimulus	Examples	Auditory Task
Words with same syllable number and different initial consonant place	big *vs* dig	Discrimination of the F2 transition from consonant into vowel.
Words with same syllable number and different final consonant place	bib *vs* big	Discrimination of F2 differences in the transition from vowel to final consonant.

language structures. When parents read books with their children, they use more complex language than during everyday routines. Children love to hear books over and over (see Chapter 14). This repetition builds auditory memory and scaffolds learning for the vocabulary and grammar used in the stories.

Telling and retelling stories is the companion to book sharing. Storytelling can begin as simply as pausing before a page is turned and asking a child, "Do you remember what comes next?" Storytelling in AVT meets several long-term goals (Robertson, Dow, & Hainzinger, 2006; Smith & Stowe, 2012): Building vocabulary, increasing auditory memory, and developing conversational skills help children create their own stories and support families to become storytellers (see Chapter 14).

Songs, Rhymes, and Fingerplays

Songs, rhymes, and fingerplays encourage auditory development in several areas: auditory memory, auditory attention, vocabulary and concepts, and phonologic awareness. Children in AVT learn the songs and rhymes that any typically developing child might learn.

Parents are likely to have songs and rhymes that they learned as children and these need to be the first ones the child learns (see Chapter 18).

Successful participation in songs, rhymes, and fingerplays requires that the child be able to follow along. We have a tendency to sing songs quickly. All this non-conversational language delivered at a fast pace can be a real challenge to any child, particularly to a child in AVT. Furthermore, the qualities that make for clear speech, e.g., slow rate and clear articulation of consonants, can get a bit blurred when singing, especially when we go quickly, so the practitioner needs to slow down and give the child time to process and understand the song.

A child's first participation in songs, rhymes, or fingerplays may be achieved through rote memory with little understanding of what he/she is singing or saying. Rote memorization can be a useful exercise for auditory memory, but gains are even greater if a child is also learning the language in these songs. Fingerplays with the song can be helpful because it is fun, the natural gestures often convey meaning, and many early songs for children include

How do Parents and Practitioners Use Children's Literature for Auditory Development?

The following, reprinted from Caleffe-Schenck (2000), describes the sequence of steps that a practitioner can follow to support auditory learning during book sharing, and how this experience is extended into the home.

"There is much to be said about the satisfaction of a parent and child reading, talking, and looking at beautifully illustrated and well-written books for children. Children's literature is one of the most powerful tools to enrich a child's auditory development while integrating listening with talking, thinking, and communicating.

"Brown Bear, Brown Bear, What Do You See? (Martin & Carle, 1968/1983) is a popular book found in many homes and classrooms around the world. The text of the book is repetitive, with the same question and answer combination being reiterated throughout the book: 'What do you see?' 'I see a [color + animal] looking at me.'

"This book may be adapted for use with children at different stages of auditory development. For younger children, the parent or listening and spoken language professional will use toy props representing the animals in the book. These props assist in maintaining the child's interest and promote the integration of audition, speech, language, and cognition. For example, a large stuffed yellow duck is related to a real duck, a realistic plastic duck, pictures, and stories about ducks. For an older preschooler, a cork can be used to represent the duck. The ultimate goal is that the phrase 'yellow duck,' which is learned through listening, represents to the child a wide array of impressions ranging from something the child sees on a pond to something the child later

discusses in a conversation with a peer or adult."

Following the principles of AVT, the practitioner will use *diagnostic teaching*, a process of individualized interactions used to assess a child's present levels of functioning in audition, speech, language, communication, and cognition to establish appropriate long-term goals and session targets. Parents incorporate these goals into their child's daily life.

The sequence of presenting auditory information while reading a book might be as follows:

- The child listens while the adult reads the text.
- The child imitates or comments on what was read.
- Props or pictures are used to reinforce the text.
- Parents expand their child's language by commenting on the story and related books or experiences.
- The child later takes the lead and spontaneously uses the spoken language prompted by the book.

Pollack, Goldberg, and Caleffe-Schenck (1997) presented a hierarchy of auditory development that has been used successfully in Auditory-Verbal Therapy and education for some years. To assist teachers, therapists, and parents in program planning and diagnostic teaching, listening and spoken language professionals use *Brown Bear, Brown Bear* (Martin & Carle, 1983) as an example for explaining specific auditory expectations using a storybook. The name "Sam" is used rather than the generic term "child." The following subsections provide a sample of the hierarchy based on the various stages of auditory development.

Auditory Awareness (Sam indicates presence or absence of sounds): Dad makes the barking sound of a dog while holding a stuffed dog under the table. Sam indicates that he hears something. Dad shows him the toy dog and hands it to Sam to explore and attach meaning to the sound. The toy is associated with the picture of the white dog in the book.

Distance Hearing and Localization (Sam hears at increasing distances and turns to the source of the sound): While walking in the park, Dad hears a dog barking a few feet away. He calls attention to this barking and shows Sam the dog frolicking in the field. (Distance hearing and localization are incorporated into each level of auditory learning once close-range hearing has been demonstrated.)

Auditory Discrimination (Sam judges whether sounds are the same or different): Mom reads, "Red bird, red bird, what do you see?" and whistles like a bird. Sam indicates by pointing to the red bird that he hears, discriminates, and remembers the differences in the whistle and the words "red bird" versus "quack, quack" and "yellow duck."

Auditory Self-Monitoring (Sam modifies speech to match what was heard): Sam demonstrates the beginning stages of auditory self-monitoring when he imitates the sounds for the animals in the book. His imitation of "ruff ruff" for the dog is different from "meow" for the cat (low pitch, short, abrupt duration vs. high pitch, long, long duration). An

example of a higher level of auditory self-monitoring is when Sam substitutes /g/ for /d/ when imitating the word *dog*. Mom acoustically highlights /d/ or uses auditory stress by babbling /da da dog/. Sam changes his speech production from /gog/ to /dog/.

Auditory Identification (Sam labels what he heard): The props or pictures used for the book are placed in front of Sam. Now it is time to put them away. Mom tells Sam, "Give me the frog." Sam picks up the frog. Then the roles are reversed, and Sam asks for the goldfish. A more advanced auditory level would be identifying "frog" versus "dog" because they are similar-sounding words.

Auditory Memory (Sam remembers what he heard): If Sam has an auditory memory for three items, he hears, listens, and remembers what he heard and picks up the "fish, sheep, and horse" from the toy props. He may be remembering and saying the repetitive phrase "I see a _____" and beginning to transfer this phrase to real life by imitating or spontaneously saying to his brother, "I see a cat," as the neighbor's cat sleeps in the sun.

Auditory Sequencing (Sam remembers in correct order what he heard): Instead of Sam picking up the toy props in random order, he hands them to his mom in the order in which she said them. He may verify or change the order in which he heard the animals by naming the animals as he picks them up. Another demonstration of sequential memory is when he recites the book from memory. Perhaps he is ready to listen to, understand, and act out a scenario such as, "Put the green frog on the rock and the goldfish in the water."

Auditory Processing (Sam thinks about what was heard and makes a cognitive judgment): At this level, just imitation, identification, or memory of what Sam heard will not be adequate for him to understand and complete the activity. He must draw upon his past experiences and knowledge of the world and use his spoken language to be an active communicator. A description game might be played, such as "I want something with fins that swims." Sam chooses the fish rather than the frog. The concepts and language structures that Sam learns through active listening evolve from simple to complex over time. The listening and spoken language professional and the parents are wise to incorporate an abundance of previously learned language targets, such as plurals, verb tenses, pronouns, conjunctions, component parts, and adjectives. More complex processing and strategies are required to understand questions such as, "What does a brown bear do when winter arrives?" Auditory closure and categorization activities encourage auditory processing. The parents and the practitioner may present incomplete statements such as, "Dogs, cats, and goldfish are pet animals. Bears, deer, and moose are wild animals." Other auditory closure tasks involve using component parts of animals, such as "A dog is covered with fur. A fish is covered with scales. A bird is covered with feathers." The possibilities for Sam to develop and practice auditory processing are limitless.

Auditory Understanding (Sam comprehends auditory information in a variety of settings with many different people): Dad and Sam are taking a walk when they notice a white dog running down the road. It reminds them of the white dog in *Brown Bear, Brown Bear*, and they discuss where the dog might be going in such a hurry. They make up their own story about the white dog. It might be a continuous story where each person tags onto what the previous person said. At home, Sam and his parents read a variety of books about dogs and compare and contrast these stories and characters.

The activities and ideas presented in the above subsections are just examples of how listening and spoken language skill levels can be developed and enhanced through use of an interesting children's book.

Conclusion

The listening and spoken language professional's successful use of children's literature as the basis of auditory development depends upon the following factors:

- Adhering to developmentally appropriate stages of auditory development to provide for and enrich successful auditory experiences for a child
- Incorporating several auditory levels within the same activity
- Integrating audition, speech, cognition, and communication at all levels
- Using books and other literary materials in creative and satisfying experiences that are motivating to a child and to the parents
- Empowering a child's parents to incorporate literature and meaningful auditory interactions throughout the day blossoms when a child is surrounded by quality books and colorful props and is engaged in meaningful interactions with adults in the child's life.

fingerplays. Acting out the songs with little toys leads even further to language comprehension.

CHAPTER SUMMARY

When a child first begins to listen with hearing technology, his/her auditory environment is perceived as a vast, undifferentiated soundscape. Innate cognitive capabilities help the child seek out regularly appearing patterns in that soundscape. The voices of the child's parents are the very first pattern that the child discovers. The acoustic and linguistic qualities of parent speech to infants and young children provide just what is needed to help the infant or young child to begin to decode the speech signal. Auditory memory and the natural inclination toward seeking regularities and patterns in the acoustic signal lead the child to further exciting discoveries in words and speech sounds that make up the phonology of his/her home language.

Children who are deaf or hard of hearing in AVT need to overcome these delays in auditory experience. Even though they are listening through less than perfect auditory systems, they follow a typical trajectory in auditory development and can attain listening skills that enable the acquisition of language for communication and learning. AVT helps make this happen by guiding the child, along with his/her parents, through typical developmental milestones and by paying attention to how a child processes sound from detection through comprehension in noise.

Practitioners and parents use conversations that provide quality input, play with sound-object associations to help a child discover first meanings and words, pay attention to the acoustic qualities of target language, and organize learning activities so a child can create semantic schema in order to support auditory development.

REFERENCES

Brooks, R., & Meltzoff, A. N. (2002). The importance of eyes: how infants interpret adult looking behavior. *Developmental Psychology, 38*(6), 958.

Brooks, R., & Meltzoff, A. N. (2005). The development of gaze following and its relation to language. *Developmental Science, 8*(6), 535–543.

Burnham, D., Kitamura, C., & Vollmer-Conner, U. (2002). What's new pussycat? On talking to babies and animals. *Science, 296*, 1435–1435.

Caleffe-Schenck, N. (2000). How do parents and practitioners use children's literature for auditory development? *The Listener*, Learning to Listen Foundation, Summer 2000, Toronto.

Cooper, R. P., Abraham, J., Berman, S., & Staska, M. (1997). The development of infants' preference for motherese. *Infant Behavior and Development, 20*(4), 477–488.

Cooper, R. P., & Aslin, R. N. (1990). Preference for infant-directed speech in the first month after birth. *Child Development, 61*(5), 1584–1595.

DeCasper, A. J., & Fifer, W. P. (1980). Of human bonding: Newborns prefer their mothers' voices. *Science, 208*(4448), 1174–1176.

Eggermont, J. J., & Moore, J. K. (2012). Morphological and functional development of the auditory nervous system. In *Human Auditory Development* (pp. 61–105). New York, NY: Springer.

Erber, N. (1982). *Auditory training.* Washington, DC: Alexander Graham Bell Association for the Deaf and Hard of Hearing.

Estabrooks, W. (1994). *Auditory-verbal therapy for parents and professionals.* Washington, DC: Alexander Graham Bell Association for the Deaf and Hard of Hearing.

Estabrooks, W. (2006). *Auditory-verbal therapy and practice.* Washington, DC: Alexander Graham Bell Association for the Deaf and Hard of Hearing.

Estabrooks, W., MacIver-Lux, K. & Rhoades, E. (2016) *Auditory-verbal therapy for young children with hearing loss and their families, and the practitioners who guide them.* San Diego, CA: Plural Publishing.

Fernald, A. (1985). Four-month-old infants prefer to listen to motherese. *Infant Behavior and Development, 8*(2), 181–195.

Fernald, A., & Mazzie, C. (1991). Prosody and focus in speech to infants and adults. *Developmental Psychology, 27*(2), 209.

Fernald, A., & Simon, T. (1984). Expanded intonation contours in mothers' speech to newborns. *Developmental Psychology, 20*(1), 104.

Gilley, P. M., Uhler, K., Watson, K., & Yoshinaga-Itano, C. (2017). Spectral-temporal EEG dynamics of speech discrimination processing in infants during sleep. *BMC Neuroscience, 18*(1), 34.

Gomes, H., Molholm, S., Christodoulou, C., Ritter, W., & Cowan, N. (2000). The development of auditory attention in children. *Frontiers in Bioscience, 5*(1), D108–D120.

Gopnik, A., Meltzoff, A. N., & Kuhl, P. K. (1999). *The scientist in the crib: Minds, brains, and how children learn.* New York, NY: William Morrow & Co.

Houston, D. M., Pisoni, D. B., Kirk, K. I., Ying, E., & Miyamoto, R. T. (2003). Speech perception skills of deaf infants following cochlear implantation: A first report. *International Journal of Pediatric Otorhinolaryngology, 67*, 479–495.

Jusczyk, P. W. (1993). From general to language-specific capacities: The WRAPSA model of how speech perception develops. *Journal of Phonetics, 21*(1–2), 3–28.

Jusczyk, P. W., & Hohne, E. A. (1997). Infants' memory for spoken words. *Science, 277*(5334), 1984–1986.

Kishon-Rabin, L., Harel, T., Hildesheimer, M., & Segal, O. (2010). Listening preference for the native language compared to an unfamiliar language in hearing and hearing-impaired infants after cochlear implantation. *Otology & Neurotology, 31*(8), 1275–1280.

Kuhl, P. K., Conboy, B. T., Padden, D., Nelson, T., & Pruitt, J. (2005). Early speech perception and later language development: Implications for the 'critical period,' *Language Learning and Development, 1*, 237–264.

Kuhl, P. K., Williams, K. A., Lacerda, F., Stevens, K. N., & Lindblom, B. (1992). Linguistic experience alters phonetic perception in infants by 6 months of age. *Science, 255*(5044), 606–608.

Kuhl, P. K. (2010). Brain mechanisms in early language acquisition. *Neuron, 67*(5), 713–727.

Kuhl, P. K. (2011). Social mechanisms in early language acquisition: Understanding integrated brain systems supporting language. In J. Decety & J. Cacioppo (Eds.), *The Oxford handbook of social neuroscience* (pp. 649–667). Oxford, UK: Oxford University Press.

Kuhl, P. K., Tsao, F. M., & Liu, H. M. (2003). Foreign-language experience in infancy: Effects of short-term exposure and social interaction on phonetic learning. *Proceedings of the National Academy of Sciences, 100*(15), 9096–9101.

Lanza, J., & Flahive, L. (2009). *Communication milestones.* East Moline, IL: Linguisystems.

Lasky, R. E., Syrdal-Lasky, A., & Klein, R. E. (1975). VOT discrimination by four to six and a half month old infants from Spanish environments. *Journal of Experimental Child Psychology, 20*(2), 215–225.

Luinge, M., Post, W., Wit, H., & Goorhuis-Brouwer, S. (2006). The ordering of milestones in language development for children from 1 to 6 years of age. *Journal of Speech, Language, and Hearing Research, 49,* 923–940.

Martin, B., & Carle, E. (1983). *Brown bear, brown bear, what do you see?* New York, NY: Henry Holt and Company. [First published in 1968]

Maxon, A. B., & Hochberg, I. (1982). Development of psychoacoustic behavior: Sensitivity and discrimination. *Ear and Hearing, 3*(6), 301–308.

McConnell, F., & Ward, P. H. (1967). *Deafness in childhood.* Nashville, TN: Vanderbilt Press.

Mehler, J., Bertoncini, J., Barriere, M., & Jassik-Gerschenfeld, D. (1978). Infant recognition of mother's voice. *Perception, 7*(5), 491–497.

Nazzi, T., Bertoncini, J., & Mehler, J. (1998). Language discrimination by newborns: Toward an understanding of the role of rhythm. *Journal of Experimental Psychology: Human Perception and Performance, 24*(3), 756.

Nazzi, T., & Ramus, F. (2003). Perception and acquisition of linguistic rhythm by infants. *Speech Communication, 41*(1), 233–243.

Neuman, S. B. (2006). The knowledge gap: Implications for early education. *Handbook of Early Literacy Research, 2,* 29–40.

Olsho, L. W., Koch, E. G., Halpin, C. F., & Carter, E. A. (1987). An observer-based psychoacoustic procedure for use with young infants. *Developmental Psychology, 23*(5), 627.

Olsho, L. W., Koch, E. G., Carter, E. A., Halpin, C. F., & Spetner, N. B. (1988). Pure-tone sensitivity of human infants. *Journal of the Acoustical Society of America, 84*(4), 1316–1324.

Parry, G., Hacking, C., Bamford, J., Day, J., & Parry, G. (2003). Minimal response levels for visual reinforcement audiometry in infants: Niveles mínimos de respuesta en la audiometría por reforzamiento visual en niños. *International Journal of Audiology, 42*(7), 413–417.

Panneton, R. P., Abraham, J., Berman, S., & Staska, M. (1997). The development of infants' preference for motherese. *Infant Behavior and Development, 20*(4), 477–488.

Paul, R. (2007). *Language disorders from infancy through adolescence: Assessment & intervention* (Vol. 324). New York, NY: Elsevier Health Sciences.

Plantinga, J., & Trainor, L. J. (2009). Melody recognition by two-month-old infants. *Journal of the Acoustical Society of America, 125*(2), EL58–EL62.

Pollack, D. (1970). *Educational Audiology for the Limited Hearing Infant.* Springfield, IL: Charles C. Thomas.

Pollack, D., Goldberg, D. M., & Caleffe-Schenck, N. (1997). *Educational audiology for the limited-hearing infant and preschooler: An auditory-verbal program* (3rd ed.). Springfield, IL: Charles C. Thomas.

Raab, M., Dunst, C. J., & Hamby, D. W. (2013). Relationships between young children's interests and early language learning. *Everyday Child Language Learning Reports, 5,* 1–15.

Ramus, F., Hauser, M. D., Miller, C., Morris, D., & Mehler, J., 2000. Language discrimination by human newborns and by cotton-top tamarin monkeys. *Science, 288,* 349–351.

Robertson, L., Dow, G. A., & Hainzinger, S. L. (2006). Story retelling patterns among children with and without hearing loss: Effects of repeated practice and parent-child attunement. *The Volta Review, 106*(2), 147–170.

Schneider, B. A., Morrongiello, B. A., & Trehub, S. E. (1990). Size of critical band in infants, children, and adults. *Journal of Experimental Psychology: Human Perception and Performance, 16*(3), 642.

Segal, O., Houston, D., & Kishon-Rabin, L. (2016). Auditory discrimination of lexical stress patterns in hearing-impaired infants with cochlear implants compared with normal hearing: influence of acoustic cues and listening experience to the ambient language. *Ear and Hearing, 37*(2), 225–234.

Segal, O., & Kishon-Rabin, L. (2011). Listening preference for child-directed speech versus nonspeech stimuli in normal-hearing and hearing-impaired infants after cochlear implantation. *Ear and Hearing, 32*(3), 358–372.

Seidl, A., & Johnson, E. K. (2006). Infant word segmentation revisited: Edge alignment facilitates target extraction. *Developmental Science, 9*(6), 565–573.

Semel, E., Wiig, E. H., & Secord, W. A. (2004). *Clinical Evaluation of Language Fundamentals (CELF) –Preschool-2*. San Antonio, TX: Pearson.

Smith, J., & Stowe, D. (2012). Why is storytelling important in Auditory-Verbal Therapy and education? In W. Estabrooks (Ed.) *101 frequently asked questions about auditory-verbal practice* (pp. 316–391). Washington, DC: Alexander Graham Bell Association for the Deaf and Hard of Hearing.

Swoboda, P. J., Kass, J., Morse, P. A., & Leavitt, L. A. (1978). Memory factors in vowel discrimination of normal and at-risk infants. *Child Development, 49*(2), 332–339.

Tharpe, A. M., & Ashmead, D. H. (2001). A longitudinal investigation of infant auditory sensitivity. *American Journal of Audiology, 10*, 1–9.

Thiessen, E. D., Hill, E. A., & Saffran, J. R. (2005). Infant-directed speech facilitates word segmentation. *Infancy, 7*(1), 53–71.

Trehub, S. E. (1976). The discrimination of foreign speech contrasts by infants and adults. *Child Development, 47*(2), 466–472.

Tuohy, J., Brown, J., & Mercer-Mosely, C. (2001). *St. Gabriel's curriculum*. Castle Hill, NSW: St. Gabriel's School for Hearing Impaired Children.

Vouloumanos, A., & Werker, J. F. (2007). Listening to language at birth: Evidence for a bias for speech in neonates. *Developmental Science, 10*(2), 159–164.

Wang, Y., Bergeson, T. R., & Houston, D. M. (2017). Infant-directed speech enhances attention to speech in deaf infants with cochlear implants. *Journal of Speech, Language, and Hearing Research, 60*(11), 3321–3333.

Wang, Y., Bergeson, T. R., & Houston, D. M. (2018). Preference for infant-directed speech in infants with hearing aids: effects of early auditory experience. *Journal of Speech, Language, and Hearing Research, 61*(9), 2431–2439.

Werker, J. F. (1989). Becoming a native listener. *American Scientist, 77*(1), 54–59.

Werker, J. F., & Tees, R. C. (1984). Cross-language speech perception: Evidence for perceptual reorganization during the first year of life. *Infant Behavior and Development, 7*(1), 49–63.

Werker, J. F., & Lalonde, C. E. (1988). Cross-language speech perception: Initial capabilities and developmental change. *Developmental Psychology, 24*(5), 672.

Werker, J. F., & Yeung, H. H. (2005). Infant speech perception bootstraps word learning. *Trends in Cognitive Sciences, 9*(11), 519–527.

Werner, L. A. (2007). Issues in human auditory development. *Journal of Communication Disorders, 40*(4), 275–283.

Wilkes, E. M. (1999). Cottage Acquisition Scales. San Antonio: Sunshine Cottage.

Zimmerman, I. L., Steiner, V. G., & Pond, R. E. (2011). *Preschool Language Scales– Fifth Edition*. Bloomington, IN: Pearson.

Appendix 9-A

LEARNING TO LISTEN SOUNDS

Karen MacIver-Lux and Warren Estabrooks

Learning to Listen Sounds (Estabrooks, 1994, 2006) is a term used by many Auditory-Verbal (AV) practitioners and parents to describe a selection of onomatopoeic sounds, ideophones, words, and/or phrases. Many of the *Learning to Listen Sounds* imitate or resemble the source of the sound or are associated with their referents such as "moo" for the cow and "choo choo" for the train (onomatopoeic sounds), are words or phrases that depict sensory information ("swish" for sudden movement of a fish) and feelings such as "ouch" for pain (ideophones), or are words and/or phrases that describe what animals and/or objects do such as "hop" for the bunny "round and round" for the spinning top. Some *Learning to Listen Sounds*, however, have been adapted from commonly used onomatopoeia, such as the *Learning to Listen Sound* for the bus ("bu bu bu" instead of "beep beep beep") or the car ("brr beep beep" instead of "vroom") so that sounds of the child's native language are represented during playful experiences with the *Learning to Listen Sounds*.

Learning to Listen Sounds, however, are *not* represented the same in all languages. They are, however, for the most part, shaped by the linguistic system of the family and used in the child's everyday environment (Bredin, 1996). For example, the Learning to Listen Sound for a clock may be *tick tock* in English, *dī dā* in Mandarin, *katchin* in Japanese, or "tik-tik" in Arabic.

Learning to Listen Sounds have specific acoustic properties. Some consist of vowels and diphthongs that have their first formants in the low- to mid-frequency range; other *Learning to Listen Sounds* consist of consonants that contain bursts of energy clustered in the mid- to high-frequency range (Estabrooks & Marlowe, 2000). By observing the child's response to each of these sounds, the AV practitioner gains valuable information about the child's functional auditory access across the speech spectrum using hearing aids, a cochlear implant, or both (see Chapter 14). The *Learning to Listen Sounds Audiogram* (Figure 9A–1) and the *Acoustics of LTLS Chart* (Figure 9A–2) are suitable references for Auditory-Verbal practitioners, audiologists, and parents. The icons on the *Learning to Listen Audiogram* represent *some* of the *Learning to Listen Sounds* and are placed *according to the location of their first and second formants/band of energy*. The child's detection and identification responses to the *Learning to Listen Sounds* can be plotted on the *Learning to Listen Sounds Audiogram* to indicate at which frequencies the child has auditory access. The *Learning to Listen Sounds* need to be presented at the intensity level of conversational speech, at a distance of 1 meter from the microphone

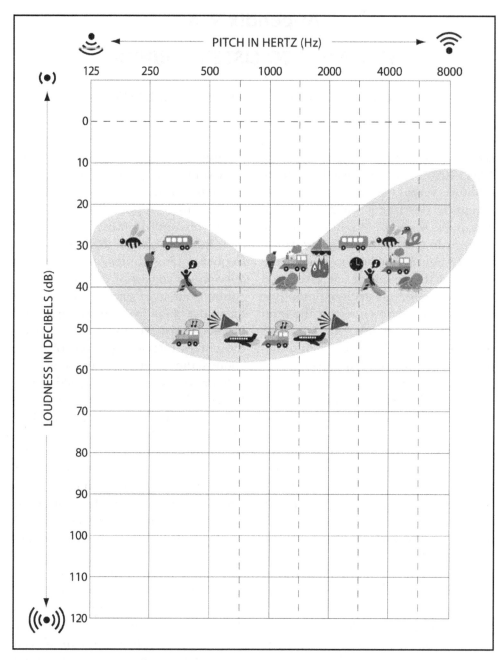

Figure 9A–1. *Learning to Listen Sounds* audiogram.

LEARNING TO LISTEN SOUNDS (LTLS) IN ENGLISH	1ST FORMANT OR BAND OF FREQUENCY	2ND FORMANT OR BAND OF FREQUENCY
/m/ "mmm" — ice-cream ("make")	250 - 350 Hz @35 - 40 dB HL	1000 - 1500 Hz @35 - 40 dB HL
/u/ "ooo" — train ("true")	430 –460 Hz @55 dB HL	1105 - 1170 Hz @55 dB HL
/tʃ, tʃ, tʃ/ "ch, ch, ch" — train (chicken)	1500 - 2000 Hz @35 - 40 dB HL	4000 - 5000 Hz @35 - 40 dB HL
/wi/ "whee" — slide (three)	370 - 437 Hz @40 dB HL	2761 -3200 Hz @40 dB HL
/ɑ/ "ahh" — airplane ("on")	768 - 1030 Hz @55 dB HL	1370 - 1551 Hz @55 dB HL
/e/ "ey!" — call out ("hay")	536 - 610 Hz @50 dB HL	2530 - 2680Hz @50 dB HL
/bʌ, bʌ, bʌ/ "buh buh buh" — bus ("bubble")	300 - 400 Hz @30 dB HL	2000 - 3000Hz @30 dB HL
/h/ "h!" — hot ("hat")	1500 - 2000 Hz @35 dB HL	
/p, p, p/ - "p, p, p" — boat ("peek")	1500 -2000 Hz @30 dB HL	
/ʃ/ "shh" — sleeping baby ("show")	1500 - 2000 Hz @40 dB HL	4500 - 5500 Hz @40 dB HL
/z/ "zzz" — bee ("zoo")	200 - 300 Hz @30 dB HL	4000 - 5000Hz @30 dB HL
/t, t, t/ "t, t, t" — ticking clock ("top")	2500 - 3500 Hz @35 dB HL	
/s/ "sss" — snake ("pass")	5000-6000 Hz @30 dB HL	

Figure 9A–2. Acoustics of *Learning to Listen Sounds.*

of the hearing technology in order to pre predict auditory access on the Learning to Listen Sounds Audiogram as accurately as possible. Most children, if provided with appropriately selected and programmed hearing devices, should find these sounds easy to hear (Estabrooks, 2006).

Some *Learning to Listen Sounds*, when spoken, contain acoustic properties that are rich in suprasegmentals that match those found in the child's native language. AV practitioners, therefore, guide parents to use infant-/child-directed speech that includes *Learning to Listen Sounds* so that spoken language sounds appealing (Shultz & Vouloumanos, 2010) and is easy to attend to (Vouloumanos & Werker, 2007) and learn (Reschke, 2002).

Learning to Listen Sounds vary in frequency, number of syllables (e.g., "bu bu bu" for the bus and "ahhh" for the airplane), and tempo (e.g., "wow!" vs. "ah"). When used in various combinations in playful scenarios, in meaningful parent-child interactions, and when listening to stories, the *Learning to Listen Sounds* help the child to discriminate, and associate spoken language to objects and meaningful experiences. For example, adult-directed speech varies in tempo across speakers and dialects, but on average consists of seven sounds per second (Krause & Braida, 2004). Parentese or infant-directed speech has a slower tempo; *Learning to Listen Sounds* typically consist of one to three sounds per second when presented in isolation. The slower tempo of infant-/child-directed speech and the presentation of the *Learning to Listen Sounds* facilitate the discrimination of sounds (Goldstein & Schwade, 2008). Furthermore, changes in pitch and tone help

gain and maintain the child's attention and facilitate auditory memory, and the understanding of the emotional content in language that promotes linguistic and social development (Kaplan, Jung, Ryther, & Zarlengo-Strouse, 1996). Therefore, *Learning to Listen Sounds* are not only easy to hear, but easy to process auditorily, enjoyable to listen to, and easy to learn (Estabrooks, 2006).

Many *Learning to Listen Sounds* are those that children typically begin producing within the first two years of life and are easy for children to say and sing (Estabrooks, 2006). For example, infants pick up the vocal cues of infant-/child-directed speech and will often pattern their own babbling after it (Goldstein & Schwade, 2008). From 12 months of age onward, children produce approximations of many of the *Learning to Listen Sounds* and phrases heard throughout their daily routines and activities, and begin to use novel combinations of *Learning to Listen Sounds* followed by words to communicate their observations, wants, and needs.

When a young child understands a variety of *Learning to Listen Sounds*, the AV practitioner and parent will say the words without using the *Learning to Listen Sounds*. The transition, therefore, to real words is often spontaneous, especially if the child has had rich auditory experiences in a variety of playful scenarios and everyday experiences with these *Learning to Listen Sounds*. Practitioners guide and coach parents to present *Learning to Listen Sounds* in creative and systematic ways, using a number of strategies described in Chapters 15 and 17, and move forward to the development of conversations as quickly and efficiently as possible.

LEARNING TO LISTEN SOUNDS AND SONGS (ENGLISH)

Sound	Activity/Toy	Song
ahh	airplane	The Airplane
oo	train	The Train
bu, bu, bu	bubbles or bus	Bubbles or The Bus
brr, beep, beep	car, truck	The Car
p, p, p	boat, popping toys	The Boat
t, t, t	clock	The Clock
ow/ouch	fall down, cut	Ouch!
ow, ow, ow	ambulance, fire truck	The Ambulance
wow	any surprise	WOW!
hee, hee, hee	monkey	Monkey in a Tree
Ha, ha, ha	clown, laughter	Funny Little Clown
g/go	running	Running, Running
Ya hoo!	cowboy	The Cowboy
Whee, whee!	slide or Chinese yoyo	The Slide or My Blue Yoyo
Mama	baby doll	Baby Doll
Hi!	mirror	The Mirror
meow	cat	Kitty Cat
ruff, ruff or bow wow	dog	The Dog
baa, oink	sheep, pig	Living on the Farm
moo, neigh	cow, horse	The Farm
quack	duck	Six Little Ducks
tongue clack	horse	Clip, Clop
hoo, hoo	owl	Mr. Owl
hop, hop	rabbit	The Rabbit
whistle	birdie	The Birds
cock-a-doodle-doo	rooster	The Rooster

Sound	Activity/Toy	Song
caw, caw	crow	Big Black Crow
round and round and round	windmill, top, wheels	The Windmill, The Spinning Top, and Wheels
mmmm	any good thing	Mmmm Good
n	"no"	No No!
d	toy shovel	Dig Dig
s	snake	The Snake
sh	sleeping games	Someone's Sleeping
La, la, la, la, la	rocking the baby	Rock the Baby
u, u, up	any "up" activity	Pick Me Up

REFERENCES

Bredin, H. (1996). Onomatopoeia as a figure and a linguistic principle. *New Literary History, 27*(3), 555–569. Johns Hopkins University Press. Retrieved February 2, 2016, from Project MUSE database.

Estabrooks, W. (1994). *Auditory-verbal therapy for parents and professionals*. Washington, DC: Alexander Graham Bell Association for the Deaf and Hard of Hearing.

Estabrooks, W. (2006). *Auditory-verbal therapy and practice*. Washington, DC: Alexander Graham Bell Association for the Deaf and Hard of Hearing.

Estabrooks, W., & Marlowe, J. (2000). *The baby is listening*. Washington, DC: Alexander Graham Bell Association for the Deaf and Hard of Hearing.

Goldstein, M. H., & J. A. Schwade. (2008). Social feedback to infants' babbling facilitates rapid phonological learning. *Psychological Science, 19*(5), 515–523.

Kaplan, P., Jung, P., Ryther, J., & Zarlengo-Strouse, P. (1996). Infant-directed versus adult-directed speech as signals for face. *Developmental Psychology, 32*(5), 880–891.

Krause, J. C., & Braida, L. D. (2004). Acoustic properties of naturally produced clear speech at normal speaking rates. *Journal of the Acoustical Society of America, 115*(1), 362.

Literary Devices Editors. (2016). *Onomatopoeias*. Retrieved February 2, 2016, from http://literarydevices.net/onomatopoeias/

Onomatopoeia. (n.d.). Dictionary.com Unabridged. Retrieved February 2, 2016, from Dictionary.com website: http://dictionary.reference.com/browse/onomatopoeia

Reschke, K. L. (2002). Ohio State University, "Baby talk." Archived August 22, 2007, at the Wayback Machine.

Shultz, S., & Vouloumanos, A. (2010). Three-month-olds prefer speech to other naturally occurring signals. *Language Learning and Development, 6*, 241–257.

Singh, L., Nestor, S., Parikh, C., & Yull, A. (2009). Influences of infant-directed speech on early word recognition. *Infancy, 14*(6), 654–666.

Vouloumanos, A., & Werker, J. F. (2007). Listening to language at birth: Evidence for a bias for speech in neonates. *Developmental Science, 10*(2), 159–164.

10

DEVELOPMENT OF THREE-DIMENSIONAL CONVERSATIONS AND AUDITORY-VERBAL THERAPY

Helen McCaffrey Morrison
and Warren Estabrooks

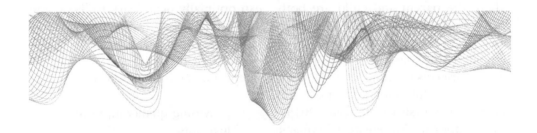

INTRODUCTION

Auditory-Verbal practitioners (practitioners) and parents endeavor to engage children who are deaf or hard of hearing in conversations, in ways that facilitate language acquisition as quickly and most enjoyably as possible. Guiding and coaching parents to engage their children in conversations form the structure and primary methodology in Auditory-Verbal Therapy (AVT), an interactive, conversation-based approach for children and their families. Conversations in AVT are child centered and intentional, stimulated and encouraged using evidence-based/informed strategies to help children acquire meaningful spoken language, primarily by listening.

Children learn language by participating in conversations. The number of adult words spoken in a child's daily environment has been found to correlate with language development (Gilkerson & Richards, 2008; Hart & Risely, 1995). Embedding those adult words in *conversational turns* between parent and child has even far greater power to impact language outcomes (Gilkerson et al., 2018; Hirsh-Pasek et al., 2015; Zimmerman et al., 2009). When children engage in conversations, they have many opportunities to practice both receptive and expressive language skills. These opportunities lead to activation of the neural firing in the Broca's area of the brain, a region linked to processes fundamental to the acquisition of receptive and expressive spoken language comprehension, such as speech production, language comprehension, and working memory (Romeo et al., 2018).

Parent–child conversational turns that are most influential on language development occur (1) in interactions where the parent and child are both focused on the same object or experience, (2) in routines, daily activities, or familiar book sharing where predictability supports learning, and (3) when parents and children take turns in the interaction (Hirsh-Pasek et al., 2015). Conversational turns create a feedback loop for parents and children that helps move a child's language forward (Romeo et al., 2018; Zimmerman et al., 2009). When parents *listen with intention* to their children they are able to fine-tune their own spoken input to better match their children's language level. Parents' responses help to extend their children's lexical knowledge and expand or refine the length and complexity of their utterances.

Practitioners and parents consciously apply strategies along three dimensions of conversation to help move children's language development forward, as illustrated in Figure 10–1.

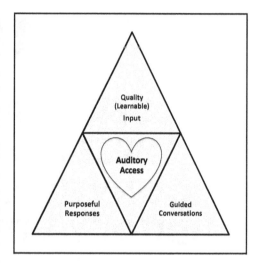

Figure 10-1. Three-dimensional conversations in Auditory-Verbal Therapy.

The first, and centermost, act in AVT is to ensure auditory access to all the sounds of speech through the use of hearing technologies so the child can optimally hear, learn to listen and talk, and become engaging partners in conversation. Parents learn to surround their listening child with three-dimensional conversations by:

- providing quality input for learning,
- guiding the child's participation in conversation, and
- responding to their child in a purposeful manner to affirm the child's attempt at conversation or to help the child improve.

We define conversation broadly, beginning at the first moments of connection between infants and parents and proceeding through dialogues that typically occur between parents and young children in everyday life. As we look more closely at how parent–child conversations function along these dimensions to facilitate language development in early childhood for typically developing children, we describe the impact of childhood hearing loss on parent–child interaction. And finally, we present evidence-based/informed conversational strategies that practitioners and parents use to engage children and help them to comprehend and use spoken language. This chapter serves as a precursor to the extensive discussion of strategies used in AVT for the development of listening, talking, and thinking, presented in Chapters 12, 15, and 17, and parent coaching, presented in Chapter 16. In addition, we provide snapshots from actual conversations that occurred among practitioners, parents, and children.

Learning to Listen in Conversation

Doreen Pollack (Pollack, Goldberg, & Caleffe-Schenck, 1997) described a child's first year following the diagnosis and fitting of hearing technology as the "Learning to Listen Year." The AV practitioner (practitioner) coaches parents to use strategies that help children achieve short-term auditory objectives, centering on detecting the sounds of life and identifying their meanings, thus connecting the infant to the world around him. The Learning to Listen sounds (see Chapter 9) are often featured in early AVT sessions to help a young child associate easily perceived speech patterns to familiar toys and experiences. The following contrasts a non-conversational approach to incorporating the Learning to Listen Sounds in AVT with one that is based in conversation.

First, as a non-conversational example, a practitioner might say the sound of a toy ("aah" for airplane, "moo" for cow, "buh-buh-buh" for bus, etc.) presenting one toy at a time, observing the child's response, passing the toy to the parent, observing the parent and child together, then discussing what happened with the parent. Presenting toys and sounds in isolation, one by one, in this manner provides a small amount of diagnostic information about the child and parent but does not engage children and parents in meaningful conversation.

Rather, AVT sessions need to focus on the ultimate goal of competence in conversation. Children learn conversation by hearing conversation and love to imitate their parents. A conversationally based approach is no longer just a test to determine if a child detects the Learning to Listen Sounds but provides a learning experience with parent and practitioner providing linguistic input during joint attention with a child, talking about the sounds that a toy makes and what that toy can do. Snapshot #1 below involves a parent, practitioner, and a toddler age 18 months. The child has auditory access to the speech spectrum with hearing aids. Listening age is 1 month.

Throughout this snapshot and the ones that follow you'll see that parent and practitioner statements have been coded along conversational dimensions:

- providing quality input
- guiding conversations
- purposeful responses

Notice how the conversation between practitioner and parent in this snapshot functions to provide input from which the child can learn. To begin, the practitioner observes that the child is attending to Mom and practitioner and not distracted by other toys.

Snapshot #1

Child: Chronological age (CA) 9 months, hearing age (HA) 3 months, severe-profound hearing loss, hearing aid user

Practitioner: I have an airplane. (*providing input*)

Parent: Oh, you do? (*providing input*)

Practitioner: You know what the airplane says, right? (*providing input*)

Parent: Right! It says "ahhhh". (*providing input*)

Practitioner: It does say "ahhhh." I like that sound. Say it again. (*providing input*)

Parent: It says, "ahhhh." (*providing input*)

Practitioner: Want to play with it? (*providing input*)

Parent: Wow! Sure. (*providing input*)

The practitioner hands the toy to the parent. The parent ensures that the child is watching the toy (*guiding conversation*). The parent then makes the airplane "fly" while saying the sound (*providing input*). Then the parent "parks" the toy on the table. The parent looks toward the child (*guiding conversation*).

Parent: Do you want to play? (*guiding conversation*)

The parent looks at the toy, waits for the child to give a verbal or nonverbal response (*guiding conversation*). The parent hands the toy to the child.

Child: Imitates flying gesture with the plane, vocalizes, and places the toy on the table.

The practitioner picks up the toy airplane.

Practitioner to child: I heard you. You said, "ahhhh" (*purposeful response*)

Practitioner to parent: Can I show you something else? (*providing input*)

Parent: Sure. (*providing input*)

Practitioner: The airplane says, "ahhhh" and it goes up, up, up and around and around and around.

The practitioner moves the plane up and then around in circles. (*providing input*)

Parent: Great idea, I can do it. (*providing input*).

The practitioner hands the toy to the parent.

Parent: I love going on airplanes that say "ahhhh." I go up, up, up and around and around.

The parent is moving the plane up and in circles. (*providing input*)

PROCESSES AND DEVELOPMENTAL MILESTONES IN EARLY PARENT-CHILD CONVERSATIONS WITH TYPICALLY DEVELOPING CHILDREN

Early parent–infant interactions evolve into conversations over the early childhood years. Children attend to adults, derive meaning from the adult signal, respond, take turns, and begin to consider the perspective of others using skills developed across a number of developmental domains—perceptual/cognitive, social, linguistic, and even motoric (Thelen, 2005) (see also Chapter 13). At the same time, parents learn to *read* their children's behaviors and communicative attempts so that they can respond in ways that support language learning (Bornstein, Tamis-Lemonda, Hahn, & Hayes, 2008). Together, children and parents co-create conversations that are contingent and sequential. An understanding of the processes and milestones in early parent–child conversations requires observation of what infants and young children do, what parents do, and the contexts in which conversations appear.

Infancy, Birth to 9 Months

Newborns listen and pay attention. In the first weeks of life infants demonstrate a preference for listening to their parents' voices by paying attention to their mothers' voices for longer durations than they do to other voices (DeCasper & Fifer, 1980) (see also Chapter 9). By 3 to 4 months of age, infant auditory preferences are influenced by their listening experience, paying attention for longer durations to their mothers' productions of infant-directed speech than to their mothers' speech delivered as though speaking to another adult (Panneton, Abraham, Berman, & Staska, 1997). These infant auditory preferences help babies *tune in* to parents and attend to linguistic input (see Chapter 9).

As well as demonstrating listening, very young infants also vocalize. Infant vocalizations during the first 2 months are reflexive, not under conscious control, and are propelled by physical states such as hunger, satiety, pain, or discomfort from a wet diaper. Reflexive vocalizations include cries, burps, coughs, grunts, and laughter (which appears at about 3 to 4 months of age). Parents can accurately interpret these vocalizations to determine the nature of their infant's state (Swain, Mayes, & Leckman, 2004) and respond with appropriate caregiving. Over the duration of the first 9 months, infants gain greater control over their vocalizations, making more speech-like sounds that parents subsequently imitate and play with during meaningful interactions with their babies. This strengthens the parent–infant bond and establishes an expectation for infants that their vocalizations will be met with parents' response, a first step toward a child's participation in conversational turn taking (see Chapter 11).

Parent–infant interactions during the first 9 months of life are *dyadic* (infants and parents respond to each other, with little reference to objects or events outside the dyad). These earliest parent–infant *conversations* take place during episodes where parents are responding to infant physical needs, providing general caregiving, engaging in daily routines, or playing (Stephens & Matthews, 2014). Parents not only talk about what they are doing but also engage in *affective speech*—comforting, soothing, and using their voices to engage the infant (Kondaurova, Bergeson, Xu, & Kitaura, 2015).

During caregiving, parents treat infant vocalizations as conversational turns, responding verbally to vocalizations and pausing for the infant to take a turn by doing what infants do—making eye contact (as early as 6 to 10 weeks), smiling, laughing, or vocalizing (Casillas, 2014). These infant responses, in turn, increase parent talk to their babies (Smith & Trainor, 2008) and build a foundation for child participation in conversational turns.

The speech directed to infants by their parents provides eminently learnable input with rich linguistic content and reference. Infant-directed speech is characterized by acoustic characteristics and linguistic features that promote speech recognition, segmentation of words and phrases, and extraction of meaning (Thiessen, Hill, & Saffran, 2005; Werker et al., 2007). Infant-directed speech is higher and more variable in pitch and creates pronounced intonational contours that communicate affect and circumscribe phrases (Fernald & Simon, 1984). Key content words appear at the end of utterances and are marked with changes in pitch (e.g., "Here's your *binkie*") (Fernald & Mazzie, 1991). Rate is slower compared with adult-directed speech, resulting in more clearly articulated phonemes (Fernald & Simon, 1984). Utterances are

---

Serendipitous Conversations

During the course of an AVT session the practitioner (below) had an "Aha!" moment that changed the direction of almost every subsequent session. This young child was bored with the activities, primarily because the practitioner wanted the child to look at a set of five cards on the table and then correctly pick out the "correct" card, after hearing the stimulus. The boy was cooperative but exhibited "yawning behaviors."

The session started off fine, capturing the child's attention with the Six Sound Test, followed by an "auditory hook" (see Chapter 15) and playing a game of "What's missing?" using a puzzle. Then came the "game" with the five cards. It was really a performance task (*aka* a test) and the practitioner thought, as an investigator, it was a good way to get the diagnostic information as quickly as possible in an "isolated" way. The practitioner slowed down the chance for developing conversation. The child yawned frequently throughout the activity and demonstrated other distracted behaviors. The practitioner had captured this child's auditory attention but not his imagination; he had not engaged the parent by handing over the activity; he had not followed the child's lead, and had not given the child anything interesting to talk about—not a good way to start or carry on a conversation. But things got better.

Conversational Scenario #2

Child: C.A 2.5 years, H.A 1.5 years, CI user on one side and hearing aid on the contralateral ear.

When the practitioner took the cards out of the box to return them to a drawer, the child looked into the box and said "Bee." Then the real learning started:

Practitioner: No, it's not a bee. (*contingent purposeful response*)
Child: Approximation for What's that?
Practitioner: It's just a piece of wool. (*providing input* with new vocabulary; *contingent purposeful response*)
Child: Wool.
Practitioner: Want to blow it? (*guiding conversation*)

The child blows the small piece of wool from the practitioner's hand. The practitioner holds a toy under the table and says, "I have a toy that spins around." (The child had demonstrated in past sessions that he knew a top was a toy that spins). The practitioner pauses, expecting the child to name the top or ask for it. (*guiding conversation*)

Child: Thank you. (expecting that this social language would gain him the toy)
Practitioner: Try again. Do you want this?

The practitioner holds out the toy, looks at the child, and waits. (*guiding conversation*)

Child: Yeah.
Parent: Then it's good to say, (name of practitioner).

The practitioner leans toward the boy expecting him to call his name (*guiding conversation*). Instead, the child kisses the practitioner on the cheek, misreading the strategy of leaning in. Then, the practitioner moved on to the next activity.

Practitioner to mother: Mommy, do you want this top? (*guiding conversation*)
Mother: Yes, sure! (*providing input*)

The practitioner hands the toy to the mother.

Practitioner to mother: Can you show us what the top can do?
Mother: It spins. It goes around and round and round. (*providing input*)
Mother to child: Would you like a turn?
Child: My turn, please.
Mother hands the child the top.
Child: (playing with top) Spin, round, round.
Practitioner: The top is going around and round. It's spinning. (*purposeful response—expansion*)
Child: Top spin. Round and round.

The child looks down at the floor and points to the piece of wool.

Practitioner: I see that. Want the piece of wool again? (*providing input, contingent purposeful response*)

The practitioner pauses and waits. (*guiding conversation*)

Child: Want blow.
Practitioner: Oh! You want to blow the wool. (*providing input, purposeful response*—expansion and extension of vocabulary)

The practitioner picks up the wool.

Then they were able to move forward with the development of a conversation moving from a small piece of wool to a toy, just because the child was now talking about something that interested him and he did not feel tested.

shorter, simpler in grammatical structure, and more concrete in semantic content (Fernald & Mazzie, 1991). Listening to infant-directed speech helps the infant build a foundation for receptive and expressive language and for the development of conversations.

The repetitiveness of parent language during routine social contexts that encompass interactive turns—caregiving, daily events, book sharing, songs, and play—lends structure and predictability to what an infant is listening to. Within the first few months of life infants learn the rhythm and sequence of interactive turns that structure the scripts of daily routines, guiding a child's participation in these same routines. By the age of 4 months, infants are so familiar with "peek-a-boo" that they become distracted and pay less attention if parents disrupt the timing and sequence of the game (Rochat, Querida, & Striano, 1999). Infants are beginning to learn when they might take a turn in any given interaction.

Late Infancy and Toddlerhood, 9 to 18 Months

The acoustic qualities in parent speech broadens during late infancy/toddlerhood. Although infant-directed speech continues to be the predominant, affective speech style for helping infants/toddlers learn language (Ramírez-Esparza, García-Sierra, & Kuhl, 2014), parents also begin to use intonational contours that are more similar to the speech of other adults (Kondaurova, Bergeson, Xu, & Kitamura, 2015). Parents use an adult-directed speech style to give simple directions that keep

their older infants/toddlers within safe boundaries, guide constructive play, and request objects or the performance of small tasks.

The routines of daily living continue to guide conversations and language learning through later infancy and toddlerhood. Routines cut a path for *word learning* (Roy, Frank, & Roy, 2012). Parents repeat the same words and phrases each time they dress, feed, diaper, or play "peek-a-boo" with their child. At the same time infants are listening to their parents' commentary, they are seeing the objects referred to and experiencing or performing the actions that are being described. The language of routines supports the formation of neural semantic networks, linking words and phrases that belong together (e.g., plates, spoons, cups, milk, are for eating; ewww, yucky, wet, wipe, nappy for diapering) (Beckage, Smith, & Hills, 2011). After 8 to 9 months of listening and participation in daily routines, infants demonstrate comprehension of their first words (Paul, 2007) and then, by the time children reach the preschool years, they are able to group words by category.

At 9 months infants engage in *joint attention* with their parents by gazing at objects or watching actions, and sharing activities together (Carpenter, Nagell, Tomasello, Butterworth, & Moore, 1998). The development of joint attention shifts parent–infant interaction from *dyadic* to *triadic* communication (Stephens & Matthews, 2014), meaning that there is now a third component—the object or activity of joint attention. The emergence of joint attention represents a significant milestone for language acquisition because it increases the number of opportunities and meaningful contexts for conversation (Carpenter, Nagell, & Tomasello, 1998; Vallotton, Mastergeorge, Foster, Decker, & Ayoub, 2017). The length of time that an infant is able to engage in joint attention with parents positively correlates with later vocabulary size and overall language development (Brooks & Meltzoff, 2008).

Parents use a variety of effective strategies to engage infants in joint attention, which in turn helps infants learn about participation in conversational turns. When parents notice what has engaged their infant's attention and then talk about the infant's focus of attention, they are better able to nurture language acquisition than if parents attempt to redirect their infant's focus to what parents want to talk about (Masur, Flynn, & Eichorst, 2005). When parents do wish to engage infants and toddlers in a joint focus of the parents' own choosing, an effective strategy is to get their child's attention and establish joint attention to an object or activity first, and then talk about what they are seeing once joint attention has been established (Estigarribia & Clark, 2007).

Parents talk to infants/toddlers during episodes of joint attention in ways that encourage their children's vocal participation and move language development forward. Parents note their child's object of attention, follow the child's lead, and respond with talk about their child's focus. Responsive comments during moments of joint attention with demonstrated impact on child language development include (Roberts, Hensle, & Brooks, 2016):

- *self-talk:* talking about what the parent is doing while both are engaged in the same activity ("I'm making my tower tall. I'm taking the block up, up, up")
- *parallel talk:* talking about what their child is doing ("You're building a tower. You're making it tall. Look at your blocks go up, up, up")
- *mirror and map:* joining in with their child by imitating their child's action and talking about the shared activity ("You're dancing! I'll dance too. Round and round")

The development of joint attention enables parents and their children to enjoy looking at books together. *Book sharing* opens an expansive world of language learning opportunities, with new words and contexts available in each new story. The repetitiveness of language each time a book is read has the same teaching power as daily routines. After listening to parents read a loved book over and over, children begin to chime in with the language of the book and even take turns "reading" some of the pages. Parents and children can have conversations about what is on the page in addition to what is printed on the page, using the pictures as a shared referent (see also Chapter 14).

Infant/toddlers, toward the end of their first year, become *active communicators*. One of the first forms of communication is pointing and gesturing (Ates & Kuntay, 2018), with first word use appearing around 11 to 12 months. Infants/toddlers from 9 to 12 months use predominantly non-verbal communicative acts to request objects or direct adults, refuse, greet or take leave, to comment, or play games. Toddlers from 12 to 18 months increase word use and add to the repertoire of their communicative acts by participating in *symbolic play* routines such as playing with dolls, pretending to talk on the phone, pushing cars or trains. Toddlers begin to engage in symbolic play, which increases the opportunities to practice conversational turns between toddlers and their parents. By 18 months toddlers have become predominantly word-users and expand their communicative intents to include requesting information (What's that? Where's Daddy?) and answering rudimentary questions (Paul, 2007).

The level and type of parents' verbal responsiveness to these early communicative attempts facilitate language development and scaffold children's participation in conversation. Responses that positively impact language development:

- occur close in time to the child's attempt
- carry a positive message
- demonstrate that the parent has listened to what the child has communicated, including imitations of the child or *contingent* statements that are related to what the child has intended to say (Renzi, Romberg, Bolger, & Newman, 2017; Vallotton et al., 2017)

Conversely, directive speech that is intrusive, negative, or prohibitive such as "no, stop, don't do that" halts conversational turns and fails to influence later language development (Renzi et al., 2017).

Toddlerhood Through the Preschool Years, Age 18 Months to 4 Years

Children's language abilities blossom as they mature from toddlerhood through the preschool years. Toddlers enter this period with a small core vocabulary and proceed to acquire new words at a steady rate. Children produce from 25 to 200 words at 18 months and from 400 to 600 words at 30 months (Braginsky, Yurovsky, Marchman, & Frank, 2016). Mean length of utterance expands from an average of 1.5 words/morphemes at 18 months to over 5 words/morphemes by age 4 years. Sentences grow in complexity and the ideas that children express are limited only by their imaginations.

Parents adapt their speech style to their children's developmental level, increasing in complexity and resemblance to adult-directed speech as children's language levels increase (Clarke, 2014; Jo & Ko, 2018; Ramírez-Esparza, García-Sierra, & Kuhl, 2014). Adult-directed intonational contours now predominate in the speech style that parents use when talking to their children. Preschoolers are more likely to learn new words from an adult-directed speech style than from infant-directed speech (Ramírez-Esparza et al., 2014).

Parents help build their children's vocabularies when they use a variety of words while talking to their toddlers and preschoolers, including unusual words, words slightly more advanced than the child's level, or playful words ("Let's make this sled go fast! Hit the accelerator!" "It's a wonkey donkey") (Huttenlocher, Waterfall, Vasilyeva, Vevea, & Hedges, 2010). Book sharing becomes an even more useful tool for parent–child conversations at this time. Parents scaffold word learning by offering new words in sentence frames that vary with the new word ("That's a _____") or in question/answer sequences where the parent asks the question and answers it ("What's that? That's a _____")

(Clark & Wong, 2002). These frames help children recognize that a new word is in play. Complete sentences are more effective than severely reduced or telegraphic speech (Bredin-Oja & Fey, 2014).

Parents' questions to their children support the integration of cognitive and language skills. "Wh" questions elicit longer utterances and more advanced words from their children (Rowe, Leech, & Cabrera, 2016). Parents use "wh" questions to guide children's narratives and help them retrieve memories of past events or retell familiar stories from favorite books (e.g., "And then what happened?" "What did Uncle Bill bring to the party?" "What happened when Goldilocks sat on Baby Bear's chair?"). Open-ended questions engage cognitive processes and lead to growth in complex language (Dickinson & Tabors, 2001) when the questions lead a child to predict ("I wonder what might happen if we drop a pebble in this pond? A leaf?"), problem-solve ("How did that kite get up there?"), or take on the perspective of others ("Why do you think that little boy is sad?").

Not all "wh" questions facilitate conversations or help nurture language acquisition at this age. Children tend to ignore or give single word answers to "wh" questions that are rhetorical or test types, or request information that is obvious to both child and parent (e.g.,

"What color is it?" "What's that shape?" "Are you bouncing your ball?").

Effective parent responses to preschool and pre-kindergarten children's communicative attempts are higher-level than those observed between parents and infants. Parent responses that were effective for facilitating toddlers' language acquisition—talking about what the child is doing, imitating the child, or labeling objects—are no longer effective when their children reach preschool age. Nevertheless, just as in infancy, preschool children learn best when parents follow their lead. Responses to preschool-aged children that *are* more likely to facilitate language development are *contingent* on what the child has said and even include some of the child's own words (Che, Brooks, Alarcon, Yannaco, & Donnelly, 2018). These include specific types of responses that help refine grammatical forms or increase vocabulary—*expansions, recasts, and extensions*:

- *Expansions* imitate the child's utterance and add a word or two (Child: "Doggie eating." Parent: "Yes! *The* doggie *is* eating") (Taumoepeau, 2016).
- *Recasts* repeat the child's words but with corrections to grammatical or speech errors (Child: "Mommy car." Adult: "Yes!

Snapshot of an Early Conversation

In the two previous snapshots the practitioner and parent provided input and guidance for a child to participate in the conversation. In this snapshot, the child is at a higher language level, using word combinations and early sentences. We observe the practitioner adding expansions as a purposeful response to help the child use more mature sentences.

Snapshot #3

Child: C.A. 3.5 years, H.A. 2 years, severe to profound hearing loss, wearing bilateral hearing aids.

Practitioner: Where's Daddy?

Child: Daddy gone.

Practitioner: Daddy's gone? Where did he go? (*contingent purposeful response*)

Child (to mother): Where Daddy?

Mommy: I don't know.

Child: I don't know.

Practitioner: Maybe he went downtown to work. (*providing input*)

Mommy: Daddy working, right. (*providing input*)

Child: Daddy working. Daddy outside.

Child: I hear a copper copper.

Practitioner: Do you?

Mommy: I hear a helicopter. (*providing input, purposeful response—recast of child word*)

Practitioner: I hear that helicopter too. (*contingent purposeful response*)

Practitioner: Listen! (*guiding conversation*)

Mommy: I hear a bird singing. (*providing input*)

Child: I hear a bird.

Practitioner: Do you hear the bird singing? (*guiding conversation, purposeful response—expansion*)

Child: Bird singing.

Warren: The bird is singing. (*purposeful response—expansion*)

Practitioner: (holds up a toy figure) Who's that?

Chile: Danta.

Practitioner: Santa Claus. (*purposeful response—expansion*) Mommy, what does Santa Claus say?

Mommy: Ho ho ho! (*providing input*)

Practitioner: Ho ho ho ho ho (*providing input*)

Child: Ho ho ho. I hear Danta.

Practitioner: You hear Santa! (*contingent purposeful response*)

Child: Danta down chimney.

Practitioner: Santa comes down the chimney. (*purposeful response—expansion*)

Child: Santa come down chimney.

Mommy's car!") (Cleave, Becker, Curran, Van Horne, & Fey, 2015).

■ *Extensions* are responses that add new information or meaning (Child: "Doggie barking." Mommy: "*He sees a kitty cat. He's excited*").

Summary

Parent–child conversations are multidimensional. Parents provide linguistic input to their children in developmentally appropriate ways that support language learning. Children listen, learn, and actively communicate, using language that grows in lexical content and complexity throughout early childhood. Parents encourage children's participation in conversation when they narrate and set up dialogues during everyday routines, play, and book sharing. Parents also observe and listen to their children's communicative attempts, respond in ways that further shape linguistic competence, and adapt facilitative responses to their children's growing sophistication in language usage.

CONVERSATIONS BETWEEN PARENTS AND CHILDREN WHO ARE DEAF OR HARD OF HEARING

Rich language environments are essential for children who are deaf or hard of hearing to develop listening and spoken language. Parent–child conversations are vital. The physical closeness between parents and young children during conversation optimizes auditory access to spoken language, essential when noise and distance degrade ambient language input. If a child does not receive consistent quality input from his parents, he is at a disadvantage compared with typically developing peers. It is helpful to identify the qualities in parent–child conversations that are most likely to help children who are deaf or hard of hearing learn language. These become a focus for parent coaching in AVT (Ambrose, Walker, Unflat-Berry, Oleson, & Moeller, 2015; Cruz, Quittner, Marker, & DesJardin, 2013; DesJardin & Eisenberg, 2007).

It is crucial that children who are deaf or hard of hearing receive, at a minimum, the typical quantity of parent talk. Computer-based analyses of day-long recordings of children who are deaf or hard of hearing reveal that the *quantity* of words spoken in their environments is similar to counts from recordings of typically developing children (Ambrose, Van Dam, & Moeller, 2014; Ambrose et al., 2015; Morrison, Lopez, & Rodriguez, 2010; Van Dam, Ambrose, & Moeller, 2012). The number of *conversational turns* between adults and children who are deaf or hard of hearing is also equivalent to counts obtained from adults and typically developing children, observed both in a large multi-site investigation of children with mild to severe hearing loss receiving a variety of intervention types (Van Dam et al., 2012) and from a program of 48 children with mild to profound hearing loss (Morrison et al., 2010). As with typically developing children, children who are deaf or hard of hearing who experience a higher rate of conversational turns in early recordings go on to develop higher language levels when assessed at later ages (Ambrose et al., 2015).

Parent–child interactions prior to the twenty-first century suggested that parents of children who are deaf or hard of hearing were more directive and used lower level language than parents of typically developing *same-age* children (Cheskin, 1981; Gallaway, Hostler, & Reeves, 1990). Current research indicates that, in reality, parents of children who are deaf or hard of hearing are *sensitive* to their children's listening and language abilities. Accordingly, the spoken language produced by parents to these children and by parents to typically developing children exhibit greater similarity when their children are matched by (1) *language level* (Cross, Nienhuys, & Kirkman, 1985; Nienhuys, Cross, & Horsborough, 1984) or (2) duration of hearing technology use, or *hearing age* (Bergeson, Miller, & McCune, 2006; Kondaurova & Bergeson, 2011; Kondaurova, Bergeson, & Xu, 2013), as opposed to matched by chronological age.

Parents' sensitivity to the abilities of their children who are deaf or hard of hearing is further demonstrated by changes in the way they talk to their children as language development progresses. When children are in the early stages of listening with hearing technology, parents use an infant-directed speech style that is similar in acoustic qualities to the infant-directed speech produced by mothers of typically developing children (Dilley et al., 2017). Also, similar to typically developing children, both the quantity and quality of infant-directed speech heard by infants and young children who are deaf or hard of hearing impact later language development (Dilley et al., 2018).

The proportion of infant-directed speech to adult-speech style decreases in parent talk as their children develop greater language skills (Kondourova et al., 2103). Once children who are deaf or hard of hearing acquire a core vocabulary and begin to use simple sentences, their parents are observed to shift to higher-level inputs and responses, including (1) increased variety of word type and mean length of utterance (DesJardin & Eisenberg, 2007), (2) parallel talk (Cruz et al., 2013), (3) expansions (Cruz et al., 2013; Szagun & Schramm, 2016), (4) recasts (DesJardin & Eisenberg, 2007), and (5) open-ended questions (DesJardin & Eisenberg, 2007; Quittner et al., 2013). Children whose parents shift to use higher-level facilitative aspects tend to demonstrate higher receptive and expressive vocabulary and more mature syntax in later years. In contrast, children's language development proceeds more slowly if their parents continue to provide input or responses that are associated with earlier stages of language development such as labeling, talking for the child's non-verbal communicative attempt, or giving directives (Quittner et al., 2013).

In summary, parents of children with hearing loss demonstrate similarity to parents of typically developing children with regard to the amount and quality of spoken language they use with their children, tailoring language to their children's language level or hearing age. The kinds of parent talk that help typically developing children learn language (e.g., parallel talk, expansions) also impact the language development of children who are deaf or hard of hearing. This is especially true when parents of children who are deaf or hard of hearing provide input and respond to their children in ways that are in synchrony with their children's listening and language levels.

CONVERSATIONAL INTERVENTION

Importantly for AVT, intervention that helps parents engage their children in conversations leads to improvements in children's language development (Burgoyne, Gardner, Whiteley, Snowling, & Hulme, 2018; Costa et al., 2019; DeVeney, Hagaman, & Bjornsen, 2017; Ferjan Ramírez, Lytle, Fish, & Kuhl, 2019; Roberts, 2019; Roberts, Kaiser, Wolfe, Bryant, & Spidalieria, 2014). Parents and practitioners apply conversationally based language interventions with all sorts of children who need help to develop communication skills. Conversationally based language intervention programs for young children with general communication delays or specific language impairment utilize strategies that are either adapted from typical parent–child interactions or designed to address the special needs of children who are developing differently. For example, some children may need assistance learning to initiate or take turns

Having a Chat

The child in the next snapshot has complete sentences, the ability to respond, and can make her own contributions in conversation. We see the practitioner applying semantic extension as a purposeful response—supplying a word that the child needs or extending her word use by adding a higher-level synonym to the child's contribution.

Practitioner: Wow, look at this animal! Do you know what this is? (*guiding conversation—establishing joint attention*).

Snapshot #4

Child: C.A. 4 years, H.A. 3 years, severe hearing loss, bilateral hearing aids

Child: A crocodile.

Practitioner: A crocodile. (*contingent purposeful response*)

Child: I'm scared.

Practitioner: You're scared? (*contingent purposeful response*)

Child: It might bite Mommy.

Practitioner: Do you think?

Child: I just put on my shoulder. Daddy just put on his shoulder.

Practitioner: Daddy will put it on his shoulder? (*purposeful response—expansion*) This one? No way, man! This is too big, but. It's a crocodile, but . . .

Child: I need a small one.

Practitioner: Well, maybe Daddy will buy you a small one. If you go shopping . . .

Child: Ya, not a big one.

Practitioner: No, just a little tiny one. Just a tiny one, okay? (*providing input, purposeful response—extension of vocabulary*)

Child: Not a big one.

Practitioner: No, not a giant one. That's for sure. (*providing input,*

purposeful response—extension of vocabulary)

Child: Small one.

Practitioner: Tiny one. (*providing input, purposeful response—extension of vocabulary*)

Look at this one. (*guiding conversation—establishing joint attention*)

Child: I see a big rabbit.

Practitioner: It is a big rabbit. Do you think this is Mommy rabbit? (*guiding conversation, contingent purposeful response*)

Child: No, baby rabbit. Where did the Mommy rabbit go?

Practitioner: I don't know. Where do you think the Mommy Rabbit went? (*guiding conversation: open-ended question*)

Child: Went to buy carrots.

Practitioner: She went to buy carrots. I think that you're right. (*contingent purposeful response*) Where? (*guiding conversation: open-ended question*)

Child: In the shopping mall.

Practitioner: Oh, she went to the shopping mall. (*purposeful responses—expansion and recast*) in conversation. Many benefit from increased and focused stimulation in conversation with language targets that are individualized to the child's needs.

Two systematic reviews of early language intervention research (Gladfelter, Wendt, & Subramanian, 2011; Roberts & Kaiser, 2011) identified effective conversational strategies for boosting language development that can be viewed along the three dimensions of conversation. Strategies with demonstrated effectiveness that *provide quality input* include:

- using an infant-directed speech style
- delivering focused or enhanced stimulation using the child's individual language targets
- talking with children during episodes of joint attention

Effective strategies for *guiding children to participate in conversation* include:

- establishing predictable home and play-based language routines
- helping children initiate conversations
- facilitating conversational turn-taking

Parents and practitioners effectively *respond to a child in a purposeful manner* when they

- respond contingently to a child's communicative attempt by reflecting the child's intent or meaning
- expand a child's utterances
- provide recasts that model a more adult form. Expansions and recasts are more likely to be effective when they target a child's individual language goals (see also

Cleave et al., 2015 for a systematic review of recast effectiveness)

Two strategies that did *not* demonstrate effectiveness in helping children with communication difficulty were:

- general language stimulation without focus on the child's individual language goals
- eliciting imitations of an adult model as a primary intervention strategy (Gladfelter, Wendt, & Subramanian, 2011)

A third systematic review of intervention with communication difficulties (Sandbank & Yoder, 2016) shows that children benefit more from *simple sentences that retain articles and other morphemes* as they naturally occur compared with listening to simplified language that does not retain these elements. For example, saying "The doggy*'s* in *his* house" is more effective in helping children learn language than, "Doggy in house." Retaining the morphemic elements of simple sentences is especially relevant for practitioners and parents of children who are deaf or hard of hearing. Not only is the natural intonational contour maintained, but children receive exposure to morphemic elements that are more difficult to hear because they are short in duration and tend to be reduced in vocal intensity.

Two intervention programs that are particularly relevant to AVT have been validated by research evidence as improving children's language outcomes: the Hanen Program (Manolson, 1992; Weitzman, 2017; Weitzman, in Van Kleeck et al., 2010) and Enhanced Milieu Teaching (EMT). Both approaches regard parents as a child's primary teacher. Parents and practitioners who use these approaches:

▪ Set child language goals that become the content for focused stimulation.

▪ Plan activities that highlight a child's language goals.

▪ Provide multiple models and repetitions of the language targets in everyday routines and play.

▪ (with infants and very young children) Provide input by using an infant-directed speech style, following the child's lead, and talking about the child's focus during episodes of joint attention.

▪ Respond purposefully to child communication efforts with expansions that are slightly above the child's mean length of utterance.

▪ Use toys and activities that *stimulate* communicative attempts: dolls, toys with lots of parts that require requesting (e.g., train cars, building blocks, clay dough), or toys in containers that are difficult to open.

▪ Use *prompts* to elicit communication that includes waiting, requests for imitation, or questions that elicit the desired language ("What do you want?" "Where did the ball go?").

In summary, evidence-based intervention with children who have communication difficulty other than hearing loss demonstrate that parents learn to use conversational strategies that help children develop spoken language. Strategies that are adapted from typical parent–child conversations are applied successfully in intervention, including following a child's lead, using child-directed speech, providing language in home and daily routines, establishing joint attention, and responding with expansions and recasts. Strategies specifically developed for the needs of other children with communication challenges can also be effectively incorporated in AVT.

GUIDANCE FOR THE AUDITORY-VERBAL PRACTITIONER

Throughout this chapter we have described a variety of conversational interactions that positively affect children's language development. Table 10–1 summarizes these interactions according to a child's chronological age and communication level, organized within the three-dimensional framework. The information in Table 10–1 can translate into five strategies used by practitioners and parents in AVT to stimulate conversations:

Listening in Conversation

The next snapshot is an example of how a conversational approach can be incorporated into an auditory task. The child is listening to clues and using auditory memory to determine what the practitioner is talking about based on the clues he hears. The practitioner gives space for the child to contribute his own comments. We see some of the strategies that appeared in previous snapshots with the addition of giving clues and using open-ended questions to keep the conversation going.

Snapshot #5

Child: CA 5, HA 3.5 years, severe-profound hearing loss, cochlear implant (CI) user

Practitioner: I heard something.

Child: Me too.

Practitioner: What was that sound?

Child: I don't know

Practitioner: It was far away. (*guiding conversation: giving clues*)

Child: I know. An airplane.

Practitioner: No, it wasn't an airplane. (*contingent purposeful response*)

Child: Yeah.

Practitioner: No, it wasn't. (*contingent purposeful response*)

Child: Yeah!

Practitioner: Did you hear It, Mommy? (*guiding conversation—providing a model*)

Mother: I heard it. It was outside. (*providing input*)

Practitioner: You know what it was? It was something you blow. (*guiding conversation—giving clues*) If there is a car in front of you and you want that car to get out of the way, you might blow your _____. (*guiding conversation—auditory closure*)

Child: Whistle! Ha, ha, ha.

(later) Practitioner: This is something that you can smell and you can pick it. (*guiding conversation: giving clues*)

Child: Apple.

Practitioner: Yes, you pick apples, but this is something else that you pick. They're beautiful and they grow in the garden. (*purposeful response—expansion; guiding conversation: giving clues*)

Child: Flowers.

Practitioner: Excellent. Yellow Flowers. (*purposeful response—expansion*) Now here's a little animal that we love at Easter Time.

Child: A bunny.

Practitioner: We love the Easter Bunny! (*contingent purposeful response*)

Child: You know what?

Practitioner: What?

Child: When I was taking Ryan home, at Ryan's house, umm umm, Ryan saw a bunny.

Practitioner: Yeah?

Child: Ryan saw a bunny and we were trying to catch it. And the bunny was hopping. He was faster and we were trying to run.

Practitioner: So, you were trying to catch the bunny? (*contingent purposeful response*)

Child: Yeah.

Practitioner: Oh cool. Did you catch him? (*contingent purposeful response*)

Child: Yeah!

Practitioner: You did?

Child: Yeah. Me and Ryan.

Practitioner: So, what did you do with him after you caught him? (*guiding conversation—open-ended question*)

Child: Ryan caught him first and he said, "Ouch!" And then he put him down on the ground and we were trying to catch him again.

Table 10–1. Three-Dimensional Interactions that Impact Language Development Child Chronological Age and Communication Milestones

Child	Parents/Practitioners		
	Birth to 9 Months: Pre-Verbal Level		
Communication Milestones	**Providing Quality Input**	**Guiding Conversations**	**Responding Purposefully**
• Prefers mother's voice, infant-directed speech style • Reflexive cries alert parents to needs • Plays with voice • Vowel-like vocalizations • Makes eye contact • Responds to adults with eye contact, smile, laugh, vocalization • Anticipates sequence and timing of verbal routines	• Use affective speech: comforting, soothing, describing infant state • Use infant-directed speech style • Routines/scripts for caregiving, daily events, games	• Engage infant with voice • Use infant-directed speech style • Routines/scripts for caregiving, daily events, games • Pause during talk to give infant a "turn"	• Affective speech: comforting, soothing, describing infant state • Use infant-directed speech style • Routines/scripts for caregiving, daily events, games • Return eye-contact • Respond to infants' vocalizations with imitation and talk

continues

Table 10–1. *continued*

9–18 Months: Pre- and Early Verbal

Child	Parents/Practitioners		
Communication Milestones	**Providing Quality Input**	**Guiding Conversations**	**Responding Purposefully**
• Learns words and phrases from routines/scripts • 9 mos: comprehends first words and phrases, joint attention emerges • 11 mos: non-verbal communicative attempts emerge • 12 mos: expresses first words • Communicative intents expressed: request objects, direct adults, refuse, greet or take leave, comment, request information	• Routines/scripts for caregiving, daily events, games, book sharing, symbolic play • Joint attention: expand topics for talk to infants beyond daily routines, refer to and narrate child's focus of attention with self-talk, parallel talk, mirror and map • Use simple, grammatically complete sentences. • Provide focused stimulation for language targets.	• Routines/scripts for caregiving, daily events, games, book sharing, symbolic play • Joint attention: follow child's focus of attention, or get child's attention to direct focus and then talk • Joint book viewing. • Entice children to initiate conversation. • Encourage children to respond in conversation, using prompts when necessary.	• Routines/scripts for caregiving, daily events, games, book sharing, symbolic play • Joint attention: respond to the child's focus of attention with self-talk, parallel talk, mirror and map • Responses to communicative attempts that are positive, timely, reflect child's intent

18 months–4 years: Development of Verbal Communication

Child		Parents/Practitioners		
Communication Milestones		**Providing Quality Input**	**Guiding Conversations**	**Responding Purposefully**
• 18 mos: uses 25–200 words, 1.5 MLU • 30 mos: 400–600 words • 4 years: 5.0 MLU • Talks about objects and events outside immediate context • Develops narrative abilities		• Increased adult-directed speech style • Provide input slightly above the child's level. • Use simple, but grammatically complete sentences. • Increase sentence complexity as child progresses. • Scaffold new words in sentence frames. • Use a variety of words, higher level words • Provide focused stimulation for language targets.	• Routines/scripts for caregiving, daily events, games, book sharing, symbolic play • Entice children to initiate conversation. • Encourage children to respond in conversation, using prompts when necessary. • "Wh," open-ended, and problem-solving questions to keep conversation going & help child with narrations	• Responses to child's statements that are positive, timely, reflect child's intent • Answer children's questions • To build child's language use expansions, recasts, extensions

- having developmentally appropriate conversations,
- starting with power conversations,
- enticing and encouraging,
- keeping it going, and
- lifting them up.

Having Developmentally Appropriate Conversations

The developmental level of the child dictates which interactions are more likely to move language forward. Parents in AVT are engaged in a developmental process as well, building the knowledge and skills they need to help their children learn to listen and use spoken language.

Coaching Parent-Child Conversations from the Beginning

Parents and children interact from the beginning of a child's life. These interactions establish a foundation for the conversational turns that are vitally important to spoken language development. Coaching parents to interact effectively with their children and establish dyadic communication in the earliest months of life has great value in AVT (see Chapters 15–17).

Tailoring Conversations to a Child's Developmental Level

Table 10–1 makes clear that parents shift their interactions as children's language and their ability to converse develop. For example, parent strategies that are effective with infants and toddlers, such as the use of infant-directed speech, are not as important to language development when a child is conversing at age 3 with a higher mean length of utterance (MLU). Narrating actions during sessions of joint attention may be effective in late infancy or when children are just beginning to understand words and phrases. It is more effective, however, to help a child express his/her own observations once the child begins to use language on his own. Accordingly, practitioners coach parents to use a variety of strategies, dependent upon the child's development, rather than to employ a fixed set of strategies that are applied across all children on a caseload regardless of developmental level.

Practitioners are advised to refer to typical development for the sequences and benchmarks for child language development, and most importantly, to use developmentally appropriate conversational strategies commensurate with the child's level of function, in pursuit of accurate diagnostic information.

Tailoring Conversations to a Child's Needs

Intervention research indicates that conversations are more effective when they emphasize a child's language goals, both in input and in the responses that adults give to children (aka focused stimulation). Practitioners are advised to choose activities and toys intentionally to help a child learn new vocabulary or grammatical forms that have been selected as learning objectives for the child, and to provide many examples for parents to replicate during play and opportunities for the child to practice.

Tailoring Conversational Strategies to Parents' Skill Development

Practitioners quickly notice the communication strategies a parent uses readily and the ones that can be increased with coaching. Practitioners take time in each AVT session to observe parents and children interacting without joining in and then collaborate with parents to help them set goals for themselves (see also Chapter 16 for parent coaching strategies).

Starting with Power Conversations

The most effective parent-child conversational turns occur in the powerful contexts of daily routines and moments of joint attention, including sharing books, during which parents can use strategies from each of the conversational dimensions.

Scaffolding Language and Conversations in Routines/ Scripts for Caregiving, Daily Events, Games, Book Sharing, and Symbolic Play

The inclusion of daily routines during AVT sessions helps parents discover many ways to narrate daily life and create opportunities for children to take a turn in the most natural contexts. If there's a need for a diaper change, then the diaper change becomes part and parcel of the session (see Chapter 17).

When a child is ready for symbolic play, acting out daily routines with dolls provides the child and parent with different roles in an action-based scenario, during which the child can take on different roles. Talking about books that portray everyday events is a powerful way to enhance natural language and expand it over the years of AVT. Table 10–2 lists sources for language routines in the home and the community that were derived from a national survey of over 3,000 parents in the United States (Dunst, Hamby, Trivette, Raab, & Bruder, 2000).

Play can become a family routine when parents are coached to play with toys in a predictable manner, saying many of the same things each time they play with a toy to create a learnable "script." For example, when using modeling clay, we can coach parents to say: "What's inside this can?" "Let's open the can," "Pull it out," "Mmm. Smell it!" Similarly, when using wind-up toys, we can coach them to say: "turn, turn, turn," "wait," "1-2-3-go!" Taking turns in play allows a child to listen to the practitioner and his parents, as well as to try out the language himself.

When planning an AVT session with conversations in mind, practitioners think ahead about the language that can be used with toys and develop short-term measurable objectives around that language. Once the routine is established, practitioners "raise the bar" so that new language can be practiced. Practitioners also repeat enjoyable learning experiences or activities from session to session. Learning proceeds from multiple exposures and therefore it may not be necessary to have a completely different session plan for each session.

Conversing during Moments of Joint Attention

Practitioners and parents provide the language for the object, event, or activity that has captured the child's attention. They talk about what they are doing (self-talk) and what the child is doing (parallel talk), and they join in and copy the child's activity while talking about what's happening (mirror and

Table 10-2. Sources for Language Routines in the Home and the Community

In the Home	Out in the Community
Preparing meals/mealtimes	Going shopping
Caring for pets	Taking walks
Bathtime/brushing teeth/washing hands	Gatherings of family or friends
Bedtime/waking up	Picnics
Picking up toys/cleaning one's room	Playdates
Toileting	Family sports
Dressing	Eating out
Looking at books	Visits to playgrounds
Cuddling	Religious practices
Riding trikes	Visits to zoos, museums
Drawing	Visits to fairs, circuses
Dancing, playing music	Going to school
Religious practices	Riding public transportation
Holiday celebrations	Children's classes: art, sports, music
Birthdays	
Having friends/family come for a visit	
Gardening	

Source: From Dunst et al., 2000.

map). This requires that practitioners and parents follow the child's lead and be mindful of the child's focus. If a box is more interesting than the toy, adults talk about the box in a way that enhances the concepts and language that the child requires. Supplying language during these serendipitous moments of joint attention takes practice. It requires being comfortable talking about one's every move or the child's every move, and using phrases appropriate in length and complexity for young children. Parents can begin to practice this skill in the privacy of their own home and, when they are comfortable and see the results, they transfer the skills anywhere, anytime.

Capturing the child's attention is especially important for children who are deaf or hard of hearing, who are likely to be missing some acoustic information in the signal, even when listening in a quiet environment with optimally fitted hearing technology. A child with hearing loss *must be ready to listen* if he is to learn from his parent's conversations. Prior to speaking, practitioners use some form of the "Listening" cue (see Chapter 15) to get a child's attention and confirm that the child is attending (e.g., cessation of activity, making eye contact).

Creating Conversations from Narrations

So far, the suggestions for language routines and episodes of joint attention have focused on parent/practitioner input. The child also needs to have a conversational turn. When parents and practitioners use language routines or scripts or share familiar books, they pause and give a child the opportunity to fill in what he knows as part of the routine (Dad: "Let's tie your shoe. Ready? Round and through and . . ." Child: "Pull!"). This strategy is especially helpful for children at the earliest stages of language development, who need the scaffolding of a language routine in order to take a conversational turn.

Parents and practitioners help the child to generate his own contributions

---

Using Imagination

The child in this snapshot is not only able to participate in conversation but can use his imagination and tell a tall tale about his vacation. The practitioner uses many strategies to expand vocabulary and prompt the child to correct a speech production.

Snapshot #6

Child: CA 5 years, HA 3.5 years, severe-profound, hearing aid user

Practitioner: Didn't you wear a bathing suit when you went to Turks and Caicos?

Child: Yup!

Practitioner: Well, what color was that one?

Child: It was Ninja Turtles!

Practitioner: Ninja Turtles? That would be nice. (*contingent purposeful response*)

Child: You know what I did? I went 'cuba diving.

Practitioner: I'm sorry? (*guiding conversation—pausing and leaning his ear toward child*)

Child: I went sssscuba diving!

Practitioner: You know, I asked Mommy about that. It wasn't scuba diving. It was snorkeling. (*purposeful response—using higher vocabulary*)

Child: AND scuba diving.

Practitioner: No . . .

Child: I went scuba diving under the water. I went scuba diving in the pool.

Practitioner: Okay, what did you see when you went under the water? (*guiding conversation: open ended question*)

Child: I saw some fish and a shark.

Practitioner: I think sharks can swim faster than you can. (*purposeful response—semantic extension*)

Child: I swam faster.

Practitioner: Than a shark? (*contingent purposeful response*)

Child: I got my motor feet on. I put them on my feet, and I went vrrrroooom up the water. And he went, "What's that? It's a boat! And he couldn't follow."

Practitioner: He couldn't follow you. You know you're lucky. (*purposeful responses—expansion and extension*)

Child: I went right on top of the water and he said, "What is that boy? He is a Motor Boat Boy."

to the conversation. Introducing problem-solving into the narration with a specific "wh" questions can promote a conversational turn. Some examples are: (1) Mom: "Let's make a peanut butter sandwich. Hmmm, now where's the bread?" Child: "Bread up there." (2) Dad: "Let's go outside. How can we keep warm?" Child: "Get our coats." Young children do not start out knowing the answers to questions, so parents and practitioners introduce questions into language routines and episodes of joint attention *before* children are able to supply the answers. We typically do not answer our own questions, especially in AVT sessions, as there is always an adult to model the answer, but if parents are alone, they may have to do just that. For example, Dad: "Here's your trike. Now, what do we need for your head? Aha! Your helmet!" Child: "Helmet head!"

Enticing and Encouraging to Guide Conversations

Practitioners and parents use a number of strategies and some handy "tricks" to encourage children to take part in conversations. Especially when children are just starting out, they *entice* children with opportunities to communicate and *encourage* them to respond to a conversational partner by using prompts.

Enticing the Child to Communicate

We create many opportunities for the child to have something to say. The following suggestions work best when applied when the child knows what is expected and is capable of attempting what he/she is asked to do. If the child doesn't communicate readily, the second adult in the session (e.g., the practitioner, the parent) provides a model to help guide the child:

(1) *Being stingy.* Parents and practitioners provide an inadequate amount of materials during play. For example, when bringing out modeling clay, they might put just a little bit on the table so that the child will ask for more. They can "joke" and give out a tiny amount each time, enticing the child to ask for bigger and bigger bits and larger portions. A word of caution—this strategy can be frustrating to a child or create power struggles if it's over-used, so it's important to be mindful that conversations need to be a source of pleasure and that conversational competence is the outcome.

(2) *Being an assistant*, by creating situations where the child needs help. For example, adults might encourage a child to say "Up" when the child wants to be picked up, or might put toys in a jar so tightly closed that a child needs to ask for help and tell the "assistant" what to do.

(3) *Taking a break in the routine.* The adult sets up a routine where the child expects certain actions, and then pauses or waits for the child to tell the adult what to do.

(4) *Giving choices.* When bringing out toys, parents or practitioners hold up two objects and ask for the one the child would like to have.

(5) *Being a saboteur*, by failing to provide the materials necessary to accomplish a task. For example,

- make a peanut butter and jelly sandwich with the child and "forget" to bring out the bread

■ make chocolate milk and bring out plates instead of glasses to drink the milk

■ set up a painting activity and provide a paintbrush that is too large for the paint pot

■ pull out vehicles with the wheels missing

(6) *Playing and acting silly.* Adults sometimes do crazy things like putting a plate of cookies on their head like a hat or trying to eat ice cream with a toy fork.

Encouraging a Child to Respond

In order to participate in a conversation, a child needs to (1) recognize that it's his turn and (2) be able to attempt the response expected. Practitioners and parents encourage and support a child to respond by *prompting*. The prompts described below are presented from the least intrusive to the most supportive. If a prompt fails to elicit vocal participation, it's helpful to be sure the child understands what he/she is being asked to do. If the child understands what to do and still has difficulty, one can move down to the next suggestion to provide a more supportive prompt. Many of these strategies are presented in a number of contexts in Chapters 12, 15, and 17; they are evidence-based/evidence-informed and particularly effective when targeting skills for the development of conversation.

(1) *Pausing or waiting for the child to join in.* The wait might take a bit of time but the "wait is worth it." Children who are deaf or hard of hearing are likely processing incom-

plete information, even with the best technology. As a consequence, they may need a bit more time to process that information and piece it together prior to responding. So, practitioners and parents relax and give themselves permission to have a bit of silence. If the child begins to turn his attention away during the wait, it is a signal to re-engage him/her with something fun.

(2) *Pausing expectantly.* Sometimes simply waiting may not provide a sufficient turn-taking cue to a child. It may be necessary to provide non-verbal cues. So, practitioners and parents pause expectantly and raise their eyebrows or widen their eyes in anticipation. They lean in toward the child and look toward what they want the child to talk about and then look back at the child. If needed, they then point to what they want the child to talk about and wait some more.

(3) *Giving clues.* If the child is asked a question and does not answer, practitioners and parents provide a clue such as "I remember what Grandma gave you" and then wait with an expectant pause. It might be necessary to provide an additional clue such as "I think she gave you something that bounces." It's important to avoid placing the child in a position of being wrong. In AVT, the practitioner and parents always will make sure the child understands the clue and its association with the word he/she is expected to use.

(4) *Giving choices.* If the child is asked a question and does not answer, some choices might be provided, such as: "What did Grandma bring

you? [expectant pause] Did she bring you a truck or a ball?" [giving choices] Adults avoid placing the child in a position of being wrong and always include the correct answer among the choices.

(5) *Anticipating auditory closure.* Adults might give the first few words and give the child an opportunity to finish the thought, such as: "We climbed up, up, up the hill. Then we got on the sled and we _____ ."

(6) *Using a conversational model.* The practitioner might ask a question of the parent so that the child can observe how the question is answered in conversation. Then, the child is asked the same question so he/she can try to respond.

(7) *Playing Round Robin.* This is a bit more structured and involves more direct imitation. Taking turns, one adult (parent or practitioner) demonstrates play and talks about a toy ("Roll, roll, roll the dough. Push!"). The other adult does and says the same thing. Then the child takes a turn.

(8) *Requesting an imitation.* This is used only if all other attempts do not work. It's important to keep everything friendly and kind and avoid making demands such as "Say _____." Rather, practitioners and parents encourage a turn ("It's my turn! Here's a cookie for Grandma. Your turn: _____") or might embed the request for imitation in an invitation ("You could say . . . It's a cookie for Grandma").

(9) *Third time's the charm.* Having a conversation should be fun. If a child does not join in or fails to understand a message, imitate a language model, or produce a sound correctly after three tries, move on. The goal is to make conversations a joy and a means for the child to make himself/herself known to the world. Backing down to an easier task so that the interaction concludes with success can help. The practitioner or parent can always come back to something more challenging later. That is diagnostic therapy and the way forward in AVT.

Keeping It Going

The timing and content of our responses to children keep conversations going. The following are some ideas to make that happen.

Making a Connection with Infants

Practitioners help parents to recognize those moments when their infant makes contact—eye gaze, laughs, vocalizations, cries of distress or discomfort—and help parents to respond accordingly. They help parents to accompany routine caregiving with rich language and an infant-directed speech style that comforts and soothes when infants are distressed, giving the infant an opportunity to tune in to the voices and words that express what he/she is experiencing. This establishes an expectation in the infant that his/her contact will be met with a response and a foundation for the conversational turns that are so important to language development.

Being Timely and Contingent with Early Communicators

Responses to a child's first words and early phrases help him/her discover the power of communication. Responding with little delay helps a child to learn that what he/she says has value and deserves a response. Language that is contingent upon, or reflects, the child's intent (Child: "Uh, uh." Parent: "You want to get *up*? You're going *up*! Now you're high *up*") encourages a child to remain in the conversation.

Avoiding Test-Type Questions

Test-type questions can put children "on the hot seat" and bring conversations to a full stop. These types of questions are frequently heard when adults attempt conversation with a young child by saying things such as: "Oh, is that your bunny?" "Are you rolling the car?" "Are you washing the baby?" The natural response for the child is simply to answer "yes" or "no" and there's nothing more to be said. In fact, these questions create missed opportunities for parents and practitioners to offer better spoken language models. It is helpful to turn these types of questions into interesting statements such as: "You have your bunny! He has such long ears." "You're rolling the car. Go car!" "You're washing the baby. Ooooh, that baby's wet."

Test-type questions can occur when adults respond to a child's comment with questions, rather than with a response that reflects a child's communicative intent. These are particularly difficult for children who are deaf or hard of hearing if they have not acquired the language to answer such questions. Some examples and alternatives are:

(1) Child: Points at his shoe. Parent or practitioner tests: "Good boy, what's that? You know what that is! Tell me." A preferred non-test alternative is: "Yes, that's your shoe. It fell off, uh oh! Let's put it back on your foot."

(2) Child: Laughs at the dog playing with its ball and says the dog's name. The parent or practitioner tests by asking: "What's the doggie doing? Tell me, who is that? What is he doing?" A better non-test alternative is: "Sammy's playing with his ball. Let's throw it for Sammy. Throw the ball."

Lifting Them Up and Helping Them Fly

Once children are using words and simple sentences, practitioners and parents apply conversational strategies to help them acquire more mature language skills. This is accomplished with rich language input and purposeful responses.

Staying in the Zone

Providing input slightly above the child's level positions that input in the child's zone of proximal development, or the level between what a child can do without help and what he/she cannot do (Vygotsky, 1987).

Using Your Words

Using a variety of words can open up a child's options for describing his/her own experience. Practitioners guide parents to use several strategies:

■ talking about categories. When parents are shopping, they might

Saying Farewell

This last snapshot is a conversation with a little girl who is about to move on from AVT. There's still some work to do, but she's ready for her next adventure in school. Notice how the practitioner is able to keep the conversation going using open-ended questions.

Snapshot #7

Child: CA 6 years, HA 4.5 years, severe-profound hearing loss, bilateral hearing aids

Practitioner: This is a special day, right? (*guided conversation: open-ended question*)

Child: My Mom and Dad are packing and me and Lise are just playing.

Practitioner: Are you? When are you leaving for Vancouver? (*guided conversation: open-ended question*)

Child: On Tuesday.

Practitioner: And what about Daddy? (*guided conversation: open-ended question*)

Child: Saturday.

Practitioner: Wow. How come you are not going with him? (*guided conversation: open-ended question*)

Child: Because it takes a long time to get there.

Practitioner: Hmmm. How are you and Mommy going out there? (*guided conversation: open-ended question*)

Child: And Lise is going with us.

Practitioner: Uh huh. How? (*guided conversation: open-ended question*)

Child: By a plane.

Practitioner: Oh, on an airplane? I wish I were going with you. Where are you going to live when you get to Vancouver? (*guided conversation: open-ended question*)

Child: In a house.

Practitioner: Have you got the house yet?

Child: Not yet.

Practitioner: Not yet? Well, that's pretty exciting. What about school? (*guided conversation: open-ended question*)

Child: Fine, we took all the pictures.

Practitioner: Mmm? (*guided conversation*)

Child: We took pictures.

Practitioner: Where? (*guided conversation: open-ended question*)

Child: In the school.

Practitioner: Oh, did you? So that you can remember all your friends! Wow, that's going to be great.

Child: And teachers!

say: "Let's find some *fruit*. What kind of *fruit* do we see? I see apples, etc."

■ talking about function. When doing the laundry with children at their side, parents might say: "Look at these clothes! They're dirty. Let's put them in the *hamper*.

The hamper *holds our dirty clothes*."

■ talking about parts of things: "Let's decorate Mom's *bike* for the parade. We'll put streamers on the *handlebars*. We'll put streamers on the *seat* and streamers on the *wheels*."

Practitioners encourage parents to become a "thesaurus" to expand their child's vocabulary. In the above examples the parent used "hamper" and "streamer" because the child already knows "box" and "ribbon." By introducing the new words, the child's vocabulary expands. Similarly, practitioners encourage parents to provide *extensions* in response to a child's contribution to the conversation, by using a child's word along with a synonym or a more advanced word. This way the child can link the new word with his/her own: Child: "Grandma gave me a ball!" Parent: "That's a wonderful ball. It's a *soccer* ball. We can kick it. Let's go outside and *kick that soccer ball*."

Expanding and Recasting

Expansions can help a child use longer and more complex sentences. When adults respond to a child by imitating what he/she says and then adding one or two more words or morphemes, they preserve the child's meaning and offer more. For example: Child: "Doggie outside." Adult: "*Our* doggie *is* outside." This is not a correction of what the child says. This is an acceptance of the child's comment and adds to it in agreement with what the child says. Recasting is another response that can help the child use more adult grammatical forms; if a child uses incorrect grammar, adults respond with the correct form while maintaining the child's original meaning. For example: Child: "He *runned* away." Adult: "Yes, he *ran* away."

An even stronger Auditory-Verbal emphasis to expansions or recasts adds a few steps. The practitioner alerts the child to "Listen," then provides the ex-

pansion or recast, and waits for the child to imitate the expansion. In this manner the practitioner is engaging auditory attention, and checking to determine if the child hears the model. This is not a demand for a perfect imitation. The intent is to diagnostically determine what the child has heard. Imitation is used with discretion so that the natural flow of conversation does not deteriorate into an adult-led demand for simple *parroting (imitating)*.

Expanding and recasting are most effective when used judiciously (see Chapter 15). These strategies are more effective if they are reserved for emphasizing an individual child's particular language targets, such as helping the child to use the present participle in expressive language: Child: "Dog jump!" Adult: "The doggie *is* jump*ing*." Expanding or recasting all of a child's utterances takes the pleasure out of conversation and does not have a significant impact on language acquisition.

CHAPTER SUMMARY

The rate of parent–child conversational turns in early childhood impacts brain development and is predictive of the level of language acquisition in later years. In Auditory-Verbal therapy, practitioners and parents use conversations between adults and children to target the development of audition, speech, language, and cognition. Observations of parent–child conversations with typically developing children and with children who are deaf or hard of hearing give us information that we can apply when coaching parents to provide quality input, develop and expand conversations, and respond in ways that develop their child's conversational competence. Of particular importance is the fact that effective parent–child conversations change with the language level of the child. Intervention research provides further information for the practice of Auditory-Verbal therapy, specifically with regard to the positive impact that is demonstrated when parents and practitioners use focused input and responses that are tailored to the speech and language targets selected for a particular child. As a consequence, we are mindful that there is no one set of conversational strategies that can, nor should, be applied to all children. Auditory-Verbal practitioners need to be continuously diagnostic and knowledgeable about a child's level of function throughout a family's journey in AVT.

REFERENCES

Ambrose, S., Van Dam, M., & Moeller, M. P. (2014). Linguistic input, electronic media and communication outcomes of toddlers with hearing loss. *Ear and Hearing, 35*(2), 139–147.

Ambrose, S. E., Walker, E. A., Unflat-Berry, L. M., Oleson, J. J., & Moeller, M. P. (2015). Quantity and quality of caregivers' linguistic input to 18-month and 3-year-old children who are hard of hearing. *Ear and Hearing, 36*(1), 48S.

Ates, B. S., & Kuntay, A. C. (2018). Sociopragmatic skills underlying language development: Boundaries between typical and atypical development. In A. Bar-On & D. Ravid (Eds.), *Handbook of Communication Disorders* (pp. 279–310). Berlin, Germany: De Gruyter.

Beckage, N., Smith, L., & Hills, T. (2011). Small worlds and semantic network growth in typical and late talkers. *PLoS ONE, 6*(5): e19348.

Bergeson, T. R., Miller, R. J., & McCune, K. (2006). Mothers' speech to hearing-impaired infants and children with cochlear implants. *Infancy, 10*(3), 221–240.

Bornstein, M. H., Tamis-LeMonda, C. S., Hahn, C., & Haynes, M. (2008). Maternal responsiveness to young children at three ages: Longitudinal analysis of multidimensional, modular, and specific parenting construct. *Developmental Psychology, 44*, 867–874.

Braginsky, M., Yurovsky, D., Marchman, V. A., & Frank, M. C. (2016). From uh-oh to tomorrow: Predicting age of acquisition for early words across languages. In *Proceedings of the 38th annual conference of the Cognitive Science Society* (pp. 1691–1696).

Bredin-Oja, S. L., & Fey, M. E. (2014). Children's responses to telegraphic and grammatically complete prompts to imitate. *American Journal of Speech-Language Pathology, 23*(February), 15–26.

Brooks, R., & Meltzoff, A. N. (2008). Infant gaze following and pointing predict accelerated vocabulary growth through two years of age: A longitudinal, growth curve modeling study. *Journal of Child Language, 35*, 207–220.

Burgoyne, K., Gardner, R., Whiteley, H., Snowling, M. J., & Hulme, C. (2018). Evaluation of a parent-delivered early language enrichment programme: Evidence from a randomised controlled trial. *Journal of Child Psychology and Psychiatry, 59*, 545–555.

Carpenter, M., Nagell, K., Tomasello, M., Butterworth, G., & Moore, C. (1998). Social cognition, joint attention, and communicative competence from 9 to 15 months of age. *Monographs of the Society for Research in Child Development, 63*(4), 1–174.

Casillas, M. (2014). Turn-taking. In D. Matthews (Ed.), *Pragmatic development in first language acquisition* (pp. 53–70). Philadelphia, PA: John Benjamins.

Che, E., Brooks, P., Alarcon, M., Yannaco, F., & Donnelhy, S. (2018). Assessing the impact of conversational overlap in content on child language growth. *Journal of Child Language, 45*(1), 72–96.

Cheskin, A. (1981). The verbal environment provided by hearing mothers for their young deaf children. *Journal of Communication Disorders, 14*(6), 485–496.

Clarke, E. V. (2014). Two pragmatic principles in language use and acquisition. In D. Matthews (Ed.), *Pragmatic development in first language acquisition* (pp. 105–120). Philadelphia, PA: John Benjamins.

Clark, E. V., & Wong, A. D. W. (2002). Pragmatic directions about language use: Offers of words and relations. *Language in Society, 31*, 181–212.

Cleave, P. L., Becker, S. D., Curran, M. K., Van Horne, A. J. O., & Fey, M. E. (2015). The efficacy of recasts in language intervention: A systematic review and meta-analysis. *American Journal of Speech-Language Pathology, 24*, 237–255.

Costa, E. A., Day, L., Caverly, C., Mellon, N., Ouellette, M., & Ottley, S. W. (2019). Parent-child interaction therapy as a behavior and spoken language intervention for young children with hearing loss. *Language Speech and Hearing Services in Schools, 50*, 34–52.

Cross, T. G., Nienhuys, T. G., & Kirkman, M. (1985). Parent-child interaction with receptively disabled children: Some determinants of maternal speech style. *Children's Language, 5*, 247–290.

Cruz, I., Quittner, A. L., Marker, C., DesJardin, J. L., & CDaCI Investigative Team. (2013). Identification of effective strategies to promote language in deaf children with cochlear implants. *Child Development, 84*(2), 543–559.

DeCasper, A. J., & Fifer, W. P. (1980). Of human bonding: Newborns prefer their mothers' voices. *Science, 208*(4448), 1174–1176.

DesJardin, J. L., & Eisenberg, L. S. (2007). Maternal contributions: Supporting language development in young children with cochlear implants. *Ear and Hearing, 28*(4), 456–469.

DeVeney, S. L., Hagaman, J. L., & Bjornsen, A. L. (2017). Parent-implemented versus clinician-directed interventions for late-talking toddlers: A systematic review of the literature. *Communication Disorders Quarterly, 39*(1), 293–302.

Dickinson, D. K., & Tabors, P. O. (2001). *Beginning literacy with language: Young children learning at home and school.* Baltimore, MD: Paul H Brookes.

Dilley, L., Wieland, E., Burnham, E., Wang, Y., Houston, D., Kondaurova, M. V., & Bergeson, T. (2017). Prosodic characteristics of speech directed to adults and to infants with and without hearing impairment. *Journal of the Acoustical Society of America, 141*(5), 3699–3700.

Dilley, L., Wieland, E., Lehet, M., Arjmandi, M. K., Houston, D., & Bergeson, T. (2018). Quality and quantity of infant-directed speech by maternal caregivers predicts later speech-language outcomes in children with cochlear implants. *Journal of the Acoustical Society of America, 143*(3), 1822–1822.

Dunst, C. J., Hamby, D., Trivette, C., Raab, M., & Bruder, M. B. (2000). Everyday family and community life and children's naturally occurring learning opportunities. *Journal of Early Intervention, 23*(3), 151–164.

Estigarribia, B., & Clark, E. V. (2007). *Journal of Child Language, 34*, 799–814.

Ferjan Ramírez, N., Lytle, S. R., Fish, M., & Kuhl, P. K. (2018). Parent coaching at 6 and 10 months improves language outcomes at 14 months: A randomized controlled trial. *Developmental Science, 22*(3), e12762.

Fernald, A., & Mazzie, C. (1991). Prosody and focus in speech to infants and adults. *Developmental Psychology, 27*(2), 209.

Fernald, A., & Simon, T. (1984). Expanded intonation contours in mothers' speech to newborns. *Developmental Psychology, 20*(1), 104.

Gallaway, C., Hostler, M. E., & Reeves, D. (1990). Speech addressed to hearing-impaired children by their mothers. *Clinical Linguistics & Phonetics, 4*(3), 221–237.

Gladfelter, A., Wendt, O., & Subramanian, A. (2011). Evidence-based speech and language intervention techniques for the birth-to-3 population. *EBP Briefs, 5*(5), 41–50. Bloomington, MN: Pearson.

Gilkerson, J., & Richards, M. A. (2008). *The power of talk: Impact of adult talk, conversational turns, and TV during the critical 0–4 years of child development.* Inforture Technical Report 01–2. Boulder, CO: LENA Foundation.

Gilkerson, J., Richards, J. A., Warren, S. F., Oller, D. K., Russo, R., & Vohr, B. (2018). Language experience in the second year of life and language outcomes in late childhood. *Pediatrics, 142*(4), 2017–4276.

Hart, B., & Risley, T. R. (1995). *Meaningful differences in the everyday experience of young American children.* Baltimore, MD: Paul H. Brookes Publishing.

Hirsh-Pasek, K., Adamson, L. B., Bakeman, R., Owen, M. T., Golinkoff, R. M., Pace, A., Yust, P. K., & Suma, K. (2015). The contribution of early communication quality to low-income children's language success. *Psychological Science, 26*(7), 1071–1083.

Huttenlocher, J., Waterfall, H., Vasilyeva, M., Vevea, J., & Hedges, L. V. (2010). Sources of variability in children's language growth. *Cognitive Psychology, 61*(4), 343–365.

Jo, J., & Ko, E. S. (2018). Korean mothers attune the frequency and acoustic saliency of sound symbolic words to the linguistic maturity of their children. *Frontiers in Psychology, 9,* 1–12.

Kondaurova, M. V., & Bergeson, T. R. (2011). The effects of age and infant hearing status on maternal use of prosodic cues for clause boundaries in speech. *Journal of Speech, Language, and Hearing Research, 54*(3), 740–754.

Kondaurova, M. V., Bergeson, T. R., & Xu, H. (2013). Age-related changes in prosodic features of maternal speech to prelin-gually deaf infants with cochlear implants. *Infancy, 18*(5), 825–848.

Kondaurova, M. V., Bergeson, T. R., Xu, H., & Kitamurab, C. (2015). Affective properties of mothers' speech to infants with hearing impairment and cochlear implants. *Journal of Speech, Language, and Hearing Research, 58*(3), 590–600.

Manolson, A. (1992). *It takes two to talk: A parent's guide to helping children communicate.* Toronto, ON, Canada: The Hanen Centre.

Masur, E., Flynn, V., & Eichorst, D. (2005). Maternal responsive and directive behaviours and utterances as predictors of children's lexical development. *Journal of Child Language, 32*(1), 63–91.

Morrison, H. M., Lopez, L., & Rodriguez, L. (2011). *Sound beginnings: Coaching families with LENA feedback.* Presented to the National Early Hearing Detection and Intervention Conference, Atlanta, GA.

Nienhuys, T. G., Cross, T. G., & Horsborough, K. M. (1984). Child variables influencing maternal speech style: Deaf and hearing children. *Journal of Communication Disorders, 17*(3), 189–207.

Panneton, R. P., Abraham, J., Berman, S., & Staska, M. (1997). The development of infants' preference for motherese. *Infant Behavior and Development, 20*(4), 477–488.

Paul, R. (2007). *Language disorders from infancy through adolescence: Assessment & intervention* (Vol. 324). New York, NY: Elsevier Health Sciences.

Pollack, D., Goldberg, D., & Caleffe-Schenck, N. (1997). *Educational audiology for the limited-hearing infant and preschooler.* Springfield, IL: Charles C. Thomas.

Quittner, A. L., Cruz, I., Barker, D. H., Tobey, E., Eisenberg, L. S., Niparko, J. K., & Childhood Development after Cochlear Implantation Investigative Team. (2013). Effects of maternal sensitivity and cognitive and linguistic stimulation on cochlear implant users' language development over four years. *Journal of Pediatrics, 162*(2), 343–348.

Ramírez-Esparza, N., García-Sierra, A., & Kuhl, P. K. (2014). Look who's talking: Speech style and social context in language input to infants are linked to concurrent and future speech development. *Developmental Science, 17*(6), 880–891.

Renzi, D. T., Romberg, A. R., Bolger, D. J., & Newman, R. S. (2017). Two minds are better than one: Cooperative communication as a new framework for understanding infant language learning. *Translational Issues in Psychological Science, 3*(1), 19–33.

Roberts, M. Y. (2019). Parent-implemented communication treatment for infants and toddlers with hearing loss: A randomized pilot trial. *Journal of Speech, Language, and Hearing Research, 62,* 143–152.

Roberts, M. Y., Hensle, T., & Brooks, M. K. (2016). More than "try this at home"—including parents in early intervention. *Perspectives of the ASHA Special Interest Groups, SIG 1, 1*(4), 130–142.

Roberts, M. Y., & Kaiser, A. P. (2011) The effectiveness of parent-implemented language interventions: A meta-analysis. *American Journal of Speech-Language Pathology, 20,* 180–199.

Roberts, M. Y., Kaiser, A. P., Wolfe, C. E., Bryant, J. D., & Spidalieria, A. M. (2014). Effects of the Teach-Model-Coach-Review instructional approach on caregiver use of language support strategies and children's expressive language skills. *Journal of Speech, Language, and Hearing Research, 57,* 1851–1869.

Rochat, P., Querido, J. G., & Striano, T. (1999). Emerging sensitivity to the timing and structure of protoconversation in early infancy. *Developmental Psychology, 35*(4), 950–957.

Romeo, R. R., Leonard, J. A., Robinson, S. T., West, M. R., Mackey, A. P., Rowe, M. L., & Gabrieli, J. D. (2018). Beyond the 30-million-word gap: Children's conversational exposure is associated with language-related brain function. *Psychological Science, 29*(5), 700–710.

Rowe, M. L., Leech, K. A., & Cabreraba, N. (2016). Going beyond input quantity: Wh-questions matter for toddlers' language and cognitive development. *Cognitive Science, 41,* 162–179.

Roy, B. C., Frank, M. C. & Roy, D. (2012). Relating activity contexts to early word learning in dense longitudinal data. *Proceedings of the Annual Meeting of the Cognitive Science Society, 34*(34), 935–940.

Sandbank, M., & Yoder, P. (2016). The association between parental mean length of utterance and language outcomes in children with disabilities: A correlational meta-analysis. *American Journal of Speech-Language Pathology, 25*(2), 240–251.

Smith, N. A., & Trainor, L. J. (2008). Infant-directed speech is modulated by infant feedback. *Infancy, 13*(4), 410–420.

Stephens, G., & Matthews, D. (2014). The communicative infant from 0–18 months: The social-cognitive foundations of pragmatic development. In D. Matthews (Ed.), *Pragmatic development in first language acquisition* (pp. 13–36). Philadelphia, PA: John Benjamins.

Swain, J., Mayes, L., & Leckman, J. (2004). The development of parent-infant attachment through dynamic and interactive signaling loops of care and cry. *Behavioral and Brain Sciences, 27*(4), 472–473.

Szagun, G., & Schramm, S. A. (2016). Sources of variability in language development of children with cochlear implants: Age at implantation, parental language, and early features of children's language construction. *Journal of Child Language, 43*(3), 505–536.

Taumoepeau, M. (2016). Maternal expansions of child language relate to growth in children's vocabulary. *Language Learning and Development, 12*(4), 429–446.

Thelen, E. (2005). Dynamic systems theory and the complexity of change. *Psychoanalytic Dialogues, 15*(2):255–283.

Thiessen, E. D., Hill, E. A., & Saffran, J. R. (2005). Infant-directed speech facilitates word segmentation. *Infancy, 7,* 53–71.

Vallotton, C., Mastergeorge, A., Foster, T., Decker, K. B., & Ayoub, C. (2017). Parenting supports for early vocabulary development: Specific effects of sensitivity and stimulation through infancy. *Infancy, 22*(1), 78–107.

Van Dam, M., Ambrose, S. E., & Moeller, M. P. (2012). Quantity of parental language in the home environments of hard-of-hearing 2-year-olds. *Journal of Deaf Studies and Deaf Education, 17*, 402–420.

van Kleeck, A., Schwarz, A. L., Fey, M., Kaiser, A., Miller, J., & Weitzman, E. (2010). Should we use telegraphic or grammatical input in the early stages of language development with children who have language impairments? A meta-analysis of the research and expert opinion. *American Journal of Speech-Language Pathology, 19*, 3–21.

Vygotsky, L. (1987). Zone of proximal development. *Mind in Society: The Development of Higher Psychological Processes, 5291*, 157.

Weitzman, E. (2017). *It takes two to talk: A practical guide for parents of children with language delays* (5th ed.). Toronto, ON, Canada: The Hanen Centre.

Werker, J. F., Pons, F., Dietrich, C., Kajikawa, S., Fais, L., & Amano, S. (2007). Infant-directed speech supports phonetic category learning in English and Japanese. *Cognition, 103*, 147–162.

Zimmerman, F. J., Gilkerson, J., Richards, J. A., Christakis, D. A., Xu, D., Gray, S., & Yapanel, U. (2009). Teaching by listening: The importance of adult-child conversations to language development. *Pediatrics, 124*(1), 342–349.

11

DEVELOPMENT OF SPEECH AND AUDITORY-VERBAL THERAPY

Helen McCaffrey Morrison

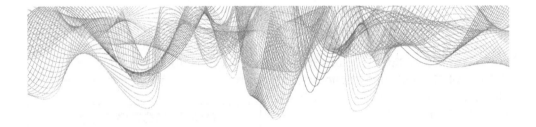

INTRODUCTION

Speech is a social act, a means for connecting with one another. Speech is language made audible by a series of precise, rapid movements. Like their typically developing peers, children who are deaf or hard of hearing in Auditory-Verbal Therapy (AVT) develop speech through maturation, multiple experiences, and learning that take place synchronously across the social, linguistic, perceptual, cognitive, and motor developmental domains (Smith & Thelen, 2003; Thelen, 1991).

Auditory access to the sounds of speech with optimally fitted hearing technology early in life, in tandem with AVT that is developmental in nature, supports the *developmental* synchrony necessary for a child with hearing loss to follow a typical trajectory toward acquiring intelligible speech. If a child receives auditory access through hearing technology later in life, however, he or she may experience developmental dyssynchrony across the previously mentioned domains. The AV practitioner understands how development occurs in each of these, and for the later-identified child, the practitioner may need to add *remedial* strategies to the developmental focus in order to devise effective learning experiences that ameliorate the dyssynchronous impact of later auditory access (Morrison & Russell, 2012).

When children learn to use speech to communicate, they learn the particular intonational contours, syllable patterns, consonants, and vowels that make up their home language. They learn the speech sound sequences that are permitted in that language (e.g., /sk/ is a permitted sequence in English but not /ks/). The system of vowels, consonants, and speech sound combinations that make up a language is the *phonology* of that language and the smallest unit of a phonology is the *phoneme*. A phoneme is a consonant or vowel that can change the meaning of a word if it is substituted with another speech sound. For example, in English, substituting the vowel /i/ with the phoneme /æ/ changes "beet" to "bat"; hence each are English phonemes. Likewise, substituting the phonemic consonant /k/ with /f/ changes "cat" to "fat." The vowel and consonant phonemes in English phonology and examples of the sounds associated with International Phonetic Association symbols can be found in Chapter 8 (Tables 8–1 and 8–2).

Phonemes are, by definition, inextricable from the larger context of the lexicon of a language. A child does not learn the phonology of his home language without acquiring a lexicon. Furthermore, in order to use speech to communicate, a child must have something to say and know the words and phrases to express it. Accordingly, attention to the development of speech in AVT takes place in communicative,

conversational contexts and learning experiences that also target language development.

This chapter offers information that the AV practitioner (practitioner) uses to assess speech skills, set short-term and long-term objectives, and implement plans for children's speech development. The contributions of social, perceptual, cognitive, language, and motor development to speech acquisition are a recurring theme throughout, beginning with a discussion of the role of sensory input for speech development and motor control. A description of sequences and milestones in typical speech development follows, leading to a further discussion of the impact of hearing loss on the expected outcomes of speech development. The suggestions regarding assessment and intervention are based on typical speech development and the impact of hearing loss on it.

THE FUNCTIONS OF SENSORY INPUT IN SPEECH DEVELOPMENT AND PRODUCTION

Sensory input establishes the speech *targets* that a child is acquiring in speech development, i.e., the suprasegmental aspects and the phonologic system in the child's home language. Sensory input is also a source of *feedback* that confirms that a child's production matches his or her targets, important for establishing and maintaining motor control to ensure accuracy and consistency of production in ongoing speech.

Auditory input is the primary sensory input for achieving speech targets. As the infant listens to words and phrases spoken by his or her parents and caregivers, the child perceives the phonemes within these utterances and, using the cognitive processes of memory and categorization, constructs a mental map of the phonemes comprised by the home language (Kuhl, 2010). This process is described in Chapter 9.

Vision is a secondary sensory input to disambiguate auditory confusions that arise under difficult listening conditions or because of inadequate auditory access. Vision cannot substitute for audition for learning the suprasegmental aspects and phonology of a language. Suprasegmental aspects are generally not visible. For example, one cannot "see" the variation in fundamental frequency that creates an intonational contour. Furthermore, a substantial number of phonemes are either (1) insufficiently visible for identification (e.g., it is generally not possible to see the tongue for production of the velar /g/) or (2) are visually impossible to discriminate (e.g., voiced/voiceless cognates such as /d/ and /t/ look alike).

A speaker does more than simply issue a motor command to move the articulators and produce a speech sound. Sensory and somatosensory feedback conveyed during speech production makes it possible to control and adjust articulatory movement to ensure accuracy. Audition and proprioception are primary sources for feedback of motor control, and tactile information is a secondary source (Guenther & Vladusich, 2012). Proprioception is neural feedback that informs the brain about articulator position, direction of movement, and velocity of movement. Tactile information is provided by articulatory

contact along the vocal tract. Together, proprioceptive and tactile information make up the somatosensory system.

Guenther's (2006; Guenther & Vladusich, 2012; Tourville & Guenther, 2011) DIVA model (Directions Into Velocities of Articulators) explains the role of feedback in the development of speech acquisition in a manner that is particularly applicable to AVT. DIVA has been validated by studies that (1) disrupt input to confirm the contributions of each type of sensory and somatosensory feedback to production and (2) identify anatomical locations in the brain associated with model components (Golfinopoulos et al., 2011; Guenther, Ghosh, & Tourville, 2006; Tourville, Reilly, & Guenther, 2008).

The DIVA model illustrates how auditory feedback, somatosensory feedback, and feedforward operate in early speech development starting with the babble period, ages 7 through 12 months. During this time, new speech sounds that an infant is learning to produce are *auditory targets* derived from listening to his home language. When an infant produces a new sound, he or she attempts to match the auditory target while listening to himself or herself. *Auditory feedback* from production enables an infant to determine whether the speech movements have reached the intended auditory target. Repetition of successful productions ultimately encode the motor commands that produce the targeted speech sound, in the infant's brain. These are *feedforward* commands that become more accurate over time as auditory feedback delivers confirmation that a production has successfully reached the auditory target. As feedforward commands become stabilized, *somatosensory feedback*, predominantly in the form of *proprioception*, enters into the speech motor control system as a means to confirm that the speech mechanism is adhering to feedforward commands. Ultimately, when feedforward commands are fully encoded, proprioception takes over as the primary feedback that a speaker uses to maintain productive control and accuracy, and ultimately reduce the role of auditory feedback in speech motor control.

Guidance for the Auditory-Verbal Practitioner

The DIVA model has several implications for speech development in AVT. Learning to listen is fundamental to phonologic acquisition and early attempts to match vocal production to adult models. Development of the auditory feedback mechanism is an important speech acquisition objective for children in AVT. In order to successfully encode feedforward commands and establish proprioceptive feedback for motor control, a child must have abundant opportunities to use speech, to listen to his or her productions, and confirm the success of such attempts. AV practitioners guide and coach parents to encourage speech communication and to respond appropriately and systematically to the child's vocal attempts. Finally, a child who transitions from hearing aids to cochlear implants will benefit from auditory learning opportunities that establish new auditory targets. Auditory learning will not only establish new auditory targets, but also will help develop an improved auditory feedback mechanism.

TYPICAL SPEECH DEVELOPMENT: AGES, STAGES, AND SEQUENCES

Infant Vocal Development (Birth to 12 Months)

From birth through 12 months, infants listen, discover how to put what they hear into motion, and use that discovery to connect with others. In the early months, the infant starts out by listening primarily to himself or herself. By the end of the first year of life the infant shows that he or she has also been listening to others and vocalizations begin to show the influence of the home language.

Finding a Voice: Reflexive Vocalizations and Cooing (Birth through 4 Months)

The social connection that motivates speech development can be observed even in the earliest weeks and months of a child's life. First moments of eye contact between parents and infants and early vocalizations that gain parents' attention are prerequisites for speech development. A child's speech and lexical development are set into motion by parents and caregivers, who engage the child, encourage him or her to communicate, and actively listen and respond as the child plays.

The oral tract in newborns and very young infants is shaped differently than in adults. The lower jaw is smaller and pulled back a bit. The palate is higher and narrower. Consequently, the infant tongue takes up more space in the oral tract and moves less easily than that of the adult. At birth, infants are able to move the tongue in and out of mouth and up and down in a general fashion. Over the first 4 to 5 months of life the palate broadens, allowing more space for exploration. The physical state of the vocal tract and the fact that much time is spent lying down serve to constrain the vocalizations produced by newborns and very young infants.

Vocalizations heard from infants from birth through about 8 weeks of age tend toward reflexive crying or vegetative sounds such as burps or sneezes, leading Oller (1980) to refer to this as the *reflexive* stage in infant vocal development. One can also hear soft vocalizations that contain pitch variations.

At around age 8 weeks, babies begin to coo, and produce backed vowel-like vocalizations with a nasalized, predominantly lip-rounded "ooo" quality. Cooing varies in duration and pitch as babies begin to explore the timing and intonational contour of vocalizations. Consonant-like sounds produced in the back of the vocal tract resemble /g/ and /k/ and are a consequence of the infant spending so much time laying on his/her back with gravity pulling the tongue back in the oral tract. These vocalizations tend to last over the duration of an exhaled breath, a foundational vocal production for speech communication.

This is a period when the infant is learning to listen to him/herself and is starting to engage in vocal play. The infant receives auditory feedback as he/she plays with the duration, intensity, and pitch of the voice. This developing ability to use auditory feedback helps the infant to refine motor control over respiration and the movements that

lead to variations in duration, intensity, and pitch, leading Oller (Oller, Eilers, Neal, & Schwartz, 1999) to designate this as the *phonation* stage in infant vocal development.

Inventing a New Game: Vocal Play (4 Months through 8 Months)

By age 4 to 5 months the larynx has descended into the neck, rendering the vocal folds more vulnerable to the supralaryngeal muscles and consequently enabling the production of a greater range of pitch production. The palate has broadened and increased room for the infant to explore the oral tract with the tongue. Increased space for movement coupled with greater motor control of tongue movement and lip closure moves infant vocalizations beyond simple exploration of the duration and pitch contour of vocal production into a period of even greater vocal play. All sorts of sounds are heard at this time while babies try out their vocal capacities, leading to this age being termed the *expansion* stage (Oller et al., 1999). They yell while exploring the coordination of the respiratory system and the larynx for intensity control. They squeal with increased control of pitch. At this age, babies are able to shut off the flow of sound in the vocal tract by constricting the tongue or the lips. They make "raspberry" sounds by sticking their tongues between the lips and blowing, and they smack their lips. They can open their mouths to create consonant-like sounds that are succeeded by vowel-like sounds, precursors to the syllables found in adult speech. These include speech-like sounds that are not present in the infant's home language.

Infants reduce the rate of nasalized vocalizations compared with vocalizations that resonate in the vocal tract (Bunton & Hoit, 2018). This is a first indicator that an infant's vocalizations are influenced not just by listening to him/herself but also by listening to the home language. An infant's "default" posture is an open passage from the nose to the lungs (open velopharyngeal port) to permit breathing. Vocalizations produced in this default position are nasalized and predominate in the first few months of life. The speech sounds in the majority of languages, however, are predominantly non-nasalized, or oral. The infant must be able to control the velum to close off the velopharyngeal port in order to produce non-nasalized sounds and match the oral resonance of the speech that surrounds the child.

Learning the Speech Game: Canonical Babble (6 through 12 Months)

Babies produce *canonical babble* from around age 6 to 7 months through the end of the first year of life. Canonical babble comprises consonant/vowel (CV) syllables that possess the regular timing characteristics of adult speech—canonical syllables are brief and consistent in duration from syllable to syllable (Davis & MacNeilage, 1995; Oller, 1980; Stark, 1980). The earliest canonical syllables tend to be reduplicative (a single syllable is repeated over and over [e.g., /didididi/]) (Oller, 1980). At around 10 months the infant expands syllable shape and control to produce variegated syllables (syllables with varied consonant/vowel combinations that are also repeated over the duration of production). This repetitiveness helps build sensorimotor integration and the establishment of proprioceptive feedback in speech motor control, described earlier in this chapter in the discussion of the DIVA model.

Canonical babble is shaped both by the ambient language and the infant's motoric abilities. Consequently, canonical babble emerges in the same period when infants begin to demonstrate the influence of the home language on speech perception (Kuhl, 2004, 2010) and to comprehend their first words (Jusczyk, 1997; Oller & Eilers, 1988). The sounds that infants babble reflect the types and proportion of speech sounds in their home language. The sounds produced during the earlier expansion stage that are not phonemic in the home language diminish in incidence, and sounds from the home language predominate in the canonical babble stage. Vowels in babble tend to represent the extremes of the vowel quadrilateral: high front, high back, low, and central (Davis & MacNeilage, 1995; Kent, Osberger, Netsell, & Hustedde, 1987). Babies who are learning English tend to babble consonants at a rate reflecting the incidence of the consonants in the language: more oral consonants than nasal consonants (Bunton & Hoit, 2018; Davis & MacNeilage, 1995; Locke, 1983), more alveolars (/d, t, l/) than labials (/b, p/) or velars (/k, g/) (Locke, 1983; Vihman, 1996).

In contrast, motor development determines how infants pair consonants and vowels to form canonical syllables. At this age, the tongue and lips move with the jaw. The jaw and tongue are not controlled independently but are tightly coarticulated (Gibson & Ohde; 2007). Consequently, the tongue configuration for the consonant in a canonical CV syllable is maintained throughout the open/closed movement of the jaw for the vowel. Front vowels tend to be combined with alveolar consonants (/ti/, /di/, /dae/), back vowels tend to be combined with velar consonants (/ku/, /gu/), and central vowels tend to be combined with labials (/bʌ/, /pʌ/) (MacNeilage & Davis 1990a, 1990b, 1993). This CV co-occurrence pattern is known as "frame-content" (MacNeilage & Davis, 1990a, 1990b). The "frame" is the tongue/jaw position, with the "content" being the various vowels and consonants that an infant might be babbling. The CV co-occurrence pattern in canonical babble is said to be "frame dominant" because the tongue position is not independent of the jaw. Frame dominance also continues in the CV co-occurrence patterns in a child's first words.

Guidance for the Auditory-Verbal Practitioner

Table 11–1 summarizes the pre-linguistic vocal developmental milestones described in this section and can be used as a reference for considering an infant's vocal progress in AVT. Vocal play occurs all throughout infancy and is very important in AVT. Practitioners can help a child play with vocal production and guide the parents to provide many opportunities for the child to listen to him/herself in addition to adult models. Imitation is encouraged as a playful, pleasurable, give-and-take. Practitioners encourage parents and children to start out by playing with all sorts of vocal sounds, without strict adherence to

Table 11-1. Summary of Prelinguistic Vocal Development

Age	Stage	Production
Birth–2 mos	Reflexive vocalizations	Crying, vegetative sounds (e.g., burps, sneezes)
2–4 mos	Phonation/cooing and gooing	Phonation with tongue toward back of oral tract, varies in pitch and duration, produced on single exhaled breath
4–6 mos	Expansion	Increased sound exploration and play with voice, tongue and lips: yells, squeals, raspberries, lip smacks, consonant-like and vowel-like sounds
6 mos	Canonical babble onset	CV or VC syllables resembling adult speech in rhythm and duration
6–10 mos	Reduplicative babble	Repeated identical CV syllables
10–12 mos	Variegated babble	CV syllables vary in consonant and vowel content

specific sounds of speech. They make sounds for animals, vehicles, and toys in playful ways to help children discover the wide range of their vocal capacity.

When we talk about the sounds and sound combinations in canonical babble, it's easy to fall into a trap of thinking that infants are building a speech system sound by sound. The infant, however, is listening to words and phrases. The most important input for learning a speech system at this age or in a period of early listening is the connected and relevant language that parents deliver in everyday routines and play. Indeed, parental response to infant and toddler vocalization more strongly affects lexical development than vocal development (Fagan & Doveikis, 2019). Infants are listening to the words that their parents say.

Phonologic Development (1 to 8 Years)

From the time children utter their first words at around age 12 months (Fenson et al., 1994; Nathani, Ertmer, & Stark, 2006; Stoel-Gammon, 1998), they build an inventory of phonemes that are mastered and can be used intelligibly in communication. Although most phonemes are incorporated into a child's phonology and mastered within the first 4 years of life, phonologic learning and refinement of production continue through about age 8 years.

Protowords, Jargon, and the First 50 Words (12 to 24 Months)

An early skill mastered by a child during the first word period is to use a specific vocalization to greet others, to request, or to refer to a specific person or object. Children must use that vocalization each time they communicate intent in order for the purpose to be understood. Toddlers may refer to their blankets or bottles by a consistent vocalization with very little resemblance to the adult form. These early consistent productions are examples of *protowords* (Menn, 1983). Toddlers have learned something very important—words are consistent references to people, objects, and emotional states. Children must say the same thing every time they request a blanket in order for the parents to understand—a foundational linguistic and cognitive achievement.

A child's first words tend to be embedded within intonational contours that resemble those that the parents produce, or *jargon* (Stark, 1981). First words are surrounded by syllables that may not be words but sound to our ears very much like speech. Rather than building speech communication sound by sound or word by word, children communicate whole ideas. Within those ideas are some words they know how to use and, in addition, some "fillers."

Children's first 50 words are similar in meaning across cultures and generally contain a variety of word types: greetings, labels, actions, and early attributes (Nelson, 1973). First words tend to be produced with many of the same sounds that were present in the child's babble repertoire, although there may be a few new additions (Vihman et al., 1985; Vihman & Velleman, 2000). First words also tend to be monosyllabic (Bat-El & Ben-David, 2017), although there is evidence that children who are learning languages with a higher proportion of multisyllabic words will more likely include those word shapes in their earliest lexical repertoire (Garmann et al., 2019).

Phonologic Mastery (2 to 8 Years)

Typically developing children experience rapid vocabulary growth around age 2 years (Bates, 1999; Locke, 1997). Vocabulary growth encourages children to attempt a greater variety of phonemes in order to produce words they are learning and to maintain acoustic contrast among words. This expands their phonetic inventory. The use of multisyllabic words increases—also as a consequence of vocabulary growth. In addition, release from frame dominance in CV co-occurrence patterns enables a greater variety of speech sound combinations (MacNeilage & Davis, 1990b). Maturation of syllable production proceeds from achievement of the canonical form to increased diversity in phonetic content and organization.

Children master the production of phonemes in a general order. The specific ages at which a particular phoneme is mastered varies across research studies for several reasons: (1) some studies consider mastery to be correct production in 75% of attempts; others use a 90% criterion, (2) some use language sampling; others use picture naming or imitation; (3) the children observed vary in social-economic background and maternal education levels, which can impact the rate of speech and language acquisition (Dollaghan et al., 1999).

Table 11–2 summarizes the sequence of vowel development from babble onset through age 2 years. Vowels are mastered earlier than consonants. Children first acquire vowels at the extremes of the vowel quadrilateral and proceed to fill in the remaining articulatory and acoustic vowel space, refining vowel production to finer movements and narrower acoustic differences in the first 2 years of life. By 25 to 29 months, children produce vowels correctly in 88% of the opportunities to use these sounds (Dodd & McIntosh, 2010). By age 3, children produce vowels correctly in words in close to 95% of provided opportunities (Dodd, Holm, Hua, & Crosbie, 2003).

Consonant mastery takes more time (Grunwell, 1987; Sander, 1972; Shriberg, 1993). The ages at which children master production of a specific consonant vary, so there is no single age for mastery, although there is an upper limit at which a strong majority of typically

Table 11-2. Sequence of Vowel Development

Age	Vowels Produced	Description
6–12 mos (babble)	i, ɪ, a/ɑ, ʊ u[1]	Represent the extremes of the vowel quadrilateral
13–18 mos	i, ɪ, ɛ, a/ɑ, ʌ, o, ʊ, u[2]	Filling in the vowel quadrilateral
18 mos–2 yrs.	i, ɪ, ɛ, a/ɑ, ʌ, o, ɔ, ʊ, u[2]	Vowel quadrilateral complete

Notes: [1]Davis & MacNeilage, 1995; Kent, Osberger, Netsell, & Hustedde, 1987; [2]Selby, Robb, & Gilbert, 2000.

Table 11-3. Early, Middle, and Late Consonant Mastery (Shriberg, 1993)

Manner	Place	Early (1–3 years)	Middle (3–6.5 years)	Late (5–7 years)
Nasal	Labial	/m/		
	Interdental/ alveolar	/n/		
	Palatal/velar		/ŋ/	
Glide	Labial	/w/		
	Palatal/velar	/j/		
Liquid	Interdental/ alveolar			/l/, /r/
Plosive/stop	Labial	/b/, /p/		
	Interdental/ alveolar	/d/	/t/	
	Palatal/velar		/g/, /k/	
Fricative	Labial		/v/, /f/	
	Interdental/ alveolar			/ð/, /θ/, /z/, /s/
	Palatal/velar	/h/		/ʃ/, /ʒ/
Affricate	Interdental/ alveolar		/dʒ/, /tʃ/	

developing children should be able to use a particular consonant in conversational speech. Shriberg (1993) categorized 24 consonants into early, middle, and late acquisition groups based on a mastery criterion of correct production in at least 90% of opportunities provided to produce that consonant, seen in Table 11–2. These early, middle, and late categories have been validated in English and in Spanish (Fabiano-Smith & Goldstein, 2010). Some general statements can be made about consonant mastery from looking at Table 11–3. There is a range of ages at which chil-dren achieve the 90% criterion for mastery of a consonant. Simple consonants, of course, precede more complex consonants. Nasals and plosives are among the earlier mastered consonant manners of production, as is the labial place of production. Fricatives and affricates tend to be mastered later. Consonant clusters or blends (e.g., /st/ as in "stop," /bl/ as in "blue") are the last consonant aspects to be acquired (Grunwell, 1981). The majority of children master consonant clusters from 6 to 7 years, with complete mastery between 8 and 9 years (McLeod & Arciuli, 2009).

Similarities in consonant mastery exist across languages, although some differences do appear. McLeod and Crowe (2018) reviewed consonant acquisition from research reports of 27 different languages. In general, almost all the consonants in the languages reviewed were acquired by age 5 years. Analysis of consonant acquisition in English, Spanish, Japanese, and Korean revealed that nasals and plosives were the earliest acquired by manner of production, with fricative and affricate acquisition appearing later.

Many typically developing children tend not to be understood by a majority of adults other than their parents until age 3 years (Flipsen, 2006). Children who are learning to talk make errors while they are mastering production and continue to make errors even beyond age 3. These errors, part of the typical acquisition process, are known as *phonologic processes*. Phonologic processes tend to affect whole categories of sounds or syllables (Grunwell, 1997). Table 11–4 lists phonologic processes and the ages at which typically developing children tend to resolve these errors. Many phonologic processes are resolved by age 3 years and most are resolved by age 5 years. Phonologic processes in typically developing children become a concern if they do not disappear at expected ages. Interpretation of this information with regard to children who are deaf or hard of hearing, however, should be applied with caution (Ling, 2002). Each example cited in Table 11–4 can be a consequence of reduced audibility of the speech aspects that are impacted by the phonologic process. It is critical, therefore, that the AV practitioner be fully informed about a child's auditory access with hearing technology and highly knowledgeable about the child's listening skills, to determine whether an error pattern is the consequence of reduced auditory access.

Guidance for the Auditory-Verbal Practitioner

When children who are deaf or hard of hearing produce protowords and embed early first words in jargon, it can be helpful to inform parents that their child is acquiring fundamental speech skills. Jargon reminds us that a child is learning to communicate using the melody of the language he/she hears. Early attempts at communication are not attempts to produce perfect syllables. The first 50 words are not perfectly spoken, nor are they necessarily produced with a wide variety of speech sounds. What's important is that the child is learning to express meaning by using a variety of nouns, verbs, modifiers, and social words. For a child to add more sounds to his/her phonologic system, the lexicon needs to move beyond the first 50 words—word learning is the basis for expanding a child's phonology.

Mastery of the vowel system precedes consonant mastery. AV practitioners and parents need to refrain from the temptation to focus on correct production of consonants if a child has only a limited number of vowels. Furthermore, some consonant error patterns are expected in the first few years of learning to talk. Children who are deaf or hard of hearing need time to learn, practice, and make natural errors and at the same time, the important adults in the their lives need to be 100% certain of the children's auditory access with

Table 11–4. Developmental Phonologic Patterns (Khan & Lewis, 2015; Shipley & McAfee, 2016)

Level	Pattern	Description/Example	Age Resolved
Syllable/word	Final consonant deletion	Final consonant in word deleted: /bæ/ for "bat"	3
	Unstressed syllable deletion	/æ-ge-tə/ for "a-lli-ga-tor"	4
	Cluster simplification	Removal of a sound from a cluster/blend: /kæp/ for "clap" /tap/ for "stop"	4 5
Segment	Devoicing	Change voiced to voiceless in final stops: /bɛt/ for "bed"	3
	Stopping	Manner change from fricative to stop: /f/ and /s/: /pæt/ for "fat," /ti/ for "see" /v/ and /z/: /bæt/ for "vat," /du/ for "zoo"	3 4
	Fronting	Place change from velar/palatal to alveolar: /ti/ for "key"	4
	Deaffrication	Manner change from affricate to fricative: /ʃer/ for "chair"	4
	Liquid simplification	Manner change from liquid to glide: /wæbɪt/ for "rabbit"	7

hearing technology. By doing so, the adults can monitor error patterns that may result from lack of acoustic access and failure to develop an auditory feedback mechanism. Subsequently, they can plan and deliver the AVT program to stimulate and develop the most intelligible speech.

THE IMPACT OF CHILDHOOD HEARING LOSS IN THE TWENTY-FIRST CENTURY

In the 1990s there was a paradigm shift for expected listening and spoken language outcomes for the majority of children who are deaf or hard of hearing. Early identification and early fitting with state-of-the-art hearing technology made auditory access to conversational-level speech more possible than at any other time in history. Much of the information regarding speech development in children who are deaf or hard of hearing that was accumulated prior to the twenty-first century was obtained by observing children who had minimal auditory access to conversational speech, or who had gained auditory access through hearing aids at later ages, resulting in significant dyssynchrony between auditory and motor development. Information regarding speech development in infants and very young children is far more robust in the twenty-first century. Accordingly, the following review focuses on twenty-first century evidence regarding speech development in infants and young children who are deaf or hard of hearing and considers only children who are learning spoken language. Two questions guide the review with regard to speech development and AVT.

(1) What is an expected developmental trajectory of children who are deaf or hard of hearing given the individual profile of auditory access with hearing technology? Auditory access to all the sounds of speech affects both audibility and discriminability of sounds in language, in phonologic acquisition and in the ability to develop auditory feedback. Contemporary research into speech development by children who are deaf or hard of hearing uses degree of hearing loss and type of hearing technology as indicators of auditory access to conversational speech. Children with hearing loss ranging from mild through severe who wear hearing aids are considered to have auditory access to conversational speech (Davis, Morrison, von Hapsburg, & Warner-Czyz, 2005; Morrison, 2012; Tomblin, Oleson, Ambrose, Walker, & Moeller, 2014; von Hapsburg & Davis, 2006), as do children with severe/profound hearing loss who wear cochlear implants (Fagan, 2014; Fulcher, Purcell, Baker, & Munro, 2012; May-Mederake, 2012). Children with severe-to-profound or profound hearing loss who wear hearing aids, are considered to have insufficient access (Davis et al., 2005; von Hapsburg & Davis, 2006) and have in most reports been determined audiologically to be candidates for cochlear implantation (Fagan, 2014; McCaffrey, Davis, Mac-Neilage, & von Hapsburg, 2000; Välimaa, Kunnari, Laukkanen-Nevala, & Ertmer, 2019).

(2) What is the expected developmental trajectory given the age at which a child begins listening with hearing technology? The age at which a child begins listening with hearing technology significantly impacts the time course of the trajectory and developmental synchrony across domains that are foundational for speech development. Researchers vary in their treatment of the time course of auditory access and the notion of hearing age (HA). Some consider the date the first hearing aid is fit or cochlear implant activated to be the first day of listening. Others recognize that not all children who are candidates for cochlear implantation are completely without auditory input during the pre-implant period and that this listening experience builds neurological auditory connections and serves as an input and feedback source for speech development. Accordingly, Flipsen and

Colvard (2016) report the date of hearing aid fitting as the start of HA and the date of cochlear implant activation as the PIA, or post-implantation age.

Prelinguistic Vocal Development

Infants with hearing loss ranging from mild through moderately severe tend to vocalize as frequently as typically developing children (Moeller et al., 2007a). Infants with severe/profound hearing loss, however, do not vocalize as often as their typically developing peers prior to implant activation. After activation these infants increase vocal output, more than double their vocalization rate and match the rate of typically developing peers within 4 months post-activation (Fagan, 2014, 2015).

The production of speech-timed syllables in canonical babble is activated by sensory input and governed by motor maturation. The greater the auditory access, the earlier the age at babble onset (Bass-Ringdahl, 2010; Colletti et al., 2005; Davis, Morrison, von Hapsburg, & Warner-Czyz, 2005; Moeller et al., 2007a; von Hapsburg & Davis, 2006). Infants who have mild-moderately/severe hearing loss and are hearing aid users, as well as infants with severe/profound hearing loss who received cochlear implants prior to the first 7 months of life, begin to babble at an age commensurate with typically developing peers. Infants with severe/profound hearing loss who wear hearing aids delay babbling onset to age 11 to 13 months and produce fewer canonical syllables in babble (Davis et al., 2005; McCaffrey et al., 2000; von Hapsburg & Davis, 2006). If such children receive cochlear implants from ages 1 to 3 years, however, a full 7 to 9 months of listening is not required for canonical babble to appear. Babble onset has been reported as early as 1 to 6 months post-activation, presumably due to motoric readiness for canonical babble among these infants and young children who are more motorically mature (Colletti et al., 2005; Ertmer & Jung, 2012; Fagan, 2015; Moore & Bass-Ringdahl, 2002; Schauwers et al., 2004; Schramm, Bohnert, & Keilmann, 2009; Välimaa et al., 2019). An additional influence of lexical development has been reported from recordings of a child who was implanted close to 4 years old. She had very few babble productions prior to cochlear implant activation and did not appear to go through a period of babble post-implantation. Rather, she incorporated newly perceived phonemes into her lexicon of words and phrases, suggesting that once a child has reached the linguistic/cognitive level of word use, babble may not be an essential aspect of speech development (Morrison, 2011).

Infants with mild-moderate/severe hearing loss babble similar vowels and consonants as typically developing infants. Vowels represent the corners of the vowel quadrilateral, in addition to some mid/central vowels. The incidence of the high front vowel /i/ and voiceless fricative consonant /s/ decreases with increasing hearing loss. The majority of consonant productions are labials, followed by alveolars and a small percentage of velars. Consonant manner of articulation includes plosives, nasals, laterals, and fricatives (Davis et al. 2005; Nelson, Yoshinaga, Rothpletz, & Sedey, 2013; von Hapsburg & Davis, 2006).

In contrast, infants with severe/profound hearing loss who wear hearing aids produce predominantly central vowels, followed in incidence by back vowels. The high front vowel /i/ is rarely produced. Vowels are frequently nasalized. Consonant place of articulation is similar to that produced by typically developing infants and infants with mild to moderately/severe hearing loss who wear hearing aids. Manner of consonant production, however, is different. There is a predominance of nasals followed by plosives (Davis et al., 2005; McCaffrey et al., 2000; Morrison, 2011; Nelson et al., 2013). Following cochlear implant activation, vowel and consonant types increase to resemble those produced by typically developing infants and those with lesser degrees of hearing loss. Representation of vowel place and height in the inventory increases and nasalization is reduced. The varieties of consonant manner of production increase, with fricatives often appearing among the first new consonants, possibly due to implant processing strategies that give emphasis to the frequency range of fricatives (Ertmer & Jung, 2012; McCaffrey et al., 2000; Morrison, 2011; Schramm, Bohnert, & Keilmann 2009).

Nevertheless, despite differences in phonetic content among typically developing children and children who are deaf or hard of hearing, syllable organization is governed by the same motor constraints across both groups. Infants combine vowels and consonants in the same way due to the coupling of the jaw and tongue in speech movement at this stage of motor development: labials with central vowels, alveolars with front vowels, and velars with back vowels (Davis et al., 2005; McCaffrey et al.,

2000; von Hapsburg, Davis, & Mac-Neilage, 2008).

Phonologic Development

Phonologic development begins with a child's first words and continues through mastery of vowel and consonant production. The evidence for phonologic development by children with hearing loss is elicited in a variety of ways: spontaneous productions during interaction, imitations of adult models, picture-naming, and performance on standardized tests. These in turn yield a variety of measures: percentage of correct productions (often referred to as "accuracy"), age equivalency, standard scores, and error patterns. Several factors are associated with proficiency in phonologic development: the amount and quality of auditory access with hearing technology, age at which hearing technology is fit, expressive vocabulary, and participation in intervention programs that have a focus on listening and the use of speech in communication (Moeller et al., 2007b; Tobey, Geers, Brenner, Altuna, & Gabbert, 2003; Tomblin et al., 2014; Yoshinaga & Sedey, 1998).

First Words

Regardless of level of auditory access, children with hearing loss tend to produce first words containing sounds that predominate in babble (Davis et al., 2005; Moeller et al., 2007b; Morrison, 2011). An exception is in productions by children whose cochlear implant activations took place just prior to first word use. Although labial and nasal consonants may have dominated the productive output prior to cochlear implant activation, alveolars and stops are the most frequently produced consonants in first words following activation (Warner-Czyz et al., 2005; Warner-Czyz, Davis, & MacNeilage, 2010). The percentage of vowels used correctly in first words is equivalent to the percentage of correct vowels in productions by typically developing children. The reported percent of correct consonants, however, is lower than in the productions of typically developing children (Moeller et al., 2007b; Warner-Czyz et al., 2005, 2010). The rate of consonant accuracy in first words is closely tied to level of expressive vocabulary (Moeller et al., 2007b).

Vowel Development

Just like typically developing peers, children who are deaf or hard of hearing master the vowel system of their language earlier than they master consonants (Ertmer & Goffman, 2011). Accuracy of vowel production is greater than consonant production through the course of phonologic development until consonant production is also mastered (Tomblin et al., 2014; Ertmer, 2001; Ertmer & Goffman, 2011; Moeller et al., 2007b; Sininger et al., 2010; Sundström, Löfkvist, Lyxell, & Samuelsson, 2018).

Rate of vowel mastery varies with the age a child begins wearing hearing technology, the quality of auditory access, the duration of listening experience, and expressive vocabulary (Moeller et al., 2007b; Yoshinaga & Sedey, 1998). Children with mild through moderately/severe hearing loss who are aided within 6 to 7 months of age produce a range of vowel types and accuracy similar to typically developing peers by ages 2 to 3 years (Tomblin et al., 2014), when typically developing children achieve accurate vowel production across the inventory. Children in this group who do not fully acquire a vowel system by 3 years tend to have hearing loss greater than 45 dB HL and a reduced expressive vocabulary. Children with profound hearing loss whose cochlear implants were activated between 12 to 36 months of age achieve close to full mastery of the vowel system from 1 to 3 years post-activation (Ertmer, 2001; Ertmer & Goffman, 2011), or at hearing ages close to the length of time that typically developing children take to listen and practice vowel production.

Children who are deaf or hard of hearing also follow a sequence of vowel mastery similar to that of typically developing children (Yang, Brown, Fox, & Xu, 2015; Yoshinaga-Itano & Sedey, 1998). Children who have auditory access with hearing aids or cochlear implants fit in infancy or early childhood make similar vowel errors, known as *developmental* errors. Vowel substitutions and deletions have been reported in productions by preschoolers ages 3 to 5 years (Eriks-Brophy, Gibson, & Tucker, 2013; Flipsen & Parker, 2008). Vowel deletions tend to be in unstressed syllables. The most frequently cited vowel substitution is between close neighbors on the vowel quadrilateral, e.g., /bɪt/ for /bit/ or /hɛd/ for /hɪd/.

Children with profound hearing loss who receive cochlear implants after age 3.5 years produce non-developmental vowel errors that are similar to those reported in times prior to the availability of cochlear implants: vowel neutralization (shift in vowel type to a more mid or central position), limited F2 range, and nasalization (Abraham, 1989; Angelocci et al., 1964; Markides, 1983; McCaffrey &

Sussman, 1994; Morrison, 2008). These *atypical* errors can continue through at least the first year of the post-activation period and, for some children, extend into later years (Morrison, 2011; Serry & Blamey, 1999).

Tonal languages, found throughout the world, use vowel pitch change, or F0 variation, to signal vowel identity in addition to height and place on the front/back dimension. Mandarin Chinese, for example, is spoken by more people than any other single global language. The acquisition of tonal phonology by children who listen with cochlear implants is of particular interest because cochlear implants do not process F0 in a conventional manner (see Chapter 6). Emerging research indicates that preschool children who received cochlear implants prior to age 2 years demonstrate tonal productions equivalent to typically developing peers (Tang, Yuen, Xu Rattanasone, Gao, & Demuth, 2019). Continuing research along these lines will inform practitioners regarding the impact of auditory access on vowel tone development.

Consonant Development

Children with early auditory access with hearing aids and/or cochlear implants produce most English consonants by age 7 (Wiggin, Sedey, Awad, Bogle, & Yoshinaga-Itano, 2013), although some may take longer to achieve full mastery (Asad, Purdy, Ballard, Fairgray, & Bowen, 2018). Some children with hearing loss who are fit with hearing technology in early childhood may not develop consonant mastery at levels equivalent to typically developing children of the same chronological age (CA), but may develop consonants in similar fashion

to typically developing children with equivalent HA (Buhler, DeThomasis, Chute, & DeCora, 2007; Flipsen & Parker, 2008) or language age (LA) (Dornan et al., 2007, 2009, 2010).

Rate of mastery, however, can vary with the age at hearing technology fitting, quality of auditory access, duration of listening experience, and vocabulary. As a group, young children with hearing aids and cochlear implants in Auditory-Verbal Therapy programs have been reported to progress at an average rate of consonant mastery from 10 to 12 months gain per year, or close to a year's growth over a year's time (Dornan, Hickson, Murdoch, & Houston, 2007; Dornan, Hickson, Murdoch, Houston, & Constantinescu, 2010; Dornan, Hickson, Thy, Aud, & Murdoch, 2009; Eriks-Brophy et al., 2013). Children who receive cochlear implants prior to age 2.5 have been observed to demonstrate early "bursts" of development in (1) receptive vocabulary during the first year after activation and (2) consonant accuracy during the first 2 years post-activation (Connor, Craig, Raudenbush, Heavner, & Zwolan, 2006). This is followed by a steady rate of progress in consonant development until mastery of the full consonant inventory is achieved. A smaller burst effect has been observed in children who received cochlear implants between ages 2.5 and 3.5 years. It was not observed in children whose implant activations were later than 3.5 years. These age effects are similar to reports of differentially sensitive periods of auditory development for children implanted prior to 2.5 years, between 2.5 and 3.5 years, and after 3.5 years (Sharma, Dorman, & Kral, 2005).

Individual differences in consonant production during early childhood can predict later speech and language outcomes. Children with aided auditory access who produced lower rates of consonant accuracy at age 2 compared with peers with equivalent hearing loss tended to also have lower speech production skills and expressive vocabulary at age 3 (Moeller et al., 2007b). Children activated with cochlear implants at age 3 years or earlier who had lower rates of consonant diversity during the preschool years were observed to also have language difficulty at age 10 (Tobey, Geers, Brenner, Altuna, & Gabbert, 2003).

The sequence of consonant mastery by children who are deaf or hard of hearing is similar to that of children with typical development (Tomblin et al., 2014; Dornan et al., 2007, 2009, 2010; Gaul Bouchard, Le Normand, & Cohen, 2007; Iyer, Jung, & Ertmer, 2017). Rate of mastery, however, can differ from those with typical development among the various consonant types. Rate of mastery for Shriberg's (1993) eight early-developing consonants (see Table 11–3) is faster than for the eight late-developing consonants (Blamey, Barry, & Jacq, 2001; Ertmer & Goffman, 2011). As the degree of hearing loss increases, the rate of consonant mastery for the late eight consonants slows even more (Wiggin et al., 2013). This difference in rate of mastery for early and late consonant groups is likely because early consonants are easier to produce and tend to have low-frequency energy, thus are more likely to fall into the range of audibility for many children with hearing loss. Conversely, the high frequency–loaded acoustic signatures of the late eight consonants are less likely to be audible and discriminable, particularly in noise and across distances.

Fricatives and affricates comprise six of the eight late-developing consonants. The most frequently reported developmental consonant error types made by children who are deaf or hard of hearing are production of these consonant types (Eriks-Brophy et al., 2013; Moeller et al., 2007a, 2007b; Wiggin et al., 2013). Children who are deaf or hard of hearing are observed to produce developmental errors that are not typical for their chronological age but may be developmentally appropriate for their hearing age (Buhler et al., 2007; Flipsen & Parker, 2008). The most frequently reported error patterns include final consonant deletions, unstressed syllable deletions, cluster simplification, devoicing of stops, velar fronting, stopping of fricatives, and liquid simplification (Buhler et al., 2007; Eriks-Brophy et al., 2013; Flipsen & Parker, 2008). These errors can also be explained by insufficient auditory access to these sounds and may be an indication of a breakdown in hearing technology or change in hearing, signaling a need to check technology and hearing. Errors that persist after age 5 years include stopping of fricatives and liquid simplification. Children who are deaf or hard of hearing make atypical, although infrequent, consonant errors, including initial consonant deletion and substitution of consonants with a glottal stop. Atypical errors are considered critical targets for intervention (Buhler et al., 2007; Flipsen & Parker, 2008).

Suprasegmentals and Vocal Production

Historically, speakers with severe and profound hearing loss who wore hearing aids exhibited atypical suprasegmental and vocal production, including monotonic speech, lack of syllabic stress, atypical rate, abnormally high or low pitch, nasal or pharyngeal resonance, breathiness, and tense or harsh vocal quality (Monsen, 1983; Osberger & McGarr, 1982; Subtelny, Whitehead, & Orlando, 1980). Children with severe/profound hearing loss who receive cochlear implants within the first 3 years of life, however, do not commonly exhibit these suprasegmental and vocal qualities (Lenden & Flipsen, 2007). Atypical suprasegmental or vocal production should alert the practitioner to confirm that the hearing technology is working properly and worn consistently, the status of the hearing has not changed, and auditory function and development of the auditory feedback loop is progressing appropriately. Children with severe/profound hearing loss who receive cochlear implants in the later years of early childhood may exhibit these vocal characteristics prior to and (for a time) post implant activation. Development of auditory function and the auditory-feedback loop can assist in remediating these characteristics.

Guidance for the Auditory-Verbal Practitioner

Much of twenty-first century research regarding speech development by children who are deaf or hard of hearing has focused on the impact of the age at which hearing technology is made available to a child. The task for the practitioner is to translate those findings into developmentally based strategies for speech assessment and intervention. The overriding message from the research validates the use of typical developmental milestones and sequences to establish short- and long-term goals for speech development for a child in AVT.

Table 11–5 summarizes this research. The information can be translated for application to AVT with the following caveats: (1) auditory access via hearing technology means auditory access across the conversational speech spectrum and (2) a range of individual variation exists across these findings.

Children's speech productions may exhibit *red flags* that call for additional assessment or *remedial* intervention. Slower than expected progress may be a consequence of issues with auditory access, consistent use of hearing technology, or a more generalized difficulty with language/phonologic learning that is exacerbated by hearing loss. Vowel and consonant error patterns that may seem to be typical and appear at expected CAs or HAs can also be a consequence of issues with auditory access or failure to develop an auditory feedback mechanism. The possibility of auditory compromise should be ruled out rather than assuming errors to be simply developmentally appropriate. Other red flags for failure to access speech through hearing include the atypical patterns listed earlier in this section plus those that have been reported in earlier years as characterizing productions by children with severe/profound hearing loss who had minimal auditory access to conversational speech: vowel nasalization and/or neutralization, monotonic voice, insufficient syllabic stress, or inappropriately low or high voice pitch.

Atypical prosodic or suprasegmental speech patterns can be indicators for difficulties with speech motor programming such as childhood apraxia of speech (CAS). CAS is rare, appearing

Table 11–5. Summary of the Impact of Hearing Loss on Speech Production by Age at Auditory Access with Hearing Technology

Auditory access at ≤ 7 months chronological age	
Babble	*Onset*: 7–9 months CA. *CV content*: similar to typically developing peers.
Vowels	*Mastery*: 3 years CA.
Consonants	*Mastery*: 7 years CA.
Auditory access ≤ 3 years	
Babble	*Onset*: 1 to 6 months HA. *CV content*: shifts over the first year HA toward more typical productions.
Vowels	*Mastery*: 1–3 years HA. *Sequence*: similar to typical development with exception of /i/, which may take longer. *Developmental errors*: unstressed syllable deletions, substitutions among near neighbors on quadrilateral. *Atypical errors*: infrequent.
Consonants	*Mastery*: 7 years CA, HA or LA, depending on auditory access. Shriberg (1993) *Rate*: Early consonants (Shriberg, 1993) mastered at faster rate than later consonants. Rapid growth in first year post-implantation. Children in AVT attain at least one-year development per year. *Developmental errors*: Stopping of fricatives and affricates most frequent. Errors are corrected at HAs or ELAs equivalent to the CA that typically developing children correct errors. *Atypical errors*: Infrequent, may include initial consonant deletion or substitution with glottal stop.
Auditory access at > 3 years chronological age	
Babble	*Onset*: 11–13 months HA *CV content*: Central and back vowels. Vowels frequently nasalized. Consonant manner nasals and plosives.
Vowels	*Mastery*: May extend beyond early childhood. *Atypical errors*: May be neutralized or nasalized. Limited F2 range with fewer or distorted front vowels.
Consonants	*Mastery*: May extend beyond early childhood *Atypical errors*: Confusions resulting from reliance on visual input: place, voice/voiceless contrasts, manner among fricatives and affricates.

in only 0.1% of the general population (Morgan, Murray, & Liégeois, 2018). The speech produced by children with CAS is characterized by three features, and all three must be present for a CAS diagnosis (ASHA, 2007): (1) inappropriate prosody, (2) inconsistency in production of words and syllables, and (3) lengthened and disrupted coarticulatory transitions. Although it can be possible for a child who is deaf or hard of hearing to also have a separate speech motor disability such as CAS, a diagnosis should only be made by a collaborative team that includes a speech language pathologist with experience in speech motor issues, a pediatric neurologist, and if possible, a geneticist (ASHA, 2007; Morgan & Webster, 2018).

The optimistic picture for speech development by children who are deaf or hard of hearing in the twenty-first century that emerges from this literature review can be misleading. The reporting describes the impact of fitting with hearing technology at various age ranges and could lead the reader to conclude that fitting with hearing technology alone is sufficient for the development of speech. The children in these studies, however, were also enrolled in intervention programs that targeted spoken language communication and many participated in AVT. Targeting speech development intentionally, therefore, needs to be an integral part of the intervention program. The next sections describe assessment and intervention practices in AVT that focus on speech development.

ASSESSMENT OF SPEECH DEVELOPMENT IN AVT

Assessment may be conducted for multiple purposes: establishing a baseline, determining intervention goals, monitoring progress, or documenting the effectiveness of intervention. A complete assessment of a child's speech production needs to include analyses of vowels and diphthongs, consonants, and intelligibility. Suprasegmental and vocal characteristics may also be part of the assessment if the child is at risk for difficulty in these areas. Speech development assessment needs to be coupled with language assessment in order to examine the interaction of development across these domains. Assessments that are normed with or designed for use with typically developing children are preferred for use in AVT. Nevertheless, children who are deaf or hard of hearing have specific needs that also influence the selection of a particular speech assessment protocol.

First Things First

Assessment of speech development begins by ensuring that a child has optimal auditory access to conversational speech with hearing technology. The AV practitioner needs current and complete audiological records, including speech perception information. If the audiological speech perception assessment includes imitation of words or identification of pictures in response to word stimuli, it is helpful for the practitioner to obtain an inventory of the words presented and the child's response to each word. Analysis of this information can suggest which speech features are more or less accessible through hearing for speech development. Regardless of the completeness of audiological information available to the practitioner, the assessment of speech production begins with the Ling Six Sound Test (Ling,

2013) to verify the integrity of hearing technology and the child's hearing status at the time of testing.

The practitioner or a colleague who is a certified speech-language pathologist needs to also conduct an evaluation of the child's oral periphery to ensure that all structures are appropriate for movement/control sufficient for speech development. Finally, assessment of speech takes place in conjunction with overall assessment of the developmental social, linguistic, perceptual, cognitive, and motor domains that support speech acquisition.

Prelinguistic Vocal Development and Babble

Today's children with hearing loss frequently enter AVT as infants, requiring AV practitioners to assess infants and very young children. This includes observation of general motor development and documentation of the feeding skills that serve as precursors to speech motor control. In addition, the communicative precursors to speech must be in place: reciprocal eye gaze, participation in daily routines, establishment of joint attention, and comprehension of first words. These are described in greater depth in Chapter 10.

Assessment of prelinguistic vocal production employs observational methods such as checklists, parent questionnaires, and descriptions/transcriptions of vocal output. The *Infant Monitor of Vocal Production* (eIMP) is an example of a parent questionnaire that can be used to establish a baseline of early infant vocal development and monitor progress until first word

use (Cantle Moore, 2014). Comprising 16 questions in an interview format, the eIMP probes the development of speech motor skills, auditory feedback, and progress toward early speech-like productions. The practitioner submits parent responses to the questions to an online analysis that generates a report of developmental status that is referenced to typical development using both chronological age and hearing age. The eIMP has been validated across several different languages and normed using typically developing infants in the first 12 months of life (Cantle Moore & Colyvas, 2018).

Assessment of the CV content in vocalizations at the onset and course of infant babble informs the practitioner about the confluence of child articulatory motor development, input from the ambient language, and a child's ability to access that input through audition. Phonetic transcription of infant babble, however, is a challenge because infants do not often produce easily recognizable phonetic units. The *Mean Babble Level* calculation (Morris, 2010) provides a means to track babble development without narrow phonetic transcription and documents the onset of babble and progression in complexity from reduplicative to variegated babble. In order to calculate the Mean Babble Level, the practitioner first records a sample of 50 of the child's utterances. Utterances for analysis are speech-like vocalizations bounded by silence, non-speech (e.g., giggle), or a parent utterance. The utterance cannot be a word or a protoword. Each utterance is scored in the following manner:

- Level 1 *Not babbled* (1 point): Composed of vowel(s) ([a]), voiced syllabic consonant(s) ([m]), or CV syllable(s) in which the consonant is a glottal stop, a glide ([j, w]), or [h].

▪ Level 2 *Reduplicative babble* (2 points): Composed of CV, VC, or CVC syllable(s) where the consonant is the same across the utterance ([bababa]). Disregard voicing differences[titidi]).

▪ Level 3 *Variegated babble* (3 points): Composed of syllables with two or more consonant types ([babadada]). Disregard voicing differences.

The number of utterances in each category is counted, then multiplied by the point value for that category. All scores are added and then divided by the total number of utterances in the sample to yield the Mean Babble Level. As a child's early speech-like utterances become more complex, the Mean Babble Level will increase.

Word Use: Assessment of Speech Sound Mastery and Error Patterns

When a toddler first begins to use words it is time to document his or her phonetic development and use of phonemes in words. Transcription of a speech sample, or even real-time listing of speech sounds produced during an AVT session, can be used to inventory the vowels/diphthongs and consonants that a child produces. Two types of speech sound inventories can be created: an independent inventory and a relational inventory (Deveney, 2019). The independent phonetic inventory is a list of the speech sounds a young child produces, regardless of whether or not these are used correctly in words. This gives the practitioner and families a notion of what a child is capable of producing and which sounds are missing that should be present for his or her chronological or hearing age. The relational phonetic inventory lists vowels and consonants that a young child uses *correctly* in words. The relational phonetic inventory demonstrates how a child has integrated his/her productive capabilities into phonologic organization.

Phonetic transcription of a connected speech sample and construction of phonetic inventories continue to be useful when a child moves beyond the first 50 words. Children's increased number and length of utterances, however, can make phonetic transcription and analysis a time-consuming endeavor. When a child is regularly using words, it is also possible to assess speech sound mastery using word-based instruments standardized on typically developing children from chronological age 3 and older. Such assessments tend to have the child name a series of pictures that depict objects, actions, and attributes. The child's production is transcribed and scored for correctness and, in some assessment instruments, for error types. The challenge at this developmental level is to find an instrument that addresses the distinct aspects of speech development by children with hearing loss, specifically slower rates of mastery of vowels and consonants, the potential for atypical error production, and delays in lexical development. Accordingly, the practitioner needs to find speech assessments that include probes of both vowel and consonant production. Unfortunately, many standardized speech assessments do not probe vowel production, due to the fact that typically developing children master vowel production early (Eisenberg & Hitchcock, 2010). An assessment also needs to include error analysis to assist with setting goals for intervention, including a means for documenting atypical error patterns that are unique to productions by children with hearing loss.

The *Diagnostic Evaluation of Articulation and Phonology* (DEAP) (Dodd, Hua, Crosbie, Home, & Ozanne, 2006) is an example of a word-based assessment normed with typically developing children ages 3 to 9 years. The DEAP screens oral motor skills, assesses vowel and consonant production, analyzes phonologic processes or error patterns, and includes protocols for collecting and assessing a connected speech sample by eliciting the narration of an illustrated sequence story. It is also possible to record atypical errors for analysis. British, Australian, and Irish versions of the DEAP include a toddler subtest that is normed on typically developing children ages 2 to 3 years (McIntosh & Dodd, 2011).

An assessment tool that is sensitive to small changes in development can help document slower progress exhibited by many children who are deaf or hard of hearing. *Identifying Early Phonologic Needs in Children with Hearing Loss* (IEPN) (Paden & Brown, 1990) is a picture-naming test that elicits early vocabulary, making it an appealing choice for assessment when a child has weak vocabulary skills. Transcription of the child's production is compared with the adult standard and scored for productive accuracy of vowel height and place, consonant manner, place and voicing, syllable number and stress, and the presence of initial and final consonants. Score points are awarded for the degree of closeness of a child's production to the particular feature. This allows for a look at the gradual trajectory that a child might take in the mastery of speech sounds. Furthermore, an analysis of speech production at the featural level makes it easier to interpret a child's production successes and errors from the perspective of speech acoustics. The IEPN is not normed using typically developing children, so the practitioner may choose to administer this assessment in conjunction with one that is normed.

Speech Intelligibility

Since a long-term goal of AVT is for children to develop intelligible speech, measurement of speech intelligibility through AVT is crucial. Higher levels of speech intelligibility are associated with successful participation in regular education classrooms (Most, 2007). A child's speech intelligibility, however, cannot be reliably inferred from transcriptions of child speech or performance on word-based articulatory assessments. Rather, speech intelligibility must be determined from unfamiliar listeners' impressions of a child's connected speech production (Ertmer, 2011).

The Intelligibility in Context Scale (ICS) (McLeod, Harrison, & McCormack, 2012) is a seven-question parent interview that surveys how well the child is understood by others: the immediate family, extended family, family acquaintances, the child's friends, the child's teachers, and strangers. Parents respond by indicating on a 5-point Likert scale the frequency with which their child is understood in each context, ranging from "never" to "always." The English version of the ICS has been normed using typically developing children ages 4 to 5 years, validated using the DEAP and developmental assessments, and demonstrates strong reliability with regard to parent reporting (McLeod, Crowe, & Shahaeian, 2015). The ICS can help the practitioner identify situations where a child might have difficulty communicating effectively and develop a plan with parents to address these. The ICS has been translated into a number of languages, all of which can be downloaded from the website in the McLoed et al. (2012) reference at the end of this chapter.

child's HA. If these are consistent with a child's HA, the child will be a candidate for developmentally based intervention with the goal of closing the gap in performance between HA and CA. Characteristics that fall below expectations for a child's HA need to be explored further for possible issues of auditory access or a need for a more structured, remedial approach to intervention, and added to intervention goals. If a child's ELA is notably below his HA, the practitioner might need to refer to speech production expectations based on the ELA in order to select targets for intervention. Any atypical vowel or consonant errors or suprasegmental/voice characteristics need to be intervention targets.

Guidance for the AV Practitioner: Interpretation of Assessment Information for Setting Goals

Table 11–6 displays the varieties of assessment information that can be used for setting speech development goals in AVT. The practitioner determines which assessment information will be collected based on the developmental level of the child. The table includes information needed to calculate CA, HA, and equivalent language age (ELA) (based on either lexical development or grammatical development as indicated by the mean length of utterance [MLU]). Speech production characteristics (e.g., vowel mastery or consonant mastery) that are consistent with the child's CA need only be monitored.

Speech characteristics that are below that expected for a child's CA need to be compared with expectations based on a

INTERVENTION FOR SPEECH DEVELOPMENT IN AVT

Intervention for speech development in AVT is geared toward helping a child listen to the language of the home, build a phonology, and master his or her sound production abilities. Speech development is integrated into the three-dimensional conversations described in Chapter 10. AV practitioners and parents provide quality input for learning speech, guide the child's vocal participation in interaction and conversation, and respond to the child in a purposeful manner that affirms the child's vocal attempts and helps the child improve. All three dimensions can be present in a single activity or interaction. The strategies presented in Chapter 10 are all relevant and important to speech development in AVT. This section will provide scenarios and evidence-based

Table 11–6. Summary of Assessment Information for Speech Development Goal-Setting in AVT

Date(s) of Assessment		Date of Birth/Chronological Age	
Date of Hearing Aid Fitting/Cochlear Implant Stimulation		Hearing Age	
Infant Development, Interaction, Prelinguistic Vocalizations			
Feeding	Eye contact		Joint reference
Reflexive vocalizations	Cooing/gooing		Vocal play
Babble onset	Reduplicative babble		Variegated babble
First Words			
Protowords	Jargon		First 50 words
Independent and Relational Phonetic Inventories			
Phonologic Organization/Articulation			
Independent and Relational Phonetic Inventories			
Missing vowels in inventories		Missing consonants in inventories	
% vowels correct		% consonants correct	
Vowel errors	Consonant errors		Atypical errors
Standard score on formal speech testing		Age equivalency on formal speech testing	
Speech intelligibility			
Age equivalency receptive vocabulary		Age equivalency expressive vocabulary	
MLU			
Suprasegmental production/voice characteristics			
Intonational contour	Syllabic stress		Atypical voice

information that expand on Chapter 10 to illustrate more explicitly how speech development can be fostered in AVT.

Infants and Toddlers

The two scenarios that follow are examples of how AV practitioners and parents provide input and guide vocal participation with their infants and toddlers. *Infancy is not a time for responding to vocalizations with corrections.* Infancy is the time to respond with joy to every vocal attempt. The recurrent language in daily routines, finger plays, silly baby rhymes, and making sounds for the baby's toys are just the sort of varied input that helps build a phonology.

Scenario #1: Baby Games

Alfonso is 4 months old and has a moderately/severe hearing loss. He was fit with binaural hearing aids at 3 months. He and his parents have been in AVT for 3 weeks and are playing Baby Games that help him learn to listen to others and to himself. Alfonso is learning to vocalize often and with varied durations, intensities, and pitches. He is also learning that his vocalizations can make things happen. Some of the games that Alfonso and his parents are playing are:

Baby Duets: When Alfonso vocalizes, Mom and Dad make eye contact, indicate that they hear him, and imitate the sounds that Alfonso makes. They pause expectantly. If Alfonso vocalizes again, Mom and Dad show their delight and take another turn. Alfonso is learning that vocal turn-taking is fun. When the time comes for intentional turn-taking and imitation, Alfonso will be familiar with this routine and will have a vocal repertoire as a foundation.

The Play's the Thing: When Alfonso engages in vocal play, he makes many of the same sounds over and over. He enjoys listening to and feeling the sensations of the sounds he can make. Repeated sound-making provides feedback from audition and proprioception to build speech motor control. Mom and Dad join in. They play with all sorts of sounds, without strict adherence to any specific speech sound types. They make a variety of sounds for the animals and toys in Alfonso's crib to help him find ways to discover the wide range of his vocal capacity.

Night-night . . . Wake up! Alfonso loves peek-a-boo and has started to expect to see his mom and dad reveal their faces. They wait for his vocalization, then uncover their faces and say, "Peek-a-boo!" As a next step, Mom and Dad generalize from peek-a-boo to help Alfonso play with vocal intensity in a routine that happens every day. Dad places a small towel over his face while Mom whispers, "Shhhhh, night-night" for a few repetitions to set the scene as a quiet place. Then, with great suddenness, Mom says loudly, "Wake up!" and Dad pulls the towel from his face and says "Hi!" to Alfonso. They play the game with the towel on Alfonso's face. Eventually, Mom and Dad wait for Alfonso to squeal loudly for his turn to tell Dad or Mom to wake up. When it's his turn to go to sleep, Alfonso pulls the towel from his face upon hearing, "Wake up!"

Establishing the Auditory Feedback Loop

The auditory feedback loop can develop naturally, even among children who are deaf or hard of hearing. Young children listen to the language around them, vocalize to try to match what they hear, monitor the results of their attempts, and make adjustments in succession. The establishment of an auditory feedback

Scenario #2: Proactive Babble

Hue is 11 months old and has a severe-profound hearing loss. She was fit with binaural hearing aids at age 4 months but her auditory access to conversational speech with hearing aids is limited. Hue has been approved for cochlear implantation at age 12 months. She and her parents have participated in AVT since she was 5 months old. Her parents have noticed that she is starting to incorporate babble into her vocalizations. She is producing /m/ plus nasalized central vowels repetitively.

Hue's practitioner and parents want to encourage her to continue to babble and help her establish productive habits that will help prevent the possibility of developing atypical patterns. The parents hold her in their laps so they can speak closely to the hearing aid microphone at conversational level so that the intensity ratio between consonants and vowels remains natural. By speaking closely to the hearing aid microphone, Hue is more likely to capture some of the essential acoustics for speech sound development.

Hue's parents play a version of "This Little Piggie," wiggling each of her fingers and babbling for each finger. They babble /mamama/ and /bababa/ so Hue has an opportunity to listen closely to the contrast between a nasal and oral consonant in a CV syllable. They hold out their fingers so she can try the game on her own. They start their syllable babble with a vowel: /aaamamama/ so that the initial vowel is not influenced by the nasal consonant. This strategy may help reduce the possibility that Hue develops a habit of nasalizing vowels prior to cochlear implant stimulation.

Hue's parents also give her an opportunity to closely listen to consonants and vowels that represent a different place of production rather than just labials. They babble /dididi/ and /gugugu/ while dancing their fingers along her arms and legs. *The vowels paired with these consonants are selected with purpose.* Young children with and without hearing loss will naturally pair a front (alveolar) consonant with a front vowel and a back (velar) consonant with a back vowel due to motor development at this age. This motor-based developmental pairing of vowels and consonants gives Hue an even greater opportunity to attempt vowels and consonants at different places of production.

loop is so fundamental to successful speech development that the practitioner and parents use specific strategies to help make listening-matching-monitoring-adjusting even more explicit. It is important to observe that a child is listening and attempting to match a model. The child's production tells the practitioner and parents something about what he or she is listening to and indicates the child's motoric capability. Feedback from the practitioner and parents regarding the closeness of a child's match to the adult form supports the development of an auditory feedback loop. Giving a child an opportunity to try again with another model helps foster the ability to adjust. As early as developmentally appropriate, the practitioner incorporates imitation of a speech model into games and casual conversation.

Establishing vocal imitation to an adult model is a fundamental skill for a child to attain, but it is __not__ the ultimate

---

Scenario #3: The Match Game

Gaia is 20 months old and has been listening with her bilateral cochlear implants for 10 months. She has started to echo her parents at home. Her AV practitioner and family have decided to incorporate an auditory feedback activity into play to build upon this emerging ability. The practitioner and parents engage in play that allows action to be combined with vocalization.

Beads on a string. The practitioner pulls beads along a string and vocalizes vowels or syllables. Mom takes a turn pulling beads and vocalizing to match the AV practitioner's model. Then Gaia takes a turn.

Rolling, rolling! Playing with modeling dough or clay provides opportunities for establishing a routine for building the auditory feedback loop. The practitioner says, "roll, roll" while rolling the dough and gives Dad and Gaia each a turn. They pass the same piece of dough from person to person to ensure that Gaia is attending to the model. Then, Dad takes a turn, makes a ring, and vocalizes some vowels and CV syllables through the ring. Gaia then takes her turn.

Making a mark. Gaia loves to scribble with markers. The practitioner takes an erasable marker and a small whiteboard and draws a long line across the board saying "ahhh." Mom takes the marker and does the same. Gaia takes a turn. Then the practitioner pokes the board with the marker, saying "dot-dot-dot, "thus providing a contrast in vocal duration between the long line and the dots. Everyone takes a turn. They run their fingers along the lines and dots on the board, playing with the different durations as they vocalize. Eventually, Gaia begins to produce this durational contrast on her own while making marks on the board.

---

goal for speech development in AVT. Although one would expect a child to imitate a model to correct production errors, once an imitation has been obtained, it's important to move from imitation to spontaneous use.

Building a Phonology

The first step in helping a child develop communicative speech is to create opportunities to communicate, seen in the scenarios above and addressed in Chapter 10. The AV practitioner and parents start by nurturing the child's desire to engage with others. When a child begins to use words, the task of speech development in AVT is to help him or her construct the productive sound system needed to communicate—the phonology of the child's home language. Developmental intervention provides focused stimulation and practice with the speech sounds in a child's language while building vocabulary in play-based conversational contexts. That is part of the exciting work and play in AVT.

The Learning to Listen Sounds

The Learning to Listen Sounds, discussed in Chapter 9, are the sounds that parents and children make for animals, vehicles, toys, and certain actions and they offer many opportunities for early speech production development. Children can say them again and again while playing, allowing for practice and the development of automaticity. The Learning to Listen Sounds are easy for the child to hear and produce early on, enabling practitioners and families to target both listening and spoken language together in play. Each family will tend to have a preferred repertoire of Learning to Listen Sounds and are generally agreed upon with the practitioner.

Vocal play using toys and sound-object associations such as the Learning to Listen Sounds can be used to facilitate the development of several speech production aspects:

Suprasegmentals: Parents and children can vary intonation and pitch when making these sounds. For example, there is a large range in pitch or intonational contour when children "meow" like a cat or pretend to be an ambulance or an airplane.

Vowels: Speech play with the Learning to Listen Sounds begins with these vowel-laden animal sounds. Animal sounds tend to be highly vowel loaded, and this appears to be true across language communities. When playing, parents give emphasis to the vowels in animal sounds. They make sure that they're not saying animal sounds with such a short duration that the vowel is not salient. They elongate the sounds such as "meowwwww, moooooo, cockadoodledooooo, whoooo, aaaarfaaaarf."

Consonants: Vehicle sounds can be consonant laden: brrrrr (raspberry), beep-beep for cars, buhbuhbuh for bus or bike, etc.

Learning to Listen Sounds that convey repeated actions increase action words in a child's lexicon. For example, a child can say "hop-hop" for a bunny, "round and round" for a top, "up up," "wheee," or "down" while playing with a toy slide. It's important to talk about the names, attributes, and associated actions when using the Learning to Listen Sounds. It's not advisable to simply pick up a toy cat and start meowing, or to start beeping as soon as one pulls a toy car from a bag. The practitioner and parents talk about the ears, eyes, and whiskers on the cat. They talk about the wheels that go around and around on the car. They engage the child by playing with items and actions used with the Learning to Listen Sounds. They feed the animals, park the vehicles, hook up train cars and make them go around a track. They put the animals in the bus and go on a little trip. All these activities help in the development of speech in AVT. A plethora of activities to foster language developed through listening and speech development in AVT can be found in session plans in Chapters 15 through 17.

Building the Lexicon

When a child has a desire to communicate, he or she must have the words needed to convey a message. To increase the use of speech and speech sound variety, the lexicon needs to increase. As a child's lexicon increases, the number of speech sounds he or she needs to use to make words clearly understandable multiplies quickly.

Scenario #4: A World of Things that "Go!"

Jaheem is 30 months old and has a moderately severe hearing loss. He was fit with binaural hearing aids at age 12 months. He loves to play with toys that move, especially vehicles. He has tended to call anything with wheels a "Go" because one of his favorite games is simply to make things "go!" Jaheem's AV practitioner and family are helping him learn the names for a variety of vehicles as well as the many actions that can be carried out while having fun with the toys, games, books, and real-life experiences associated with them.

This new vocabulary is not taught or learned as a series of single words. To be sure that Jaheem is developing intonational contours and voice quality, target words appear in meaningful, short phrases that show the function and meaning of those words. For example, rather than simply holding up a car, giving it a name, and asking his parents and Jaheem to imitate the label name, Jaheem experiences "car-ness" and a variety of phrases in enjoyable, age-appropriate play. Jaheem is not only listening to or telling his parents to "Go, car!" He's also experiencing and practicing "Stop car. That's my car, Momma, push the car. Uh-oh, the car's broken." The practitioner and parents may then present a mat with a road, a train track, and a pond. As play proceeds, a train, a boat, a truck, and an airplane appear. Language expands to include "on the track, in the water, up in the air." *Jaheem is using all sorts of different vowels and consonants in connected speech with natural intonational contours while spending time with his favorite toys. This is how speech develops in AVT.*

Focused Stimulation

Focused stimulation provides auditory exposure and practice with targeted speech sounds in words and phrases. The AV practitioner and parents immerse a child in words and phrases containing targeted sounds. They engage in language experiences, day-to-day routines, conversations, book sharing, and songs that give the child multiple opportunities for listening and cumulative practice in using words and phrases that contain the sound. Focused stimulation activities enable the practitioner and parents to target language goals simultaneously with speech goals.

Providing opportunities for a child to listen to and produce a variety of words that contain the targeted sound not only gives intensive exposure but also productive experience with the targeted sound in a variety of phonemic contexts and in a variety of positions within the word. This in turn strengthens the flexibility of feedforward motor commands for production of the targeted speech sound. Focused stimulation is used when a child demonstrates the following: awareness response to sound, spontaneous vocalization and vocalization on demand, an attempt to imitate a vocal model, the ability to identify some Learning to Listen Sounds, and the understanding and use of a few functional words (Caleffe-Schenk & Baker, 2008). The practitioner and parents select the vowel or consonant to receive the stimulated focus from the child's specific short-term objectives in speech.

Doreen Pollack first introduced focused stimulation in AVT with her "Babble Units" (Pollack, 1970, 1997). Her concept was expanded by Nancy Caleffe-Schenk and Diane Baker, who called the approach *auditory bombardment* and created a guide for developing consonant production (Caleffe-Schenk & Baker, 2008). The Caleffe-Schenk and Baker consonant guide was followed by a guide for auditory bombardment with suprasegmentals and vowels (Eskridge, et al., 2011). In auditory bombardment, parents and practitioners engage the child in language experiences using words and phrases containing the speech target for a two-week cycle and providing intensive meaning-based exposure to the sound. Turn-taking during language experiences allows for guided stimulation with the sound as well as practice in production. The cycle can be repeated after a few other sounds receive attention if the child needs more experience in order to start to incorporate it into production.

Focused stimulation and auditory bombardment are also two approaches for the treatment of speech delay and phonologic disorders in the practice of speech-language pathology. Evidence for the effectiveness of focused stimulation has been demonstrated with children with cleft lip and palate (Kaiser, Scherer, Frey, & Roberts, 2017; Pushpavathi, Kavya, & Akshatha, 2017). The effectiveness of the more specific cycles approach found in auditory bombardment has been demonstrated with children with cochlear implants (Encinas & Plante, 2016) and as a cyclic approach with children with phonologic disorders (Arabi, Jalilevand, & Marefati, 2017).

Responding with Purpose in Conversation

Speech development in AVT expects the same purposeful responses described in Chapter 10 to help move the child's development forward. Purposeful responses to a child's speech attempts give a child feedback with regard to accuracy of production, supply information to help a child improve accuracy, and keep a child at a level of success. Some strategies that can be applied are as follows:

Imitate the production to figure out the source of error. At times it is difficult to figure out just what a child is doing when he produces a speech sound. The practitioner needs to discern what needs to be changed to make the production more accurate. Thus, imitating what the child is doing helps the practitioner to discover how that production differs from what should be done.

Apply a hierarchy of corrective responses to errors. Sometimes it may seem as though there are just too many aspects in a child's production that need correction. The application of a hierarchy to corrective responses helps keep the conversation going. The practitioner needs to determine the lowest developmental level of a child's error and then model correct production. For example, if a child has both vowel and consonant errors, the adult models correct vowel production and works on that first. A suggested hierarchy is: (1) syllable number and stress,

(2) vowels/diphthongs, (3) consonant manner, (4) consonant place, (5) consonant voicing, and (6) clusters, or blends.

Use acoustic highlighting. Acoustic highlighting that helps children acquire speech gives emphasis to those features that are in error, thus helping a child recognize what he or she needs to change:

- Increase duration of vowels in words and "sing" or give an intonational contour to the vowel. This will help the child track the vowel formants.
- Whisper voiceless phonemes: /p, t, k, s, ʃ, f, θ, h/. The entire word that contains the phoneme should be whispered.
- Increase the duration of continuants: /s, ʃ, f, θ, ð, m, n, ʒ, z, h, v/, e.g., "MMMine!" "shhhoe"
- Bounce initial plosives: /p, b, t, d, k, g/. This highlights the plosive in isolation (b-b-b-bus, d-d-d-dog). Repeat the plosive slowly and then produce the word. Refrain from overuse of this highlighting strategy to avoid a tendency to call everything a "b-b-b-bus" or "d-d-d-dog."

Break it down and build it up. If a child is unable to correct a production with acoustic highlighting as input, he or she may benefit from being guided through the movements needed to produce that sound. Isolate the word with the error and have the child imitate the correct word. If still incorrect, isolate at the syllable level. Once a child makes correct production or one that is close to correct, build back up in level—from sound to syllable to word.

Listening first and last (see Chapter 15). Sometimes historically referred to as "putting it back into hearing" and the "auditory sandwich," *listening first and last* is used in response to errors, and not as a first strategy for providing input for speech learning. If there is an error, first give an auditory model as a corrective response and request that the child try again. If the child's imitation of the model is incorrect, use acoustic highlighting in an auditory model to make the target more salient. If the imitation continues to be incorrect, add additional sensory information such as visual cue. Once the child succeeds, model the production again, through listening only, without acoustic highlighting and encourage the child to imitate the model. This final step is essential. The child needs to hear the natural model once he has achieved correct production. This will help him learn to associate the correct production with the auditory model, strengthening the auditory feedback loop.

Three times a charm. If a child fails to produce a sound correctly after three tries, the practitioner moves down to an easier task so the interaction concludes with success. If a child is unable to correct a production after three tries to correct it, it is likely that he is simply not ready and needs more input and practice.

REMEDIATION: TWENTY-FIRST CENTURY LING

Ling's seminal book on teaching speech to children with hearing loss was first introduced over 40 years ago in 1976 (Ling, 1976), reissued in 2002. Ling followed the 1976 publication in 1988 with a book that offered further explanations and additional information about intervention in a conversational context. These books remain a resource for AV practitioners who seek remedial strategies for eliciting production and helping a child practice the movements needed for accurate and consistent speech production.

In 1976, the understanding of auditory brain development did not exist to the extent that it does today. Children were identified on average around 4 years of age, used body-worn hearing aids predominantly, and cochlear implants were not available. Speech development was slower and more tedious. The Ling approach guides children carefully through small teaching steps toward speech development. Today, the Ling approach is often recommended as a remedial approach for those children who are late entries in intervention programs and/or who require more specific structure due to the presence of additional challenges.

Assessment and teaching in the Ling approach are based on a seven-stage model of speech development that involves both phonologic and phonetic levels (Ling, 1988). Speech development at the phonologic level proceeds as a child uses words, phrases, and sentences. The phonetic level pertains to the articulatory movements that create

the sounds of speech. The phonologic level of intervention takes place at the level of words and connected speech. Phonetic-level intervention incorporates syllable-based skill development and subsequent practice. The phonologic and phonetic hierarchies are presented here in Table 11–7.

Ling recommended a sequence that consonants and vowels needed to be targeted in intervention (Ling, 1976, 2002), seen also in Table 11–7. This sequence was organized based on his observations of the order that children who are deaf or hard of hearing master speech sounds, ease of articulation (proceeding from simple to more complex), and audibility. Audibility was based primarily on the aided auditory access with hearing aids by children with severe/profound hearing loss in the late 1970s. Although the developmental hierarchies and teaching sequence in Table 11–7 are not based on data from typically developing children, they are compatible with typical development.

Ling recommended that the first teaching approach be conversationally (phonologically) based and is indeed how AV practitioners and parents today follow daily routines and language experiences that provide focused auditory stimulation and spoken language practice with incorporated speech targets. If this conversational phonologic approach does not provide sufficient information and practice for a child to develop speech targets, he recommended moving to a more structured phonetic approach, breaking down the speech target into smaller steps for practice.

If a child requires phonetic work to develop a speech target, it is developed first by *eliciting* the speech sound, then moving the child through phonetic-level

Table 11-7. Teaching Order from Ling (1976, 1988)

Phonologic	Phonetic	Speech Targets (1976)
Vocalizes communicatively.	Vocalizes spontaneously and on demand.	Vocalize spontaneously Vocalize in imitation or with cue
Consistent communicative vocalizations.	Uses suprasegmental patterns.	Vocal duration, intensity and pitch
Approximates words with vowels.	Uses a range of vowels with vocal control.	Step 1: /ɑ/, /i/, /aʊ/, /aɪ/ Step 2: /ɔ/, /ɔɪ/, /ɛ/, /ʊ/, /ɪ/ Step 3: /ae/, /ʌ/, /o/, /eɪ/ Step 4: r-colored vowels
Some clear words.	Consonant repertoire varies in manner; used with most vowels.	Step 1: initial and final /p or b/, /w/, /f or v/, /θ or ð/, /h/, /m/
Some clear phrases.	Consonant repertoire varies in manner and place; used with most vowels.	Step 2: initial and final /d or t/, /j/, /l/, /s or z/, /ʃ or ʒ/, /n/ Step 3: initial and final /g or k/, /r/, /tʃ or dʒ/, /ŋ/
Some sentences said clearly.	Consonant repertoire varies in manner, place, and voicing; used with most vowels.	Step 4: /p, b/, /t, d/, /k, g/, /f, v/, /θ, ð/, /s, z/, /tʃ, dʒ/
Intelligible and natural sounding speech.	Uses initial and final blends.	Word Initial Step 1: 2-organ sequential /sm, sp, sw/ Step 2: 1-organ sequential /sk, sl, sn, st, θr/ Step 3: 2-organ co-produced /bl, br, fl, fr, kw, pl, pr, tw/ Step 4: 1-organ co-formulated /dr, gl, gr, kr, ʃr, tr/ Step 5: complex /skr, kw, spr, str/ Word Final Step 1: continuant-continuant (e.g. /-nz/) Step 2: continuant-stop (e.g. /-lp/) Step 3: stop-continuant (e.g. /-aeps/) Step 4: stop-stop (e.g. /-aekt/) Step 5: complex (e.g. /-aekts/)

subskills that a child masters to progress toward the final phonetic target. The child works toward *automaticity* of targeted speech sounds and patterns through practice that can include syllable drill and building proprioceptive speech motor control. The practitioner and the parent help the child *generalize* targeted speech sounds or patterns to new contexts. If a speech target is clearly and automatically produced in one syllable type, practice begins in another syllable. For example, if a child can produce /s/ in syllables that include front vowels, he or she moves to production of /s/ in back vowels. The final stage in phonetic-level training is *carry-over* into everyday spoken language through focused stimulation.

CHAPTER SUMMARY

As an aspect of expressive language development in AVT, speech development takes place in meaningful interactions and conversations. It is the product of development across multiple domains—social, linguistic, perceptual, cognitive, and motor. The development of auditory feedback is an essential trigger for speech development, to enable the child to *tune in* to adult input, match what he or she hears, and adjust production to improve the model. Abundant opportunities to produce speech strengthen the accuracy and control of speech production by building auditory feedforward through proprioceptive feedback.

Typically developing infants begin to build speech control in the first months of life when they begin to play with the suprasegmental aspects of phonation. Prior to the end of the first year, infant vocalizations begin to sound speech-like with the onset of canonical babble. True phonologic organization takes place as children begin to use their first words, and phonologic development is closely linked to a child's expanding lexicon. Vowel mastery precedes consonant mastery. Typically developing children tend to make some of the same kinds of errors as they master speech accuracy, and resolve these errors at similar ages.

Children who are deaf or hard of hearing in AVT follow similar sequences to develop the sounds of speech. The age at mastery of speech sounds varies with the age at which a child acquires optimal auditory access to spoken language through hearing technology. Children in AVT also make developmental errors similar to those of typically developing children and resolve them, dependent upon age at consistent auditory access. Some children who are deaf or hard of hearing, however, produce errors that are atypical, usually as a consequence of late fitting with hearing technology or deficits in auditory access.

It is expected that children in AVT will follow the speech development of typical children. Typical speech development, therefore, is used as the model for assessing speech development and needs to be viewed from such a perspective. It is important, however, to have an assessment protocol that allows for assessment of slower speech development and accommodates for possible reduced lexicons. Today's children with hearing loss in AVT learn to use speech in meaningful conversational contexts with interactional intervention by AV practitioners and parents who provide focused stimulation with abundant opportunities for the child to talk. Speech is, in fact, listening set into motion. Today's children who are deaf or hard of hearing are part of a new and exciting generation, and through AVT they have many opportunities to acquire highly intelligible speech, commensurate with that of their typically hearing peers. Such development of intelligible speech, of course, is one of the many desired outcomes attainable by children who are deaf or hard of hearing through Auditory-Verbal Therapy.

REFERENCES

Abraham, S. (1989). Using a phonological framework to describe speech errors of orally trained, hearing-impaired schoolagers. *Journal of Speech and Hearing Disorders, 54,* 600–609.

Angelocci, A. A., Kopp, G. A., & Holbrook, A. (1964). The vowel formants of deaf and normal-hearing eleven- to fourteen-year-old boys. *Journal of Speech and Hearing Disorders, 29,* 156–170.

American Speech-Language-Hearing Association. (2007). Childhood apraxia of speech [Position statement]. Available from http://www.asha.org/policy

Arabi, A., Jalilevand, N., & Marefati, A. (2017). A review of evidence-based treatment in phonologic interventions with emphasis on cycles approach. *Journal of Modern Rehabilitation*, 195–200.

Asad, A. N., Purdy, S. C., Ballard, E., Fairgray, L., & Bowen, C. (2018). Phonological processes in the speech of school-age children with hearing loss: Comparisons with children with normal hearing. *Journal of Communication Disorders, 74,* 10–22.

Bass-Ringdahl, S. M. (2010). The relationship of audibility and the development of canonical babbling in young children with hearing impairment. *Journal of Deaf Studies and Deaf Education, 15*(3), 287–310.

Bat-El, O., & Ben-David, A. (2017). Developing phonology. In A. Bar-On & D. Ravid (Eds.), *Handbook of communication disorders: Theoretical, empirical, and applied linguistic perspectives* (pp. 63–87). Boston, MA/Berlin, Germany: de Gruyter.

Bates, E. (1999). Language and the infant brain. *Journal of Communication Disorders, 32*(4), 195–205.

Blamey, P. J., Barry, J. G., & Jacq, P. (2001). Phonetic inventory development in young cochlear implant users 6 years postoperation. *Journal of Speech, Language, and Hearing Research, 44,* 73–79.

Buhler, H., DeThomasis, B., Chute, P. & DeCora, A. (2007). An analysis of phonologic process use in young children with cochlear implants. *The Volta Review, 107*(1), 55.

Bunton, K., & Hoit, J. D. (2018). Development of velopharyngeal closure for vocalization during the first 2 years of life. *Journal of Speech, Language, and Hearing Research, 61*(3), 549–560.

Caleffe-Schenck, N., & Baker, D. (2008). *Speech sounds: A guide for parents and professionals.* Sydney, Australia: Cochlear Corp.

Cantle Moore, R. (2014). The infant monitor of vocal production: Simple beginnings. *Deafness & Education International, 16*(4), 218–236.

Cantle Moore, R., & Colyvas, K. (2018). The Infant Monitor of vocal Production (IMP) normative study: Important foundations. *Deafness & Education International, 20*(3–4), 228–244.

Colletti, V., Carner, M., Miorelli, V., Guida, M., Colletti, L., & Fiorino, F. G. (2005). Cochlear implantation at under 12 months: Report on 10 patients. *The Laryngoscope, 115*(3), 445–449.

Connor, C. M., Craig, H. K., Raudenbush, S. W., Heavner, K., & Zwolan, T. A. (2006). The age at which young deaf children receive cochlear implants and their vocabulary and speech-production growth: Is there an added value for early implantation? *Ear and hearing, 27*(6), 628–644.

Davis, B. L., & MacNeilage, P. F. (1995). The articulatory basis of babbling. *Journal of Speech & Hearing Research, 38,* 1199–1211.

Davis, B. L., Morrison, H. M., von Hapsburg, D. & Warner-Czyz, A. D. (2005). Early vocal patterns in infants with varied hearing levels. *Volta Review, 105*(2), 151–173.

DeVeney, S. L. (2019, March). Clinical challenges: Assessing toddler speech sound productions. *Seminars in Speech and Language, 40*(2), 81–93.

Dodd, B., Hua, A., Crosbie, S., Home, A., & Ozanne, A. (2006). *Diagnostic Evaluation of Articulation and Phonology* (DEAP). San Antonio, TX: Pearson.

Dodd, B., Holm, A., Hua, Z., & Crosbie, S. (2003). Phonologic development: A normative study of British English-speaking children. *Clinical Linguistics & Phonetics, 17*(8), 617–643.

Dodd, B., & McIntosh, B. (2010). Two-year-old phonology: Impact of input, motor and cognitive abilities on development. *Journal of Child Language, 37*(5), 1027–1046.

Dollaghan, C. A., Campbell, T. F., Paradise, J. L., Feldman, H. M., Janosky, J. E., Pitcairn, D. N., & Kurs-Lasky, M. (1999). Maternal education and measures of early speech and language. *Journal of Speech, Language, and Hearing Research, 42*(6), 1432–1443.

Dornan, D. I., Hickson, L., Murdoch, B., & Houston, T. (2007). Outcomes of an auditory-verbal program for children with hearing loss: A comparative study with a matched group of children with normal hearing. *The Volta Review, 107*(1).

Dornan, D., Hickson, L., Thy, B. S., Aud, M., & Murdoch, B. (2009). Longitudinal study of speech perception, speech, and language for children with hearing loss in an auditory-verbal therapy program. *The Volta Review, 109*(2–3), 61–85.

Dornan, D., Hickson, L., Thy, B. S., Aud, M., Murdoch, B., Constantinescu, G., & Path, B. S. (2010). Is auditory-verbal therapy effective for children with hearing loss? *The Volta Review, 110*(3), 361–387.

Eisenberg, S. L., & Hitchcock, E. R. (2010). Using standardized tests to inventory consonant and vowel production: A comparison of 11 tests of articulation and phonology. *Language, Speech, and Hearing Services in Schools, 41,* 488–503.

Encinas, D., & Plante, E. (2016). Feasibility of a recasting and auditory bombardment treatment with young cochlear implant users. *Language, Speech, and Hearing Services in Schools, 47*(2), 157–170.

Eriks-Brophy, A., Gibson, S., & Tucker, S. K. (2013). Articulatory error patterns and phonologic process use of preschool children with and without hearing loss. *The Volta Review, 113*(2), 87.

Ertmer, D. J. (2001). Emergence of a vowel system in a young cochlear implant recipient. *Journal of Speech, Language, and Hearing Research, 44*(4), 803–813.

Ertmer, D. J. (2011). Assessing speech intelligibility in children with hearing loss: Toward revitalizing a valuable clinical tool. *Language, Speech, and Hearing Services in Schools, 42*(1), 52–58.

Ertmer, D. J., & Goffman, L. A. (2011). Speech production accuracy and variability in young cochlear implant recipients: Comparisons with typically developing age-peers. *Journal of Speech, Language, and Hearing Research, 54*(1), 177–189.

Ertmer, D. J. & Jung, J. (2012). Prelinguistic vocal development in young cochlear implant recipients and typically developing infants: Year 1 of robust hearing experience. *Journal of Deaf Studies and Deaf Education, 17*(1), 116–132.

Eskridge, H., et al. (2011). *Speech sounds vowels: A guide for parents and professionals in English and Spanish.* Sydney, Australia: Cochlear Corp.

Fabiano-Smith, L., & Goldstein, B. A. (2010). Early-, middle-, and late-developing sounds in monolingual and bilingual children: An exploratory investigation. *American*

Journal of Speech-Language Pathology, *19*(1), 66–77.

Fagan, M. K. (2014). Frequency of vocalization before and after cochlear implantation: Dynamic effect of auditory feedback on infant behavior. *Journal of Experimental Child Psychology, 126,* 328–338.

Fagan, M. K. (2015). Why repetition? Repetitive babbling, auditory feedback, and cochlear implantation. *Journal of Experimental Child Psychology, 137,* 125–136.

Fagan, M. K., & Doveikis, K. N. (2019). What mothers do after infants vocalize: Implications for vocal development or word learning? *Journal of Speech, Language, and Hearing Research, 62*(8), 2680–2690.

Fenson, L., et al. (1994). Variability in early communicative development. *Monographs of the Society for Research in Child Development,* i–185.

Flipsen, P., Jr. (2006). Measuring the intelligibility of conversational speech in children. *Clinical Linguistics & Phonetics, 20*(4), 303–312.

Flipsen, P., Jr., & Colvard, L. G. (2006). Intelligibility of conversational speech produced by children with cochlear implants. *Journal of Communication Disorders, 39*(2), 93–108.

Flipsen, P., Jr., & Parker, R. G. (2008). Phonologic patterns in the conversational speech of children with cochlear implants. *Journal of Communication Disorders, 41*(4), 337–357.

Fulcher, A., Purcell, A. A., Baker, E., & Munro, N. (2012). Listen up: Children with early identified hearing loss achieve age-appropriate speech/language outcomes by 3 years-of-age. *International Journal of Pediatric Otorhinolaryngology, 76*(12), 1785–1794.

Garmann, N. G., Hansen, P., Simonsen, H. G., & Kristoffersen, K. E. (2019). The phonology of children's early words: Trends, individual variation and parents' accommodation in child-directed speech. *Frontiers in Communication, 4,* 10.

Gaul Bouchard, M. E., Le Normand, M. T., & Cohen, H. (2007). Production of consonants by prelinguistically deaf children with cochlear implants. *Clinical Linguistics & Phonetics, 21*(11–12), 875–884.

Gibson, T., & Ohde, R. N. (2007). F2 locus equations: Phonetic descriptors of coarticulation in 17- to 22-month-old children. *Journal of Speech, Language, and Hearing Research, 50*(1), 97–108.

Golfinopoulos, E., Tourville, J. A., Bohland, J. W., Ghosh, S. S., Nieto-Castanon, A., & Guenther, F. H. (2011). fMRI investigation of unexpected somatosensory feedback perturbation during speech. *Neuroimage, 55*(3), 1324–1338.

Grunwell, P. (1981). The development of phonology: A descriptive profile. *First Language, 2*(6), 161–191.

Grunwell, P. (1987). *Clinical phonology* (2nd ed.). Baltimore, MD: Williams & Wilkins.

Grunwell, P. (1997). Natural phonology. In M. J. Ball & R. Kent (Eds.), *The new phonologies: Developments in clinical linguistics* (pp. 35–75). San Diego, CA: Singular Publishing.

Guenther, F. H. (2006). Cortical interactions underlying the production of speech sounds. *Journal of Communication Disorders, 39*(5), 350–365.

Guenther, F. H., Ghosh, S. S., & Tourville, J. A. (2006). Neural modeling and imaging of the cortical interactions underlying syllable production. *Brain and language, 96*(3), 280–301.

Guenther, F. H., & Vladusich, T. (2012). A neural theory of speech acquisition and production. *Journal of Neurolinguistics, 25*(5), 408–422.

Iyer, S. N., Jung, J., & Ertmer, D. J. (2017). Consonant acquisition in young cochlear implant recipients and their typically developing peers. *American Journal of Speech-Language Pathology, 26*(2), 413–427.

Jusczyk, P. W. (1997). Finding and remembering words: Some beginnings by English-learning infants. *Current Directions in Psychological Science, 6*(6), 170–174.

Kaiser, A. P., Scherer, N. J., Frey, J. R., & Roberts, M. Y. (2017). The effects of enhanced milieu teaching with phonologic emphasis on the speech and language skills of young children with cleft palate: A pilot study. *American Journal of Speech-Language Pathology, 26*(3), 806–818.

Kent, R. D., Osberger, M. J., Netsell, R., & Hustedde, C. G. (1987). Phonetic development in identical twins differing in auditory function. *Journal of Speech and Hearing Disorders, 52*(1), 64–75.

Khan, L. M. L., & Lewis, N. P. (2015). *Khan-Lewis phonological analysis* (3rd ed.). New York, NY: Pearson.

Kuhl, P. (2004). Early language acquisition: Cracking the speech code. *Nature Reviews: Neuroscience, 5,* 831–843.

Kuhl, P. K. (2010). Brain mechanisms in early language acquisition. *Neuron, 67*(5), 713–727.

Lenden, J. M., & Flipsen, P., Jr. (2007). Prosody and voice characteristics of children with cochlear implants. *Journal of Communication Disorders, 40*(1), 66–81.

Ling, D. (1976, 2002). *Speech and the hearing-impaired child: Theory and practice.* Washington, DC: Alexander Graham Bell Association for the Deaf and Hard of Hearing.

Ling, D. (1988). *Foundations of spoken language for hearing–impaired children.* Washington, DC: Alexander Graham Bell Association for the Deaf and Hard of Hearing.

Ling, D. (2013). What is the Six-Sound Test and why is it so important in auditory-verbal therapy and education? In W. Estabrooks (Ed.), *101 frequently asked questions about Auditory-Verbal practice* (pp. 58–62), Washington, DC: Alexander Graham Bell Association for the Deaf and Hard of Hearing.

Locke, J. L. (1983). *Phonologic acquisition and change.* New York, NY: Academic Press.

Locke, J. L. (1997). A theory of neurolinguistic development. *Brain and Language, 58*(2), 265–326.

Lenden, J. M., & Flipsen, P., Jr. (2007). Prosody and voice characteristics of children with cochlear implants. *Journal of Communication Disorders, 40,* 66–81.

MacNeilage, P. F., & Davis, B. (1990a). Acquisition of speech production: Frames, then content. In M. Jeannerod (Ed.), *Attention and performance 13: Motor representation and control* (pp. 453–476). Hillsdale, NJ: Lawrence Erlbaum Associates.

MacNeilage, P. F., & Davis, B. L. (1990b). Acquisition of speech production: The achievement of segmental independence. In *Speech production and speech modelling* (pp. 55–68). Dordrecht, Netherlands: Springer.

MacNeilage, P. F., & Davis, B. L. (1993). Motor explanations of babbling and early speech patterns. In *Developmental neurocognition: Speech and face processing in the first year of life* (pp. 341–352). Dordrecht, Netherlands: Springer.

Markides, A. (1983). *The speech of hearing-impaired children.* Manchester, UK: Manchester University Press.

May-Mederake, B. (2012). Early intervention and assessment of speech and language development in young children with cochlear implants. *International Journal of Pediatric Otorhinolaryngology, 76*(7), 939–946.

McCaffrey, H. A., Davis, B. L., MacNeilage, P. F., & von Hapsburg, D. (2000). Multichannel cochlear implantation and the organization of early speech. *The Volta Review, 101,* 5–29.

McCaffrey, H. A., & Sussman, H. M. (1994). An investigation of vowel organization in speakers with severe and profound hearing impairment. *Journal of Speech and Hearing Research, 17,* 938–951.

McIntosh, B., & Dodd, B. (2011). *Toddler Phonology Test.* London, UK: Pearson.

McLeod, S., & Arciuli, J. (2009). School-aged children's production of consonant clusters. *Folia Phoniatrica et Logopaedica,* *61,* 336–341.

McLeod, S., & Crowe, K. (2018). Children's consonant acquisition in 27 languages: A cross-linguistic review. *American Journal of Speech-Language Pathology, 27*(4), 1546–1571.

McLeod, S., Crowe, K., & Shahaeian, A. (2015). Intelligibility in Context Scale: Normative and validation data for English-speaking preschoolers. *Language, Speech, and Hearing Services in Schools, 46*(3), 266–276.

McLeod, S., Harrison, L. J., & McCormack, J. (2012). *Intelligibility in Context Scale.* Bathurst, NSW, Australia: Charles Sturt University. Retrieved from http://www.csu.edu.au/research/multi lingual-speech/ics.

Menn, L. (1983). Development of articulatory, phonetic, and phonologic capabilities. *Language Production, 2,* 3–50.

Moeller, M. P., et al. (2007a). Vocalizations of infants with hearing loss compared with infants with normal hearing: Part I— Phonetic development. *Ear and Hearing, 28*(5), 605–627.

Moeller, M. P., et al. (2007b). Vocalizations of infants with hearing loss compared with infants with normal hearing: Part II— Transition to words. *Ear and Hearing, 28*(5), 628–642.

Monsen, R. B. (1983). Voice quality and speech intelligibility among deaf children. *American Annals of the Deaf, 128*(1), 12–19.

Moore, J. A., & Bass-Ringdahl, S. (2002). Role of infant vocal development in candidacy for and efficacy of cochlear implantation. *Annals of Otology, Rhinology & Laryngology, 111*(5 suppl.), 52–55.

Morgan, A. T., Murray, E., & Liégeois, F. J. (2018). Interventions for childhood apraxia of speech. *Cochrane Database of Systematic Reviews* (5), CD006278.

Morgan, A. T., & Webster, R. (2018). Aetiology of childhood apraxia of speech: A clinical practice update for paediatricians.

Journal of Paediatrics and Child Health, 54(10), 1090–1095.

Morris, S. (2010). Clinical application of the mean babbling level and syllable structure level. *Language, Speech, Hearing Services in Schools, 41,* 223–230.

Morrison, H. M. (2008). The locus equation as an index of coarticulation in syllables produced by speakers with profound hearing loss. *Clinical Linguistics and Phonetics, 22* (9), 726–240.

Morrison, H. M. (2012). Coarticulation in early vocalizations by children with hearing loss: A locus perspective. *Clinical Linguistics and Phonetics, 26*(3), 288–309.

Morrison, H. M., & Russell, A. (2012). What does it really mean that AVT follows a developmental approach to speech rather than a remedial approach? In W. Estabrooks (Ed.), *101 frequently asked questions about auditory—verbal practice.* Washington, DC: Alexander Graham Bell Association for the Deaf and Hard of Hearing.

Most, T. (2007). Speech intelligibility, loneliness, and sense of coherence among deaf and hard-of-hearing children in individual inclusion and group inclusion. *Journal of Deaf Studies and Deaf Education, 12*(4), 495–503.

Nathani, S., Ertmer, D. J., & Stark, R. E. (2006). Assessing vocal development in infants and toddlers. *Clinical Linguistics & Phonetics, 20*(5), 351–369.

Nelson, K. (1973). Structure and strategy in learning to talk. *Monographs of the Society for Research in Child Development, 38*(1–2, Serial No 149), 136.

Nelson, R., Yoshinaga-Itano, C., Rothpletz, A., & Sedey, A. (2007). Vowel production in 7-to 12-month-old infants with hearing loss. *The Volta Review, 107*(2), 101–121.

Oller, D. (1980). The emergence of the sounds of speech in infancy In: G. Yeni-Komshian, C. Kavanagh, & C. Ferguson (Eds.), *Child phonology I: Production* (pp. 93–112).

Oller, D., & Eilers, R. (1988). The role of audition in infant babbling. *Child Development, 59*(2), 441–449.

Oller, D. K., Eilers, R. E., Neal, A. R., & Schwartz, H. K. (1999). Precursors to speech in infancy: The prediction of speech and language disorders. *Journal of Communication Disorders, 32*(4), 223–245.

Osberger, M. J., & McGarr, N. S. (1982). Speech production characteristics of the hearing impaired. In *Speech and language* (Vol. 8, pp. 221–283). New York, NY: Elsevier.

Paden, E., & Brown, C. (1990). *Identifying Early Phonologic Needs in children with hearing loss (IEPN)*. Innsbruck, Austria: Med El.

Pollack, D. (1970). *Educational audiology for the limited hearing infant.* Springfield, IL: Charles C. Thomas.

Pollack, D., Goldberg, D., & Caleffe-Schenck, N. (1997). *Educational audiology for the limited hearing infant and preschooler: An Auditory-Verbal program* (3rd ed.). Springfield, IL: Charles C. Thomas.

Pushpavathi, M., Kavya, V., & Akshatha, V. (2017). Efficacy of focused stimulation in early language intervention program for toddlers with repaired cleft palate. *Global Journal of Otolaryngology, 9*(1).

Sander, E. K. (1972). When are speech sounds learned? *Journal of Speech and Hearing Disorders, 37*(1), 55–63.

Schauwers, K., Gillis, S., Daemers, K., De Beukelaer, C., & Govaerts, P. J. (2004). Cochlear implantation between 5 and 20 months of age: The onset of babbling and the audiologic outcome. *Otology & Neurotology, 25*(3), 263–270.

Schramm, B., Bohnert, A., & Keilmann, A. (2009). The prelexical development in children implanted by 16 months compared with normal hearing children. *International Journal of Pediatric Otorhinolaryngology, 73*(12), 1673–1681.

Selby, J. C., Robb, M. P., & Gilbert, H. R. (2000). Normal vowel articulations between 15 and 36 months of age. *Clinical Linguistics & Phonetics, 14*(4), 255–265.

Serry, T. A., & Blamey, P. J. (1999). A 4-year investigation into phonetic inventory development in young cochlear implant users. *Journal of Speech, Language, and Hearing Research, 42*, 141–154.

Sharma, A., Dorman, M. F., & Kral, A. (2005). The influence of a sensitive period on central auditory development in children with unilateral and bilateral cochlear implants. *Hearing Research, 203*, 134–143.

Shipley, K. G., & McAfee, J. G. (2015). *Assessment in speech-language pathology: A resource manual.* Nelson Education.

Shriberg, L. D. (1993). Four new speech and prosody-voice measures for genetics research and other studies in developmental phonologic disorders. *Journal of Speech, Language, and Hearing Research, 36*(1), 105–140.

Sininger, Y. S., Grimes, A., & Christensen, E. (2010). Auditory development in early amplified children: Factors influencing auditory-based communication outcomes in children with hearing loss. *Ear and Hearing, 31*(2), 166.

Smith, L. B., & Thelen, E. (2003). Development as a dynamic system. *Trends in Cognitive Sciences, 7*(8), 343–348.

Stark, R. E. (1980). Stages of speech development in the first year of life. In G. H. Yeni- Komshian, J. F. Kavanagh, & C. A. Ferguson (Eds.), *Child phonology: Volume 1, production* (pp. 73–91). New York, NY: Academic Press.

Stark, R. E. (1981). Infant vocalization: A comprehensive view. *Infant Mental Health Journal, 2*(2), 118–128.

Stoel-Gammon, C. (1998). Sounds and words in early language acquisition: The relationship between lexical and phonologic development. *Exploring the Speech Language Connection, 8*, 25–52.

Subtelny, J. D., Orlando, N. A., & Whitehead, R. L. (1981). *Speech and voice characteristics of the deaf.* Washington, DC: Alexander Graham Bell Association for the Deaf and Hard of Hearing.

Sundström, S., Löfkvist, U., Lyxell, B., & Samuelsson, C. (2018). Prosodic and segmental aspects of nonword repetition in 4- to 6-year-old children who are deaf and hard of hearing compared to controls with normal hearing. *Clinical Linguistics & Phonetics, 32*(10), 950–971.

Tang, P., Yuen, I., Xu Rattanasone, N., Gao, L., & Demuth, K. (2019). The acquisition of Mandarin tonal processes by children with cochlear implants. *Journal of Speech, Language, and Hearing Research, 62*(5), 1309–1325.

Thelen, E. (1991). Motor aspects of emergent speech: A dynamic approach. In: N. Krasnegor (Ed.), *Biobehavioral foundations of language* (pp. 339–363). Hillsdale, NJ: Erlbaum.

Tobey, E. A., Geers, A. E., Brenner, C., Altuna, D., & Gabbert, G. (2003). Factors associated with development of speech production skills in children implanted by age five. *Ear and Hearing, 24*(1), 36S–45S.

Tomblin, J. B., Oleson, J. J., Ambrose, S. E., Walker, E., & Moeller, M. P. (2014). The influence of hearing aids on the speech and language development of children with hearing loss. *JAMA Otolaryngology–Head & Neck Surgery, 140*(5), 403–409.

Tourville, J. A., & Guenther, F. H. (2011). The DIVA model: A neural theory of speech acquisition and production. *Language and Cognitive Processes, 26*(7), 952–981.

Tourville, J. A., Reilly, K. J., & Guenther, F. H. (2008). Neural mechanisms underlying auditory feedback control of speech. *Neuroimage, 39*(3), 1429–1443.

Välimaa, T. T., Kunnari, S. M., Laukkanen-Nevala, P., & Ertmer, D. J. (2019). Vocal development in infants and toddlers with bilateral cochlear implants and infants with normal hearing. *Journal of Speech, Language, and Hearing Research, 62*(5), 1296–1308.

Vihman, M. M. (1996). *Phonologic development: The origins of language in the child.* New York, NY: Blackwell Publishing.

Vihman, M., Macken, M., Miller, R., Simmons, H., & Miller, J. (1985). From babbling to speech: A re-assessment of the continuity issue. *Language, 61*(2), 397–445.

Vihman, M. M., & Velleman, S. L. (2000). The construction of a first phonology. *Phonetica, 57*(2–4), 255–266.

Von Hapsburg, D., & Davis, B. L. (2006). Auditory sensitivity and the prelinguistic vocalizations of early-amplified infants. *Journal of Speech, Language, and Hearing Research, 49*(4), 809–822.

Warner-Czyz, A. D., Davis, B. L., & Morrison, H. M. (2005). Production accuracy in a young cochlear implant recipient. *The Volta Review, 105*(2), 151–173.

Warner-Czyz, A. D., Davis, B. L., & MacNeilage, P. F. (2010). Accuracy of consonant–vowel syllables in young cochlear implant recipients and hearing children in the single-word period. *Journal of Speech, Language, and Hearing Research, 53*(1), 2–17.

Wiggin, M., Sedey, A. L., Awad, R., Bogle, J. M., & Yoshinaga-Itano, C. (2013). Emergence of consonants in young children with hearing loss. *The Volta Review, 113*(2), 127–148.

Yang, J., Brown, E., Fox, R. A., & Xu, L. (2015). Acoustic properties of vowel production in prelingually deafened Mandarin-speaking children with cochlear implants. *Journal of the Acoustical Society of America, 138*(5), 2791–2799.

Yoshinaga-Itano, C., & Sedey, A. (1998). Early speech development in children who are deaf or hard of hearing: Interrelationships with language and hearing. *The Volta Review, 100*(5), 181–211.

12

THE DEVELOPMENT OF PLAY AND AUDITORY-VERBAL THERAPY

Rosie Quayle, Louise Ashton, and Warren Estabrooks

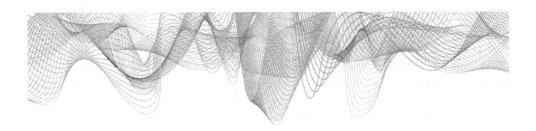

INTRODUCTION

Play has been described as such a "fundamental necessity" to child development that it is now recognized as a human right in article 31 of the United Nations Convention on the Rights of the Child (Yogman et al., 2018). Dating back to ancient times (Frost 2010), play is part of almost every culture. Defined as "the act of engaging in an activity for enjoyment rather than a practical purpose" (Oxford English Dictionary, 2015), play is viewed as a fun and spon-taneous way to learn, especially when there is active engagement with a play-mate and when the "reward" of play is intrinsic (Yogman et al., 2018).

It is well documented that play is an essential vehicle for developing skills in cognition, attention, literacy, language, speech, motor skills, social skills, math-ematical ability, meta-cognition, Theory-of-Mind, executive functioning, and self-concepts (Moyles, 2015; Weisberg, Hirsh-Pasek, Golinkoff, Kittredge, & Klahr, 2016; Yogman et al., 2018). In fact, Yogman and colleagues (2018) link brain development with the function of play and calls play "building brain circuitry," a way *to build a prosocial brain that can interact effectively with others*. The Center on the Developing Child at Harvard University informs that play in early childhood, and in fact, across the life span, is an effective way of supporting responsive relationships, strengthening core life skills, and reducing sources of stress (2019). This fits perfectly well with the "work" of Auditory-Verbal Therapy (AVT) practitioners.

The value of play and its key role in childhood development and in the fostering of the above-mentioned skills have evolved greatly in the twenty-first century and so have most global systems of education. Today's children who are deaf or hard of hearing who engage in AVT are expected to participate in more *formal learning* from a younger age (Moyles, 2015). Practitioners guide and coach parents of very young children who are deaf or hard of hearing to become their child's first playmates and engage in play as the primary way to facilitate the development of interaction, listening, language, speech, spoken conversation, and literacy. In AVT, all forms of play are valued and encouraged because children learn as they play, and most importantly, during play, children in AVT, like their typically hearing peers, learn how to learn (Donaldson, 1993).

THE IMPORTANCE OF PLAY IN AUDITORY-VERBAL THERAPY

During interactive play, children practice and rehearse ways to engage and interact with others and learn new skills through unintentional events. Children learn to collaborate with others by practicing a variety of social communication skills such as making choices, sharing and negotiating, and expressing wants and needs. Children also learn to use their imagination and communication skills to solve problems and resolve conflicts. They exercise decision-making skills, discover unique interests, confront fears, regulate emotions, and develop new competencies that enhance resilience, confidence, and self-advocacy (Moyles, 2015). These are all essential skills for living a meaningful adult life, and part of the grander scheme and expected outcomes of AVT.

The literature presents a number of schemas and models that describe various types of play at different ages. A challenge for the practitioner and the parents may be how to transfer the knowledge of these models into creating play opportunities for children that are fun and motivating and enable their children who are deaf or hard of hearing to learn most effectively and efficiently.

Play in AVT with Joey

Joey, 2 years, 6 months old has been receiving intervention services from a local speech-language pathologist (SLP) following the diagnosis of hearing loss and fitting of hearing aids shortly after he was born. His parents and SLP feel Joey is not making the expected progress, despite his hearing technology giving him full access to all speech sounds, and he now exhibits behavioral challenges in the intervention sessions. At the last session, the SLP:

- prepared an activity with colored stickers to reinforce learning of colors.
- presented bright, engaging pictures to encourage Joey's understanding of two-word utterances.
- hid different objects beginning with the sound /d/ around the room for Joey to find to target correct phoneme production in single words.
- asked the parents to sit in the corner of the room to avoid being a distraction.

Joey entered the room and screamed when he saw the stickers. He refused to sit on the chair and closed his eyes when he was shown the cards. He kicked each object when he found it, instead of playing with it.

- The SLP suggested the parents investigate parenting classes to "rethink how they discipline Joey."
- The SLP, worried about his behavior and progress, decided to refer Joey to a few specialists.

One of those specialists was an Auditory-Verbal practitioner (practitioner) and Joey and his parents met the practitioner for an introductory session. In the first AVT session:

- The practitioner asked the parents to join Joey and him around a table and asked the parents to sit on either side of Joey, so that they could play and communicate with him as the practitioner coached them.
- Joey played with a toy chosen from a toy box, and the practitioner asked the parents what Joey enjoyed playing with and what they most wanted from the session. They indicated they just wanted to see their son enjoy his session and find ways that they could help him.
- The practitioner and parents noticed that Joey selected trains, tracks, and little people who could fit on the train. The practitioner got down on the floor with Joey and encouraged the parents to join them, where they *played* for the remainder of the session.
- The practitioner demonstrated ways to play with the train tracks to check Joey's auditory access to the Ling Six Sounds and to do some targeted speech babble.
- Each time they got a new piece of track, they enjoyed making a sound with it that Joey could imitate.
- Then Joey used the piece to build the track and after a few turns the parents selected the track piece themselves and presented sounds for Joey to imitate.

All of this was done as they played with the train, train tracks, and the little people. The practitioner and parents observed that Joey was successfully accomplishing the short-term objectives and he even started to join in singing about the train. He was able to demonstrate auditory closure abilities, such as: "Uh-oh! We need . . . (more!)" and he demonstrated understanding of some two directions ("We need a man and a baby!" "Man. Sit down! Girl come off!"). The practitioner coached the parents to introduce interesting problems (e.g., a track breaking, a cow on the tracks) to encourage Joey's thinking and to give him something to really talk about. Joey left the session with a smile on his face, wanting to know when he could come again to play! The parents commented that Joey enjoyed the session and that they had strategies and ideas to support his learning through play at home. The practitioner demonstrated Joey's ability to learn, and as a result, his abilities were highlighted while everyone was engaged in playing.

As seen from the above, purposeful play was used to deliver an AVT session (see Chapter 17) where the practitioner follows the principles of AVT by coaching the parents; to help their child use hearing as the primary sensory modality in developing listening and spoken language; to become the primary facilitators of their child's listening and spoken language development through active consistent participation in individualized Auditory-Verbal Therapy; to create environments that support listening for the acquisition of spoken language throughout the child's daily activities; and to help their child integrate listening and spoken language into all aspects of the child's life (AG Bell Academy for Listening and Spoken Language, 2007) (see Chapters 1, 15, 16, 17).

Moyles (2015, p. 852) wrote that "performance-type *activities can look like play, without actually being play . . . but if it's a teacher-driven activity, it may be playful teaching, but it may not be play in the child's eyes.*" Play in the AVT session needs to feel like one big play session to the child and the adult playmates. An engaged child who is paying attention and playing will benefit from a myriad of learning opportunities. In AVT, parents learn that the fewer "performance-type activities," the better.

By the end of the session, Joey's parents were using some strategies to target the six goals of many AVT sessions (see Chapters 15, 16, 17):

Six Goals of the Listening and Spoken Language Specialist (LSLS) Cert. AVT for the AVT Session*

Goal #1: Create a listening environment.

Goal #2: Facilitate auditory processing.

Goal #3: Enhance auditory perception of speech.

Goal #4: Promote knowledge of language.

Goal #5: Facilitate spoken language and cognition.

Goal #6: Stimulate independent thinking.

(*Adapted from Estabrooks, MacIver-Lux, & Rhoades, 2016)

In the examples of AVT activities and Tips presented in this chapter, the authors have indicated goals from the above list that can be targeted in various play activities. For a comprehensive discussion of evidence-based and evidence-informed strategies for listening, talking, and thinking used in AVT, and those used in coaching parents, the reader is encouraged to see Chapters 15 and 16.

PLAY AND THE CHILD WHO IS DEAF OR HARD OF HEARING

There is limited research that documents the relationship between hearing loss and play, although a number of studies in the twentieth century demonstrated that some children who are deaf or hard of hearing are vulnerable to delays in their play, which may be secondary to associated delays in language and/or limitations of world knowledge and experience (Spencer & Deyo, 1993). Spencer (1996) found that in children with hearing loss and language delay, higher language levels were associated with better sequences and play. Even today's generation of children with hearing loss, who are implanted young and may never have a language 'delay,' is vulnerable to play that is delayed compared with children with typical hearing because they play in noisy classrooms and daycare settings with limited opportunities to overhear (Cole & Flexer, 2008). This results in a hiatus in their world knowledge that can have a significant impact on play (Brown, 1999).

Spencer and Meadows-Orlans (1996) found that children with hearing loss born to parents with typical hearing had delayed skills in preplanned play at 18 months compared with children with typical hearing and Deaf children born to Deaf parents. They also found an association between mater-

nal responsiveness and children's play at this age, suggesting that there is a major role for AVT in helping parents to know how to play with their children at different ages. In a small sample of preschoolers whose language during play in a preschool setting was statistically analyzed, Brown, Prescott, Rickards, and Paterson (1997) found that children who are deaf or hard of hearing used a higher degree of literal language and current action (as opposed to scripted play) language than their peers with typical hearing. Both these studies make the case for practitioners to plan, deliver, and evaluate AVT sessions to help parents prepare their children to play in partnership with peers with typical hearing (see Chapter 17).

PURPOSEFUL PLAY IN AUDITORY-VERBAL THERAPY

In AVT, the practitioner knows to work within the child's zone of proximal development (Vygotsky, 1978), because the child is motivated to play. The practitioner coaches parents to enhance their child's play at or just above, the child's zone of proximal development even if the child has delayed play skills. Play needs to be purposeful and have intrinsic rewards so that the child thinks, remains motivated and attentive, and is able to achieve the short-term objectives outlined by the practitioner and the parent. For example, rather than immediately turning over a piece of paper that keeps rolling up, the practitioner encourages the child to problem solve by using language such as: "Oh no! It keeps rolling up. That's a problem. I wonder what we can do!" Following strategies presented in Chapter 16, the family waits for a response and then verbally suggests ideas of their own, such as "We could stick it down!" or "We could put something heavy on it!" The child has an opportunity to think, problem solve, and then see the satisfaction of what comes of it. This keeps the child busy and engaged in meaningful play for a prolonged time and provides key skills for everyday living. Practitioners observe children in therapy sessions primarily with adults rather than peers and therefore adults are not only play partners but the primary agents of change in the development of their children by targeting learning through play. Active engagement of the parents, therefore, is essential because *"children should be taught to play as intentionally and systematically as you would teach literacy or math"* (Leong & Bodrova, 2012). Active and intentional parental behaviors such as turn-taking, modeling, verbal suggestions, contingent commentary (Brown, 1999), and explicit teaching (Leong & Bodorva, 2012) rather than passive observation have a significant positive effect on play development. This is playing the Auditory-Verbal way and is substantiated by Smith (1990), who proposes that adults who intervene in a sensitive way can enhance and show new possibilities and opportunities in the child's play. Moyles (2015) states that practitioners need to model play and become play partners. Weisberg et al. (2016) sees 'guided play' as a combination of adult initiation and child direction. Guided play incorporates adult structuring of the play environment, but the child maintains certain control in the environment. In order for new learning to take place, adults need to scaffold play (Goal #5) chosen by the child in such a way that the child can experience cumulative practice in language learning in conversational contexts.

Play in AVT—Back to Joey

- It is clear that the practitioner used guided play that was purposeful with Joey and his parents.
- First, the practitioner discovered the toys Joey enjoyed so that he would be motivated to play and followed his lead.
- Second, the practitioner provided additional objects and more ideas to make the play purposeful.
- Next the practitioner used sabotage to stimulate for Goal #6 by hiding a few tracks so that Joey had a reason to ask for more. (This demonstrates how the practitioner structured the play environment, where he could coach the parents to use acoustic highlighting and modeling to help Joey ask for more by using two-word utterances to stimulate for Goals #2, #3, and #5.)
- Once the track was built, Joey started to play with the little people by putting them in the train and going around the track (directed the play). (After a short time, it became obvious that "going around the track" was repetitive, risking Joey's quickly losing interest.)

- The practitioner coached the mother to ask Joey to pretend to be the little person who looks like the mother and that the people needed to buy tickets before boarding a train. (The practitioner made suggestions to move the play to a different level so that additional opportunities for language development and interaction emerge.)

- Joey started looking around for a structure to resemble a payment booth and pretended to buy some tickets. He said he wanted to visit his grandfather. (The child kept playing.)
- Father and Joey jointly decided to visit Granddad on the farm and then buy ice cream at the park. (The adult followed the child's lead, kept the play going, and purposefully extended it.)

In AVT, young children typically learn about specific schemas for play scenarios (e.g., going shopping, going to the library, going on holiday) through parental modeling. When they become *more experienced players*, and generate their own schemas and scenarios, they subsequently develop higher levels of listening, language, and learning. There are a number of tips for creating or extending play demonstrated in Play in AVT with Joey (above):

- Create a problem (don't have enough track out).
- Add another idea ("They need to buy tickets!").
- Talk for the characters ("I want a ticket!").
- Add an object ("I wonder what this box could be . . . an engine shed? or a station?").
- Pose a question to prompt their imagination ("I wonder where the train is going").
- Assign roles ("Who can I be?").
- Invite others to play ("I wonder who Mom would like to be").

COMMON ISSUES IN WORKING THROUGH PLAY

"Play is a child's work" (Piaget, 1977), *and to a child it must not feel like work.* As indicated in the literature, some children who are deaf or hard of hearing may have delayed play. It is relevant, therefore, that the practitioner accurately identifies the child's level of play in order to select developmentally appropriate activities so that the child is engaged and experiences an abundance of successful learning opportunities. There are many stories reported by both practitioners and parents about children who throw toys, refuse to engage with an activity, or are finished after one minute of exploration with a new toy. This may be the result of an inappropriately determined level of play or the child may not understand the potential of the toy or the activities (Brown, 1999). Practitioners, therefore, need to accurately identify a child's play level and this can be done in the following ways:

(a) formal assessment of the child's play skills through a standardized test such as the Symbolic Play Test (Loewe & Costello, 1976);

(b) observation of the child playing independently or with a parent prior to the session in the clinic, the home, or preschool; and/or

(c) engagement in an AVT session that encourages play at the child's current level and zone of proximal development. Identification of the child's current stage of play ensures the child progresses in accordance with the milestones within an age group and that practitioner and parent know when it's time to move on to the next stage of play skills development.

Most children who play within the zone of proximal development engage with a play activity for a significant period of time. Some children with other challenges such as a gross or fine motor delay or sensory integration difficulties, however, may have difficulty playing at their cognitive level. For example, children with sensory seeking behaviors may want to attend to a task but their sensory needs may prevent them from focusing. Support from allied health partners or members of the children's intervention team may be required (Estabrooks et al., 2016).

TYPICAL DEVELOPMENT OF PLAY

To set appropriate short-term and long-term goals for play skills, the practitioner needs to have a thorough understanding of play development in children with typical hearing. The following sections highlight the stages of play development for children with typical hearing from birth to 5 years. A brief overview of the key features of each stage is provided in tandem with specific evidence-based milestones. The ages attributed to these stages are guidelines. A child with delayed play skills needs encouragement to consolidate each stage before the next stage is started. Sample activities for the practitioner and the parent are offered and are related to the *six goals of the practitioner* that are required in most AVT sessions (see Chapter 16). Also, Chapter 17 presents a number of AVT session snapshots at a variety of ages that demonstrate the use of strategies used in play in AVT to target the six goals.

The Birth to 6-Month-Old Child Playing

Baby Kezia wants nothing more than to look into her mother's eyes. She studies her face intently and when mother sings, her face lights up. She is slowly learning to stretch out her legs and uncurl her fingers, yet her movements mostly appear random. Kezia wants to be close to her mother as she encounters her new world.

The first 12 weeks of a baby's life are now referred to as the fourth trimester (Isaacs, 2018), during which the baby and caregivers are adapting to each other. Like any new parents, these parents may be trying to cope with sleep deprivation, a child that who has colic, establishing feeding, weight gain, fussy periods, and nappies, in addition to dealing with the shock and grief many parents report when their child is diagnosed with a hearing loss. Parents need time and space to talk, and the practitioner needs to actively listen to support them in observing their baby's communication attempts. The practitioner can suggest and demonstrate activities that can easily fit into their everyday routines. Many parents report that the early AVT sessions gave them hope— by showing them things their baby could do and could learn, and by giving them practical suggestions that were easy to do at home. The basic needs of the baby are food and physical contact with parents and caregivers. They want to be picked up, held, carried around, and cuddled during most waking hours (van der Rijt & Plooij, 2013). The best "toys" are the caregiver's face, touch, and voice! The practitioner coaches caregivers to talk and play with their babies in a purposeful way, use parentese with lots of pausing and waiting, singing and humming. Baby massage, rocking, and singing provide caregivers with many opportunities to introduce rhythm and auditory attention to speech sounds. At about 3 to 4 months, babies begin to gain more control over their bodies. They start to lift their heads, sit independently, and start to roll. Cognitively, they become interested in toys they can grab, hold, and take to their mouths (Faure & Richardson, 2014). From 3 months of age, they begin to understand and anticipate some everyday social routines (Sheridan, 2006). This is the ideal time to help caregivers learn how to talk before, during, and after actions or experiences with their babies to promote knowledge of language (see Chapter 15). Table 12–1 lists the developmental play milestones that develop over the first six months, along with some for interaction and communication during AVT sessions and at home.

Table 12–1. Development of Play 0 to 6 Months

Developmental Progress	Evidence Base	Suggested Activities
"Fourth Trimester"—want to be picked up, held, be carried around and cuddled	Van der Rijt & Plooij (2013)	• Talking to baby using parentese and lots of pauses. • Baby massage, rocking and singing
Look at lights, focus on objects with light and dark contrast. Look at slow moving objects and enjoy listening to interested in lights and high frequency sounds	Van Huyssteen (2014)	• Follow the child's gaze and talk about what they see using L2L's, parentese and pausing. • Books with high contrasting pictures of baby faces, touchy-feely books and flap books (see textbox for more information)

continues

Table 12-1. *continued*

Developmental Progress	Evidence Base	Suggested Activities
Enjoy spoken language more than environmental sounds	Van Huyssteen (2014)	• Telling baby the plans ahead of time • Singing and rhymes
Reflexively imitate adult facial expressions (e.g., sticks out tongue) from birth	Meltzoff & Moore, (1983) Nadel et al. (1999)	• Watch baby carefully and respond to every unintentional imitation as if it is intentional communication.
Gaze intently at mother's face and can recognize her voice	Trevarthan (1979) Sheridan (2009)	• Feeding • Using parentese with pausing and singing
Prefer to look at human faces over other stimuli until 3 months	Rosser (1994) Van de Rijt & Plooij (2013)	• Facial expressions • Respecting the child's nonverbal contributions as valid and providing a follow-up
Lay on gym play mat under a mobile	Faure & Richardson (2014)	• Talking about what the baby is looking at using L2L's and acoustic highlighting
Reach out for toy, grasp, mouth, shake and bang start to develop from 4 months	Sheridan (2006)	• Nesting cups, balls that can shake, shakers, rattles, blocks. • Using shake shake shake vs stop as auditory contrast • Uh oh when it falls as auditory hooks
Enjoy vocal and facial expression during interaction with caregivers		• Vocal turn taking by copying the sounds they make • Action songs: Start singing before doing the actions
Anticipate every day routines	Faure & Richardson (2014) Sheridan (2006)	• Talking ahead about what will happen and using L2L's for everyday routines (feeding, bath time, story time, naps). • Playing finger games and rhymes (e.g., this little piggy). • Start leaving gaps in songs/rhymes

Tips for Playing with 0- to 6-Month-Olds in AVT

▪ Talk *before* performing an action (e.g., "time to pick you up, up, up"), daily routines (e.g., "it's time to eat"), or play with toys that can be associated with Learning to Listen Sounds (LTLS) (see Chapter 15) (e.g., "let's find the doggie that's barking . . . woof woof!") (Goal #4).

▪ Stimulate auditory attention by using auditory hooks, parentese, and pausing, and especially before engaging in facial expressions or verbal turn taking games (Goal #2) (see Chapter 15).

▪ Give the baby unconditional positive regard as an individual with thoughts and feelings of its own to communicate. Support caregivers to become keen observers of the baby's unintentional gestures and movements that can be nurtured to become intentional communication.

▪ Use many books. Newborns enjoy looking at books with black and white, high-contrast pictures or baby faces. From 6 weeks and on, babies enjoy bright and colorful pictures and photographs of babies. From 3 months on, babies like touchy-feely books, and from 4 months, babies enjoy "lift the flap" books with simple repetitive stories (see Chapter 14).

▪ Sing songs that incorporate actions where parents can use hand-over-hand to help their babies make the actions (see Chapter 18). Sing first before doing the action (Goals #1 and #2).

▪ From about 4 months, some babies who have experienced much repetition can demonstrate auditory closure when parents leave off the last word of the phrase (e.g., if you see a crocodile don't forget to _____ (wait for the baby to scream) (Goals #2 and #3).

▪ Recite rhymes and demonstrate finger plays using popular children's songs. Use rattles to shake, blocks to bang, and objects to mouth. These help the baby notice auditory contrasts when one talks about the action they make (e.g., "Shake, shake, shake" versus "Stop!") (Goals #2 and #3).

The 6- to 12-Month-Old Child Playing

Arthur loves being busy! At almost 8 months of age, he sits securely for extended periods and manipulates toys in new ways. He babbles reduplicated syllables such as "baba-baba" as he bangs his stacking cups against each other. They fall away and he barely glances at them, and then leans forward to retrieve the next toy. He studies it carefully, passing it between his hands, before he bangs it too. At the sound of his father calling, he turns to him, smiles, and moves his whole body in excitement. He pays close attention to his dad's movements when he sings "If you're happy and you know it clap your hands."

The 6- to 12-month period is an exciting time of rapid motor development in babies (Faure & Richardson, 2014), and it is useful for the practitioner to include a lot of physical activities during the AVT sessions and for the parents to do the same at home. Babies at this age just love things in motion, including themselves and their caregivers. Table 12–2 highlights expected milestones and appropriate activities for this age group.

One of the most noticeable areas of development during these months is the transition from being stationary to physically moving around. Babies typically roll from their backs to their sides at about 4 to 5 months, and vocally move from cooing noises to using first words. Many babies start to crawl between 6 to 10 months, pulling up against furniture at around 10 to 11 months and often take their first independent steps around their first birthday (Faure & Richardson, 2014), often in synchrony with their first words. With each passing month they gain more mobility and show great enjoyment in games where they can explore with all their senses. Sensory play, shaking, banging, kicking, splashing, filling, emptying, clapping hands, singing action songs, listening to nursery rhymes, and dropping toys happen at around 6 months, and all these activities are used in AVT sessions and at home. As soon as they are up on their feet, they are ready for push-and-pull toys and fetch-and-bring games. They start to anticipate familiar routines, songs, and events, and at 9 months they demonstrate knowledge of object permanence (Sheridan, 2006). They start to relate to themselves by looking in a mirror (Faure & Richardson, 2014) and associate everyday actions to objects (e.g., wiping the table with a cloth) and they find great pleasure in opening and closing and packing and unpacking. Children with typical hearing at this age start to vary their babbling and may be quite vocal when they are playing. In AVT, creative and intuitive practitioners find interesting ways to make the most of this *sound play* in functional and fun ways as they establish the foundations for understanding language and enhancing the development of the auditory feedback loop.

Tips for Playing with a 6- to 12-Month-Old Child in AVT

The practitioner plans, delivers, and evaluates every AVT session with focus on facilitating auditory processing, enhancing auditory perception, and promoting knowledge of language (see Chapters 15 and 17).

- Grab, squeeze, and wash toy animals such plastic ducks in a bowl of water. The ducks can swim, dive and splash, dry off, walk around, look up and down, go to sleep, run around. Name it and ducks can do it, just like all the other things that children at this age love.
- Use the ducks to sing "Five little ducks went swimming one day" and leave a gap at the end for them to fill in the Learning to Listen Sound for a duck (Goals #2, #3, and #4).
- Introduce sensory play by filling a container with different texture/sensory items and rotating these. Water, foam,

Table 12-2. Development of Play 6 to 12 Months

Developmental Progress	Evidence Base	Suggested Activities
Development of cause and effect—shake a rattle deliberately to make a sound	Sheridan (2006) Faure & Richardson (2014)	• Games that allow them to make a lot of noise such as shaking noisy toys, banging pots and pans with a wooden spoon. • Pop-up toys where they can be expected to use their voice to make something happen or start using their auditory feedback loop to shape their utterances. • Dropping toys from the high chair. Use this to awaken auditory attention and auditory feedback loop (see main text).
Interested in the sensation of different textures and explore objects by touching, stroking and patting them	van Huyssteen (2014) Faure & Richardson (2014)	• Sensory play: Various containers with different texture/sensory items (water, foam, sand, jelly, cooked spaghetti, edible paint, shaving cream, balls of different sizes). Introduce a range of verbs (in, out, feel, squeeze, mix, stamp, throw, splash, roll) descriptive concepts (wet, dirty, soft, hard) and free exploration. • Patting and stroking soft toys whilst taking about the sounds they are making or singing songs with animals (e.g., Old MacDonald). • Looking at textured books and talking about what they are seeing and feeling.
Search for a partially hidden object	Sheridan (2006)	• Partially hide a familiar toy under a blanket or in a container—talk about the object you are looking for (using L2L or label) and the action needed to retrieve the object (e.g., pull).

continues

Table 12-2. *continued*

Developmental Progress	Evidence Base	Suggested Activities
Object permanence has developed—loves peek a boo games	Sheridan (2006) Adamson et al. (1996)	• At around 9 months they develop object permanence and start to enjoy peek-a-boo games with parents or toys disappearing. Use an auditory hook (uh oh) to indicate something is gone and hooking the child in. Start working on questions (e.g., Where is daddy?) and pointing when you find him (There he is!). • Hide behind furniture and call baby to crawl to find you. Let him follow your voice to develop auditory location.
Development of early play schemas—takes objects in and out of containers, opens and closes doors	Sheridan (2006)	• Allow children to unpack a cupboard with plastic bowls, spoons and containers. Sing a tidy up song when you pack it all away and leave gaps for them to fill as they become familiar with this. • Provide a bit of sabotage—nothing in the cupboard that usually contains the plastic bowls or a door that is stuck. Guide them to start to use a verbal response to ask for help or saying uh oh to indicate there is a problem.
Does actions in simple play routines, e.g., waving bye-bye, pat a cake	Sheridan (2006)	• Show children how to use the 'bye-bye' for social greeting, but also as a strategy to communicate when they are done with a toy or their food instead of throwing it or pushing it away. • Start leaving gaps during routine rhymes and finger play and wait with a look of expectation if the child uses a gesture to support some verbal response.
Relates objects to one another—puts a spoon in a bowl, keys in the door	Sheridan (2006	• Early pretend play when acting on a book to pretend to feed/wipe the baby in the photographs from 10 months.

sand, jelly, cooked spaghetti, edible paint, shaving cream, balls of different sizes can be exciting to stimulate function words and other verbs (in, out, feel, squeeze, mix, stamp, throw, splash) and descriptive words (wet, dirty, soft, hard). Parents can determine how to engage children in the home and community environments to achieve short-term objectives related to Goals #4, #5, and #6 (see Chapters 15 and 17).

■ Blow bubbles and use other cause and effect toys to motivate children in this group to use their voices purposefully and to begin shaping their imitations through auditory perception and facilitating spoken language and cognition (Goal #5).

■ Enjoy games that allow babies to make a lot of noise (e.g., shaking noisy toys, banging pots and pans with wooden spoons, clapping hands). In AVT sessions the practitioner encourages games where all participants shake, wave, dance, bang, clap, push, and pull.

Nursery rhymes and actions/songs also work well for these.

■ Drop toys from the high-chair or cot, listen for the sound (Goal #1), invite the parent to pick it up or pretend that it's gone, and then search for it (Goals #3 and #5). These are opportunities for stimulating auditory attention and adding more language (e.g., "Uh oh! Did you hear that?" "*What* did you hear?"), using auditory contrast and a gap for them to fill in (e.g., "We need to pick it up, up, up—we need to pick it up") (Goal #3).

■ Add surprise elements to everyday events by turning a dropped toy into a hide-and-find game or playing peekaboo (Goals #1, #5, and #6).

■ Copy games where babies look at themselves in the mirror. Talking about who they are seeing and looking at different body parts (Goals #5 and #6).

■ Share books with baby faces and demonstrating pretend play relating actions and objects using the baby face (e.g., "Baby's mouth is dirty—let's wipe her face") (Goals #1, #2, and #5).

The 12- to 18-Month-Old Child Playing

Maddie's mother is thrilled at how her 15-month-old is toddling around on her own two feet, starting to exert independence by wanting to hold the cutlery herself, and rapidly developing language. Maddie seems to love the word "No!" Today is her first play date with Muhammad, who is 17 months old. When they arrive, Maddie begins to interact with and investigate the little boy. Muhammad picks up a toy feather duster and pretends to dust the shelf with toys. This duster is one of Maddie's favorite toys. In a flash, she pushes Muhammad and grabs it from his hands while saying "No!" Crying, Muhammad responds by holding on tightly to the duster. One of the adults intervenes by giving Maddie a baby doll and a spoon with which to feed her. Maddie feeds the doll, wipes its mouth, and pretends to put it to sleep. It's not long before the two toddlers are both grabbing and yelling for the same toy again, and the adults intervene again, by taking the ball over which they were fighting and rolling it back and forth between them. After a few minutes Muhammad toddles off toward the kitchen and proceeds to open the cupboards to investigate what he can find. Maddie is pretending to be asleep and is looking to see if her mommy will play along by saying

"Wake up!" Muhammad's mother tries to get him back to the playroom, but he is adamant that he wants to play in the kitchen with the plastic cutlery and pans he has found. He is trying to stack them on top of each other and see if they will fit if he pushes them together. He enjoys pretending to play drums and attempts to sing a song his mother usually sings with him. He throws a tearful tantrum when he is removed and it's only when the adults start showing the children how they can play "chase" with each other by running and catching that he leaves the kitchen, giggling and joining in.

The above scenario is typical play of the first half of the second year for toddlers. They play independently from one another, often in parallel, and might imitate older children and adults. They are very curious to investigate their playmates and to explore their environment to learn what they can do within boundaries. As they experience everything from their viewpoint, they are, of course, the center of the universe and cannot understand about sharing toys. They are no longer babies; they are toddlers, trying to make sense of a grown-up world while expressing some independence. Their motor skills and language skills continue to develop rapidly and from the above scenario it is clear that *toddlers need adults to be reading their thought bubbles*, modeling the words they need, and supporting their playful interactions with others. This is a particularly challenging time for parents of children with typical hearing, but even more so for children in AVT who may be compromised by various hearing

challenges. Table 12–3 documents the developing milestones with some ideas of play for this age group.

Tips for Playing with 12- to 18-Month-Olds in AVT

- Collect clean, empty shampoo bottles, soap, and cream containers for bathroom cupboards, and plastic cutlery, pots, pans, and wooden spoons for kitchen cupboards so that children can explore freely. Talk about the many attributes of these items and their functions.
- Create real-life scenarios with the items, such as pretending to cook food. Demonstrate how to play with them and how to imagine they might be other things such as a pot being a boat or a car (Goals #4, #5, and #6).

▪ Play tea parties with a teddy bear, a doll, and yourself and the child. Show the toddler how to give all the participants a cup by saying words such as, "Here is a cup for you." Pretend to pour tea in each cup and pretend the bear is drinking. Tell the child that the bear spilled some tea and he or she needs to wipe it up. Then demonstrate it, coach the mother or father to do it, and then observe as the child takes his/her turn. Just like in any AVT session for a young child, the focus is on playing and moving forward by achieving the short-term objectives for each session.

▪ Pretend to fall asleep and wait for the child to shout "Wake up!" before opening your eyes. Show the child how he or she can make you sleep again by saying "Shhhh." Take turns waking someone up and putting the person to sleep (Goals #2, #3, and #5).

▪ Create processes—fill a toy truck with sand, drive it to a bowl, and dump the sand in it. Pretend to hide something and look for it together—load it in the truck and drive off to the next place (Goals #4, #5, and #6).

▪ Introduce painting in two or three steps: dip the paint brush in paint, paint on the paper, then Daddy has a turn (Goal #5).

Table 12–3. Development of Play 12 to 18 Months

Developmental Progress	Evidence Base	Suggested Activities
Between 12–15 months a lot of the play consist out of exploring and investigating		• Have books with flaps, everyday pictures and patterns on a low shelf that are accessible for them to pull out and explore while you might need to make an important phone call or cook dinner • See main text for more ideas
Real objects are used according to their function, e.g., sweeping the floor.	Sheridan (2006) Brown (1999)	• Involve them in sweeping, wiping, packing away, cleaning, washing, drying, brushing, dressing. Use these verbs and talk about why you are doing it using adjectives (e.g., we are washing because the cups are dirty)

continues

Table 12-3. *continued*

Developmental Progress	Evidence Base	Suggested Activities
Acts on self (e.g., pretending to drink) 12–14 months	Adamson (1996)	• Show them how to pretend to feed themselves or brush their hair when playing with toy items. Use the L2L+relevant verb
Decentered play (15 months); begin to pretend on others	Sheridan (2006)	• Start to introduce personal pronoun (e.g., you and me) to show them that they can pretend to give you (for me) a bottle and then themselves (for you) a bottle
Early pretend play on objects (progress from decentered play on real people to pretending with an object), e.g., feeding dolly, putting teddy to sleep.	Adamson (1996)	• See main text
Begin to take turns with adults	Brown (1999)	• Take turns playing peek-a-boo • Pretend to chase your toddler, e.g., mummy is going to catch you—here I come—run run run. • Take turns being chased and chasing • See main text
Play becomes more sequenced with 3 steps around 12–15 months	Loewe et al. (1976)	• Show your toddler how to scoop sand in a bucket and turn it over and lift it off, to make a sandcastle • Put water in a watering can, carry it to the plants and water them • See main text

Table 12–3. *continued*

Developmental Progress	Evidence Base	Suggested Activities
Self-pretend play is the first step to develop imaginative play and starts at around 14–15 months. Pretending to sleep when they are awake (can start when they are supposed to nap and part of understanding boundaries!)	Van Huyssteen (2014)	• Show them how to expand this pretend play by pretending be dirty and need to be washed without having all the props • Show them how they can pretend to be a dog that walk on all fours and barks • Playing "sleeping bunnies"

The 18- to 24-Month-Old Child Playing

Isla enjoys taking her doll with her wherever she goes. Now that she is 20 months of age, she insists on bringing along the doll's diaper bag containing a toy bottle, blanket, diaper, wash cloth, and spoon. Mother is busy washing dishes when Isla puts her doll in the highchair. Talking to the doll, she says, "*Open mouth*" and with her toy spoon pretends to feed the doll and then wipe its mouth. Then she takes the doll from the highchair and pretends to go for a walk, holding the doll's hand and saying, "*Walk outside*." She pretends to give the doll milk from the toy bottle and to wrap the doll in the blanket. Isla says, "*Shhh Shh Shh.*" When her mother moves to the living room, she gives Isla some little toy people and a bus to play with. Isla picks up each person, names them (e.g., Mommy, Daddy, Isla) and tells them to "*Sit down*" before placing them in the bus. She pushes the bus around trying to sing the song "Wheels on the Bus." Her mother joins in and at the end of the song Isla tells the people to "*Get out*" and "*Go sleep*" followed by giving each a kiss.

This is a very exciting period in typical play development—as the child moves from a very busy, exploratory play (Piaget, 1977) toward constructive play (Smilansky, 1968). This often means that parents can observe their child beginning to engage with the same toy for a longer period of time and performing a number of actions on it. Table 12–4 shows the key areas of play that develop over this six-month period, along with some ideas/activities to enhance the child's play and attention in the AVT session and at home.

Along with more detailed pretend play sequences with dolls, vehicles,

Table 12-4. Development of Play 18 to 24 Months

Developmental Progress	Evidence Base	Suggested Activities
Begins to substitute objects in pretend play, e.g., a brick can be used to represent a car, a hairbrush or an ice cream!	Casby (2003) Belsky et al. (1981)	• Bricks of different shapes and sizes • Loose parts box (Nicholson 1971) containing open ended play objects, e.g., corks, balls, string, lids, feathers
Actions on dolls and other people become increasingly sequenced and less linear, e.g., pours water in a cup, gives doll a drink, wipes its mouth—all actions on the same doll before moving onto the next thing	Casby (2003) Brown (1999)	• Play with dolls or soft toys including feeding, bathing, changing • Pretend picnics/tea parties • Washing cars—wash with bubbles, rinse, dry
Imitates everyday parent activities in play, e.g., sweeping the floor, dusting, talking on the phone	Sheridan (2006)	• Toy kitchen with saucepans • Pretend fruit that can be cut up
Transitions from larger objects to small world play figures, initially with simple sequences, e.g., putting small people in and out of a bus		• Small world figures with familiar objects they can go in and out of e.g., little people and a bus, train, or aeroplane
Begins to use words to talk directly to the play objects, e.g., telling doll to "sit down" or saying "night night."		• Play through familiar everyday routines with the toys
More exercise-based play is seen as the child becomes steadier on his feet and so is able to explore the physical world more thoroughly	Parten (1932)	• Space—studies show that more exercise based play occurs in less spatially dense environments • Assault courses with opportunities to climb, crawl, carry objects etc. Ideally with problem solving elements built in—should we go under or over the log?

and soft toys, the toddler becomes interested in small world figures, initially representing familiar adults such as "Mommy," and "Daddy," and performs familiar, predictable routines on these figures. The child enjoys having them sit on chairs, go to bed, or drive a car and begins to ask for a "man" if given an empty car.

At this stage, children who are deaf or hard of hearing in AVT may follow similar patterns to those of typically hearing children in terms of how they act on the toys, but there may be a noticeable difference in their expressive language depending on the age of diagnosis, fitting of hearing technology, and commencing AVT. Sometimes, even children with age-appropriate language have had fewer opportunities to overhear how their peers play in noisy environments. So, these children may not have learned any significant verbal play through overhearing. At this time, the Symbolic Play Test might be accompanied by informal observation, followed by recording the words the children used while playing. This might demonstrate a difference from their typically hearing peers.

As children become steadier walkers, they access more of the world, and consequently need more space to move about during play. Early rough and tumble play can account for 8% of adult–child interaction (Jacklin, DiPietro, & Maccoby, 1984) and so it is key that in the AVT session environment, and in the home and community, opportunities are created to integrate AVT objectives into such robust physical play. The practitioner needs to ensure that play becomes, and remains, a collaborative auditory-verbal and physical experience.

Tips for Playing with 18- to 24-Month-Olds in AVT

- ▪ *Present* with a simple problem to "re-engage" children with a toy when they tire of a current sequence. For example, if they finished feeding baby, enhance auditory attention and processing (Goal #2) by presenting a new idea (suggest that it has a soiled nappy, needs a bath, or is tired).
- ▪ Substitute an object in play— give the child a brick and say that it's milk for the baby. This can facilitate spoken language and cognition (Goal #5).
- ▪ Model how to talk to small world toys—and even "Boss them around!" Tell them to "Sit down" as they get in the bus, or to go "Up" (Goals #5 and #6).
- ▪ Coach parents to involve the children in household tasks with the associated problems of these tasks. Doing laundry is a classic example (Goals #3, #5, and #6).
- ▪ Suggest a trip to the park, the zoo, the library, the supermarket, the pond, the beach, the shopping mall, et al. The goals remain the same, but the environment changes.

The 2- to 3-Year-Old Child Playing

Youssif is often found crouched on the floor with a small figure in each hand. He does the same scenarios again and again—one figure climbs up onto the slide, says "My turn" and slides down. Then the other figure pronounces "My turn" and has a go. After a while the sequence changes—one of the characters pushes the other over! Youssif speaks for the other character by saying "No pushing!!" and equips the original character to say "Sorry!" At 2½ years old, Youssif loves when his older sister plays shopping with him. He likes pretending to be the shopkeeper and to scan the pretend food with a "beeper" and then shout, "I need money!"

The third year of life marks significant development in the complexity of the child's pretend play. He or she is no longer content to merely act upon an object but wants to be the object or for it to take on the role of another. These are opportunities for the child to consolidate the emerging language structures and vocabulary by taking on roles and repeating or rehearsing scenarios seen in everyday life. For the 2-year-old, this begins by taking on roles in small world play—actually talking for the characters, allowing them to use and rehearse everyday language, such as, "My turn!" "Push me!" "Mommy come here!"

As they move toward 2½ years, children begin to take on the roles of people they observe regularly in everyday life. Multiple repetitions of familiar role play sequences such as going shopping or making tea are often demanded of parents and caregivers! As children become more familiar with these everyday scenarios, they begin to venture outside their comfort zone and begin to act out scenes of other people they have seen—pretending to be the doctor, the postman, a mechanic, the hair stylist, the bus driver, et al. As they approach their third birthday, children begin to move toward increasingly imaginary scenarios and characters—copying some simple attributes of a superhero or a character in a familiar story. This is preparation for the transition into the imaginary world of the 3- to 4-year-old.

Development of play in the third year needs to be closely monitored in the child in AVT as he or she moves toward more collaborative play. Children need to know appropriate scripts and world knowledge to join in role play when initiated by another child, and to initiate the play by themselves! Opportunities to play in quiet environments where the child can hear the scripts for these role play scenarios prepare the child to listen ahead and fill in gaps in the noisy daycare or preschool classroom. Parents and practitioners need to know the favorite play scenarios of the nursery or classroom so that they can provide children with experience using relevant vocabulary—"train" may not be enough if the children are talking about "engines" and "locomotives."

Table 12–5 developmental milestones at 2 to 3 years lists the key areas of development in this period.

Tips for Playing with 2- to 3-Year-Olds in AVT

- Show the child how to talk *for* a doll by modeling. For example, you can have your doll say, "It's my turn!" or "I want bubbles!" (Goal #5).
- Find a quiet environment (Goal #1) to play shopping with another child and give the children a simple script to imitate (e.g., "Hello!" "I want

a banana! How much money?"
"Thanks! Bye!") (Goal #5).

■ Spend time in childcare settings observing children playing games (Doctors and nurses? Hair stylists? Drivers? Salespeople? Mommies and Daddies?) (Goal #4).

■ Make sure the children experience the vocabulary and world knowledge needed to

join in these popular scenarios (Goal #4).

■ Coach parents to use books to introduce increasingly imaginative scenarios, particularly familiar fairy tales such as "The Three Bears" and "The Billy Goats Gruff."

■ Create intrigue in play by adding urgency, misbehaving characters, and problems to solve (Goal #4 and #5).

Table 12–5. Development of Play 2 to 3 Years

Developmental Progress	Evidence Base	Suggested Activities
Pretend to be another agent, e.g., a doll or teddy, taking on their role	Sheridan (2006) Casby (2003)	• Showing them how to talk FOR the toy, e.g., doll saying "I want milk!"
Acts out short sequences of familiar everyday activities, e.g., making a cup of tea, going to the shops	Sheridan (2006)	• Kitchen with tea set and toy food • Till and shopping bag for playing shops or cafes
Transition through the second half of the year to less familiar play sequences such as going to the doctor or car garage	Sheridan (2006)	• Doctor's kit • Pretend petrol pump • Making a bus out of chairs
Use words to describe pretend worlds or scenarios, e.g., "The monster in the corner is eating all the food!" and provides a meaningful running commentary of their play with toys	Saarni (1999) Sheridan (2006)	• Duplo/playmobil small world toys with houses/shops/restaurants/playgrounds • Books with accompanying toy sacks, e.g., Billy Goats Gruff, The Three Bears, The Tiger Who Came to Tea
Talk through toys— toys have increasing personalities or characters	Brown (1999)	• Small world people who can "misbehave," e.g., pushing people over, running away, climbing up something!
Play sequence still follows a logical order	Brown (1999)	

The 3- to 4-Year-Old Child Playing

Ellie is 3 years and 2 months old and loves to pretend. She loves the story of "Rapunzel" and is desperate to explore it in her imaginary play. She doesn't need the right toys anymore—a few bricks can make a tower for Rapunzel, shoelaces are her hair, and the "witch" is a small toy man from her toybox. She is keen to involve others in her play and tells her mom, "*You be the witch, and I'll be Rapunzel.*" She wants to explore again and again the threat of the witch: "*If you escape, I'll put a spell on you!*" She shows increasing empathy for how the characters are feeling—and comforts them by saying, "*Don't worry Rapunzel, we will rescue you!*" and by telling off the naughty witch. Ellie's play is transporting her to an imaginary world, well outside of the "here and now" and keeps her engaged for long periods of time.

Carl Jung (1865–1971), the Swiss psychiatrist and psychoanalyst, said, "Without this playing with fantasy, no creative work has ever yet come to birth. The debt we owe to the play of imagination is incalculable." The fourth year of childhood is characterized by play that moves increasingly out of the "here and now" into imaginary worlds. The everyday scenarios of a 3-year-old play give way to 4-year-old play that centers on imaginary worlds and characters. For children who are deaf or hard of hearing to join in with their peers, they need to have:

- heard sufficiently what the plan for the play is. For example, "Let's play princesses—you be the princess and I'll be the wicked witch!"
- sufficient world knowledge to understand how to cope in an imaginary world.
- knowledge of the kind of "script" and voices of the characters in that world and the language of pirates, princesses, superheroes, and villains.

Opportunities for children who are deaf or hard of hearing in AVT to do this in quiet environments is key. Reading good books can provide much of the necessary background and world knowledge. The practitioner helps by coaching parents, caregivers, and others to focus on helping the child to join in and to initiate this kind of play, and to help the child to problem solve and use appropriate repair strategies when the play breaks down.

The fourth year is a transition for children in learning to take part in games that are increasingly rule based, often with a set order and multiple steps that need to be followed. Three-year-olds begin to display this in play, and specific ideas emerge. More complex direction takes place between children. For example, a child might say, "You're the bad guy so you need to come and catch us!" Experimenting with rules and conventions lays the groundwork for the 4-year-old to follow the rules of games such as "snakes and ladders" or for the 6-year-old who enjoys chess.

Table 12–6 presents some key developmental milestones that children pass through during this fourth year.

Table 12-6. Development of Play 3 to 4 Years

Developmental Progress	Evidence Base	Suggested Activities
Regularly take on play themes beyond their own personal experience (e.g., pretending to be a fireman)	Sheridan (2006)	• Exposing children to a range of themes through books, outings, a home corner, and play invitations. • Occupations
Plays cooperatively with other children, negotiating roles, e.g., "you be . . . I'll be . . . "	Ginsberg (2007) Garvey (1984)	• Opportunities to play in quiet environments with smaller groups of children. • Working on the language of negotiation—assigning roles, problem solving, advocating for themselves, offering turns to others.
Able to create completely imaginary scenarios, including imaginary friends.	Taylor et al. (2004)	• Ask questions to encourage imaginary thinking "whose in your buggy?" when no one is there. • Generate multiple ideas of what you can do with an empty box—"It could be a . . . or a . . ."
Role-play becomes increasingly fantasy based—pretending to be knights, princesses or superheroes.	Sheridan (2006)	• Rich diet of literature to introduce fantasy scenarios such as fairy tales. • Ensuring they have the language and world knowledge of the current fads—movies, books etc.
Dress up in imaginary play.	Sheridan (2006)	• Range of costumes and props • Language of description and negotiation to decide who is going to wear what!
Uses different voices for characters, which reflect the age, gender or key characteristics of the character.	Garvey (1984)	• Adults reading aloud stories, modelling these voices. • Opportunity to practice making voices through imitation (without cognitive load of having to think what they're actually going to say initially).
Plan cooperatively with other children, using language.	Ginsburg (2007)	• Opportunities to practice key language areas in cooperative play (see main text).

Tips for Playing with 3- to 4-Year-Olds in AVT

- Create "invitations" for children to play increasingly imaginative scenarios by providing toys and books that support the themes. For example, make a ship and have eye patches and treasure to play pirates (Goals #5 and #6).
- Ask questions to encourage imaginary thinking, such as "Who's in your buggy?" when no one is there, or "Where are you going?" or "What do you think will happen next?" (Goals #3, #4, and #6).
- Read aloud often and voice different characters and encourage the child to imitate that character (Goals #2, #3, and #6).
- Play simple board games such as lotto, memory, snap, snakes and ladders, to begin to expose them to "rules" within the play (Goals #5 and #6).

The 4- to 5-Year-Old Playing

At almost 5, Levi is a stickler for the rules! Whether it's playing snakes and ladders or cops and robbers, he's keen that everyone do things the right way, and that no cheating happens (unless he's the one doing it, of course!). The game of "cops and robbers" has an intricate set of rules, with clearly defined places in the playground that serve as jail and police station. Robbers are arrested using some words from a script he has heard on television and there is no negotiation in handing out jail sentences!

In the fifth year, there is a shift in the way children play. Play is increasingly more verbally based with fewer physical toys needed and a greater reliance on interaction with others to facilitate the play. The 4- to 5-year-old demonstrates much more complexity in play, as the child develops rich miniature worlds (Sheridan, 2006) that may have their own rules. Adults who join in the play of a 4-year-old are more likely to be told they're getting it wrong! ("Mommy, fairies don't go there, they have to sit on the toadstool and wait for the unicorns to come!") This reflects both increased world knowledge and the transition to understanding the rules of the world and of the play/games of older children. By age 6, the child is able to take part in complex board games with multiple steps and rules.

Play also provides great opportunities for such children to experiment with some of the more complex Theory-of-Mind concepts that they are beginning to understand, particularly that of truth/lies and deception (see Chapter 14). The complex worlds and scenarios they build allow them to experiment with characters who deceive one another, good ones and bad ones. Table 12–7 presents the key developmental milestones in children's play from 4 to 5 years.

SELECTING TOYS TO COMPLEMENT PLAY IN THE AVT SESSION

Today's generation of children is exposed to a lot of electronic toys that often require minimal adult input or

Table 12-7. Development of Play 4 to 5 Years

Developmental Progress	Evidence Base	Suggested Activities
Create miniature worlds in their play that are rich in narrative and story structure	Sheridan (2006)	• Making up stories with a couple of simple prop/pictures
Increased use of emotion based language and schemas in their play	Saarni (1999)	• Prompt questions "I wonder how . . . is feeling? What could we do to help? • Reading books rich in theory of mind concepts and complex emotions
Reliably judge "fact" versus "fiction"	Woolley et al. (2006)	• Magic tricks • Stories where characters are telling lies—can the child recognise this?
Play complex games requiring literacy/numeracy skills	Ramani et al. (2008)	• Board games with rules

---

Tips for Playing with 4- to 5-Year-Olds in AVT

■ Encourage the child to create pretend scenarios without supporting toys—make up talking stories (Goals #3, #4, #5, and #6).

■ Give suggestions to get started (e.g., "Shall we pretend to be knights or superheroes?") (Goal #6).

■ Help the child develop a script for the characters by reading and sharing books and by role-playing (Do they know how a queen talks vs how a robber talks?) (Goals #2 and #6).

■ Introduce concepts such as deception into the play and give the child time to problem solve (Who is telling the truth/lying? How can we find out?) (Goals #5 and #6).

---

other interaction from peers. Practitioners and parents carefully consider the use of electronic toys in their interaction with children. Playing with electronic toys decreases opportunities to hear varied and complex language (Zosh et al., 2015). Language use with these toys is often repetitive (*"Push this button"*; *"Push that button again"*) *and of lower quality language* (Zosh et al., 2015). Parent talk is often less about the intended function of the toy and creating opportunities for joint thinking and problem solving, and more about the features of the toy itself—which does not always support carryover. Playing with electronic toys is also associated with less pretend play and with less expansion of play to include higher level language or thinking, less engagement from adults, and more distraction (Plowman & Stephen, 2005)—so typically, children play only with the toy for a short while before becoming bored and needing something else. Playing with electronic toys can lead to isolated play and less need for interaction. The big question to answer when selecting toys and games is "Do these toys promote joint play, thinking, and communication?"

A number of toys have screens that children are required to look at for periods of time. The American Academy of Pediatrics (AAP) indicates that for children younger than 18 months, use of screen media other than video-chatting should be discouraged, and that parents of children 18 to 24 months of age who want to introduce digital media should choose high-quality programming/applications (apps) and use them together with children; but letting children use media by themselves should be avoided (AAP, 2019).

WHAT DOES PLAY THAT IS DELAYED LOOK LIKE?

Practitioners work from a developmental perspective rather than from a remedial one and as such, need to be familiar with the norms for each age and stage of play in child development so that children who do not make the expected progress or appear to follow an unusual trajectory in play can be identified as early as possible.

Brain research (Yogman et al., 2018) has shown commonality in the areas of the brain linking play, behavior, and sensory integration, so practitioners may need to join other members of the child's team to make a differential diagnosis for the above-mentioned children. There may be many questions to answer, such as: Is the play being affected by the child's behavior, underdeveloped sensory integration, or something else? The practitioner will consider particular characteristics and learning styles of each child, as he or she would do in considering the same of parents:

- The passive child: fails to reach play milestones; uninterested in age-appropriate toys; shows little interest with play or interaction with toys.
- The "accidental" offender: throws toys; gets frustrated after a short time; snatches or gets physical with parents/siblings/peers; does not like sharing toys.
- The active child: mismatch of cognition and the expected play level; gets easily frustrated; bores quickly; wants to be in control; demonstrates very short joint attention span for interaction or games; flits between activities.

Reduced opportunities for children who are deaf or hard of hearing to overhear means they may not "catch" the play ideas their typically hearing peers overhear. If children have delayed language, this can cause many of the issues outlined above, and as they get older, these children may exhibit play as follows:

- No story plot or play plot. The child is not able to see the potential in a toy because he/she cannot generate a plot about it. This means that after manipulating and exploring the toy, the child has no further use for it.

- Stuck in a play loop (e.g., boy pushing car back and forth). The child might not know a sequence of what a toy can do, or the potential of the toy—he or she may think a car is just for moving, and not know that a car may involve people, roads, gas stations, traffic lights, etc. This may be due to the child's lack of world knowledge for a variety of reasons, including limited overhearing.
- Experience the toy as a challenge and not know how to go about solving the problem (e.g., a wind-up toy) and subsequently throw it across the room.
- Focus on the outcome rather than the process. May not understand the sequence involved in preparing for, doing, or finishing an activity.
- Often can't get started, because the child does not know where the play is headed and may not be able to play jointly.
- Not able to negotiate due to lack of language and is often described as "difficult to share or play with others and likes to control the toys."

WHAT TO DO WHEN IT ALL GOES WRONG!

Lilly is 3½ and comes to the AVT session with her mother. Her mother notes that Lilly tries to play shopping with her older sister but gets bored quickly and often ends up throwing something or just walking away. She says that Lilly always wants to be the one who pushes the shopping cart around. She does not understand the exchange of money when her sister is behind the cash register and will often just move the trolley up and down the room, throwing things in and taking them out. She enjoys having a purse but has a meltdown if there is no pretend money in it. Lily would benefit from using language to join another's thoughts and exchange ideas and from thinking of ways to solve problems by herself.

The parent can *present new language* to aid Lilly's play development by becoming her play partner (Moyles, 2015), being explicit about modeling the play (Leong & Bodrova, 2012), and using guided play (Weisberg et al., 2016). Practitioners can help parents with evidence-based and evidence-informed strategies (see Chapter 16) so that their children can become competent play partners, participate in a range of scenarios, demonstrate flexibility within the play, and have play that is sufficient to stimulate thinking and language. The practitioner can establish problems (sabotage) and solutions throughout the play to motivate children who are stuck in a loop or have no play plot and facilitate their independent thinking (Goal #6). This can move play forward and gives the child a reason to use words. The following three elements may be used to re-engage the child to become interested in the problem:

- Support the child to spot the problem using audition and wait for the child to join you, showing he or she has noticed the problem. In Lilly's case she might think about the problem of the money that is not in the purse.

- Use the appropriate word/sentence for the developmental stage of the child to label the problem.
- Allow some pausing for the child to process the language and start thinking how to solve it.
- Scaffold an appropriate solution and support the child to verbalize this perception.

In AVT, most practitioners will playfully create problems that are age appropriate. Different problems will be interesting at different ages. Table 12–8 shows some appropriate problems and solutions to consider for children of different ages.

As children become older, their play becomes highly verbal, and they bring extensive general knowledge to the play scenario. Adults can scaffold a play plot by using a little process (Leong & Bodrova, 2012) such as:

- Planning; where the adult jointly makes a plan with the child or the adult suggests a plan. (For Lilly this might be "Let's tell your sister you want to play shopping.")

- Having different roles for different people. (Lilly can be supported to think about the various roles in a shopping game—e.g., the customer, the shop assistant, the person behind the cash register.) The adults can model how to assign roles to different people and talk with her about the different roles and what they will do.
- Providing language or a script to develop a scenario or co-ordinate the actions of different players. (If Lilly's role is the person coming to buy groceries, she needs to have the language to ask a shop assistant where she might find a certain product [another problem in the session!], or how much all her groceries cost.) (If Lilly is to be the person behind the cash register, she needs language to tell the customer how much the shopping costs and perhaps ask if he or she would like a bag and the receipt.) New ideas can be incorporated by being explicit and giving her a small script by modeling when she is the customer.

Table 12-8. Problems and Solutions for Different Ages

Age	Problem	Solution
0–6 months	• Comment on obvious problems—e.g., oh dear! It stopped!" "Let's make it swing, swing" • Use routine events—such as nappy change, feeding, bath time to hook the child in—e.g., "*uh oh—are you hungry?*"	• Let's make it "*swing swing swing*" • *Let'eat—yumm yumm*
6–12 months	• Allow the child time to explore the toy and use relevant comments, e.g., "*oh it's stuck*," "*Uh oh, it's all gone!*" • Ask questions: "*Where's that monkey oo oo oo . . . ?*" • Talk about things that fell down—"*Uh oh—it fell down!*"	• "*We need to push,*" *Let's get more!*" • Point to the monkey and say "*There!*" • Show the child that you can get it back up by say—"*up up up*"
12–18 months	• Toys are closed, stuck, wet, dirty. • Dolls/teddies are hungry, sleepy, thirsty, hurt	• They need to be opened, pushed, wiped, washed • Dolls/teddies can eat, go to bed, drink, given a plaster
18–24 months	• Pretend baby is crying "*Wah wah wah, baby needs to eat, can you find her something for eating?*"	• While giving the child an option of two objects (one being something for eating and one being another object not related to eating)
2–3 years	• Arts and craft items might be lost, broken, empty • Have situations where people don't want the things they offer—e.g., "*Daddy does not want tea, he does not like tea, what shall we do?*"	• Pretend to make something • Ask other's where things are you need • Stick torn paper. • Show children how to make and verbalize different plans when things does not quite go as they have hoped
3–4 years	• Children might not want the role they are given, want to change the game or play something different • Playground politics around who is first, who gets to play, etc.	• Negotiate roles, e.g, do you want to be . . . • Negotiate around turn taking; me first then you • Negotiate using rock, paper, scissors
4–5 years	• Higher level, TOM problems—someone wants to change rules of a game or play miniature worlds differently.	• Negotiate rules

CONCLUSION

This chapter has provided an overview of brain development through play from the AVT perspective, based on the milestones of play for children with typical hearing (the benchmark for AVT). Play the Auditory-Verbal way needs to be purposeful and exciting, and mostly it is a social engagement. Play is the essence of AVT for very young children who are deaf or hard of hearing and their parents who engage them, interact with them, stimulate them, take turns, and add more language in all AVT sessions, at home, in the child's community, at the child's cultural event, and everywhere the child goes.

Listening and spoken language as the desired and expected outcomes of AVT are mostly for socialization and occur best in an "environment of relationships" that is crucial for the development of a child's *brain architecture*, which lays the foundation for later outcomes such as academic performance, mental health, and interpersonal skills. Growth-promoting relationships are based on the child's continuous give-and-take ("serve and return" interaction) with a person who provides what nothing else in the world can offer—experiences that are individualized to the child's unique personality, build on his or her own interests, capabilities, and initiative, shape the child's self-awareness, and stimulate the growth of the child's mind. That is play the Auditory-Verbal way.

I tried to teach my child with books,
He gave me only puzzled looks.
I tried to teach my child with words.
They passed him by—often unheard.
Despairingly I turned aside.
"How shall I teach this child" I cried.
Into my hand, he put the key.
"Come," he said, "Play with me."
(Unknown)

REFERENCES

Adamson, L. B. (1996). *Communication development during infancy*. Madison, WI: Brown & Benchmark.

AG Bell Academy for Listening and Spoken Language. (2007). Retrieved September 25, 2019 from http://www.agbellacademy.org/principles-of-lsl-specialists/

American Academy of Pediatrics. (2019). Retrieved from http://www.healthychildren.org/English/media/pages/default.aspx

Belsky, J., & Most, R. K. (1981). From exploration to play: A cross-sectional study of infant free play behaviour. *Developmental Psychology, 17*, 630–639.

Brown, M. (1999). Early development in deaf and hard of hearing children: The state of play. *Australian Journal of Education of the Deaf, 5*, 27–36.

Brown, P. M., Prescott, S. J., Rickards, F. W., & Paterson, M. M. (1997). Communicating about pretend play: A comparison of the utterances of 4-year-old normally hearing and deaf or hard-of-hearing children in an integrated kindergarten. *The Volta Review, 99*(1), 5–17.

Casby, M. (2003) Developmental assessment of play: A model for early intervention. *Communication Disorders Quarterly, 24*, 175.

Cole, E. B., & Flexer, C. A. (2008). *Children with hearing loss developing listening and talking birth to six*. San Diego, CA: Plural Publishing.

Donaldson, O. F. (1993). *Playing by heart: The vision and practice of belonging*. Deerfield Beach, FL: Health Communications.

Estabrooks, W., MacIver-Lux, K., & Rhodes, E. (2016). *Auditory-Verbal Therapy: For young children with hearing loss and their families, and the practitioners who guide them.* San Diego, CA: Plural Publishing.

Faure, M., & Richardson, A. (2014). *Baby sense: Understanding your baby's sensory world—the key to a contented child.* Cape Town, South Africa: Metz Press.

Frost, J. L. (2010). A *history of children's play and play environments: Toward a contemporary child-saving movement.* New York, NY:Routledge.

Garvey, C. (1984). *Children's talk.* Fontana, UK: Oxford University Press.

Ginsburg, K. R., Shifrin, D. L., Broughton, D. D., Dreyer, B. P., Milteer, R. M., Mulligan, D. A., . . . Smith, K. (2007). The importance of play in promoting healthy child development and maintaining strong parent-child bonds. *Pediatrics, 119*(1), 182–191.

Greenberg, J., & Weitzman, E. (2005). *Fostering peer interaction in early childhood settings.* Hanen Early Language Programme, Ontario, Canada.

Isaacs, D. (2018). The fourth trimester. *Journal of Paediatrics and Child Health, 54,* 1174–1175.

Jacklin, C. N., Dipietro, J. A., & Maccoby, E. E. (1984). Sex-typing behaviour and sex-typing pressure in child/parent interaction. *Archives of Sexual Behaviour, 13,* 413–425.

Leong, D. J., & Bodrova, E. (2012). Assessing and scaffolding make-believe play. *National Association for the Education of Young Children. 67(1). 28–34*

Loewe, M., & Costello, A. (1976). *Symbolic Play Test (SPT).* Windsor: NFER-Nelson.

Meltzoff, A. N., & Moore, M. K. (1983). Newborn infants imitate adult facial gestures. *Child Development, 54*(3), 702–709.

Meltzoff, A. N., & Moore, M. K. (1997). Explaining facial imitation: A theoretical model. *Early Development and Parenting, 6,* 179–192.

Meltzoff, A. N. (2005). Imitation and other minds: The "Like Me" hypothesis. Cited in S. Hurley & N. Chater (Eds.), *Perspective on imitation: From neuroscience to social science* (Vol. 2, pp. 55–77). Cambridge, MA: MIT Press.

Moyles, J. R. (Ed.). (1994). *The excellence of play.* Berkshire. UK: Open University Press.

Moyles, J. R. (Ed.). (2015). *The excellence of play* (4th ed.). Berkshire. UK: Open University Press.

Nadel, J., & Butterworth, G. (Eds.). (1999). *Imitation in infancy. Cambridge studies in cognitive perceptual development.* New York, NY: Cambridge University Press.

National Scientific Council on the Developing Child. (2004). *Young children develop in an environment of relationships: Working Paper No. 1.* Retrieved September 25, 2019 from http://www.developingchild.harvard.edu

Nicholson, S. (1971). How not to cheat children: the theory of loose parts. *Landscape Architecture, 62,* 30–34.

Oxford English Dictionary. (2015). Stevenson A. (Ed.). Oxford, UK: Oxford University Press.

Parten, M. (1932). Social participation among preschool children. *Journal of Abnormal Psychology, 27,* 309–314.

Piaget, J. (1951). *Play, dreams and imitation in childhood.* London, UK: Routledge & Kegan Paul.

Piaget, J. (1977). *Insight and illusions of philosophy.* New York, NY: Routledge.

Plowman, L., & Stephen, C. (2005). Children, play, and computers in pre-school education. *British Journal of Educational Technology, 36*(2), 145–157.

Ramani, G. B., & Siegler, R. S. (2008). Promoting broad and stable improvements in low-income children's numerical knowledge through playing with number board games. *Child Development, 79*(2), 375–394.

Rosser, R. (1994) *Cognitive development: Psychological and biological perspectives.* Boston, MA: Allyn & Bacon.

Saarni, C. (1999). *Developing emotional competence.* New York, NY: Guilford.

Sheridan, M. (2006). *From birth to five years: Children's developmental progress.* Oxon, UK: Routledge.

Smilansky, S. (1968). The effects of socio-dramatic play on disadvantaged preschool children. In *Drama in education.* New York, NY: Wiley.

Smith, P. K. (1990). The role of play in the nursery and primary school curriculum. In C. Rogers & P. Kutnick (Eds.), *The social psychology of the primary school.* London, UK: Routledge.

Spencer, P. (1996) The association between language and symbolic play at two years: Evidence from deaf toddlers. *Child Development, 67*(3), 867–876.

Spencer, P. E., & Deyo, D. (1993). Cognitive and social aspects of deaf children's play. In M. Marschark, & M. D. Clark (Eds.), *Psychological perspectives on deafness* (pp. 65–92). Hillsdale, NJ: Lawrence Erlbaum Associates. Cited in Brown, M. (1999) Early development in deaf and hard of hearing children: The state of play. *Australian Journal of Education of the Deaf, 5*, 27–36.

Spencer, P., & Meadows-Orlans, K. (1996). Play, language and maternal responsiveness: A longitudinal study of deaf and hearing infants. *Child Development, 67*(6), 3176–3191.

Taylor, M., Carlson, S. M., Maring, B. L., & Charlye, C. M. (2004). The characteristics and correlates of fantasy in school-age children: Imaginary companions, impersonation, and social understanding. *Developmental Psychology, 40*(6), 1173–1187.

Trevarthan, C. (1979). Communication and cooperation in early infancy: A description of primary intersubjectivity. Cited in M. Bullowa (Ed.), *Before speech: The beginning of interpersonal communication* (pp. 321–347). New York, NY: Cambridge University Press.

Van de Rijt, H., & Plooij, F. (2013). *The wonder weeks.* Kiddy World Publishing. First published in 1992 as Oei, ik groei! By Zomer & Keuning boeken BV, Ede and Antwerp, Nertherlands.

Van Huyssteen, L. (2014). The *practical guide to individual stimulation.* The Van Huyssteen Family Trust, South Africa.

Vygotsky, L. (1978). *Mind in society. Development of higher psychological processes.* Cambridge, MA: Harvard University Press.

Weisberg, D. S., Hirsh-Pasek, K., Golinkoff, R. M., Kittredge, A. K., & Klahr, D. (2016). Guided play: Principles and practises. *Current Directions in Psychological Science, 25*(3), 177–182.

Woolley, J., & Van Reet, J. (2006) Effects of context on judgments concerning the reality status of novel entities. *Child Development, 77*(6), 1778–1793.

Yogman, M., Garner, A., Hutchinson, J., Hirsh-Pasek, K., Golinkoff, R. M., & AAP Committee on Psychosocial Aspects of Child and Family Health, AAP Council on Communications and Media. (2018). The power of play: A paediatric role in enhancing development in young children. *Paediatrics, 142*(3), e20182058.

Zosh, J. M., Verdine, B. N., Filipowicz, A., Golinkoff, R. M., Hirsh-Pasek, K., & Newcombe, N. S. (2015). Talking shape: Parental language with electronic versus traditional shape sorters. *International Mind, Brain and Education Society and Wiley Periodicals, 9*(3), 136–144.

13

THE DEVELOPMENT OF COGNITION AND AUDITORY-VERBAL THERAPY

Frances Clark and Warren Estabrooks

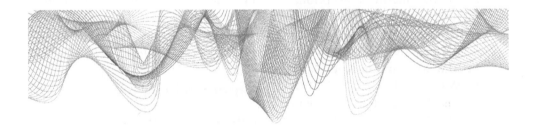

INTRODUCTION

"Thought is not merely expressed in words; it comes into existence through them." (Vygotsky, 1978)

Cognitive development is accepted as the emergence of a child's ability to think and understand (Bjorklund & Causey, 2018). Traditionally there is a distinction between the development of language and intelligence (i.e., verbal and non-verbal abilities). Auditory-Verbal practitioners coach and guide parents to help their children who are deaf or hard of hearing in the processes of developing listening and language, talking, and thinking. Research in cognitive psychology falls largely into the following categories: **Piagetian cognitive development**, the **information-processing approach**, and **psychometric conception** (Carr, 2006). **Vygotsky**'s model of conceptualizing cognition in fundamentally social terms has further influence on a child's development of interactions. In addition to these models, an understanding of **Executive Functioning (EF)** and **Theory of Mind (ToM)** is crucial to ensure that a child is fully equipped with the abilities to plan, remember, focus, problem solve, and successfully interact with other people.

These models and an understanding of both EF and ToM are critical influences in the development of listening, language, talking, and thinking in every Auditory-Verbal Therapy (AVT) session and throughout the child's entire Auditory-Verbal journey.

This chapter addresses the role of the practitioner in supporting parents to help their children who are deaf or hard of hearing to develop thought processes so they can be expressed through spoken language. The authors will:

- describe the development of cognition with regard to the models of Piaget, Vygotsky, the Information-Processing Approach, and Psychometric Conception;
- identify how these models relate to hearing loss and AVT;
- define EF, how it relates to hearing loss, and how it relates to AVT;
- discuss ToM (particularly cognitive ToM) and how it relates to hearing loss and AVT;
- outline typical development of EF;
- relate cognition to specific etiologies of hearing loss (e.g., meningitis and cytomegalovirus); and
- identify red flags and how to make appropriate referrals for additional services.

MODELS OF COGNITIVE DEVELOPMENT

Piaget

For most of the twentieth century, cognitive development was based around the work of Jean Piaget, who theorized that the development of cognition relied on the reorganization of mental processes that occurred through biological maturation and a child's interaction with his or her environment (Assmusen et al., 2018). Piaget's theory was formulated through thousands of observation hours of children in both natural and artificial situations such as clinical experiments or assessments. He regarded cognitive growth to be reliant on a child's active attempt to adapt to the world, assimilate new knowledge into previously established schemas, and/or accommodate new knowledge by changing schemas (Carr, 2006). He concluded that children's cognitive development could be described through four progressive stages as outlined in Table 13–1 (Assmusen et al., 2018). How does this relate to AVT?

Sensorimotor Stage

In the **sensorimotor stage** from birth to 2 years, children's object knowledge is influenced by *joint attention*—their ability to share attention with others. Joint attention develops in the first year of life and is a key ability in ToM development (Charman et al., 2000). Adults facilitate joint attention by drawing a baby's focus to something through visual and auditory cues. During an AVT session with a baby or young child, parents are coached to facilitate joint attention by *pointing* to a specific object, *waiting* for their child to join the adult's thinking by looking at that object, and then providing the child with the auditory input for that object. For example, the parents may be coached to draw their child's attention to a monkey toy on the table. The parents learn to talk

Table 13-1. Progressive Stages of Cognitive Development in Children (Assmusen et al., 2018)

Age	Stage	Type of Thinking	Abilities of Child by the End of the Stage
Birth–2 years	Sensorimotor	Exploration and learning through senses and movement.	*Object permanence*: the understanding that objects are separate from oneself and continue to exist when out of sight/sound/touch.
2–7 years	Pre-operational	Acquisition of motor skills, development of language, memory and imagination.	Understands and communicates through symbols, evidenced by use of language. Can make predictions that may be logical or illogical. Thinking is largely egocentric and revolves around the self.
7–11 years	Concrete operational	Logical thinking begins. More concrete and less egocentric.	Understands the logic behind cause and effect and arithmetic and can apply this to concrete problem-solving.
11–16 years	Formal operational	Hypothetical problem solving. Abstract	Can make and test hypotheses.

about the toy first, then point to it, wait for the child to look at the monkey, and then say, *"Look! It's the monkey."* The practitioner coaches the parent, in a number of ways, to use acoustic highlighting and other evidence-based strategies (see Chapter 15) that are in tandem with the child's development. These strategies vary depending on the chronological and hearing ages of the child. For example, a child who is waiting to get cochlear implants may need to hear "*Looook at the oo oo oo*," whereas a child who has better auditory access

may be able to understand, "*Look at the monkey!*" The practitioner coaches the parent to look for *triangulation*, which typically develops at around 9 months, and use this as a moment of communication opportunity. An example of triangulation is when a child looks at a toy and then back at his or her parent and then back at the toy. This demonstrates that the child is thinking about that toy. The parent can "seize the moment" to provide the child with stimulating auditory input (the word or *learning to listen sound* associated with that object). For example, when they look toward the toy airplane, the input might be "*Oh it's an airplane. It goes up up up. It says Ahhhhhhhh.*"

Children's object knowledge and cognition are advanced by learning to label objects. This occurs in children with typical hearing between 9 and 24 months of age (Assmusen et al., 2018). Label learning that is facilitated by joint attention impacts on: children's attention to salient features of the object they are observing; understanding the function of the object and awareness of the features that the object shares with other objects (Gelman, 2003 in Assmusen et al., 2018). In AVT sessions, the practitioner coaches the parents to use *learning to listen sounds* to facilitate these key cognitive factors, e.g., "*mmm mmm, your spoon, mmm mmm*" or they may say "*mmm mmm*" relating to milk (see Chapters 15, 16, 17). The child subsequently learns that "*mmm mmm*" relates to something that he or she is eating or drinking. Assmusen et al. (2018) highlight the need for early intervention to "*promote the importance of object manipulation and exploration during the first six months of life.*" All early AVT sessions and the subsequent generalization of the short-term objectives at home are golden opportunities for the child to explore objects and their features while the adults stimulate the child's auditory cortex and the development of listening skills.

It is evident at each of Piaget's stages of development that audition is required in order to mediate the interaction with the environment and move to the next cognitive stage. For a child under the age of 2 years it is important to: develop the understanding that sound carries meaning and understand that sound is made by people and objects separate to oneself and that the people or objects continue to exist when the sound ceases— for example, understanding that an ambulance will continue to exist when the siren can no longer be heard. During an AVT session, this may occur when an adult says "*bye bye*," indicating that he or she is leaving. By coaching adults to *talk ahead*, the practitioner supports them to help their child demonstrate an understanding of language and his or her thinking (e.g., if the parent says "*bye bye*" before waving or getting up to go, the child may demonstrate understanding by waving to the parent or looking toward the door). *Object permanence* occurs when the child indicates awareness that the person has exited and continues to look at the door for his or her return. Object permanence is a milestone that points to the interaction between linguistic and cognitive development and is typically developed by the end of the first year of life (Siegler, Deloacher, & Eisenberg, 2011). This stage highlights the overlap between thinking and language. In order for the practitioner to coach parents to use the word "gone," the child first needs to develop the concept of object permanence (Gopnik & Melzoff, 1987 cited in Carr, 2006). For example, a child may be playing with a toy car that falls off the table. The practitioner coaches the parent to point to the table (see Chapter 16) and say "*uh oh! It's gone!*" The child will demonstrate object permanence if he or she is looking toward the place where the car fell off the table.

Pre-Operational Stage

Piaget's pre-operational stage, from two to seven years, refers largely to the development of language—both concrete and abstract. It is an important stage for memory and imagination. Children are egocentric during this stage and they have difficulty thinking outside of their own viewpoints (Marcin, 2018). During this stage the practitioner can help children to start thinking about the perspectives of others by coaching parents to talk about how people have different likes and dislikes and by talking about the language of ideas. In AVT sessions, the practitioner can model by asking each person sitting at the table or on the floor about his or her ideas and this will demonstrate differences in thinking. A 2-year-old will benefit from hearing what each person likes (e.g., when choosing a snack, *"I like apples," "I like bananas," "I like cookies"*). As children get older, parents are coached to encourage them to inquire about others' thinking (e.g., *"Ask Alice what her idea is?"* or *"Ask Alice what she thinks"*). Younger children may require modeling such as, *"Alice, what is your idea?"* or *"Alice, what do you think?"* Typically, the young child will follow by repeating the stimulus and when Alice replies with an idea, the child learns that this question provides information about someone else's thinking.

Many authors indicate that according to Piaget, the main achievement of this stage is thinking about things symbolically. This can be promoted in AVT sessions through play (e.g., pretending that a banana is a telephone, a wooden block is a car). As language develops, more words are used to represent objects. Developed symbolic capabilities during this stage are also evident through children's drawing. Between the ages of 3 and 5, children's drawings demonstrate conventional symbols such

as a big circle for a cat's body, a small circle for its head and triangles for its ears. Parents can help their children to develop this symbolism by talking about how to draw (e.g., *"to draw a cat, we make a big circle for the body, a small circle for the head and triangles for the ears"*). Talking first and then drawing makes this task auditory and drawing provides the child with visual symbolic representation.

In this stage, children learn best by doing. Encouraging interaction with books, people, games, and objects stimulates perspective and the development of symbolic thought. Encouraging children to ask questions helps them to understand that they can acquire information through the minds of others. Sometimes this is acquired readily by a model from the parent when he or she poses a question to the practitioner. Often, the practitioner will pause expressing a *thoughtful look* and think about a response. Subsequently, the child may follow the parent's lead and repeat the question. Asking questions may require scaffolding (e.g., *"if you don't know how this game works, you can ask: **how** do you play?"*; *"if you don't know what this word means, you can ask: what does_____ mean?"*) and, once again, waiting for the child to ask unassisted to acquire the information. The strategy of waiting is encouraged across the entire Auditory-Verbal journey to give the child time to process the received information and formulate a response.

Concrete Operational Stage

Children are less egocentric during the **Concrete Operational** stage between the ages of 7 and 11 years. A discussion of this stage is offered simply as a continuum, since most children in AVT and their families have "graduated" by this time. This stage is marked by more logical and methodical manipulation of symbols. The main goal is for the child to start working things out mentally "in his or her head." This is referred to as operational thought and enables the ability to solve problems without physically encountering objects (Marcin, 2018). To apply this stage to cognitive and language development, the parents and the child's teachers would: focus on open-ended questions; use riddles and brain teasers to foster analytical thinking; have hypothetical "what if?" conversations; design experiments and hypothesize on the outcomes (Marcin, 2018).

Formal Operations

The stage of formal operations, the summit of Piaget's stages of development, includes the ability to think abstractly, discuss a hypothesis, and apply reason to it (synthesis) (Siegler et al., 2011). To apply this stage to cognitive and language development, the adults offer step-by-step explanations of concepts. It is suggested that charts and visual aids are useful at this stage too (Marcin, 2018).

The practitioner, who is likely playing a consultative role at this late stage, may encourage parents and teachers to explore hypothetical situations that can be related to current events or social issues.

Piaget's stages have been criticized for underestimating the abilities of children at different ages. However, a major implication regarding teaching children that is relevant for AVT is that all the adults in the child's life need to be cognizant of distinctive ways of thinking at various ages and apply strategies that best suit those stages (Siegler et al., 2011).

Vygotsky's Zone of Proximal Development

Another significant contributor to cognitive theory is Lev **Vygotsky**. People use language primarily to share information, thoughts, and feelings with others, and Vygotsky believed that children's thinking and their ability to make meaning is socially constructed and emerges out of their social interactions and their environment (Vygotsky, 1978). Duncan, Kelly, and Hooper (2005) presented on *"Giving new meaning to the 'V' in AV: Vygotsky"* by forwarding the idea that *"ideally in daily practice, Auditory-Verbal practitioners work within a theory of human learning and development."*

In order to understand Vygotsky's theories/constructs, it is necessary to understand that Vygotsky considered language to be the driver of cognitive development, with language being the interface between children's thinking and social environments (Owens, in Duncan, Kelly, & Hooper, 2005). Children's learning is facilitated by interacting with other children, parents, and educators (Kaufman, 2004) and thus this social interaction theory can be used as a framework in AVT sessions to serve as a guide in coaching, goal setting, and decision making in the moment. Vygotsky's constructs can form the backbone of an AVT session and an entire AVT treatment plan (see Chapter 17).

The **Zone of Proximal Development (ZPD)** is the distance between a learner's actual developmental level and his or her potential developmental level that can be achieved with the help of a competent adult (Carr, 2006). The ZPD is fundamental to the AVT session outlined in Principle 7: *Guide and coach parents to use natural developmental patterns of audition speech, language, cognition and communication* (see Chapter 1). During AVT sessions, the practitioner and parent jointly observe and evaluate a child's current abilities to identify the next developmental step that the child is capable of achieving (see Chapter 17). As the adults adjust their level of input according to the child's abilities, **scaffolding** takes place (see Chapters 15, 17). Scaffolding provides support to progress to a new developmental level through direction, guidance, demonstration, explanation, modeling, and providing feedback (Kaufman, 2004). Scaffolding occurs in the AV session when the practitioner/parent completes the initial part of a sequence of actions, subsequently enabling the child to complete the action. After several repetitions, the practitioner or parent reduces the amount of input, and the child can carry out more of the sequence each time, until independence is achieved (see Chapter 15).

Scaffolding can be used in play development, language development, phonological awareness, and any number of aspects of AVT. Listening, however, underpins the development in all of these and auditory scaffolding stimulates such development. For example, if the adults were to scaffold the expression of a new word such as "pour," they would: *talk ahead*—telling the child about pouring before he or she sees the action; *use acoustic highlighting "poooouuuur"* to provide more acoustic properties; *model "pouuuur,"* then *wait* while pointing to the jug. This may prompt the child to use the new word in an appropriate context.

Practitioners identify a child's ZPD, and subsequently plan, deliver, and evaluate meaningful learning tasks, rich in listening and language learning, and coach parents to scaffold for the child to move to the next developmental stage (see Chapter 17).

As children mature, *internal scaffolding* develops. This refers to children's ability to self-monitor in order to take responsibility for what they are learning (Kaufman, 2004). Internal scaffolding relates to metacognition (the understanding of one's own thinking) and metalinguistic awareness (the ability to talk about, analyze, and think about language) (Bjorklund & Causey, 2018; Duncan et al., 2005).

The practitioner facilitates internal scaffolding/self-talk by coaching parents to help their children to indicate when they have not understood something, express what they have not understood in spoken language, and become aware of how they may facilitate their own learning (see Chapter 15). For example, if it is evident that a child doesn't understand a word in an instruction such as *"trace your hand on the page,"* the practitioner/parent may provide the child with the necessary steps for finding the information required (e.g., *"if you don't understand what trace means, you can ask. You could say: 'can you tell me what trace means?'"*). This further relates to cognitive ToM, which is discussed later in this chapter.

Duncan et al. (2005) applied Vygotskian theory to evidence-based practice in AVT through 10 steps. The components of each step are suggested as essential in providing intervention that has functional and diagnostic principles at its roots.

Applications of Vygotsky for the AV Practitioner in 10 Steps (Duncan et al., 2005)

Step I

Obtain comprehensive child/student/family information.

The practitioner does this by taking a case history. Some practitioners may surmise an indication of the child's ZPD from information obtained by phone prior to the initial consultation. This helps in the planning and delivery of the initial AVT sessions (see Chapter 17).

Step II

Observe the child in a variety of communicative contexts.

Information regarding communication at home/daycare/education settings, etc. can provide a more holistic view of the child and the family.

Step III

Conduct the first AVT session to establish baseline of contextualized functional communication.

Obtain diagnostic information about a child's audition, receptive and expressive communication, thinking and problem solving, pragmatics/social skills, speech and sensory and motor development.

Step IV

Complete qualitative data analysis.

Detailed observations provide the platform for goal setting and for establishing the most efficient and effective coaching strategies.

Step V

Complete standardized assessment.

Standardized language assessment informs the practitioner about the child's language age compared with chronological age and can signal *red flags* early.

Step VI

Establish Zone of Proximal Development (basal and ceiling) and use this information to set goals.

The child's ZPD is obtained from the qualitative data and the assessment so that goals can be set with parents.

Step VII

Plan the AVT session based on the short-term objectives established in tandem with the ZPD and the Auditory-Verbal treatment plan (see Chapter 17).

Step VIII

Plan, deliver, and evaluate the AVT session by using scaffolding, as stated above, and a number of other evidence-based strategies for listening, talking, and thinking that are appropriate for the child's Zone of Proximal Development (see Chapters 15, 16, 17).

Step IX

Modify the AVT session based on ongoing diagnostic observations of the child's behavior.

Step X

Repeat the cycle as often as required.

This process using Vygotsky's model promotes an evidence-based structure for all AVT sessions and the AV treatment plan in its entirety (see Chapter 17).

INFORMATION-PROCESSING APPROACH (IPA) AND AVT

Another model of cognition is the information-processing approach (IPA). The IPA is described by a computer metaphor, looking at the processes that occur between input and output in order to solve problems (Carr, 2006). The input is the information that the child receives from his or her senses, and the output is the expressive language or how the child acts upon the information received. Siegler (2011) discusses how memory is crucial to everything we do as human beings. The skills that we employ to engage in any task, the language that we use when speaking or writing, and our feelings in relation to a specific situation all depend on learning acquired from past experience and are reliant on memory. Each AVT session comprises skills, language, feelings, and learning and each one is memory dependent.

The key components of memory relating to the IPA are as follows:

1. **Sensory memory**, where visual/auditory/tactile or other sensory information is retained for less than a second. The information is then either identified and moved to working memory or it is lost. The brain recruits different areas according to the sensory modality that is being activated. For example, the visual cortex is active in memory for what is seen, and the auditory cortex is activated for memory of what is heard (Siegler et al., 2011). Providing children in AVT with increased auditory input early on is, therefore, fundamental in the development of the auditory cortex.

2. **Short-term memory**, where data is retained for a few seconds.

3. **Working memory**, where information from short-term memory is processed using strategies including rehearsal, organization, and elaboration (for more information, see the section "Executive Functioning").

4. **Long-term memory** and automatization.

5. **Retrieval**.

Information-processing capacity develops with age. In a study conducted by Davidson et al. (2019), children with cochlear implants scored significantly lower than children with normal hearing on assessment of working memory, after accounting for mother's age and education. There were clearer differences between the groups for verbal working memory compared with visual spatial working memory. One might consider how each of these components occur for a child when he or she is processing a new skill during an AVT session and this leads to the question: what do the AV practitioner and the parents need to do to promote age-appropriate development of the verbal working memory?

Two of the most common forms of memory strategies for children are *rehearsal and organization*. Bjorklund (2005, 2018) discusses how active *rehearsal* enables the ability to see relationships between items that one is attempting to remember. This leads to *clustering* (grouping items together), which positively impacts on the ability to recall them later. For example, when attempting to remember what one needs to buy at the grocery store, organizing the items by category will impact on recall (e.g., vegetables, fruits, beverages, cleaning products). Facilitating the ability to categorize during the AVT session provides the child with an organizational strategy that enables him or her to cluster items in the brain and influence short-term memory, long-term memory, and retrieval.

Automatization and strategy building particularly affect cognitive development. In the early stages of acquiring a new skill, much information processing is taken up with attention to individual components but with repetition and rehearsal, automaticity occurs, and spare capacity becomes available for developing strategies for further skills or refinement. For example, a child who has learned to ride a bicycle and no longer has to focus on pedaling has spare capacity to consider the route he or she may want to ride (Carr, 2006). This is useful in considering the activity provided during an AVT session. If an activity is cognitively challenging, the child may have more difficulty learning the associated language but once the activity is mastered, there will be more capacity available to learn the targeted vocabulary, grammar, or social language. For example, it may be difficult for a child at 2 years of age to equally divide six cupcakes between three people while learning to use the pronouns "*me* and *you*." Providing the child with one cupcake at a time may be less cognitively challenging and he or she can focus on using the language "*for you*" as the cupcake is handed over to someone.

Building *auditory memory* through rehearsal needs to be an important feature in AVT sessions, until the task becomes automatic for the child (for example, planning an activity and rehearsing the steps through listening): "*We are going to bake a cake. First, we are going to stir, then cook, then ice.*" In AVT, auditory memory also plays a starring role in the development of speech sounds. Even though, children in AVT today typically have very intelligible speech, they have learned the sounds of speech through a great deal of practice until the sounds of speech become automatic. Speech sounds need to be rehearsed to the level of automaticity in order to be used without having to think about those sounds (see Chapter 11).

Autobiographical memory is a particular type of long-term memory consisting of a special collection of memory scripts that focus on the self and identity (Carr, 2006). Fivush (2011) discusses the link between the development of *autobiographical memory* and the quality of conversation parents have when reminiscing with their children. From an information-processing perspective, the assistance with retrieval and rehearsal that parents provide impacts on the ability to form long-term memory. Autobiographical memory is strongly linked to ToM as it forms the basis of understanding one's own identity. It is also linked with social competence as it promotes the ability to share *personal event narratives* (Westby & Culatta, 2016). These are the narratives that recount the child's whereabouts, experiences, and feelings about those experiences. These narratives form much of the foundation of conversation and social interaction with others. These are the narratives adults use when meeting with a friend or chatting to a colleague over lunch. They consist of the stories of their weekends, holidays, day-to-day experiences: their lives. Developing the ability to share these types of narratives is therefore essential in developing children's language and especially conversational skills (See Chapter 11).

Judith Hudson (1990, cited in Bjorklund, 2005, p. 260) states that "remembering can be viewed as an activity that is at first jointly carried out by a parent and a child and later performed by the child alone." Many parents of children who are deaf or hard of hearing simplify their conversations in the early years in an attempt to help their children develop concepts and vocabulary that their children may need to learn in order to "catch up."

The practitioner's role in promoting autobiographical memory is to facilitate three-dimensional conversations between parents and children early on (see Chapter 11). Using photo albums, experience books, and children's literature in the early years is an excellent springboard into conversation for all children and in particular for children in an AVT session and at home (see Chapters 14 and 17). Enriched conversations include relating these to mental state terms, including those of affect (emotion words such as *sad, happy, excited*) and cognition (*thinking* words such as *remember, wonder, know*). For example, a parent and child are looking at a family picture of a trip to the zoo during an AVT session. The practitioner coaches the parent to say, "*remember when we went to the zoo, but we forgot the umbrella and it rained! You were cross because you were wet. I thought the umbrella was in my bag, but I left it at home. I decided to use a plastic bag to keep my hair dry. You thought that was funny.*" Parents may be coached in ways to re-enact some of these events to help younger children recall them. When the practitioner is willing to act these events out in the session, the parent is more at ease and will follow the model (e.g., putting an umbrella up inside, putting a plastic bag on his or her head and laughing at the humor of it all). Many scenarios such as this can promote the development of memory, mental states, and engaging conversations.

Problem Solving and AVT

Another aspect of information processing theory is the assumption that children are active problem solvers (Siegler et al., 2011). Problem solving always involves a goal, an obstacle that prevents the goal from being met, and a strategy to use for overcoming the obstacle and achieving the goal (Siegler et al., 2011). Problems that are presented in the children's ZPD can be very interesting, can promote interaction in order to reach a solution, and can achieve a number of short-term objectives quickly if they have high interest for the child and the parent.

To link the information processing approach with Piagetian theory, Piaget described the 1-year-old as "the child as a scientist" because at this stage he or she becomes actively engaged in how objects can be used. Sometimes, parents may consider it negative behavior if a child repeatedly drops toys or food on the floor. Piaget, however, saw this as active experimentation and created problems to see how the child could solve them (Siegler et al., 2011).

AVT sessions use problems from very early on in order to facilitate the strategy of "turning on the voice." For example, when a child drops a toy on the floor, the practitioner coaches the parent to say, "uh oh!" or "oh dear!" These *auditory hooks* indicate there is a problem. The practitioner models the language that is appropriate for the action and the parent follows by pointing to the toy and making sure the child is also focused on it. Then, they wait for the child to vocalize, indicate that he/she wants the toy, and then use words such as "up up up" *in synchrony with the movement* (see Chapter 15).

As children get older, problems start to become increasingly more interesting, particularly around the age of 18 months, when the practitioner helps the parent to help the child solve the problem. For example, as well as using an auditory hook to indicate the problem, the parents talk about the problem by saying, "*Uh oh!! It's wet. We need to dry.*" The practitioner coaches the parent to leave gaps such as "*uh oh, it's . . . we need to . . .*" *and then wait* to give the child time to think and to respond with language that he or she knows in order to understand the problem and find a solution.

Sabotage, the creation of a problem or the presentation of something out of the ordinary such as entering the therapy room to discover all the chairs are upside down, (outlined in depth in Chapter 16) is a highly valued and often-used strategy in AVT sessions. This strategy attracts the child's interest when he or she notices something is wrong, consequently, the child needs to communicate with someone in order to solve the problem (Rosenzweig, 2015). One of the earliest forms of sabotage is to ask a child to open a container that is too tight. A parent may scaffold the word "open!" for the child to request that another adult open it. As he or she matures, the scaffolding may change to the child using his or her own words, such as "help me" or "help me open."

For older children who demonstrate conversational competence, the practitioner and the parent may set up a scenario of a joint art project that might be done at school. The sabotage might include broken crayons, missing paint brushes, no scissors or other tools, or not enough information on what to do. This can yield language such as "*May I borrow your scissors, mine are broken?*" and/ or "*I am not sure what we have to do, can you explain?*" This also helps to promote and develop self-advocacy skills.

Another way practitioners and parents can follow Information-Processing Theory is by playing board games with the children. Siegler and Ramani (2008, 2009 in Siegler et al., 2011) demon-strated that playing board games such as "snakes and ladders" with preschoolers improved their numerical knowledge and ability to answer arithmetic problems. A child's numerical knowledge at the start of kindergarten predicts his or her academic achievement in mathematics throughout later school years (Duncan, Kelly, & Hooper, 2005; Stevenson & Neweman, 1996 in Siegler et al., 2011). Furthermore, board games stimulate the child's ability to rehearse and retrieve rules, and can have a big impact on language and auditory memory (e.g., "*if you land on a snake then you go down, if you land on a ladder, then you go up*"). Playing board games provides many problem-solving opportunities. For example, "There are four people but only two counters. What can you do?"

As previously discussed, information processing involves many active processes, including *encoding, storing,* and *rehearsing* information. As children actively problem solve, they stimulate thinking skills. In order to progress cognitively, they need to incrementally develop active thinking. However, sometimes inhibiting active thoughts is as important as activating them. *Inhibition* is crucial in the development of cognition and can be part of the active learning during an AVT session. In order to solve problems, therefore, children in AVT, like their hearing peers, need to demonstrate inhibition and cognitive flexibility, both components of executive functioning.

EXECUTIVE FUNCTIONING AND AVT

Executive Functioning (EF) is an essential factor in examining and developing cognition, and hence, an important understanding in order to plan, deliver, and evaluate an AVT session. Executive functions are the basic cognitive processes that control thought and actions, feelings, and behaviors (Benedek, 2014). The National Scientific Council on the Developing Child describes EF as the "air traffic control system" that controls, filters distractions, prioritizes tasks, sets and achieves goals, and inhibits thoughts. Tests measuring different types of EF abilities indicate that these begin to develop shortly after a child is born and that the ages of 3 to 5 are a window of opportunity for their most effective development (Center on the Developing Child, 2012). Practitioners who work with families of children this age will benefit greatly from understanding the development of these skills. EF is considered a determining factor in quality of life, school, math, reading competence, and job success (Davies et al., 2010, Morrison et al., 2013, Bailey, 2007 in Diamond, 2013).

EF is typically understood to consist of the following components (Diamond, 2013): cognitive flexibility; working memory, and inhibition control. Children are not born with these abilities, but they are born with the potential to develop them. Researchers have found that children's early experiences and environments shape their *brain architecture*, the very foundation of how their brain is going to function. Furthermore, early experience and environments affect whether genes activate, which results in ongoing brain behaviors. If children do not receive what they need from their environments and their relationships with adults, or if there is toxic stress received, their development can be adversely affected (Center on the Developing Child at

Harvard University, 2017) (see Chapter 24). Toxic stress results from major, frequent, and/or ongoing adversity and usually occurs when there is inadequate support from the adults around a child (Fickenscher, 2019). Repeated activation of the brain's fight or flight response can deplete it from the energy it requires to make healthy neural connections.

The Center on the Developing Child at Harvard University points to Three Core Principles to improve outcomes for children and their families: (1) Support responsive relationships; (2) Reduce sources of stress; (3) Strengthen core life skills. The critical factors in developing a strong basis for the development of EF are children's relationships and their living, learning, and playing environments. The practitioner can influence all of these factors.

Supporting relationships is critical to developing brain architecture, creating neural connections, and laying a strong foundation for learning (Hearing First, 2016). A major building block for this is the principle of "serve and return," the back and forth communication between a young child and adult. Hearing First (2016) provides a useful article developing serve and return experiences for children with hearing loss. Practitioners can guide and coach parents to: recognize when their child is "serving" communication through movement, gesture, and speech and expand on the child's communication, providing pausing and waiting and expectant looks to facilitate a return.

Regarding relationships, children are more likely to develop effective EF if their caregivers:

- Model the skills the child is required to carry out.

- Support children's efforts.
- Engage in activities where they can practice their skills.
- Ensure a constant reliable presence.
- Guide them from relying on the adult to relying on the self.
- Protect them from stress (Center on the Developing Child, 2012).

Once again, The Center on the Developing Child (2017) suggests factors to facilitate stress reduction for families. These are applicable to the LSLS Auditory Verbal Therapy program:

- Provide therapy in well-regulated, friendly environments that reduce stress for parents and children.
- Guide, coach, and support parents in developing a stable home environment with consistent and predictable routines.
- Ask about major stressors affecting the family as part of the assessment process and check in on a regular basis.
- Provide practitioners with support to manage their caseload/workload, ensure responsive supervision and mentoring, opportunities to debrief, and skill development, so they can manage their own stress in order to provide the best service to families.

A child's "work" is play and by developing meaningful play that is stress free and facilitates "serve and return," the practitioner is strengthening brain architecture and therefore EF ability (see Chapter 12). The practitioner plays an important role in guiding and coaching parents to foster these skills particularly by modeling, supporting their efforts and providing age-appropriate activities. By demonstrating activities that can easily fit into the child's home environment, the practitioner affects the environment and helps the parent in developing the child's self-reliance and independence (e.g., an AVT session around making the child's own snack and then washing his or her hands is natural and fits into a number of environments). The components of EF are further discussed below with specific reference to AVT.

Cognitive Flexibility

This involves mentally shifting from one task to another or from one set of rules to another. In an AVT session for example, a child and the adults are playing a game when someone knocks on the door. The practitioner observes whether the child can shift his or her attention attention to talk to the person at the door and then return to the game. As the child matures, he or she needs to develop greater cognitive flexibility (e.g., tolerate a new rule that is introduced halfway through the game).

Working Memory

This involves the amount of information that one can hold in short-term memory and the ability to manipulate this information to solve problems. Working memory could be considered a kind of mental notepad that stores information for everyday activities such as remembering what to buy at the store and following directions and instructions

(Gathercole, 2008). Working memory comprises many different interacting subsystems, including verbal memory and visuospatial memory material, and an attentional component that controls activity within working memory (Baddeley, 2000).

Poor working memory skills occur fairly frequently in childhood and have a significant impact on children's development and learning (Gathercole, 2008). As mentioned in the cited research on information processing, children with cochlear implants performed less well on working memory tasks than children with typical hearing.

Updating forms part of working memory. This is the ability to use working memory to control attention. For example, during an AVT session, at home, or in preschool (see Chapter 20), if a child is drawing a picture of a man, he or she may check back on another picture to see if his or hers looks like a person. Working memory is used to hold information in the mind when working out a math problem mentally. For example, when children are playing soccer and counting the goals, they are required to tally up the score mentally after a few minutes of play.

Considering how working memory difficulty may be manifested in the classroom, consider the following example of Matthew, who is nearing graduation (discharge) from AVT. He has had bilateral cochlear implants since the age of 1 year and has age-appropriate language on the assessments in AVT. At school, however, he is struggling with many classroom activities. He often fails to follow instructions such as "*Put your books on the shelf, pencils in the box and sit on the floor for story time.*" Typically, Matthew only completes the initial part of the instruction and then doesn't proceed any further. His peers are learning to add two numbers together in their minds, but Matthew is finding this task very difficult. His teacher thinks that he cannot hear the instructions, she says he has a short attention span and is easily distracted by other children. He often repeats steps/words in a sequence (such as rehearsing the months of the year) or leaves something out completely, like writing his name at the top of a page, something the children are required to do often.

Working memory is generally useful and flexible, but information held in working memory can be easily lost through distraction or overload (Gathercole, 2008). For Matthew, too much background noise and classroom activity overloads his capacity to remember, even though he may have initially heard the instruction. One of the ways that his teacher can enhance his working memory is by using the strategy of auditory closure. For example, she might say, "*Put your books on the_____, pencils in the_____, and come and sit on the_____.*" Another effective strategy is to ask him to repeat the instructions.

Gathercole (2008) reports that many studies regarding working memory indicate that children with problems in this domain are rarely described by their teachers as having memory problems; instead, they typically report the children as having problems with attention and listening, seeming to "zone out." This is important to consider when working with children in AVT as challenges with memory might not be considered but assumed to be characteristic of hearing loss. What may occur for these children is that they have listened to and heard incoming information, but their working memory becomes so overloaded that it is no longer able to store the information required to complete the activity. If a child with good auditory access displays difficulties such as Matthew, assessing EF through a referral to an occupational therapist or educational psychologist may help in fostering his working memory.

Gathercole (2008) also cites the following red flags concerning children with working memory challenges:

- Normal social relationships with peers but reserved in group activities.
- Poor progress in literacy and math.
- Problems learning activities that require remembering as well as processing.
- Struggling to follow instructions.
- Difficulty keeping place ("starting where they left off").

Inhibition Control

Inhibition control concerns the extent to which one can suppress or regulate desires and inhibit a response to incoming sensory information. This is also used to focus attention. Difficulty with inhibition can be seen in the AVT session when a child is unable to supress a desire to play with a particular toy or talk about a particular topic. It is important that the child learns to do this within the context of the AVT session as it is fundamental to being accepted socially (e.g., suppressing the need to talk loudly at the cinema).

Holt (2019) asserts that inhibition control is essential for psychosocial de-

velopment and academic success and is interlinked with language development. Inhibiting attention to an incoming stimulus is particularly important when there is a degraded speech signal and a child must focus and attend carefully to the speech, such as a preschool teacher's voice, and ignore interfering background noise (Stenback et al., 2016 cited in Holt, 2019). Children who are deaf or hard of hearing, more than children with typical hearing, must depend on inhibition control when processing speech, even in quiet, as some of these children have degraded speech perception and less developed higher-level language skills (Castellanos, Kronenberger & Pisoni, 2018). Hence, in AVT sessions, the adults prepare children to face these challenges from early on. Hearing speech through appropriate hearing technology (see Chapters 4–8) and using spoken language help children in AVT to develop executive functions to attend to, concentrate on, and process temporally unfolding signals in working memory, and to use self-talk to regulate behavior and emotional stability (Alderson-Day & Fernyhough, 2015; Conway et al., 2009 cited in Holt, 2019).

A number of studies have indicated that children with hearing loss have increased risk of weak EF. Most of these studies indicate that language and EF are inextricably related, and therefore delayed language due to hearing loss could impact cognition. Beer et al. (2014), who conducted the first study on executive and organizational-integrative processes (listed above), showed that preschoolers with cochlear implants showed significantly poorer performance on inhibition control, concentration, and working memory than their peers with typical hearing.

The authors suggest that the development of EF processes may be impacted by a period of auditory deprivation, followed by initial degraded auditory input through cochlear implants, placing children with hearing loss at risk.

This discussion suggests that EF needs to be explicitly examined by the practitioner. The Center on the Developing Child at Harvard University (https://developingchild.harvard.edu) provides a detailed resource on understanding and providing activities for EF in young children. This resource and a chart entitled *"Hierarchy of Social/ Pragmatic Skills as Related to the Development of Executive Function"* (https:// nyspta.org/wp-content/uploads/2017 /08/Conv17-305-Executive-Functions -Hierarchy-Handout-Peters.pdf) created by Kimberly Peters, PhD, LSLS Cert AVT, were used to devise Table 13–2. The table discusses the developmental stages of EF and the activities the practitioner can incorporate in the early years to facilitate development of EF.

THEORY OF MIND (TOM) AND AVT

Theory of Mind (ToM) is discussed in greater detail, primarily in Chapter 12 on the topic of Play in AVT. It is important here as well, because ToM is directly related to AVT in general. The broad definition of "Theory of Mind" is the ability to understand that others have thoughts, feelings, and perspectives that differ from one's own. Increasing research indicates that ToM is delayed in children who are deaf or hard of hearing (of hearing parents) with *delayed language development* regardless of communication approach (Peterson & Siegal, 2000, 2006; Figueras-Costa & Harris, 2001; Woolfe, Want, & Siegal, 2002; Peterson, 2009; Peterson & Wellman, 2013).

The key words here are *delayed language*. Controlled comparisons carried out by Moeller and Schick (2006) indicated that mothers who hear talk *less* about mental states with their children who are deaf or hard of hearing than they do with their children who hear 90% of the language that children learn through overhearing (Cole & Flexer, 2011), meaning that children who are deaf or hard of hearing are at a disadvantage for *hearing* about the feelings and thoughts of others when conversations are not directed at them. Limited access to conversations with others as a result of hearing loss influences the development of ToM skills (Wellman, 2014). Often, hearing technology does not permit the overhearing of arguments and disputes, particularly in school, because of noise and distance. Overhearing encourages the development of ToM, in that the child can perceive and try to understand two or more differing perspectives.

Westby and Robinson (2014) made an important distinction between cognitive and affective ToM that is summarized in Table 13–3.

A review of the literature by Tyskiewicz and Clark (2016) indicated that the underpinnings of ToM include: social interaction with siblings and familiar peers; social play; exposure to mental state language and "mind mindedness"—the way in which the parent is mentally attuned to his or her child's feelings or thoughts. These factors will be briefly discussed to establish

Table 13–2. Developmental Stages of EF and Activities for Facilitation

Age	EF Development/Tasks Requiring EF	Strategies for Developing EF
0–3 months	Behavior designed to meet immediate needs Cognitive flexibility not emerged	• Face to face interaction
3–6 months	Turn taking develops through "vocal volley" and imitating facial expression	• Vocal turn-taking with care-providers • Facial expressions: tongue protrusion, "oh," raspberries. • From three months show baby faces in a board book to develop attention
6–9 months	Early inhibitory control emerges; basic response to inhibition (able to refrain from touching something told not to touch) Joint attention; tolerates longer delays and still maintains simple, focused attention **Working memory**; remembers that hidden objects are still there (e.g., toy hidden under a cloth); learns to sequence two actions (e.g., remove cloth, grab toy)	• Play peek-a-boo with baby faces book, toys and people • Partially hide objects for baby to find • Completely hide objects or remove them so baby can track where they went • Draw attention to pictures in books such as faces and acting upon them (e.g., touching them)
9–12 months	**Inhibitory control:** inhibits reaching immediately for a visible but inaccessible reward (e.g., a toy on the other side of the window.) Delays a moment to reach around the barrier. **Working memory:** can look in one place and act on another (e.g., look at mother while reaching for a toy)	• Singing/finger plays/nursery rhymes—learn to practice the sequence of the songs and match listening to the physical action • Routines such as patty-cake and "this little piggy" • Lap games such as routines and nursery rhymes stimulate working memory and have particular sequences and rules the child learns to follow • Stack blocks and wait to knock them down • Wave goodbye when someone leaves

Age		
	Cognitive flexibility: develops different methods to retrieve objects beyond reaching for what is directly in view Understands step of communication for action (e.g., can use gestures and words before crying)	• Push toys/food away; shakes head for "no" (modeling saying "no" and shaking your head) • Model how to play with objects (e.g., feed a picture of baby with a spoon) (introduces the concept of using symbols for real objects) • Joint attention activities—pointing to and commenting on what the child is looking at; (this increases the child's ability to maintain attention to the object, develops memory for what is said, and maps words onto objects and actions.
12–18 months	Can inhibit certain behaviors Can change responses according to a change in the environment Some self-monitoring and emerging ability to identify errors Impulsive behaviors reflect immature attentional system, distractibility, and undeveloped inhibitory control	• Model single words for age-appropriate functions (e.g., "more" "open") • Play routines (play with a doll, pretend to talk on the phone, push trucks). Add a step to child's play sequence (e.g., if child feeds doll over and over again. Show them how you can feed doll and then wipe its mouth.) • Put toys out of reach but in sight for child to request with voice • Make objects/toys/food "wait" so child can see them but can inhibit need to have them immediately • Hide object without showing the child where you hid it (he or she will develop working memory of searched locations)

continues

471

Table 13–2. continued

Age	EF Development/Tasks Requiring EF	Strategies for Developing EF
18–24 months	Can inhibit certain behaviors and shift to new response sets Some self-monitoring and inconsistent early ability to identify errors Impulsive behaviors reflect immature attentional system, distractibility, and undeveloped inhibitory control Begins to identify correct vs. incorrect block constructions (compared to designs) but unable to "fix" incorrect version.	• Songs with sequenced actions such as "Heads Shoulders Knees and Toes" or "Wind the Bobbin Up" • Alert child to problems (e.g., "uh oh its broken")
24–30 months	Demonstrates knowledge of rules but unable to shift or alter behaviors; demonstrates perseveration Begins to use language to regulate behavior Able to keep verbal rules in mind Can follow verbal directions Better problem solving as language continues to develop	• Target emotion words for emotional regulation • Use imaginative language (think, feel, wonder) • Tease ("that's silly")—important for regulation • Problem solve (things are wet, broken, dirty—how do you solve the problem?) • Sort and match toys according to categories (e.g., all the square things, all the things that have wheels)
30–36 months	Most choices made by chance Unable to delay gratification but emerges near 36 months: less impulsive and more flexible **Working memory:** can hold two rules in mind simultaneously and act according to these rules (e.g., "red goes here, yellow goes here") Acts in light of a conscious plan	• Games that require active inhibition (e.g., musical statues where children have to "freeze") • Song games that require the child to start and stop, or slow down and speed up (e.g.) Jack in the Box; Popcorn or Ring Around the Rosie

36–42 months	Increased attention, self-control, concentration, and inhibition, but not mature Gradual decline in impulsivity, although still present Occasional perseverative behavior Incremental improvements in verbal fluency Gradual improvements in processing speed and accuracy on impulse control tasks Demonstrate knowledge of rules and emerging ability to shift behaviors, but only for one rule necessary for task success	• "What's missing" game with 3+ items • Give at least two tasks before child has game he or she wants to play (e.g., "first we will read a story, then draw a picture and then you can play football") • Elaborate conversations ("tell me about what happened at school today"—may need to model this type of conversation) • Retell simple stories/developing chain narratives • Games that have differing rules such as "snakes and ladders"
42–48 months	Runs simple errands ("get your shoes from the bedroom") Tidies bedroom with some assistance Performs simple chores and self-help tasks with reminders Inhibits behaviors (don't run in the street, don't hit your friend, etc.)	• Retell simple stories or sequences (such as how to brush teeth) in correct order • Sequence three to four pictures and then describe the events • Determine which "step" is missing in a three- to four-step event ("What comes next?" "What do you do before you cut the sandwich?") • Report to parent what happened in therapy/school/activity (child needs support for this—experience book) • Predict what comes next in a story • Self-talk (e.g., rehearse a shopping list or how to complete a task • Attention through quieter activities such as jigsaw puzzles or, connect the dots

continues

Table 13–2. *continued*

Age	EF Development/Tasks Requiring EF	Strategies for Developing EF
48–60 months	Can process 2- to 3-step units of information (48 mo.) and 4-step units of information (60 mo)	• Change the rules of a game half way through
	Begins to demonstrate ability to shift and flex between two simple task requirements, but continue to have difficulty when response sets increase in complexity	• Songs/word games that repeat and add on words (e.g., "I went to the market and I bought an apple. I went to the market and I bought an apple and a sausage . . .")
	Begins to have more successful task completion due to increase in mental flexibility and rapid switching between two simple response sets	• Cook to practice inhibition when waiting for instructions
	Begins to make more advantageous choices	• Enhance working memory while holding complicated directions in mind and focus attention when measuring and counting
	Generates new concepts and ideas	
	Response speed and verbal fluency improve	
	Inhibitory control: reduced perseveration (persistence of a rule/idea even when the rules change, or game has shifted)	
	Can delay eating a treat	
	Working memory: understands that appearance does not always equal reality (e.g., an eraser that looks like candy is not edible.)	
	Cognitive flexibility: Can shift actions according to changing rules (e.g., takes shoes off at home, leaves shoes on at school, puts sports shoes on during sports lessons)	

Table 13-3. Distinction Between Cognitive and Affective ToM

	Interpersonal (relationships between people)	**Intrapersonal (relationship and understanding of oneself)**

Cognitive Theory of Mind	• Understand that others can have thoughts, feelings, and desires differing to one's own.
	
	• Abilities:
	  ○ to make inferences and draw conclusions about the mental states of others.
	  ○ to assume behavior based on thoughts (e.g., infer that someone who needs a spoon is going toward the drawer because they think the spoons will be found inside).
		Awareness of one's own thoughts, feelings, and desires
		
		Ability to plan one's own behavior
		
		Use metacognitive learning strategies (thinking about thinking and learning)
		
		Relate to Vygotsky's *self-talk*.

Affective Theory of Mind	• Abilities:
	  ○ to identify the emotions of others
	  ○ to infer the feelings of others.
	  ○ to make inferences and draw conclusions about the feelings of others.
	  ○ to have empathy for others.
		Awareness of one's own feelings/emotions
		
		Ability to control one's own emotions that are appropriate to a specific situation.

strategies that the practitioner can use to guide and coach parents to help develop their child's ToM.

Ages 0 to 12 Months

Parenting behaviors during the first year of life that are associated with later ToM abilities include the following (Assmusen et al., 2018):

Joint attention commenting: joining in attention about what the child is seeing and talking about and how he or she thinks or feels with reference to his or her internal states. In an AVT session, the practitioner might coach the parent to follow the child's line of vision, comment on it, and then comment on his or her emotional reaction to it (e.g., if the child is looking at a jumping toy and laughing, the parent may say *"it's jumping . . . that's funny!"*).

Mindful facilitation: engaging a child's attention in activities he/she finds interesting and sustaining the interest. By working in a child's Zone of Proximal Development as discussed earlier, the practitioner and the parent find activities suitable to the child's developmental level of interest. The practitioner coaches the parent to capture the child's attention through auditory highlighting and auditory hooks. *Problems* become particularly interesting when a child is about 18 months of age. Using an auditory hook such as *"uh oh"* or *"oh no!"* gets his or her attention and draws them toward the problem and a solution—a springboard for conversation and the development of conversation. For a young child this could be that something is wet/dirty/broken. For an older child, this might be a social problem, such as there are not enough plates for everyone who wants cake.

Pacing: regulating the pace of the interaction so that the child is not over- or understimulated during the activity. The parent and practitioner can slow the activity down or "up the energy" depending on signals provided by the child. By discussing what the child needs with the parent, the practitioner facilitates the attunement between parent and child.

In Cejas and Quittener (2019), "An Intervention to Improve Parent-Child Interactions and Communication," the authors cite that observational studies showed that relative to mothers with hearing children, hearing mothers of children with hearing loss asserted more control in their verbal and non-verbal interactions (Quittner et al., 2007), they spent less time in coordinated joint attention with their child (Spencer & Waxman, 1995), and are less likely to respond appropriately to the child's emotional and behavioral cues (Swisher, 2000). These factors result in less secure attachment, difficulties with sustained attention and exerting behavioral control, and slower development of communicative competence (Bornstein, 2000; Bornstein et al., 1998, Lederberg & Prezbindowski, 2000). These factors relate to both EF, as discussed above, and ToM.

Affect catching: displaying attunement to the child's emotions by sharing positive or negative affect. The practitioner can facilitate this by commenting on a parent's natural instinct to do this and reinforcing the reasons why it is important for the child. For example, if a child accidentally hurts himself or herself during an AVT session, the parent's natural instinct is to acknowledge it and comfort the child. Affect catching involves labeling the emotions for the child, e.g., "you are really sore."

When 2-year-old Jack came for an AVT session with his mother, he wanted to have a cookie. His mother was adamant that he could have one, but only after the session.

She knew from experience that the sugar would overexcite him. Jack became angry and threw all the toys off the table. Jack's mother asked the practitioner if she should give in and provide Jack with a cookie, to save the session. The practitioner coached her to label Jack's emotions for him: *"I know you want a cookie. You can have one later. That makes you cross! You are really cross."*

Ages 12 to 24 Months

Research shows that, in the second year of life, mental state conversations primarily involve people's desires (Assmusen et al., 2018). At 18 to 24 months children begin to use "want" to describe their desires (Lahey, 1988 in MacIver-Lux et al., 2016). The practitioner coaches parents to facilitate the development of this for children, through modeling and scaffolding, and to use mental state terms such as *"you like that one."* For example, if everyone was choosing a cookie from a plate and the child reached for a particular cake, the parent might say *"mmm, you like that one."*

During an AVT session, one of the activities was a tea party. Grace, aged 20 months, who has a severe hearing loss and wears bilateral hearing aids, and her mother are playing. The practitioner coaches Grace's mother to talk about what she likes when choosing something to eat. She reaches into a tin and says, *"I like the sandwich,"* takes it and puts it on her plate. The practitioner then reached in and said, *"I like pie,"* taking a pie. Grace was then offered a choice and when she said

"cake," her mother scaffolded *"you can say, I **like** cake."*

Ages 24 to 36 Months

Studies indicate a relationship between parents' use of mental state terms and children's later ToM abilities (Tompkins et al., 2018). A longitudinal study that tracked children from 15 to 33 months found that maternal "mind speak" (use of mental state terms) during the early years was the most effective predictor of a child's use of mental state terms, therefore directly impacting cognitive ToM development. Quality supersedes quantity. "Causal explanatory talk" about what is happening in the mind has the most influence on kindergarten children's ToM development. Causal explanatory talk relating to cognitive ToM includes the subjectivity of mental states and includes the *reason* behind these, e.g., "I didn't *know* because you didn't tell me" "I'm *guessing* it's a . . . because . . ." "I don't *understand* because . . ." To facilitate ToM Development, the practitioner models for parents, then coaches them to:

- use mental state terms pertaining to thoughts (e.g., *"I have an idea . . ." "I think . . ." "I wonder. . . ." "I know . . ." "I understand" "I forgot"* (e.g., *"I forgot how to play this game"*)
- encourage the use of these terms by their child, so that *self-talk* begins to develop (e.g., *"do you remember? If you don't remember you can say, I forgot!"*)
- use causal explanatory talk—providing both *mental state*

terms and the *reasons* for them (e.g., *"I was happy because I won a prize!"*)

- provide explanations about events and relate to stories including a number of conversational turns pertaining to the explanations linked to ToM development (e.g., *"Baby bear was crying because he was sad," "He was sad because his chair was broken," "Mummy, when are you sad?"*)

Parents play the key role in developing ToM from both an affective and a cognitive perspective and the practitioner can be a facilitator of the attunement between the parent and the child.

PSYCHOMETRIC APPROACH

The psychometric study of intelligence started when Binet attempted to develop a method of testing children's abilities in order to inform educational settings (Deary, 2000 in Carr, 2006). Assessments were devised and normative data were used to assign *mental ages* to children. One of Binet's valuable insights was that the most useful way to assess intelligence is to view people's actions on tasks that require a number of different intellectual skills such as memory, problem-solving, language comprehension, and spatial reasoning. Modern intelligence tests provide information on all of these skills as well as other aspects of intelligence (Siegler et al., 2011).

Wechsler moved away from the idea of "mental age" by defining an IQ of 100 as the mean score of the standardization sample at any age. For the purposes of

this chapter, the author mentions psychometric conception/testing to support referrals to clinical or educational psychologists for a measure of non-verbal IQ. The Stanford-Binet intelligence test and the Weschler intelligence scales are the most widely used measures for preschoolers, children, and adults. When referring a child to an educational psychologist for a cognitive assessment, it is useful to know that the Wechsler test measures five domains: *Verbal Comprehension*; *Visual spatial*; *Fluid reasoning*; *Working memory*; *Processing speech* (Wechsler, 2012).

ETIOLOGY, RED FLAGS, CONSIDERATIONS FOR AVT

Essential to examining cognition is the consideration of what may be affecting it. This leads to a brief discussion about: etiology of hearing loss and how etiology may be linked to cognition; some *red flags*, and some considerations for AVT sessions and the AVT plan (see Chapter 17).

Estimates indicate that 25 to 40%, or more, of children who are deaf or hard of hearing have additional challenges that may be evident at birth or develop over time (Hitchins & Hogan, 2018) (see Chapter 22). Some of the major causes of deafness also affect cognition. It is important for practitioners to be aware of the key patterns present in these etiologies in order to address them during therapy and to make appropriate referrals to other key professionals in the multidisciplinary team.

Meningitis and septicemia can cause brain injury and consequently affect the ability to use and develop cognitive skills including attention, memory, concentration, reasoning, and problem solving. Owing to localization of mental functions in different parts of the brain, some but not necessarily all of these skills may be impacted. Given that the brain develops throughout life, these difficulties may not be evident immediately after the illness. Children generally retain skills that were developed prior to this but may develop other challenges later on (Meningitis Now, 2017).

Congenital Cytomegalovirus

Congenital cytomegalovirus (cCMV) infection during pregnancy has been recognized as a cause of sensorineural hearing loss (SNHL) in children for a significant period of time. Congenital CMV presents with many associated difficulties, however, and an understanding of these is essential for the practitioner (Hogan et al., 2015).

Cognitive difficulties relating to CMV include (Inscoe & Nikolopoulos, 2004; Inscoe, 2009):

- *dyscalculia* (difficulty with number sense, memory pertaining to numbers, accurate and fluent calculation and number reasoning) (American Psychiatric Association, 2013)
- *dyslexia* (difficulty with letter sense, memory pertaining to letters shapes and fluency with reading and writing) (Siegler et al., 2011)
- sequencing difficulties (particularly grasping time concepts)

Incorporating numeracy and literacy concepts in AVT sessions including reading

and writing of numbers and letters may indicate signs of dyscalculia and dyslexia. Again, an effective collaboration with an educational psychologist will benefit the child and his or her family.

Seventy percent of children who are deaf or hard of hearing also exhibit sensory difficulties (Bharadwaj, Matzke & Daniel, 2012; Rhoades, 2001). Sensory difficulties particularly affect children who have had a history of CMV and meningitis. Sensory integration therapy provides sensory, motor, and problem-solving opportunities which can have an impact on the brain's ability to process information. This provides a foundation for learning and cognitive development (Schaaf & Mailloux, 2015). Effective referral and liaison with a Sensory Integration practitioner is therefore another important collaboration when supporting a child through AVT (Estabrooks et al., 2016).

Red Flags

Cognitive *red flags* have been discussed throughout this chapter. The practitioner's job is diagnostic in all developmental domains. With regard to cognition, the following factors need to be considered as cognitive *red flags* during the preschool years, according to the Leeds, Grenville, and Lanarck council (2007) in a published document for Red Flags in children. Red flags:

- Delayed language after Auditory-Verbal intervention.
- Slow to process auditory information.
- Slow to process visual information—slow to track objects, slow to follow a point/wave/gesture

- Slow to read social cues.
- Slow growth in vocabulary, particularly relating to concepts such as body parts, shapes, numbers.
- Poor attention span.
- Difficulty following directions.
- Difficulty following routines.
- Difficulty interacting with peers.
- Memory impairments (auditory and visual).
- Problem solving difficulties (planning, organizing and initiating tasks).

Cognitive challenges in school-age children are diagnosed by a psychologist who assesses: auditory and visual perceptual skills, processing speed, organization, memory (short- and long-term storage and retrieval), fine motor skills, gross motor skills, attention, abstractions (interpreting symbolism), and social interaction (Leeds et al., 2007).

The practitioner is usually not authorized to administer a standardized assessment of cognition. Standardized assessment is more sensitive than milestone case history taking and often age ranges relating to milestones are broad (Dosman et al., 2012).

Dosman et al. (2012) present a red flag milestone checklist with the published age limits and refers to gross motor, fine motor, speech and language, cognitive and social emotional skills. *The Integrated Scales of Development* published in Listen, Learn, and Talk (2003) outline typical stages of development regarding listening, language, speech, cognition, and pragmatics. The cognitive sections of these checklists are summarized in Table 13–4.

Table 13-4. Cognitive Checklist (Integrated Scales of Development, 2003; Dosman et al., 2012)

0–3 months	Turns to visual stimuli
	Shows preference for contrast (black and white)
	Shows preference for human faces, particularly eyes
	Looks at people and objects briefly
	Visually follows a horizontal arc
4–6 months	Explores the environment visually
	Visually interested in hands
	Searches room with eyes to find caregiver
	Recognizes familiar people
	Anticipates routine, e.g., starts sucking when bottle is being made up
	Brings objects toward mouth
	Bangs objects together
	Looks toward where objects have fallen on the floor

Table 13-4. *continued*

7–9 months	Imitates a physical action such as banging on the table
	Places objects in one hand and then the other hand
	Holds one object and takes another one
	Shows objects to adults
	Gives objects to adults
	Begins to point
	Shows developing object permanence develops
	Searches for hidden objects
	Pulls rings off a stick
10–12 months	Demonstrates trial and error of cause and effect toys (e.g., pushing a button to activate a mechanical toy)
	Looks for an object that's out of sight
13–15 months	Builds a tower with two blocks
	Uses objects functionally (e.g., a brush to brush their hair)
	Imitates adult action (e.g., kissing dolly)
	Removes lid to find toy or food in a container
16–18 months	Points to pictures in books
	Begins to turn pages
	Retrieves toys from behind an obstacle
19–24 months	Demonstrates symbolic play (e.g., using a toy broom to sweep the floor, feeding dolly)
	Imitates the order of nesting cups
	Uses two toys together (e.g., stirring with a spoon in a cup)
	Completes puzzle with pull out pieces
	Activates mechanical toys by pulling strings/pushing buttons.
25–30 months	Turns one page at a time when reading
	Connects two parts of a whole (e.g., a puzzle, a toy with two parts)
	Imitates vertical and horizontal lines
	Draws a circle
	Matches identical pictures and shapes
	Understands the number concepts of one and two

continues

Table 13-4. *continued*

31–36 months	Sorts and categorizes toys
	Names an object when part of it is show in a picture (e.g., names a car when the tire and door are shown)
	Adds two missing body parts to a drawing
	Develops an interest in drawing and writing (drawings begin to resemble the objects they represent)
	Pretends in symbolic play (e.g., uses a block to represent a car)
37–42 months	Correctly names familiar colors
	Understands the idea of same and different
	Begins size comparisons
	Pretends and fantasizes more creatively
	Remembers parts of a story and retell it
	Understands time (e.g., morning, afternoon, night)
	Counts, and understands the concept of counting
	Sorts and compares objects by shape and color
	Completes age-appropriate puzzles
	Recognizes and identifies common objects and pictures
43–48 months	Makes simple drawings (bodies, houses)
	Understands more time concepts (today, tomorrow, yesterday)
	Matches patterns
	Makes inferences
	Does self-talk in problem solving
	Understands use of objects

CONCLUSION

It is vital that Auditory-Verbal practitioners have a comprehensive understanding of cognitive development in order to provide a solid learning foundation for children who are deaf or hard of hearing. This chapter has examined cognition with regard to the major approaches in the field of psychology: Piaget, Vygotsky, Information-Processing Approach, and Psychometric testing. Viewing these approaches through the lens of the practitioner provides insight into their applications in the AV session and across the duration of the AV treatment plan. Auditory-Verbal Therapy provides a strong foundation for children who are deaf or hard of hearing and their families, by using developmental building blocks for listening, receptive language, spoken language, and cognition.

Since Executive Functioning and Theory of Mind further underpin a child's ability to learn, a sound knowledge of the development and potential red flags in these areas can help the practitioner to ensure that children are referred to appropriate professionals, so that any cognitive difficulties are diagnosed and treated as efficiently and effectively as possible, in tandem with the AV treatment plan. Vygotsky says, "*it is through thoughts that we develop into ourselves.*"

REFERENCES

American Psychiatric Association. (2013). *Diagnostic and statistical manual of mental disorders* (5th ed.). Washington, DC: American Psychiatric Association.

Assmusen, K., Law, J., Charlton, J., Acquah, D., Brims, D., Pote, I., & McBride, T. (2018). *Key competencies in early cognitive development: Things, people, numbers and words*. Early Intervention Foundation, Public Health England.

Baddeley, A. D. (2000). The episodic buffer: A new component of working memory? *Trends in Cognitive Sciences, 4*, 417–423.

Beer, J., Kronenberger, W. G., Castellanos, I., Colson, B. G., Henning, S. C., & Pisoni, D. B. (2014). Executive functioning skills in preschool-age children with cochlear implants. *Journal of Speech, Language, and Hearing Research, 57*, 1521–1534.

Benedek, M., Jauk, E., Sommer, M., Arendsy, M., & Neubauer, A. C. (2014). Intelligence, creativity, and cognitive control: The common and differential involvement of executive functions in intelligence and creativity. *Intelligence, 46*, 73–83.

Bharadwaj, S. V., Matzke, P. L., & Daniel, L. L. (2012). Multisensory processing in children with cochlear implants. *International Journal of Pediatric Otorhinolaryngology, 76*, 890–895.

Bjorklund, D. F. (2005). *Children's thinking, cognitive development and individual differences* (4th ed.). Wadsworth.

Bjorklund, D. F., & Causey, K. B. (2018). *Children's thinking, Cognitive development and individual differences* (6th ed.). London, UK: Sage Publications.

Bornstein, M. H. (2000). Infancy: Emotions and temperament. In A. E. Kazdin (Ed.), *The encyclopedia of psychology* (Vol. 2, pp. 278–284). New York, NY: American Psychological Association and Oxford University Press.

Bornstein, M. H., Haynes, M. O., & Painter, K. M. (1998). Sources of child vocabulary competence: A multivariate model. *Journal of Child Language, 25*(2), 367–393.

Carr, A. (2006). The *handbook of child and adolescent clinical psychology. A contextual approach*. London, UK and New York, NY: Routledge.

Castellanos, I., Kronenenberg, W., & Pisoni, D. (2018). Questionnaire-based assessment of executive functioning. *Psychometics Applied Neuropsychology: Child 7*(2), 93–109.

Cejas, I., & Quittner, A. L. (2019). PEARLS: An intervention to improve parent-child interactions and communication. *The impact of hearing loss on childhood development and family constellation*. Presented to the AG Bell Association Symposium, Madrid, Spain.

Center on the Developing Child. (2012). Executive function (In brief). Retrieved from http://www.developingchild.harvard.edu

Center on the Developing Child. (2017). Three principles to improve outcomes for children and families. Retrieved from http://www.developingchild.harvard.edu

Charman, T., Baron-Cohen, S., Swettenham, J., Baird, G., Cox, A., & Drew, A. (2000). Testing joint attention, imitation, and play as infancy precursors to language and theory of mind. *Cognitive Development, 15*(4), 481–498.

Cole, E., & Flexer, C. (2011). *Children with hearing loss developing listening and talking, birth to six.* San Diego, CA: Plural Publishing.

Davidson, L. S., Geers A. E., Hale, S., Sommers, M .M., Brenner C., & Spehar, B. (2019). Effects of early auditory deprivation on working memory and reasoning abilities in verbal and visuospatial domains for pediatric cochlear implant recipients. *Ear and Hearing, 40*(3), 517–528. doi: 10.1097/AUD.0000000000000629

Diamond, A. (2013). Executive functions. *Annual Review of Psychology, 64*, 135–168.

Dosman, C. F., Andrews, D., & Goulden, K. J. (2012). Evidence–based milestone ages as a framework for developmental surveillance. *Paediatrics & Child Health, 17*(10), 561–568. doi:10.1093/pch/17.10.561

Duncan, J., Kelly, A., & Hooper, K. (2005). *Giving new meaning to the "V" in AV: Vygotsky.* Canada Listens, Auditory-Verbal International Conference, Toronto, July 8–9, 2005.

Estabrooks, W. MacIver-Lux, K., Rhoades, E., & Lim, S. (2016). Auditory-verbal therapy: An overview. In W. Estabrooks, K. MacIver-Lux, & E. Rhoades (Eds.), *Auditory-verbal therapy for young children with hearing loss and their families, and the practitioners who guide them* (pp. 1–23). San Diego, CA: Plural Publishing.

Figueras-Costa, B., & Harris, P. (2001). Theory of mind development in deaf children: A nonverbal test of false-belief understanding. *Journal of Deaf studies and Deaf Education, 6*(2), 92–102.

Fivush, R., Habermas, T., Waters, T., & Zaman, W. (2011) The making of autobiographical memory: Intersections of culture, narratives and identity. *International Journal of Psychology, 46*(5), 321–345.

Fickenscher, S. (2019). *Resilience, breakthrough impacts on brain architecture.* Presented at AGBELL Symposium July 2019, Madrid, Spain.

Gathercole, S. E. (2008). Working memory in the classroom. *The Psychologist, 21,* 382–385.

Hearing First. (2016). LSLS strategies to support serve and return. Retrieved September 5, 2019 from: https://hearingfirst.org/-/media/Files/Downloadables/HF_ServeReturn_Checklist.pdf

Hitchins, A. R. C., & Hogan, S. C. (2018). Outcomes of early intervention for deaf children with additional needs following an auditory verbal approach to communication. *International Journal of Pediatric Otorhinolaryngology, 115,* 125–132.

Hogan, S., Shaw, L., Stokes, J., & White, C. (2015). *Congenital cytomegalovirus—more than hearing loss alone.* Presented at BCIG Conference March 2015, Bristol, UK.

Holt, R. F. (2019). *Family environment contributions to children's neurocognitive development.* Presented at AGBELL symposium 2019 Research Forum: The Impact of Childhood Development and Family Constellation.

Inscoe, J. M. R., & Nikolopoulos, T. P. (2004). Cochlear implantation in children deafened by cytomegalovirus: Speech perception and speech intelligibility outcomes. *Audiology and Neurotology, 25*(4), 479–482.

Inscoe, J. M. (2009). *CMV deaf children using cochlear implants-outcomes.* Oral presentation CMV study day Ear Foundation, Nottingham, UK .

Kaufman, D. (2004). Constructivist issues in language learning and teaching. *Annual Review of Applied Linguistics, 24,* 303–319. doi: 10.1017/S0267190504000121

Lederberg, A. R., & Prezbindowski, A. K. (2000). Impact of child deafness on mother-toddler interaction: Strengths and weaknesses. In P. E. Spencer, C. J. Erting, & M. Marschark (Eds.), *The deaf child in the family and at school: Essays in honor of Kathryn P. Meadow-Orlans* (pp. 73–92). Mahwah, NJ: Lawrence Erlbaum Associates Publishers.

Leeds, Grenville, and Lanarck Council. (2007). *Red flags: Early identification red flags—for children birth to six years.* Retrieved from http://healthcareathome.ca/south east/en/care/Documents/Red–Flags –Guide.pdf. Accessed on: 25 July 2019.

Listen, Learn, and Talk (2003). *Integrated scales of development.* Sydney, Australia: Cochlear Limited.

MacIver-Lux, K., Lim, S., Rhoades, E., Robertson, L., Quayle, R., & Honck, L. (2016). Milestones in Auditory-Verbal development. In W. Estabrooks, K. MacIver-Lux, & E. Rhoades (Eds.), *Auditory-verbal therapy for young children with hearing loss and their families, and the practitioners who guide them.* San Diego, CA: Plural Publishing.

Marcin, A. (2018). *What are Piaget's stages of development and how are they used?* Retrieved May 23, 2019 from https://www .healthline.come/health/piaget-stages-of -development~stages

Meningitis Now. (2017). Retrieved July 24, 2019 from https://www.meningitisnow .org/meningitis-explained

Moeller, M., & Schick, B. (2006). Relations between maternal input an TOM understanding in deaf children. *Child Development, 77,* 751–766.

Peterson, C. C. (2009). Development of social-cognitive and communication skills in children born deaf. *Scandinavian Journal of Psychology, 50,* 475–83.

Peterson, C. C., & Siegal, M (2000). Insights into Theory of Mind from deafness and autism. *Mind and Language, 15,* 123–145.

Peterson, C. C., & Siegal, M. (2006). Deafness conservation and Theory of Mind. *Journal of Psychology and Psychiatry, 36,* 459–474.

Peterson, C. C., & Wellman, H. M. (2013). Deafness, thought bubbles, and theory of mind development. *Development Psychology, 49,* 2357–2367.

Rhoades, E. A. (2001). Language progress with an auditory-verbal approach for young children with hearing loss. *International Pediatrics, 1*(16), 1–7.

Rhoades, E., Estabrooks, W., Lim, S., & MacIver-Lux, K. (2016). Strategies for listening, talking and thinking. In W. Estabrooks, K. MacIver-Lux, & E. Rhoades (Eds.), *Auditory-verbal therapy for young children with hearing loss and their families, and the practitioners who guide them.* San Diego, CA: Plural Publishing.

Rosenzweig, E. (2015) *Playing tricks in therapy.* Retrieved July 18, 2019 from https:// auditoryverbaltherapy.net/2015/04/01 /playing-tricks-in-therapy/

Schaaf, R. C., & Mailloux, Z. (2015). *Clinician's guide for implementing Ayres Sensory Integration. Promoting participation for children with autism.* Bethesda, MD: Aota Press.

Siegler, R., Deloacher, J., & Eisenberg, N. (2011). *How children develop.* New York, NY: Worth Publishers.

Spencer, P., & Waxman, R. (1995). Joint attention and maternal attention strategies. *Nine, 12,* 18.

Swisher, M. V. (2000). Learning to converse: How deaf mothers support the development of attention and conversational skills in their young deaf children. In P. E. Spencer, C. J. Erting, & M. Marschark, *The deaf child in the family and at school: Essays in honor of Kathryn P. Meadow-Orlans* (pp. 21–39). Mahwah, NJ: Lawrence Erlbaum Associates Publishers.

Tompkins, V., Benigno, J. P., Kiger Lee, B., & Wright, B. M. (2018). The relation between parents' mental state talk and children's social understanding: A meta-analysis. *Social Development, 27*(2), 223–246.

Tyskiewicz, E., & Clark, F. (2016). *Theory of mind in day to day therapy.* Presented at AGBELL convention July 2016, Denver, CO.

Vygotsky, L. S. (1978). *Mind in society: The development of higher psychological processes.* Cambridge, MA: Harvard University Press.

Wechsler, D. (2012). *Wechsler Preschool and Primary Scale of Intelligence* (4th ed.). San Antonio, TX: Psychological Corporation.

Wellman, H. M. (2014). *Making minds. How theory of mind develops.* Oxford, UK: Oxford University Press.

Westby, C., & Culatta, B. (2016). Telling tales: Personal event narratives and life stories. *Language Speech and Hearing Services in Schools, 47*(4), 1.

Westby, C., & Robinson, L. (2014). A developmental perspective for promoting theory of mind. *Topics in Language Disorders, 34*(4), 362–382.

Woolfe, T., Want, S. C., & Siegal, M. (2002). Signposts to development: Theory of mind in deaf children. *Child Development, 73*(3), 768–778.

14

DEVELOPMENT OF LITERACY IN AUDITORY-VERBAL THERAPY

Lyn Robertson and Denise Wray

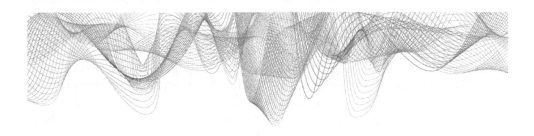

"The foundations of learning to read are set down from the moment a child first hears the sounds of people talking, the tunes of songs, and the rhythms of and repetitions of rhymes and stories. Children who have not been regularly talked to, sung to, or read aloud to from birth find life at school much more burdensome than they otherwise might. In particular, learning to read becomes a major stumbling block rather than a surprising delight." (Fox, 2008, pp. 18–19)

INTRODUCTION

All children thrive in settings where meaningful listening and talking are valued and nurtured. Learning to listen, the precursor for learning to talk, is the capability that paves the way for the development of reading, writing, and thinking that take place throughout the child's life. For the child with hearing loss, the focus on hearing and listening must begin as soon as possible and the principles and practices of Auditory-Verbal Therapy (AVT) today can prepare the child for the development of literacy, defined in this chapter as reading and writing.

The Auditory-Verbal pioneers created the foundations of this approach in ways to help children who are deaf or hard of hearing become conversant in the *hearing world*. Had they set out explicitly to foster emergent literacy skills, along with a love of language, reading, and writing, they would not have needed to do anything different. The first step in AVT is also the first step toward literacy: helping parents to help their child learn to listen as quickly and efficiently as possible with the most effective hearing technology. Much depends upon the quantity, quality, and timing of their receptive and interactive auditory experiences, throughout infancy and the toddler years. In a white paper discussion of the Logic Chain, Flexer lays out the necessary connections between and among brain development, language development, hearing technology, early intervention, and literacy development by summarizing Kral and Sharma (2012) concerning the importance of brain development to eventual literacy acquisition:

"The brain is a dynamic self-organizing system that develops based on reciprocal experiences between neural activity and stimulation from the environment. Auditory experience provides temporal patterns to the developing brain which could be important for developing sequential processing abilities such as pattern detection, sequential memory, and sustained attention in general. As a result, limitations in auditory experience during development might affect neuro-cognitive functioning well beyond spoken language." (Flexer, 2018, p. 10).

To listen is to learn, and to learn is to organize and reorganize the brain (see Chapter 2). Organizing and reorganizing are inherent functions of the brain and are essential to the development of spoken language and learning. Indeed, if all children, including those with typical hearing, were presented with the dynamism of Auditory-Verbal environments, there would be fewer reading and writing problems. In AVT, children are immersed in so much meaningful *listening and spoken conversation* that they develop a complete mastery of the spoken languages they hear as they interact meaningfully with people in their daily lives. A caveat, however, is that while spoken language is necessary for the development of literacy in young children, that in itself is not always sufficient. Some individuals with or without hearing loss do experience processing difficulties that interfere with reading and writing, despite the presence of a well-developed spoken language base. Likewise, some children, with or without hearing loss, have difficulties learning spoken language for reasons unrelated to hearing and listening. These are beyond the scope of this chapter.

A BRIEF HISTORY OF READING ACHIEVEMENT AMONG INDIVIDUALS WITH HEARING LOSS

When children experience spoken language deprivation, we can see what happens by looking at the trajectory of studies that have attempted to gauge the academic and literacy levels of children who are deaf or hard of hearing. Such studies are available from the beginning of the twentieth century (Pintner & Paterson, 1916) and are reported in some detail by Robertson (2014). Spoken language maturity figures prominently in the progression of studies of literacy development in *students with hearing loss*. Individuals who heard better, individuals who had spoken language exposure prior to hearing loss or to intensive therapy that made use of their residual hearing, and individuals who made use of well-fitted hearing technologies began to emerge in the studies as more successful in reading as measured by standardized tests. As these outcomes increased, so did theories about reading development in individuals with typical hearing that pointed increasingly to the relationship between spoken language capability and reading achievement. In addition, parents and Auditory-Verbal practitioners began reporting that the dire predictions about low levels of reading and academic achievement they had received at the time of their child's diagnosis were not happening (Robertson, 2014). More recently, a study to be published about Swedish children who use cochlear implants (CIs) found them to be functioning in ways comparable to their peers with typical hearing. That particular study states: "The results of this study suggest that orthographic learning and reading fluency in children with CI are strongly dependent on similar cognitive and linguistic skills as in typically hearing peers. Efforts, therefore, need to support phonological decoding skill and

vocabulary in this population." (Wass et al., 2019).

COMPREHENSION: THE GOAL OF LITERACY PROCESSES

The most important place to begin when thinking about literacy, hearing, and hearing loss is to specify comprehension as the goal of reading and writing. In global professional training Warren Estabrooks often states, "we need to begin with the end in mind." In general, comprehension takes place because the reader uses his or her array of prior knowledge to construct a logical sense about a passage of text and is able to store that understanding in memory for later use. The flip side of reading for comprehension is the production of writing that makes sense to the writer and to others. To create a spoken utterance or a passage of writing meaningful to another, the child needs to learn to think about what she or he knows and wants to express, and what the recipient of the message will recognize and connect with.

Reading and writing, two receptive and expressive processes we cluster under *literacy*, depend on the individual making use of letter, word, and sentence structure knowledge simultaneously with content knowledge drawn from first-hand and symbolic or virtual experiences in the world. Taken together, these processes produce the *click of recognition* one feels during a successful reading episode and the feeling of satisfaction when one has completed a writing task and receives validation from someone who reads it.

Comprehension is an ongoing task of constructing meanings, and the mastery of literacy is a continuous process. Learning to read and write involves far more than learning to look at the print on the page and pronounce it or learning to spell words and then transfer them to paper. The National Council of Teachers of English states:

"Learning to read is a life-long process. People begin developing knowledge that they will use to read during their earliest interactions with families and communities. In their pre-school years children learn to understand and use spoken language and learn about their world through meaningful interactions with others. Children also learn about written language as more experienced readers provide meaningful demonstrations of reading and writing." (Commission on Reading of the National Council of Teachers of English, 2004, para 7)

As seen in the guidelines offered in this chapter, learning to read is a gradual process that increasingly connects a person's spoken language capabilities and knowledge of the world gained through actual and virtual experiences to the words printed on the page. All reading is interpretation because comprehension is created based on what one already knows and can say. Given such complexity, preparing children who are deaf or hard of hearing to become literate adults capable of functioning in every part of society has been a daunting task. Over many decades, and even before the advent of appropriate hearing aids, AVT enabled many children to become ready for literacy. And now, an exciting new era of advancing hearing technologies is fostering the development of excellent listening skills and enhancing the prior knowledge necessary for literacy to emerge.

PREREQUISITE KNOWLEDGE FOR LITERACY DEVELOPMENT

Literacy involves complex interactions among the components of spoken language: first-hand knowledge of the world combined with vocabulary and word meanings (semantics), phonological awareness and knowledge (phonology), language structure and word order (syntax), word functions (grammar), intonation, conventional ways of speaking and writing (pragmatics and discourse), and sound-symbol relationships. When children are learning to listen and talk, they are also learning to shift attention between short-term (working) memory and long-term memory, to recognize sequencing and cause and effect, to make predictions and confirm or disconfirm them, to identify affirmation and negation, to make comparisons and contrasts, and to draw inferences. The growing ability to use all of these aspects of language in listening and talking is critical for literacy acquisition; the beginning reader must first be able to use language and demonstrate the kind of thinking she or he will encounter in reading and writing experiences.

Firsthand Knowledge of the World: Content and Process Schemas

First-hand knowledge of the world is built from experiences, and the wider the world of the child, the more background knowledge he or she has in terms of both content and processes. The experiences children have with language and its connections to what they see, hear, touch, taste, and feel, as well as to their emotions, create their knowledge base. Experiences in the home, school, community, and society at large provide access to commonly held knowledge about objects, actions, descriptors, relationships, and interpretations, as well as the referential, culturally appropriate language used to talk about them. Interacting in meaningful ways with as many people as possible about the full range of such experiences is essential to developing comprehension. Virtual knowledge constructed through indirect experience such as photos, images in books and electronic devices, stories and descriptions, and pretend play is also vital. Other important kinds of knowledge include how to carry out particular processes and how to name and interpret feelings.

First-hand, virtual, and procedural knowledge combine and come to represent a child's knowledge base that becomes the foundation of all future learning. In cognitive psychology, each such memory structure is called a schema (see Anderson, R., 2004, for an interesting discussion of this robust theory). Schemas, or schemata (an alternate plural), overlap and connect everything the child stores away in memory; the ability to tap into one's memory network in the presence of new experiences is what enables the child to learn. Every child's understanding of the world informs and is informed by the ever-growing network of bits of memory connected by the brain in ways accessible to that person. Simply put, throughout our lives, we learn a great deal when we enlarge or revise our schemas and when we discover new ways to connect them in our memory network.

Comprehension, whether through listening, reading, or using one's senses, and expression, whether through talking or writing, depend upon connecting this base of common knowledge to the language that represents its many parts. Auditory-Verbal Therapy serves children well in that it encourages many experiences and meaningful conversations about them, thereby enabling them to apply spoken words to their schemas and to store them in their memory networks.

Vocabulary and Word Meanings

Children learn words when their parents narrate experiences before, during, and after they happen. Children set up networks of related words and concepts in memory and build upon them quickly. For over 20 years, the effects of spoken language deprivation on children with typical hearing have been known in a specific, quantifiable way (Hart & Risley, 1995; Hart & Risley, 1999). While Hart and Risley focused on children with typical hearing, their findings carry salient implications for intervention with children who are deaf or hard of hearing. Their interest was in quantifying the amount of spoken language in the home environments of children, hypothesizing that at least one cause of the general differences in school progress among children from homes where the parents were professionals, working class homes, or homes where the family was on welfare might be the sheer number of words the children encountered during their earliest, language-acquisition years. On a monthly basis, they tape recorded the language used in these homes and extrapolated estimates of the number of words, repetitions included, each group of children had heard by age 4. The differences were substantial: the children of the professionals had had access to 45 million words, the children of parents in the working class had had 26 million words, and the children of parents on welfare had had 13 million. Hart and Risley observe, "parents who talked a lot . . . or only a little ended up with 3-year-olds who talked a lot, or only a little" (1999, p. 12). This phenomenon associated with parental style in talking with their children has been termed the 30 Million Word Gap, and this knowledge is being used as the basis for programs aimed at enriching the language abilities of children unfortunate enough to be born into the chaos that poverty often creates (Suskind, Thirty Million Words Initiative, http://thirtymillionwords.org/). Hart and Risley's work dealt with vocabulary development and was not about identifying socioeconomic strengths and weaknesses; indeed, in some families with few resources, the prevalence of talking was rich and productive. The point of their findings highlights the importance of talking with children, so they enter school with an extensive vocabulary and rich facility with spoken language. Such knowledge is connected directly to the progress a child can make with reading; it has been established that a child's spoken language ability at preschool age has a direct relationship to the child's reading ability in second grade (Scarborough, 1989) and beyond. The more spoken words the child recognizes, understands, and

uses, the better chance the child has of excelling in reading and writing.

The implications of these findings for children who are deaf or hard of hearing need to be stressed emphatically. During the early years when the brain is most receptive for language development, the child with hearing loss whose hearing is not increased by hearing technology is in a similar and damaging situation to that of the child who hears typically but has little opportunity to listen and speak. Consistent access to increasingly complex interactions using spoken language is imperative for creating the conditions for emerging reading. For a child with hearing loss, any decrease in the number of spoken words heard completely and in connected, meaningful contexts jeopardizes the development of many aspects of spoken language needed for reading.

Parents introduce their children who are deaf or hard of hearing to the world by using many words that describe people, places, things, and experiences. When parents use language the child already knows and *slip in* new words and expressions, they expand their child's repertoire. A trip to the playground with a toddler might sound like this:

- Let's go to the playground! It's just down the street. What do you want to play on today? [wait for an answer] The swings? Oh, you liked swinging the last time, didn't you?
- Put on your jacket. First, your right arm goes into your right sleeve. And, then your left arm. Are your shoes tied? Let's make sure the laces are

tight enough, but not too tight. Are they okay? [wait for an answer]

■ We open the door and go out on the porch. Can you close the door? Thank you! Now, down the steps we go! One, two, three . . .

■ The sidewalk is nice and wide. See where the playground is? [wait for an answer] Yes, there it is!

■ Here's the swing. I'll lift you up and put you in the chair. Hang on to the chains, and I'll push. Here we go! Up and down, up and down!

■ Let's go on the slide now. This one is just your size. Climb up the steps. I'll hold your hands while you slide down. Whee! Isn't this fun? [wait for an answer]

■ Time to go home!

■ At home: What did you like best today? [wait for an answer] I liked that, too! Shall we go again soon? [wait for an answer]

Phonological and Phonemic Awareness and Knowledge

During the past two decades, research has pointed to a connection between insufficient phonological skill, specifically phonemic awareness, and an increased risk of reading difficulties in children with typical hearing (Catts, Fey, Zhang, & Tomblin, 2001; Schuele & Boudreu, 2008; Yopp, 1997), and this knowledge has obvious implications for children who are deaf or hard of hearing. In the United States, The National Reading Panel (Eunice Kennedy Shriver National Institute of Child Health and Human Development, NIH, DHHS, 2000) identified phonemic awareness as a key building block in reading acquisition. Children with phonological awareness sensitivity recognize the sound structure of a spoken language and can manipulate this sound structure of spoken words at the syllable, onset-rime, and phoneme levels (Gillon, 2004). Phonological awareness sensitivity enables the child to make the connection between the letter (the graphemic symbol) and the letter sound (the phonemic vocalization), thus supporting skills in word decoding that help the child connect written symbols with spoken language that is stored in memory. An awareness of the phoneme as it relates to the spoken sound structure supports reading acquisition and is necessary to discovering the logic of the written system (Yopp, 1999). Such awareness must precede phonics instruction; otherwise the instruction does not make sense to the emerging reader. The development of alphabetic awareness begins with the child's discovery of one written letter and its sound, and proceeds to working out the multiple relationships between sounds and their written symbols (Adams, 2002). This is the goal of many of the alphabet books created for very young children. Linking visible letters to audible sounds is not, however, the entire story because many words in English do not follow general pronunciation rules ("have" and "cave" do not rhyme), and children must learn that rules are often just guidelines that offer approximations.

Phonological awareness and phonemic awareness require full auditory access to the entire speech spectrum.

In the past, as described above, this requisite skill underlying literacy development posed major obstacles for children who are deaf or hard of hearing due to poor auditory accessibility to all the sounds of speech. The current combination of early identification, state-of-the-art hearing technologies, and early Auditory-Verbal Therapy intervention can ameliorate the debilitating factors that hearing loss poses, thereby opening the door to age-appropriate listening, talking, reading, writing, and thinking skills that define literacy achievement.

Mastery of Language Structure

For the child with hearing loss, the absence or instability of phonological knowledge is highly problematic, because so much is conveyed by the sounds in phonemes (the smallest units of speech), syllables, words, phrases, sentences, and longer utterances represented as paragraphs and chapters. For the beginning reader, a growing ability to listen and then segment a phrase into words, a word into syllables, and a syllable into phonemes is needed in order to begin to make sense of how words are put together. As the child hears, listens, and uses more spoken language, she or he becomes better prepared to identify words and word parts in print. Such phonological discovery takes place in the presence of spoken language, and we have known for decades that most children with typical hearing learn to recognize and produce the sounds spoken around them by the time they are 6 or 7 (Fry, 1966). The American Speech-Language Hearing Association list of milestones for 4- to

5-year-olds includes: "Hears and understands most of what she hears at home and in school" and "Says all speech sounds in words" (American Speech-Language-Hearing Association, 2019). Lindfors (2008) observes that most children with typical hearing have mastered listening, conversing, and using spoken language simply by interacting every day with adults and other children. Opper (1996) cites Lindfors in writing that by ages 5 to 6 "virtually every child acquires an abstract and highly complex system of linguistic structure and use." For the typical learner, then, first grade is a reasonable time for most children to begin receiving formal instruction in reading, and it is highly desirable to prepare children who are deaf or hard of hearing to do the same. Scarborough (2001) documents that many studies have demonstrated that "preschoolers with language impairments are, indeed, at considerable risk for developing reading disabilities (as well as for continued spoken language difficulties) at older ages." Formal instruction that includes word identification strategies (both *"sounding out"* and *"whole word"*) is comprehensible to the child at this time, because it depends upon the auditory and semantic language base of the child. Learning to read, in the presence of both formal reading instruction and informal instruction at home, helps children fill in the sounds and words they have not already mastered (Adams, 2002; Goswami, 2000). This is particularly advantageous for the child with hearing loss who may have some gaps, but attempting to teach letter sounds to children who cannot already listen and talk, with the goal of their learning to identify written words, is not recommended.

Geers and Hayes (2011) report results of a longitudinal study that followed the performance of language-related skills in 184 students who had severe-to-profound hearing loss and who received cochlear implants prior to age 5. Without differentiating among students who received AVT and those who did not, they followed these students throughout elementary school and were able to reassess the reading, writing, and phonological processing skills of 112 of those original subjects in high school. They found that, depending on the test, between 47% and 66% performed within or above the average range for reading in comparison to hearing peers, an encouraging outcome in view of previous research findings. However, two areas remained challenging for the subjects, that of written expression and phonological processing. Such processing skills are so important that they have been found to be critical predictors of high school literacy skills. More research is needed focusing on and comparing reading achievement of children who have followed AVT or other approaches and children with typical hearing.

Predictions and Confirmations

In AVT, skills associated with listening and talking are typically learned in a naturalistic manner. For instance, while engaged in the natural activity of reading aloud, the parent and child can apply some of the strategies suggested in guided reading and shared reading coaching tools (Byrd & Westfall, 2015; Spears, 2015). Prediction and confirmation of predictions can be nurtured using strategies involving questions used by the parent prior to, during, and after reading an engaging picture book (Spears, 2015). Questions that encourage the child to utilize illustrations in the book to make predictions and support hypotheses can be posed while prompting the child to look at the cover and the pictures and predict what the plot of the story may be. To garner meaning, the practitioner and parent can encourage the child to use echo reading or imitation of the parent using expression while reading. After completing the story, they can compare and contrast the predictions made beforehand with the actual events in the story. Sequencing, explanations and descriptions can be promoted using the Language Experience Book (LEB), as discussed by Robertson (2014). Daily events illustrated by the child and the parent can be recounted, sequenced, and recalled using various words, expressions, verb tenses, and complex sentences. The parent and practitioner can design the language in at least two ways: language that is entirely within the child's experience and language that stretches just a bit beyond the child's experience. LEBs motivate children to sequence and discuss events experienced personally in their own daily lives. The internet is replete with many appealing websites that support increasingly complex thinking such as making inferences, identifying affirmation and negation, and comparing and contrasting. Super Duper Publications (http://www.superduperinc.com) offers "fun decks" that explore the topics of inference, prediction, and comprehending negation. Instructional /educational websites such as http://www.teacherspayteachers.com provide motivating printable activities accessed by simply typing in the language target area desired. For printable stories and graded books, often accompanied by comprehension questions, some of the most popular websites include http://www.readinga-z.com, http://www.dltk-teach.com, http://www.1-2-3learncurriculum.com, http://www.turtlediary.com/kids-stories.html, as well as http://www.storybook.com, in which the student can create his or her own stories. These are all appropriate for Auditory-Verbal Therapy.

velopment. The practitioner needs to provide evidence of each child's progress through the stages, chart the findings, and provide coaching and guidance for mastering the next stage. Table 14–1 provides a general checklist that can help the practitioner in monitoring a child's progress. By realizing the progression of literacy development, we can "keep the end in mind."

KNOWING WHAT TO EXPECT

The practitioner possesses knowledge of typical milestones in language and literacy development, as these are benchmarks for AVT. These benchmarks are integral in coaching and guiding the parents in ways that can help the child with hearing loss benefit from interacting with children with typical hearing. Noted researcher Jean Chall (1983) developed a list of age-appropriate evidence-based behaviors foundational to literacy development that span from birth to adulthood, and these are instructive for practitioners and teachers as they work with children both with and without hearing loss (see Table 14–1). Again, elements of the Logic Chain (Flexer, 2018) are evident in the progression depicted from learning to listen to mature uses of literacy in capable adulthood: brain development, language development, hearing technology, early intervention, and literacy development. For the child with hearing loss, the critical matter is establishing hearing and using it in developing the ability to listen. The brain is developing at every step along the way, and each subsequent literacy stage represents progressive complexity in cognitive de-

PRACTICAL APPROACHES FOR BUILDING A FOUNDATION FOR LITERACY

Moving from theory into practice is the exciting task of the practitioner and the parent. Table 14–2 links the LSLS Domain 9 and literacy theory with AVT and demonstrates how it is intentional in fostering emerging literacy. The focus of Domain 9 is the development of the auditory and language skills that underlie and support the acquisition and advancement of literacy.

The underlying reason for the practical approaches offered in this section is the fostering of auditory memory in order to facilitate auditory-based thinking, another goal of Auditory-Verbal Therapy. A critical element in auditory processing involves phonological memory. The combination of phonological awareness, phonological memory, and phonological retrieval comprises a cluster of requisite skills for learning to read and read fluently (Justice, 2006); these skills underlie the ability to become aware of, store, and retrieve phonologically encoded information in words and sentences, including that found in extended discourse (Catts & Kamhi, 2005).

Table 14-1. Age-Appropriate Literacy Behaviors: Evidence-Based Expectations and Norms

Pre-reading/ Emerging Literacy Birth–6 years Chall, J. (1983).	Birth–2 years • Learns to listen and begins to speak • Enjoys word play and being read with by an adult
	2–4 years • Continues to learn to listen and speak • Enjoys word play and being read with by an adult • Names some items in books • Enjoys and responds to Language Experience Books • Enjoys rhyming games • Exhibits book handling skills • Identifies some logos and symbols encountered in daily life • Enjoys scribbling
	4–6 years • Continues to learn to listen and speak • Demonstrates knowledge of basic concepts about print • Enjoys word play and being read with by an adult • Enjoys and responds to Language Experience Books • Enjoys retelling simple stories • Draws lines and shapes • By the end of this stage, child 　◦ knows and uses the structures of his/her spoken language 　◦ converses in complete sentences 　◦ comprehends, remembers, and formulates stories 　◦ interacts with some printed words 　◦ pretends to read and write 　◦ understands thousands of spoken words, but can read only a few of them 　◦ has established a beginning level of phonemic awareness
Initial Reading 6–7 years First grade and into second	Age-appropriate behavior: evidence-based expectations and norms • Learns alphabetic principle • Learns to read simple text, make predictions, construct meaning • Enjoys being read from texts more difficult than s/he can read • Develops more advanced language, vocabulary, concepts • By the end of this stage, child understands at least 4000 spoken words and can read about 600 words

continues

Table 14-1. *continued*

Confirmation and Fluency 7–8 years	Age-appropriate behavior: evidence-based expectations and norms • Reads simple, familiar stories with increasing fluency • Consolidates decoding, sight vocabulary, and meaning • Listening remains more effective than reading • By the end of this stage, child understands at least 9000 spoken words and can read and understand about 3000 words
Reading for Learning 9–13 years	Age-appropriate behavior: evidence-based expectations and norms • Reads to learn new ideas, gain new knowledge, experience new feelings, learn new attitudes, usually from one point of view • Reads texts whose complexity is increasing • By the end of this stage, reading and listening comprehension are about equal • Reads with more efficiency
Multiple Viewpoints 15–17 years	Age-appropriate behavior: evidence-based expectations and norms • Teenager reads a wide range of materials from multiple viewpoints and for multiple purposes • At this stage, reading comprehension of difficult material is better than listening comprehension of the same material
Construction and Reconstruction 18+ years	Age-appropriate behavior: evidence-based expectations and norms • Adult reads for personal and professional purposes • Adult reads to create new knowledge by adding the knowledge of others to his/her own knowledge • Adult reads efficiently

INTENTIONAL DEVELOPMENT OF PHONOLOGICAL AWARENESS

Research has demonstrated that intervention can positively influence phonologic awareness skills and has documented improvement in word iden-tification and decoding skills (Schuele & Boudreu, 2008). Numerous reports suggest that phonological instruction must be initiated in preschool and no later than kindergarten (Schuele & Boudreu, 2008); AVT begins such instruction even earlier. It is important that the practitioner and the parents of young children with hearing loss recognize a hierarchy of phonological awareness knowledge

Figure 14–2. Linking LSLS Domain 9 and Literacy Theory with Auditory-Verbal Therapy

LSLS Domain 9	Literacy Theory: National Reading Panel Category	Auditory-Verbal Therapy: Practices
a. Reciting finger plays and nursery rhymes	Phonemic awareness Phonics Fluency Vocabulary Comprehension	Targeted listening practice • Example: Discriminating between 1- and 2-syllable words whose phonemes differ by one (ex: mat-bat, bat-bam, batter-matter, batter-badger) • Exposing child to melody, expression, rhythm, rhyme, intonation • Using repetition
b. Telling and/or retelling stories	Vocabulary Comprehension	Targeted listening practice • Responding with spoken language • Waiting for and requiring child to use spoken language • Daily interactive read-aloud with the child • Positioning close to the microphone • Using acoustic highlighting • Pausing, waiting (providing thinking time for the child) • Changing voices for characters • Asking and answering questions in a conversational manner • Using classic literature, songs, nursery rhymes
c. Activity and story sequencing	Vocabulary Comprehension	Targeted listening practice • Responding with spoken language • Waiting for and requiring child to use spoken language

continues

Figure 14–2. *continued*

LSLS Domain 9	Literacy Theory: National Reading Panel Category	Auditory-Verbal Therapy: Practices
d. Singing songs and engaging in musical activities	Phonemic awareness Phonics Fluency Vocabulary Comprehension	Targeted listening practice • Exposing child to melody, pitch, expression, rhythm, rhyme, intonation • Using repetition
e. Creating experience stories/experience books	Vocabulary Comprehension	Targeted listening practice • Developing conversations using natural interactions • Highlighting vocabulary • Paying attention to word order • Changing words by adding prefixes and suffixes
f. Organization of books (e.g., cover; back; title; author page)	Vocabulary Comprehension	Incorporating book-reading vocabulary during shared reading
g. Directionality and orientation of print	Vocabulary Comprehension	Incorporating book-reading vocabulary during shared reading

h. Distinguishing letters, words, sentences, spaces, and punctuation	Phonemic awareness
	Phonics
		Targeted listening practice
		• Acoustic highlighting
		  ○ Suprasegmental
		  ○ Segmental
		• Asking, "What did you hear?"
		Pointing out and talking about letters, words, sentences, spaces, and punctuation

i. Phonics (e.g., sound-symbol correspondences and letter-sound correspondences)	Phonemic awareness Phonics	Targeted listening practice • Preparing a child who listens for formal instruction that leads to understanding the alphabetic principle
j. Phonemic awareness (e.g., sound matching; isolating; substituting; adding; blending; segmenting; deleting)	Phonemic awareness Phonics	Targeted listening practice • To one's own speech • Six-Sound Test • Nursery rhymes • Music and singing
k. Sight word recognition	Fluency	Allowing sight word identification to develop naturally during read-aloud without focusing directly on this aspect of reading during the emergent reading period

l. Strategies for the development of listening, speaking, vocabulary, reading and writing	Phonemic awareness Phonics Fluency Vocabulary Comprehension	Targeted listening practice
		• Focus on building
		  ◦ auditory memory
		  ◦ receptive and expressive spoken language
		Providing the child with mature models of spoken and written language structure and function
		Playtime alone, with parent, and with other children

m. Contextual clues to decode meaning	Vocabulary Comprehension	Having frequent conversations with the child in the course of daily activities fosters meaning making
n. Oral reading fluency development	Fluency	Having frequent conversations with the child in the course of daily activities fosters fluency in spoken language and reading

continues

Figure 14–2. *continued*

LSLS Domain 9	Literacy Theory: National Reading Panel Category	Auditory-Verbal Therapy: Practices
o. Text comprehension strategies (e.g., direct explanation; modeling; guided practice; and application)	Vocabulary Comprehension	Narrating life as it happens Bringing sounds to life through meaningful experiences Having frequent conversations Learning through exposure • Semantics • Morphology • Syntax Learning to • Turn statements into questions, exclamations, etc. • Apply words to objects, actions, relationships modifiers, and ideas • Use pragmatic aspects of language • Apply memories of experiences to text
p. Abstract and figurative language (e.g., similes; metaphors)	Vocabulary Comprehension	Focusing on abstract and figurative language with the child during • Frequent conversations • Daily shared reading
q. Divergent question comprehension (e.g., inferential questions; predictions)	Vocabulary Comprehension	Asking divergent questions of the child during • Frequent conversations • Daily shared reading

that moves from the global to the specific so that appropriate intervention can take place in a timely fashion (Adams, 1990). Particular emphasis needs to shift focus progressively toward the level of the phoneme, as intervention that leads the child from phonological to phonemic awareness promotes the child's use of strategies for effective decoding and spelling (Price & Ruscher, 2006). Since children with hearing loss in AVT have early access to hearing the full speech spectrum, formal attention to phonological awareness can realistically begin in preschool. In fact, Johnson and Goswami (2010) conclude that early cochlear implantation is associated with improved phonological awareness skills as well as improved spoken language and auditory memory. Studies have demonstrated that sequential acquisition of these skills is similar for children with and without typical hearing, and instruction can be conducted in small group or one-on-one settings.

The following hierarchy of phonemic awareness levels is recommended:

1. Rhythm and Rhyme: the ability to recognize, complete, and produce word patterns and detect spoken syllables;
2. Parts of a Word: the ability to blend, segment, and delete syllables;
3. Sequencing of Sounds: the ability to recognize initial and final sounds;
4. Separation of Sounds: the ability to segment sounds in words and blend sounds; and
5. Manipulation of Sounds: the ability to add, delete, and/or substitute sounds (Fitzpatrick, 1997; Yopp & Yopp, 2000).

Price and Ruscher (2006) suggest a naturalistic approach that provides pho-

nological awareness instruction within the context of children's picture books and literature; this instruction is consistent with the principles first described by Justice and Kaderavek (2004). Such instruction promotes explicit and hierarchical phonological awareness training while providing socially meaningful encounters with literacy experiences throughout the day complemented by structured lessons that target specific emergent literacy goals. Price and Ruscher's *embedded-explicit approach, quite applicable to AVT*, suggests the following sequence of instruction for phonologic awareness skills:

1. Instruction progresses in the following order at these sound unit levels:
   a. Syllables
   b. Rhyming with onset-rime
   c. Sound-symbol associations and alliteration
   d. Phonemes
2. Within these sound unit levels, instruction about tasks and operations progresses in the following order:
   a. Blending
   b. Segmenting
   c. Counting
   d. Deleting
   (Price & Ruscher, 2006, pp. 23–77).

Important intervention tenets supported by evidence-based research include the following:

▪ Explicit instruction is systematic.
▪ Intervention occurs within authentic reading and writing contexts and class curriculum.
▪ Phonemic awareness skills are causally related to word decoding and spelling.

- Instruction is done in small groups.
- Focus is on a small set of skills (for example, blending or segmenting) rather than a large number of operations at once.
- Total instruction should occupy approximately 20 hours spread across a 10-week period (Carson, Gillon, & Boustead, 2013).
- Strongest effects will occur during the preschool and/or kindergarten years.
- Close collaboration is necessary between the speech language pathologist and the teacher.
- Students at risk must be identified early, with identification followed by instruction tailored for each student.
- Instruction needs to be organized in a logical order from easier to more difficult skills (e.g., blending, segmenting, counting, and deleting) within each of the sound unit levels of syllable awareness, rhyming with onset-rime, sound-symbol identification/alliteration, and finally, phoneme awareness (Justice, 2006).

Over two decades of research suggest that children with and without hearing loss can benefit from intense phonological awareness instruction, that such instruction matters in reading acquisition, and that it must occur early and intensively with attention given to the challenges facing the individual child. Tailored to meet the needs of the child, an explicit and systematic plan can be implemented with positive impact on word identification, decoding, spelling, and comprehension

(Carson et al., 2013; Price & Ruscher, 2006; Schuele & Boudreu, 2008; Yopp & Yopp, 2006). The child receiving Auditory-Verbal Therapy can benefit greatly from such intervention.

Using the classic children's book *Brown Bear, Brown Bear, What Do You See?* by Bill Martin Jr. and Eric Carle (1967) (also found in Chapter 9), the following demonstrates how various phonological awareness skills may be employed in a natural shared reading setting:

- Rhyme: The ability to recognize rhyme, complete rhyme, and produce rhyme. Example: Does *sheep* rhyme with *bear*? Does *dog* rhyme with *frog*?
- Syllables: The ability to blend, segment, and delete syllables. Example: *chil-* and *-dren* together says *children*. Example: Clap the sound parts in *teacher*. (2 claps) Example: Say *goldfish*. Now say it without saying *gold*. (*fish*)
- Phonemes: (1) The ability to recognize individual sounds in words, beginning with the initial and final sounds. Example: What is the first sound in the word *bear*? (b) Example: What is the last sound in the word *dog*? (g); or (2) The ability to blend onset and rime. Example: What is this word? "c-at" (cat); or (3) The ability to blend, segment, and delete phonemes. Example: "h-or-s." What's the word? (horse) Example: What are the sounds you hear in *dog*? /d/ /a/ /g/ Example: Say *red* without the /r/. (ed) Example: Say *sheep* without the /p/. (she)

▪ Phoneme Manipulation: The ability to add and/or substitute phonemes. Example: Say /at/. Now add /k/. (cat) Example: Replace the first sound in *duck* with /b/. (buck) Example: Replace the last sound in *bird* with /n/. (burn) (Zgonc, 2000).

SHARED READING EXPERIENCE

Reading aloud with children has been identified as one of the most important activities for promoting the skills that lead to their eventual success in reading alone (Trelease, 2015). Initially, it is not so important to teach the child *how* to read, but rather to encourage the child to *want* to read.

"When we get involved in reading aloud to [and *with*] and other children, we often forget entirely that we *should* be reading aloud. We have such a rollicking good time, and we relate so warmly to our kids as we read together, that it becomes a delicious 'chocolate' kind of experience." (Fox, 2008, p. 11)

Such reading entices the child to want to *break the code* of squiggles (*letters*) on the page. Consequently, reading, just like Auditory-Verbal Therapy, becomes a *labor of love*, not a struggle. In Auditory-Verbal Therapy, spoken language needs to be "easy to hear, easy to listen to, easy to say, easy to use in conversations in everyday life, and subsequently become easy to read, and to write."

Research suggests that guided and shared reading experiences with a child can have a significantly positive impact on the child's early language development and subsequent ability to read. Whitehurst and his research team suggest that adults need to create a highly interactive reading experience, similar to a *dialogue* in which the adult invites and maintains the child's active participation while reading both *to* and *with* the child (Whitehurst et al., 1988). Specific strategies that define *dialogic reading* include the following:

▪ Labeling objects and events.
▪ Presenting simple *wh-* questions.
▪ Posing more complex *what* questions about function and attributes.
▪ Repeating the child's verbal attempts.
▪ Requesting that the child imitate verbally.
▪ Offering praise.
▪ Providing verbal expansions.
▪ Posing open-ended questions.

Williams (2006) suggests an integrated approach, *Enhanced Dialogic Reading* (EDR), which integrates instruction in phonological sensitivity (associated with decoding skills) and spoken language (associated with comprehension skills) while engaging with the child. The goal of EDR is to encourage the two precursors of reading to become interactive, so that phonological sensitivity and spoken language will create fluent, accurate readers.

Similarly, Marsha Spears's work *Shared Reading Coaching Tool* (2015) promotes print conventions such as directionality, picture cues, letter activities, and phonemic awareness while simultaneously focusing on spoken language skills such as asking the child to predict, self-monitor, guess vocabulary meaning, retell and repeat story elements, and note repetitive patterns in the language of the text. Spears's step-by-step process to teach shared reading uses an intense three-day protocol.

Steps in a Shared Reading Experience

It is vital that the practitioner coach parents so they feel assured that their child *gets something* from a book during each shared reading experience. The child and/or adults may do something such as this:

1. Choose three books: a favorite, a familiar, and a new one.
2. Examine the favorite book together and talk about its cover, its pictures, and what the child thinks will happen in the book.
3. Ask the child questions about the story and wait for responses.
4. Read the book aloud and check in with the child to monitor whether he or she is paying attention and what is being understood. Talk about the story in ways that feel natural.
5. After reading the book, ask the child to tell you the story, and prompt with appropriate questions where the child falters or cannot come up with relevant language. This can be done in conversation, so that the child is not feeling "tested."
6. Keep a log in the child's chart of what the child is able to say about the book over repeated readings.
7. Proceed to the familiar book and then to the new book in the same

way during the same session if the child is enjoying it.

The child, however, must be interested and have something to talk about, so it is counter-productive to push the child too much. Many of the strategies outlined in Chapters 15, 16, and 17 will be of great value during shared reading experiences. The sequence of events over time is "reading aloud—reading along—reading alone."

Monitoring of shared reading (Moore, Perez-Mendez, & Boerger, 2006) suggests a *4-Squares Technique* that analyzes parents' readings of favorite stories with their child. The experience is videotaped while the parent follows a discussion framework with a facilitator afterward. The observation instrument includes strengths of the caregiver and the child, as well as the next steps to be taken by both the parent and the child. For example, a parent's strengths might include pointing to familiar letters, using emotion while reading, and waiting for the child to respond. *These strategies are all familiar to the practitioner.* Strengths of the child might include turning the pages and watching intently, asking various questions, and pointing to pictures. Next steps for the parent might include asking the child to predict the rest of the plot and retell the story, while relating the story to the child's everyday life. The child's subsequent steps may include filling in words that appear in the story, something that encourages the child to continue talking about the story or retelling the plot.

These shared reading paradigms demonstrate that there is no best, invariant way to teach children to read.

Using the popular children's book *The Hat* (Brett, 1997), an integrated approach to reading aloud demonstrating dialogic reading, enhanced dialogic reading, and shared reading strategies may proceed when the practitioner coaches the parents in the following way:

■ Can you show me the front of the book? Where's the title? Yes, and the title is *The Hat*.

■ Do you know what these words are? It's the author's name. Jan Brett wrote this book. Look at the picture on the front cover, and tell me what you think this story is about.

■ Turn to the first page of the book. Look . . . inside it says Jan Brett wrote this book for Sara and Joshua Carty. I wonder who they are, maybe her niece and nephew.

■ While we read this book, I may ask you to say a sentence after me. You'll be my "echo." Do you remember what season it is in this story? Yes, winter.

■ The girl in the story named Lisa looks like she's searching. How did I know that?

■ Turn to the second page. Something is happening . . . the sock blows away. Do you think Lisa knows? Why not?

■ This is an unusual farm animal. Have you ever seen a hedgehog? Show me the word. "Hedgehog" begins with the same letter as your name . . . Hannah! I hear it . . . /h/ . . . /h/ . . . hedgehog. They say his fur is prickly. What animal does he resemble or look similar to? Perhaps a mouse? Can you guess what will happen next?

■ You were right! Hedgie climbed into the sock and he got stuck! Do you think the hen will help Hedgie? Look at the right side of the page. Yes, there's another farm animal called a "gander" or a large goose. Turn to the fourth page . . . there it is! That picture on the right told us what animal is next. Do you see another word that begins with /h/? Yes, there it is . . . "honk" begins with /h/. I hear it!

■ There's the next farm animal . . . the cat. What sound do you hear at the beginning of "cat"? What rhymes with "cat"?

■ Can you guess what animal I'm saying . . . /d/-/a/-/g/? Yes, I said, "dog."

■ Is anyone helping Hedgie? Why do you think they all run away after seeing Hedgie? The hen ran, the gander ran, the cat ran, and the dog ran. They all disappeared. (Acoustically stress the irregular verb tense and articles)

■ Here's the last page of the book. Was there a problem in the story? What did Lisa think was so silly in the book? What did Lisa and Hedgie say? "Animals should never wear clothes!" What do you think about that?

Rather, an integrated approach that prepares a child for the demands of phonological sensitivity (decoding/bringing sound to print) and comprehension (bringing meaning to spoken language) increases the probability that a child with hearing loss will develop the requisite skills for a successful reading acquisition experience and will go on to become a lifetime reader.

Enhancing Auditory Skills in Shared Reading Experiences

For the child with hearing loss, the best signal-to-noise ratio occurs when the child is sitting on the caregiver's lap. While listening and discussing the details shared in children's books, the adult and child can explore lands never traveled and discuss narratives with intriguing story lines. The conversation that ensues between the reader and the listener strengthens conversational competence and encourages the child's inferential and critical thinking skills.

Engaging the child in interactive shared reading experiences expands auditory attention and memory (Trelease, 2015). Exposing children to literature is motivating for both the child and the adult and can be both emotionally bonding and intellectually stimulating. The child's personal Language Experience Book (LEB) can be used for shared reading and story retelling in the same ways. The use of the child's own language makes the familiar narrative and the written language that represents it accessible and more memorable. That the LEB is about the child's own experience facilitates parent–child interactions involving the story, including recall of facts, feelings, and predictions (Robertson, 2014). Repetitive reading of the LEB stories also contributes to developing fluency in speech and in reading aloud (Rasinski, 2010).

Reading and auditory recall can also be promoted by creating and introducing a *Poetry Notebook* containing various kinds of poetry and rhymes, song lyrics, famous speeches, jump rope chants, cheers, jokes, and movie scripts. Initially, the task involves auditory memory, and then it is used to encourage children to actually see and read the words in the text as they develop fluency in guided reading practice (Rasinski, 2010). Each passage in the notebook can be accompanied by an object or a picture that represents the main feature. This demonstrates the connection between spoken and written language and plants the seeds of fluency and phonemic awareness. Reading with significant others is encouraged daily, and the child is asked to obtain *signatures* from the listeners of her/his *Poetry Notebook*.

An excellent example of using the children's book *Brown Bear, Brown Bear, What Do You See?* (as cited earlier) by Bill Martin Jr. and Eric Carle (1967) in helping children through the hierarchy of auditory development is provided by Caleffe-Schenck (The Listener, 2000) and can be found in detail in Chapter 9.

Story Retelling

Story retelling strategies (Robertson, Dow, & Hainzinger, 2006) involve the child interacting with the reader of the story while engaged in shared reading. A study by Robertson, Dow, and Hainzinger (2006) demonstrated that a sample group of children with hearing loss who were following AVT did as well at remembering and using the words and concepts in a book as children with typical hearing. As the child gains more competence in listening, remembering, and talking, he or she begins to repeat words and sentences that are presented verbally, and verbatim utterances become possible. Comprehension builds as the child learns how to make sense

> For example, in a story, Kellie says, *"The trip to the zoo will be the first time I see tigers!"* This might prompt the adult to ask, *"What does Kellie want to see?"* The child will learn over time and progress in using language associated with the reading from saying, *"See tigers!"* to *"First time see tigers!"* to *"This will be the first time Kelly will see tigers!"*

of what he or she hears in a story, and spoken language develops accordingly. This can easily be encouraged at home between the parent and child during shared readings of children's literature. Using toy figures to relate narratives is highly motivating, and the resulting speaker-listener dialogue involves auditory memory recall.

Guided Reading

Byrd and Westfall (2015) outline several strategies for use in guided reading; these appear in their *Guided Reading Coaching Tool*. The use of these strategies involves listening, talking, and learning about books and stories.

In addition, there are guided reading suggestions involving decoding unfamiliar and frequently occurring words that enhance every child's ability to recall and comprehend many genres of text. These practical suggestions can lead children in Auditory-Verbal Therapy on their journey toward literacy in a motivating and engaging manner. When teaching book handling and directionality, ask the child:

- Show me the front of the book.
- Point to the title.
- Open the book.
- Which page do we read first?
- Point to the first word we will read.
- In which direction should we turn the page?
- Where do our eyes go next after we get to the end of the line?

To teach the child how to gain information from the illustrations, ask the child:

- Who do you see in the picture?
- Tell me all of the names that Jackie [a character] could be called (e.g., girl, daughter, princess, sister, classmate, etc.).
- How is the character feeling?
- What details do you see in the background?
- Where is the story taking place?
- What will happen next? [Can you make any predictions from this picture?]
- Does it look like there may be any problems in this story?

To teach the child to use background knowledge to make sense of the text, ask the child and then prompt with related questions:

- Remember when we went to the _____? What did you see? What did it look like? Did it smell good?
- What happens when you _____?
- Have you ever _____?

To draw the child's attention to visual cues, words, and sentence structure, say to the child:

- Does ____ make sense in that sentence?
- Try a new word that may make more sense.
- When you said ___ did it make more sense?
- Let's use our common sense to determine what this means.
- Does that new word look right and sound right?
- Does the sentence make sense when you hear it?

SHARED WRITING

Calkins (1994) and Graves (2003) explain that children often engage in writing prior to or along with their experiences with reading, and it is often the writing experience that incites a desire to learn to read. Graves suggests reading and writing are "synergistic," with each feeding off the other's characteristics.

A Framework for the Writing Process

Newman (2001) identifies four concepts in the writing process that provide a framework when analyzing children's writing: intention, organization, experimentation, and orchestration. In *intention,* the child writes with purpose or meaning. The child is intent on conveying a meaningful message. A child learns to communicate verbally to express desires, needs, requests, denials, or refusals, and likewise learns that the written word manipulates the environment as well. In *organizatio*n, the

child displays awareness that writing has various formats to which it must adhere. In English, there are three directional principles to be learned: we read and write top to bottom, left to right, and return quickly from the right to left and begin again (Clay, 1987, 2010). In *experimentation,* the child explores punctuation conventions she or he may see but not fully understand. Risk-taking is an integral part of experimentation, and the child is attempting to learn what she or he can control in the writing process. Last, the child learns that writing is a matter of *orchestration.* The child learns the necessity of juggling many aspects of writing at once, such as spelling, grammar, printing, and meaning, while simultaneously making decisions about prioritizing those aspects. When they receive responses to their writing from others, children learn that writing is a powerful, complex process.

The Language Experience Book and Writing

In helping the child understand the relationship between reading and writing, the LEB offers an excellent vehicle by which a child who is deaf or hard of hearing in Auditory-Verbal Therapy can experience the process of writing and its power to function as another form of communication. Because children are developmentally egocentric, participating in the writing of the LEB can fascinate the child and help him or her to recall actions, narratives, concepts, and feelings, along with the words that represent them. As a way of chronicling daily activities, the LEB compiles and illustrates step-by-step details of the child's experiences. The development of sequencing can be helped along and extended by using the LEB. Documenting daily events in a notebook provides purpose for the child and parent to interact using shared writing as they record events and ideas important to the child. The parent helps to foster the child's desire to share with others using a form that goes beyond speaking—writing words down on paper.

In fostering writing, the following incentives need to be used routinely with eager young authors:

▪ Weekly surprises are always literacy based: pens, markers, crayons, notepads, diaries, books, printable books, or props such as popsicle stick pointers to follow words of songs, finger plays, or nursery rhymes; all can be found at home, at flea markets, or as freebies from family and friends.

▪ Writing needs to be a social experience. On different occasions the practitioner and the parent model the writing process by writing alongside the child on the floor, at the table, or wherever it is comfortable. It is not surprising when children imitate, as imitation is the way children learn from experienced writers.

▪ Adults might create their own Language Experience Books as well as expecting the children to participate in doing so. Children love to hear the adults share their weekly challenges and dramas. They love to listen and laugh at life experiences chronicled in the LEBs.

▪ Parents need to be involved throughout the sharing of the LEB to demonstrate the importance of making reading and writing a part of everyday living. Once they observe the motivation of the LEB, they recognize the contribution that writing makes in creating a lifetime reader and writer in their child.

Ways to use the LEB approach to literacy development change as the child changes. The practitioner and parent guide the child through a progression that shifts the production of spoken and written language from the adult to the child. They focus on the child's experiences so that the basic language is in the child's experiential vocabulary and new language is introduced as it fits the situation. The general progression begins with the adult as writer and moves over time toward the child becoming the writer. At every step, the adult and child read and talk about what is on the page, and the adult intentionally expands the child's responses to it by asking questions, supplying and eliciting additional words, and assisting with editing.

1. The adult puts a drawing, picture, or souvenir on a page in the LEB and writes sentences about it.
2. The child chooses or makes a drawing, picture, or souvenir for a page in the LEB, and the adult writes what the child says about it.
3. The child chooses or makes a drawing, picture, or souvenir for a page in the LEB, and tells the adult what to write about it.

4. The child chooses or makes a drawing, picture, or souvenir and writes the words and/or sentences with the help of the adult.

5. The child chooses or makes a drawing, picture, or souvenir for the LEB and writes words and sentences *without the help of the adult.*

6. The child keeps a journal for personal and study purposes, and the adult weighs in about it as the child/teenager seeks his/her input. (Robertson, 2014)

The LEB commits authentic daily activities to a written format so the child can relive experiences at a later time with significant others. Excursions provide motivating and relevant topics that may be entered into the LEB. The LEB can be used to present both known and new information, new words, language structures, and ways to use language. An example of a common activity might be an outdoor nature walk. During this event, the child can collect objects he discovers on the walk. The parent can take the bag of nature mementos to the practitioner to review and enter a passage in the LEB. A sample script can be seen in the text box below.

Digital Literacy

The question of whether and how to use digital, electronic devices with children is becoming increasingly frequent,

---

- "So, Emily, you went on a walk with Daddy? Let's write that in your book." (Acoustically highlight past verb tense inflections and age-appropriate adjectives) Write: Dad and I went for a walk in the woods on a windy day. We looked for interesting things to put in our nature bag.

- "Do you know what treasures you discovered outside? I see a pinecone, a feather, a stick, a piece of bark, a buckeye, a stone, and green moss. Wow! Cool treasures! What did you find?" Child: "I found a pinecone, I found a stone, some bark, a feather, and I found a buckeye and a stick, and I found moss."

- "Let's put your treasures in piles of soft, hard, smooth, rough, light, and heavy." (Follow up by categorizing the items into the various adjective descriptors in order to build a schema network. Tape all objects into the book while leaving room on the page for written text.)

- "Now let's write what you found in your book." Write: I found a soft feather and soft moss. I found a rough pinecone and a rough piece of bark. I found a smooth stone and smooth stick. I found a light feather and green moss and a heavy stone.

- "Emily, what should we call our walk outside today? Let's give our day a name or a title." Child: "Let's call it Our Fun Trip Outside." "How about a bigger word for 'fun' and 'trip'? How about 'Our Exciting Adventure Outside'? I'm so glad you like it. Now let's write the title in our book so you can share this adventure with Nana, Papa, your brother Sean, Uncle Joe, and Aunt Maria."

as we are experiencing a profound change in the ways we record, store, and retrieve information. Digital technology is powerful and useful. Some embrace the idea of using it with children, thinking it will work wonders, and others will not let their children near it, fearing it will damage them. Its potential benefits for children are being studied, and the current summary of the National Association for the Education of Young Children and the Center for Early Learning and Children's Media at Saint Vincent College includes:

"Special considerations must be given to the use of technology with infants and toddlers. The statement recommends prohibiting the passive use of television, videos, DVDs, and other non-interactive technologies and media in early childhood programs for children younger than 2 years of age, and it discourages passive and non-interactive uses with children ages 2 through 5. Any uses of technology and interactive media in programs for children younger than 2 years of age should be limited to those that appropriately support responsive interactions between caregivers and children and strengthen adult-child relationships." (Fred Rogers Center, 2012 p. 2)

The American Academy of Pediatrics (2016) recommends creative play away from digital media for infants and toddlers. Carefully constructed media can be introduced around 18 months, but parents should participate with their children in watching it so they can assist the children in understanding it.

The concerns associated with exposing children to digital media range from sleep and behavior problems to diminished academic achievement to a lesser development of language and social skills. Of particular concern is non-interactive technology, as it hampers both physical and linguistic activity. From an Auditory-Verbal Therapy point of view, the major worry concerning using digital media with children is that it can interfere with language acquisition and the learning of social skills. If a caregiver believes that use of such media can substitute for the presence of and the interaction with an adult, then precious time with the child who needs more spoken language input than children with typical hearing is lost, never to be regained. Anything that gets in the way of spoken language learning likely limits the acquisition of literacy, so if *screen time* replaces listening and talking, the child will not make the same progress she or he would if someone were engaging the child in conversations about interesting experiences.

Used in ways that stimulate interactions, digital media can bring the outside world to a child in enriching ways. Photographs, videos, and interactive programs can offer much to a child, and the best use of them is in the presence of an adult who uses well-formed language to talk about what is appearing on the screen. Such use is similar to using traditional materials for reading or writing with a child. For example, there are phone and tablet apps where language experience books can be created with a child.

In reporting on a study done in British classrooms with children ages 3 to 4, 4 to 5, and 7 to 13, Flewitt, Messer, and Kucirkova (2014) distinguish between closed and open content in apps being used with children. Closed content apps assume a transmission model of learning that attempts to fill the learner with particular knowledge. Such knowledge often includes phonics and vocabulary, and the approach of such apps is one of drilling and rewarding correct responses. Children often tire of this quickly, whether it is presented on paper or by electronic means.

Open content apps assume that children learn through extensive interaction; they invite children's creative engagement in activities such as composing stories, and they support children as they learn how to develop ideas and the words for them. Children learn how to use a particular electronic device by using it, regardless of the open or closed character of instruction. Flewitt, Messer, and Kucirkova (2014) observed older children exhibiting enthusiasm for complex planning while using tablets to collaborate in writing a play, acting out their writing, and then using a camera to preserve their work. They conclude that such use of electronic devices can provide "a rich platform for language and communication, collaborative problem-solving, negotiating meanings and sharing experiences" (p. 302), but they caution that "unless 'new' digital devices are woven innovatively into the fabric of classroom practice, their potential positive use could easily become no more than a device for delivering repetitive curriculum content, albeit with added interactive multimedia appeal" (p. 303). These same writers challenge practitioners to explore and develop interactive ways to use the technology offered by phones, tablets, and computers so that children's language and vocabulary grow in ways that support literacy.

In AVT, the interactions between an adult who provides high quality narration and the child who is jointly engaged with the adult is critical for the child's learning regardless of the medium used. Rather than focusing on the technology, parents, teachers, and practitioners focus on the content that children can learn and use in multiple interactive ways. This content can come in real life experiences or in virtual (digital) experiences, but it is the spoken and written language provided by the adults that makes the difference; "the most logical conclusion to be drawn from the existing scholarly literature is that it is the educational content that matters—not the format in which it is presented" (Wainright & Linebarger, 2006, p. 3). In summary, the position of the NAEYC and the Fred Rogers Center offers suitable guidance for those who work with and care about young children with hearing loss:

"Technology and interactive media are tools that can promote effective learning and development when they are used intentionally by early childhood educators, within the framework of developmentally appropriate practice (NAEYC, 2009a), to support learning goals established for individual children." (p. 5)

CONCLUDING WHERE WE BEGAN: BECOMING LITERATE IS A LIFELONG PROCESS

We conclude where we began. Drawing on the immense literature concerning literacy processes and practices, we remind ourselves that becoming literate begins with listening, and listening must begin as early in a child's life as possible.

The ability to read and write at proficient levels carries with it the enormous access to human knowledge, the world of work, creativity, personal growth, and enjoyment. Reading and writing are important means to thinking, and children who are deaf or hard of hearing have the need, indeed the right, to become part of the literate world.

In conclusion, literacy is a major goal of Auditory-Verbal Therapy, and as such:

■ Reading and writing are thought processes associated with and dependent upon listening and talking.
■ The active construction and communication of meaning are the purposes of literacy.
■ Knowledge of spoken language is the prerequisite for becoming literate in that language.
■ Literacy involves mastery of complex interactions among the components of spoken language.

Where it was once exceedingly rare, it is now commonplace to find highly literate young adults with hearing loss who have used hearing technology all their lives. These individuals have few communication difficulties and are working as professionals alongside and in sustained communication with people with typical hearing. These young adults are doctors, lawyers, psychologists, information technology experts, teachers, and so on; indeed, they can be found throughout the world of work (Robertson, 2014). The primary difference between mature and diminished literacy development is the degree to which the child learns to listen and use spoken language. In Auditory-Verbal Therapy, we aim to set children who are deaf or hard of hearing on their way toward emerging literacy by helping them establish a solid foundation in spoken language on which to build a lifetime of learning and linguistic discovery.

REFERENCES

1-2-3 Learn Curriculum. (n.d.). Retrieved from http://123learncurriculum.info/

Adams, M. (1990). *Beginning to read*. Cambridge, MA: MIT Press.

Adams, M. (2002). Alphabetic anxiety and explicit, systematic phonics instruction: A cognitive science perspective. In S. Neuman & D. Dickinson (Eds.), *Handbook of early literacy research* (pp. 66–80). New York, NY: Guilford Press.

Alexander Graham Bell Association for the Deaf and Hard of Hearing. (2015). The Academy for Listening and Spoken Language. Retrieved September 21, 2015 from http://www.listeningandspokenlanguage.org/AcademyDocument.aspx?id=563

American Academy of Pediatrics. (2016). American Academy of Pediatrics announces new recommendations for children's media use. Retrieved October 15, 2019 from https://www.aap.org/en-us/about-the-aap/aap-press-room/Pages/American-Academy-of-Pediatrics-Announces-New-Recommendations-for-Childrens-Media-Use.aspx

American Speech-Language and Hearing Association. (2019). Retrieved January 5, 2019 from https://www.asha.org/public/speech/development/45/

Anderson, K. L. (2004). *Auditory skills checklist. Success for kids with hearing loss*. Retrieved from https://successforkidswithhearingloss.com/resources-for-professionals/early:intervention-for-children-with-hearing-loss

Anderson, R. (2004). Role of the reader's schema in comprehension, learning, and memory. In R. Ruddell & N. Unrau (Eds.),

Theoretical models and processes of reading (5th ed., pp. 594–606). Newark, DE: International Reading Association.

Brett, J. (1997). *The hat.* New York: G.P. Putnam's Sons.

Byrd, D., & Westfall, P. (2015). *Guided reading coaching tool.* Jacksonville Beach, FL: Professional Development Resources.

Calkins, L. (1994). *The art of teaching writing* (2nd ed.). Portsmouth, NH: Heinemann.

Caleffe-Schenck, N. (2000). Literature for listening and learning. *The Listener* (pp. 59–60).

Carson, K. L., Gillon, G. T., & Boustead, T. M. (2013). Classroom phonological awareness instruction and literacy outcomes in the first year of school. *Language, Speech, and Hearing Services in Schools, 44,* 147–160.

Catts, H. W., Fey, M. E., Zhang, X., & Tomblin, J. B. (2001). Estimating the risk of future reading difficulties in kindergarten children: A research-based model and its clinical implementation. *Language, Speech, and Hearing Services in Schools, 32,* 38–50.

Catts, H. W., & Kamhi, A. G. (Eds.). (2005). *Language and reading disabilities* (2nd ed.). Boston, MA: Allyn & Bacon.

Chall, J. (1983). *Stages of reading development.* New York, NY: McGraw–Hill Book Company.

Clay, M. (2010). *How very young children explore writing.* Hong Kong: Heinemann Publishers.

Clay, M. (1987). *Writing begins at home: Preparing children for writing before they go to school.* Hong Kong: Heinemann Publishers.

Commission on Reading of the National Council of Teachers of English. (2004). On reading, learning to read, and effective reading instruction: An overview of what we know and how we know it. Retrieved November 5, 2018 from http://www2.ncte.org/statement/onreading/www.dltk-teach.com

Estabrooks, W. (Ed.). (2012). *101 frequently asked questions about auditory-verbal practice.* Washington, DC: Alexander Graham Bell Association for the Deaf and Hard of Hearing, questions 1, 24, 25, 26, 33, 58, 67, 68, 69, 70, 71, 78, 79.

Eunice Kennedy Shriver National Institute of Child Health and Human Development, NIH, DHHS. (2000). *Report of the National Reading Panel: Teaching Children to Read: Reports of the Subgroups* (00-4754).

Fitzpatrick, J. (1997). *Phonemic awareness: Playing with sounds to strengthen beginning reading skills.* Cypress, CA: Creative Teaching Press.

Flewitt, R., Messer, D., & Kucirkova, N. (2014). New directions for early literacy in a digital age: The iPad. *Journal of Early Childhood Literacy, 15*(3), 289–310.

Flexer, C. (2018). Start with the brain and connect the dots. Retrieved from https://hearingfirst.org/downloadables/logic–chain

Fox, M. (2008). *Reading magic.* Orlando, FL: Harcourt.

Fry, D. (1966). The development of the phonological system in the normal and the deaf child. In F. Smith & G. Miller (Eds.), *The genesis of language: A psycholinguistic approach* (pp. 187–206). Cambridge, MA: MIT Press.

Geers, A., & Hayes, H. (2011). Reading, writing, and phonological processing skills of adolescents with 10 or more years of cochlear implant experience. *Ear and Hearing, 32,* 49S–59S.

Gillon, G. T. (2004). *Phonological awareness: From research to practice.* New York: NY: Guilford Press.

Goswami, U. (2000). Phonological and lexical processes. In M. Kamil, P. Mosenthal, P. D. Pearson, & R. Barr (Eds.), *Handbook of reading research* (Vol. III, pp. 251–267). Mahwah, NJ: Lawrence Erlbaum.

Graves, D. (2003). *Writing: teachers and children at work* (2nd ed.). Portsmouth, NH: Heinemann.

Hart, B., & Risley, T. (1995). *Meaningful differences in the everyday experience of young American children.* Baltimore, MD: Brookes.

Hart, B., & Risley, T. R. (1999). *The social world of children learning to talk*. Baltimore, MD: Brookes.

Johnson, C., & Goswami, U. (2010). Phonological awareness, vocabulary, and reading in deaf children with cochlear implants. *Journal of Speech, Language, and Hearing Research, 53*, 237–261.

Juel, C. (2006). The impact of early school experiences on initial reading. In D. Dickinson & S. Neuman (Eds.), *Handbook of early literacy research* (Vol. 2, p. 423). New York, NY: Guilford Press.

Justice, L. M. (Ed.) (2006). *Clinical approaches to emergent literacy intervention*. San Diego, CA: Plural Publishing.

Justice, L. M., & Kaderavek, J. N. (2004). An embedded-explicit model of emergent literacy intervention for young at-risk children: Part I. *Language, Speech, and Hearing Services in Schools, 35*, 201–211.

Kral, A., & Sharma, A. (2012). Developmental neuroplasticity after cochlear implantation. *Trends in Neurosciences, 35*(2), 111–122.

Lindfors, J. (2008). *Children's language: Connecting reading, writing, and talk*. New York, NY: Teachers College Press.

Manley, J. (2016). *Speech perception instructional curriculum and evaluation* (2nd ed.). St. Louis, MO: Central Institute for the Deaf.

Moog, J. S., Biedenstein, J. J., & Davidson, L. S. (1995). *Speech perception instructional curriculum and evaluation*. St. Louis, MO: Central Institute for the Deaf.

Moore, S. M., Perez-Mendez, C., & Boerger, K. (2006). Meeting the needs of culturally and linguistically diverse families in early language and literacy intervention. In L. M. Justice, *Clinical approaches to emergent literacy intervention* (pp. 29–70). San Diego, CA: Plural Publishing.

NAEYC and Fred Rogers Center (2012.) A joint position statement of the National Association for the Education of Young Children and the Fred Rogers Center for Early Learning and Children's Media at Saint Vincent College (2012). Retrieved October 17, 2019 from https://www.fred rogerscenter.org/wp-content/uploads /2018/03/KeyMessages-NAEYC-FRC-Posi tion-Statement-Mar-6-2012.pdf

National Council of Teachers of English. (2004). A call to action: What we know about adolescent literacy and ways to support teachers in meeting students' needs. Retrieved November 26, 2019 from http://www.ncte.org/positions/state ments/adolescentliteracy

National Council of Teachers of English. (2018). Parents as Partners in Promoting Writing among Children and Youth (English Version). Retrieved November, 26, 2019 from http://www.ncte.org/positions /statements/howtohelpenglish

National Institute of Child Health and Human Development (NICHD). (2000). *Report of the National Reading Panel. Teaching children to read: An evidence-based assessment of the scientific research literature on reading and its implications for reading instruction: Reports of the subgroups* (NIH Publication No. 00-4754).Washington, DC: US Government Printing Office. Also available on-line from http://www.nichd.hih .gov/publications/nrp/report.htm

Newman, J. (2001). *The craft of children's writing* (2nd ed.). Spring, TX: Absey & Company.

Opper, S. (1996). *Hong Kong's young children: Their early development and learning*. Hong Kong: Hong Kong University Press.

Pintner, R., & Paterson, D. (1916). Learning tests with deaf children. *Psychology Monographs, 20*.

Price, L. H., & Ruscher, K. Y. (2006). Fostering phonological awareness using shared book reading and an embedded-explicit approach. In A. van Kleeck (Ed.), *Sharing books and stories to promote language and literacy* (pp. 15–77). San Diego, CA: Plural Publishing.

Rasinski, T. V. (2010). *The fluent reader: Oral & silent reading strategies for building fluency, word recognition & comprehension*. New York, NY: Scholastic.

Reading, A-Z. (n.d.). Retrieved from https://www.readinga-z.com/

Robertson, L. (2014). *Literacy and deafness: Listening and spoken language* (2nd ed.). San Diego, CA: Plural Publishing.

Robertson, L., Dow, G., & Hainzinger, S. (2006). Story retelling patterns among children With and without hearing loss: Effects of repeated practice and parent-child attunement. *Volta Review, 106*(2), 147–170.

Scarborough, H. (1989). Prediction of reading disability from familial and individual differences. *Journal of Educational Psychology, 81*(1), 101–108.

Scarborough, H. S. (2001). Connecting early language and literacy to later reading (dis)abilities: Evidence, theory, and practice. In S. Neuman & D. Dickinson (Eds.), *Handbook for research in early literacy* (pp. 97–110). New York, NY: Guilford Press.

Schuele, C. M., & Boudreau, D. (2008). Phonological awareness intervention: Beyond the basics. *Language, Speech, and Hearing Services in Schools, 39*, 3–20.

Spears, M. (2015). *Shared reading coaching tool* (rev. ed.). Jacksonville, FL: Professional Development Resources.

Story Book. (n.d.). Retrieved from https://storybook.js.org/

Super Duper Publications. (n.d.). Retrieved from https://www.superduperinc.com/

Suskind, D. (2016). *Thirty million words initiative.* Retrieved November 26, 2019 from https://cri.uchicago.edu/portfolio/thirty-million-words/

Trelease, J. (2015). *The read-aloud handbook* (7th ed.). New York, NY: Penguin Books.

Turtle Diary. (n.d.). Retrieved from https://www.turtlediary.com/

Walker, B. (2009). *Auditory learning guide.* Retrieved November 26, 2019 from https://www.psha.org/member-center/pdfs/auditory-learning-guide.pdf

Wainright, D., & Linebarger, D. (2006) cited in National Association for the Education of Young Children and the Fred Rogers Center for Early Learning and Children's Media at Saint Vincent College. Retrieved from http://www.naeyc.org/files/naeyc/file/positions/PS_technology_WEB2.pdf

Wass, M., Anmyr, L., Lyxell, B., Ostlund, E., Karltorp, E., & Lofkvist, U. (2019). Predictors of reading comprehension in children with cochlear implants, *Frontiers of Psychology, 10*, 2155. Retrieved November 23, 2019 from https://www.frontiersin.org/articles/10.3389/fpsyg.2019.02155/full

Whitehurst, G., Falco, F. L., Lonigan, C. J., Fischel, J. E., DeBaryshe, B. D., Valdez-Menchaca, M. C., & Caulfield, M. (1988). Accelerating language development through picture book reading. *Developmental Psychology, 24*, 552–559.

Williams, A. L. (2006). Integrating phonological sensitivity and oral language instruction into enhanced dialogic reading. In L. M. Justice, *Clinical approaches to emergent literacy intervention* (pp. 261–294). San Diego: Plural Publishing.

Yopp, H. K. (November 1997). *Research developments in phonemic awareness and implications for classroom practice.* Presentation at the Research Institute at the annual meeting of the California Reading Association, San Diego, CA.

Yopp, H. K. (1999). Phonemic awareness: Frequently asked questions. *The California Reader, 32*, 21–27.

Yopp, H. K., & Yopp, R. H. (2000). Supporting phonemic awareness development in the classroom, *The Reading Teacher, 54*, 130–143.

Yopp, H. K., & Yopp, R. H. (2006). *Literature-based reading activities* (4th ed.). Boston, MA: Pearson Education.

Zgonc, Y. (2000). *Sounds in action: Phonological awareness activities & assessment.* Peterborough, NH: Crystal Springs Books.

Part IV

THE PRACTICE OF
AUDITORY-VERBAL THERAPY

Part IV

THE PRACTICE OF AUDITORY-VERBAL THERAPY

15

STRATEGIES FOR DEVELOPING LISTENING, TALKING, AND THINKING IN AUDITORY-VERBAL THERAPY

Karen MacIver-Lux, Elaine Smolen,
Elizabeth Rosenzweig, and Warren Estabrooks

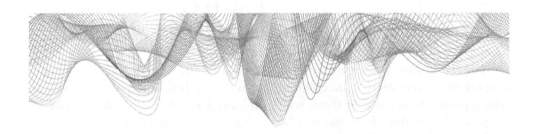

INTRODUCTION

The Auditory-Verbal Therapy (AVT) practitioner (the practitioner) coaches and guides parents to use a wide range of strategies that facilitate the development of listening, receptive and expressive language, and thinking skills in AVT sessions and, most importantly, during active family living. These evidence-based/evidence-informed strategies help the important adults in the child's life to:

■ Promote language development using natural activities, routines, and play in everyday life.
■ Tune In to the child's interests, Talk More to increase vocabulary and spoken language development, and Take Turns (Suskind,

Suskind, & Lewinter-Suskind, 2015), as they follow the child's lead while sharpening their observation and reporting skills.

- Adjust ways of talking to help the child's language grow as quickly as possible through *serve and return* events.
- Enhance listening and spoken-language interactions that lead to conversational competence among all those who engage with the child who is deaf or hard of hearing.

> **Six Goals of the Auditory-Verbal Practitioner***
>
> 1. Create a listening environment.
> 2. Facilitate auditory processing.
> 3. Enhance auditory perception of speech.
> 4. Promote knowledge of language.
> 5. Facilitate spoken language and cognition.
> 6. Stimulate independent learning.
>
> (*Adapted from Rhoades, Estabrooks, Lim, & MacIver-Lux, 2016)

A *strategy* is a plan of action, a method, an approach, or put very simply, "a way" or a combination of ways to achieve a desired outcome, such as any short-term objective (STO) determined by the practitioner and the parent. The positive application of any strategy in AVT is highly dependent on the learning styles of the child and the parents, on effective planning, delivery, and evaluation by the practitioner, and on generalization of "strategy use" in challenging hearing environments of everyday life.

The strategies presented in this chapter are often used with children with typical hearing and/or those with language delays/disorders, and can be easily woven into the fabric of everyday lives of children who are deaf or hard of hearing, whose parents, the primary agents of change in the development of their children, have chosen to pursue their desired outcomes through AVT. Each strategy promotes capturing the child's interest and the parents' imagination, as they become engaged in naturalistic intervention (child centered, play based following the child's interests, and incidental and responsive engagements) that is embraced by practitioners (Esta-

brooks, MacIver-Lux, & Rhoades, 2016). Each strategy is used to address one or more of the *six goals of the AV practitioner* for every AVT session (Rhoades, Estabrooks, Lim, & MacIver-Lux, 2016).

STRATEGIES USED IN AVT TO FACILITATE LISTENING, TALKING, AND THINKING

Presented in alphabetical order, followed by a brief example, the authors discuss a number of evidence-based/-informed strategies that are widely used in AVT to facilitate listening, talking, and thinking. There may be a number of additional strategies used by practitioners, and by no means do the authors suggest that a practitioner limit her/himself to those found here (see Table 15–1).

Accepting and Making Mistakes

Excessive background noise, unfamiliar topics or vocabulary, and/or less-than-clear

Table 15–1. Strategies and Goals of the AV Practitioner

Goals/ Strategies	Strategies Used in AVT and Goals Targeted					
	Goal #1 Create a Listening Environment	Goal #2 Facilitate Auditory Processing	Goal #3 Enhance Auditory Perception of Speech	Goal #4 Promote Knowledge of Language	Goal #5 Facilitate Spoken Language and Cognition	Goal #6 Stimulate Independent Learning
Accepting and Making Mistakes					◐	◐
Acoustic Highlighting		◐	◐	◐	◐	
Adjusting and Modifying the Listening Environment	◐	◐	◐			
Asking Stage-Appropriate Questions					◐	
Asking "What did you hear?"		◐			◐	

continues

Table 15–1. *continued*

Goals/Strategies	Goal #1 Create a Listening Environment	Goal #2 Facilitate Auditory Processing	Goal #3 Enhance Auditory Perception of Speech	Goal #4 Promote Knowledge of Language	Goal #5 Facilitate Spoken Language and Cognition	Goal #6 Stimulate Independent Learning
Connecting the Familiar with the Unfamiliar				◐		
Creating the Unexpected				◐	◐	◐
Emphasizing Actions, Relations and Attributes				◐		
Focusing on What the Child Knows		◐		◐		
Imitating Child's Vocalizations		◐	◐		◐	
Leaning Forward with an Expectant Look					◐	

Making Sound-Object Associations		●	●	●	●
Positioning Within Earshot	●	●	●		
Presenting a Listening Look with Verbal Prompt or an Auditory Hook		●			
Prompting for Auditory Closure		●		●	●
Prompting for Listening First and Last		●			
Recasting, Expanding, and Expatiating Child's Words and Utterances				●	
Scaffolding for Language Production					●
Signaling with Objects					●

continues

Table 15–1. *continued*

Goals/Strategies	Goal #1 Create a Listening Environment	Goal #2 Facilitate Auditory Processing	Goal #3 Enhance Auditory Perception of Speech	Goal #4 Promote Knowledge of Language	Goal #5 Facilitate Spoken Language and Cognition	Goal #6 Stimulate Independent Learning
Speaking Language from the Child's Angle and View				●		
Speaking Parentese		●	●	●		
Taking Turns				●	●	
Talking Before, During, and After the Action or Object Is Presented				●		
Transitioning Beyond the Comfort Zone				●		
Waiting for the Child's Response		●			●	

Source: Adapted from Estabrooks, MacIver-Lux, & Rhoades (2016), pp. 288–289.

diction make spoken messages difficult for children who are deaf or hard of hearing (Bellis & Bellis, 2015; Smaldino & Flexer, 2012). As a result, such children are at higher risk of experiencing communication breakdowns with conversational partners due to mishearing (Erber, 1981). Repeated listening and communication difficulties have been shown to have a negative impact on the child's self-concept, social communication, and social adjustment, and may increase feelings of powerlessness, frustration, anger, self-pity, and withdrawal from social interaction (Tye-Murray, 2020; Wong et al., 2018).

In AVT, parents learn that when *they lean in and get within earshot*, they demonstrate positive listening behaviors that promote social communication success. Parents also learn to celebrate their child's hearing and listening successes (e.g., "Yay! You heard the birds in the tree!").

When parents find spoken messages difficult to hear, they are encouraged to share this fact openly with their child. For example, "I heard Grandma, but she spoke so softly. I couldn't understand what she said. What about you?" Children eventually learn that factors other than hearing loss can cause listening difficulties and communication breakdowns. The practitioners encourage parents and children with hearing loss to observe other adults around them who are experiencing listening difficulties and taking steps to resolve them. Children begin to realize that the success of all communicative interactions is in part dependent on their ability to advocate for their listening needs and to use repair strategies that effectively resolve communication breakdowns (Antia, Reed, & Shaw, 2011; Suranata,

Atmoko, Hidayah, Rangka & Ifdil, 2017; Tye-Murray, 2020).

As children grow older, parents learn to take a "back seat" to allow their child time to process what was heard (to allow for internal auditory rehearsal and auditory closure) and to determine what steps need to be taken to repair any communication breakdown. When parents take a "back seat" during difficult interactions, they demonstrate for their child that they have confidence in his/her listening and communication abilities. This show of confidence gives children with hearing loss the courage they need to take risks that bring about rewards of communication success. This stimulates independent learning.

Accepting and making mistakes also applies to other domains of development, not just listening. Learning occurs daily through trial and error; especially during the first few years of life. Studies have found that learning is enhanced in children when trials are

---

Example

A practitioner brought out a musical toy and played it for 3-year-old Annika and her mother. When the musical toy stopped, the practitioner whispered, "I like this song. I've heard it before. Have you?" When the child looked at the practitioner but did not say anything, the mother leaned toward the practitioner and said, "I'm sorry, what did you say?" The practitioner smiled and repeated the statement and question. Mother nodded her head and replied, "Yes, I have. It's one of my favorite songs." Annika joined the conversation by saying, "I like it too!"

difficult and mistakes are made (Kornell, Hays, Jensen, & Bjork, 2009). Although mistakes and failures are difficult to endure, the practitioners and parents help children to realize that when times are challenging, opportunities for learning and resilience building are boundless.

Acoustic Highlighting

Acoustic highlighting is a group of strategies used to make a spoken message easier to hear, process, understand, and respond to. One or several acoustic highlighting strategies might be used for one sound, word, or phrase and include: elongating a sound; putting additional stress on a sound, word, or phrase; pausing; chunking; slowing the rate of speech; and whispering. The selection of an acoustic highlighting strategy is largely driven by the practitioner's knowledge of speech acoustics and the child's degree of auditory access to sounds across the speech spectrum.

When a child has difficulty hearing an unstressed word in a sentence (e.g., a, the, it) or a particular speech sound (e.g., s, f), the practitioner will *elongate* the key sound or word, instead of saying it louder. For example, a child may say "buh" for "bus." The practitioner would then say, "bus" and extend /s/. Two reasons for this are: many high-frequency consonant sounds and unstressed words in sentences *go by very quickly* and are easily missed by children who are deaf or hard of hearing who may have a young central auditory nervous system (CANS) that does not rapidly process speech. When the practitioner elongates the missing sound, the young CANS will be able to "catch" the sound, process

it efficiently, understand it, and use it. *Reducing the rate of speech* has a similar effect. Secondly, some consonant sounds and unstressed words are typically higher in frequency and more difficult to hear. Many well-meaning adults speak louder, thinking that it will help the child hear better, when in fact it does the opposite. Today's hearing technologies have various signal processing strategies to increase the audibility of soft speech sounds and compress (make softer) loud environmental sounds. If a speech sound is spoken loudly, the hearing technology may "interpret" it as an environmental noise, consequently making it barely intelligible or distorted sounding. Therefore, it is better for the speaker to use a conversational level of speech and elongate the misheard or unheard sound.

Whispering is used to acoustically highlight voiceless consonant sounds in words. Voiceless consonant sounds tend to get *drowned out* by louder lower frequency sounds due to upward spread of masking (see Chapter 9). When the speaker whispers a word (e.g., map, sat, pass, off) the voiceless consonant sounds are more acoustically salient.

Singing is used to acoustically highlight unstressed vowels/nasals in words or unstressed words in phrases. Singing helps to highlight the suprasegmentals that contribute to natural, pleasant, and melodic sounding speech.

Pausing may be important before modeling an important grammatical feature. Pausing uses negative space (silence), rather than changes in intensity or pitch, to emphasize the syntax in a phrase or sentence. This unexpected change in the adult's prosody captures the child's auditory attention and clues the child that important information is coming. In addition, having time to process what was said before, pausing helps the child's brain refocus on a new syntactic feature and hold new words as a chunk in his/her auditory memory (Jones, 2012). A practitioner might begin a sentence with familiar words, pause for a few seconds, and then say the unfamiliar word or words. For example, to model the past perfect progressive tense during book sharing, the practitioner might say, "The big dogs [pause] had been playing outside." Pausing before the verb construction allows the child time to chunk the words together and hold them in his/her auditory memory for later use. Parents use pausing for emphasis to model target language and to recast their child's words. If the child comments, "Mama going store," the parent can respond, "Right! Mama is going [pause] to the store." The pause emphasizes the new words added to the sentence without exaggerating the pitch or intensity of those words.

Adjusting and Modifying the Listening Environment

Practitioners guide parents in incorporating modifications to the child's daily environment so that it is quieter and less reverberant (with less echo) (Smaldino & Flexer, 2012), particularly for young listeners. Environments with poor listening conditions compromise children's ability to accurately perceive speech and learn new language (Newman, Chatterjee, Morini, & Remez, 2015). There is also an abundance of evidence that demonstrates that poor acoustics in the child's daily learning environments can create negative learning effects not only for children who are deaf or hard of hearing (Nelson & Soli, 2000) but also for children with typical hearing (Shield & Dockrell, 2003). Children younger than 7 years do not have the full complement of auditory processing skills required for spoken-language understanding and learning in non-ideal listening environments such as a daycare or preschool classroom (Bellis & Bellis, 2015).

Background noise in an unoccupied room should not exceed 30 dB (A-weigh), with reverberation less than 0.4 seconds and signal to noise ratio = +15 dB, to minimize auditory load during learning opportunities (Crandell & Smaldino, 2001). Using highly rated sound-absorbing materials such

---

Example

Five-year-old Louisa is helping her father wash the family's car. Louisa's father said, "It's really tricky to get the dirt off the tires. This sponge doesn't work!" Louisa replied, "That sponge does work. How about water?" Noting Louisa's confusion between *does* and *doesn't*, her father decided to emphasize the difference using the acoustic highlighting technique of pausing. Louisa's father replied, "Water sounds good. But did you say that the sponge does work or the sponge [pause] doesn't work?" The pause allowed Louisa to listen to the correct form, and she replied, "The sponge doesn't work." Louisa's father laughed and said, "Okay. Forget about the sponge!"

Example

In the house, there is carpet in the living room and the child's bedroom. There is tile in the foyer, but the ceilings are low and there are paintings on the walls. The kitchen has fabric place mats on the tables, and there are wooden blinds at the windows. The television and radio are off to reduce background noise.

---

need to be avoided (Seep et al., 2000) because when exposed to hearing technology, these can create external noise that distracts the *listening child* and interferes with comprehending speech. Lastly, parent(s) learn to control the noise level in their home environment by ensuring that noises from household appliances and television/radio are kept to a minimum, particularly when engaged in conversations and experiences that provide rich language learning opportunities.

as ceiling tiles, throw rugs, corkboard bulletin boards, and window blinds reduce reverberation. Sources of mechanical noise such as fluorescent light bulbs and air conditioning/furnace noise

Conversely, the practitioner and the parent may choose to introduce background sounds and/or noise to challenge the child's auditory processing skills. The type of noise, the source (location),

Table 15–2. Levels of Difficulty for Figure Ground Tasks that Facilitate Development of Auditory Processing Skills

Figure Ground (Presence of Noise)	Easier	More Difficult	Most Difficult
Source (location)	Noise presented on opposite side of better ear at a distance of 12 ft or more.	Noise presented on midline (center) of the listener's head at a distance of 12 ft or more.	Noise presented on side of the better ear, at a distance of 6 ft. or less.
Type	Consistent fan-type noise (e.g., white noise).	Intermittent environmental sounds (e.g., sound of cutlery being used in a restaurant; background music).	Speaker babble and multiple talkers (e.g., multiple conversations at dinner table and in a restaurant).
Loudness	Softer than conversational speech.	Same as conversational speech.	Louder than conversational speech.

and the position of the listener in relation to the person speaking can be manipulated to increase or decrease the complexity of listening tasks (see Table 15–2).

Asking Stage-Appropriate Questions

Stages in all developmental domains are perceived to be hierarchical, integrative, and universal. This means that children rely on previously learned skills to fine-tune and develop new linguistic skills and despite differences in cultures and environments, children seem to proceed through the stages of language development in the same order. When children demonstrate the linguistic competence to understand and answer stage-appropriate questions, parents can seize valuable opportunities to ask questions that facilitate the development of higher-level skills in listening, spoken language, and critical thinking. But the key is knowing how to ask stage-appropriate questions that *keep the conversation going* (Pepper & Weitzman, 2004). There is evidence to suggest that parents naturally adjust the type and complexity of their questions as their children grow (Kuchirko, Tamis-LeMonda, Luo, & Liang, 2016). While questions form an integral part of any conversation, questions that are poorly matched to children's language level do not help them grow their language skills.

When children exhibit language delays, many parents ask endless questions, eliciting labels, yes/no answers, or already known information (e.g., an adult who is eating asks the child, "Am I eating?" when it is obvious that she is),

confusing this with true language facilitation. These types of questions often put children on the defensive, and they end up talking less and engaging less during parent–child interactions (Pepper & Weitzman, 2004).

The practitioner encourages parents to first observe their child, wait, and listen to what he/she has to say (Pepper & Weitzman, 2004). When all is quiet, then the parents are encouraged to make a *self-statement* (e.g., "I'm hungry. I am going to eat your yummy looking cupcake!"). Such a statement may elicit a protest from the child. Then the adult asks stage-appropriate questions to keep the conversation going (e.g., "Why can't I eat your cupcake?"), being careful to match the child's interests. Practitioners encourage parents to ask sincere questions they don't know the answer to. Other strategies, such as "*pretending that objects are something else, creating the unexpected (sabotage), talking with imaginary friends,*" hook children into conversations that grow listening, spoken communication, and cognitive skills.

Asking "What Did You Hear?"

Promoting self-advocacy skills, even for very young children, is crucial in AVT. One way practitioners and parents encourage children to take responsibility for their own listening is by asking, "*What did you hear?*" When a child requests clarification, does not respond to a question, or experiences another communication breakdown, it might seem natural simply to repeat the message. However, asking "*What did you hear?*" engages children in active listening

---

Example

Two-year-old girl Sutha, who was recently diagnosed with a moderate sensorineural hearing loss, attended her first AVT session with her father, who admitted that he was feeling anxious about Sutha's current receptive and expressive language skills. The practitioner asked him to tell her more about Sutha's current skills and what the parents wanted to get out of AVT sessions. Sutha found a doll and a box of doll-sized clothing. The father quickly joined Sutha on the floor and asked several questions one after the other: "What's that?" "Is that a dolly?" "What color is this dress?" Sutha got up and moved to the other side of the room where she found a boat. The practitioner suggested to her father that it was best to let Sutha lead the conversation. The practitioner quietly joined Sutha and observed her play and invited the father to join his daughter. The practitioner caught Sutha's gaze and she *leaned in* and *looked expectantly*. Sutha said, "Boat go!" The practitioner smiled and said, "Yes, the boat is going. I wonder where the boat is going?" Sutha smiled and said, "Boat go home!" Father looked relieved. Upon the practitioner's signal, Sutha's father joined the conversation by saying, "The boat is going home. Can I come?" Sutha giggled and said, "No, you stay here!"

---

and encourages them to trust their own hearing. It allows them to think about what parts of the message were and were not understood and attempt to fill in any "blanks" in the conversation. Asking children to repeat the part of the message they understood also helps the practitioner or parent to diagnose what the child hears. Based on the child's answer, the adult can assess where the breakdown in listening occurred and track patterns in the child's listening comprehension across settings. Rosenzweig and Smolen (2018) found that certified Listening and Spoken Language Specialists were significantly more likely to report using this advanced strategy than non-certified practitioners. The practitioner and or caregiver first assesses the listening environment. If distance or background noise (e.g., a passing ambulance, a loud television) may truly have prevented the child from hearing, the adult will repeat the message. However, if the adult judges that the child likely missed only part of the message or requested repetition because he/she was not confident in listening, asking *"What did you hear?"* is very helpful.

Connecting the Familiar with the Unfamiliar

Childhood is an exciting time—there is so much new to see, do, and learn. For practitioners and parents, helping children who are deaf or hard of hearing to learn all the new words and language structures they need can seem overwhelming. A developmental approach, however, simplifies the process because skills build upon each other. *Children learn best through connecting the familiar—words, syntax, concepts—to*

Example

While preparing dinner, Jeffrey's mother asked, "Can you ask Daddy to get a knife?" Jeffrey responded, "Huh?" His mother asked, "What did you hear?" in an encouraging tone. Jeffrey replied, "I heard 'Can you ask Daddy to get a nice?' which, of course does not make sense." Jeffrey's mother made a mental note of the confusion of /s/ and /f/, two high-frequency sounds, as well as his ability to use top-down processing to realize that what he heard could not be right. Jeffrey's mother then used *acoustic highlighting strategies* to emphasize the final /f/ in *knife* and consequently helped him to identify clues from the context (food preparation) to fill in the missing auditory information (promote auditory closure).

---

the unfamiliar. Vygotsky (1978) theorized that children learn from interacting with adults who model language that is just above the language children can produce on their own. Using familiar vocabulary to teach new sentence structures or explain *unfamiliar words connects the familiar to the unfamiliar* and ensures that language input is appropriate and meaningful (Huttenlocher, Vasilyeva, Cymerman, & Levine, 2002).

Practitioners use this strategy when planning and delivering AVT sessions that introduce a new language target or concept. Using known farm animals and colors when introducing the combination of an attribute and an entity, for example, encourages the child to focus on the unknown (the new two-word utterance) without struggling with the known (the familiar color and animal vocabulary). Being thoughtful about the balance between known and unknown items in a session sets the child up for success while being challenging. Parents *connect the familiar to the unfamiliar* when they explain new concepts using familiar ones (e.g., explaining the new category word *dessert* by giving known examples—*cookies, ice cream, pudding*—and descriptors—*sweet, chocolate, lemon*). They might also prompt the child to engage in a new dramatic play routine like cooking, which might be abstract, by discussing real experiences cooking, looking at familiar pictures, or reading a familiar book.

Example

Bella is a 3-year-old who loves to draw pictures. She drew pictures of the different flavors of ice cream she had enjoyed earlier. Bella's mother purposely withheld a few crayons that were varying shades of pink. Bella asked for a pink crayon. Bella's mother replied, "I have so many different shades of pink crayons. This one here is bubblegum pink. This one is fuchsia. Which one do you prefer?" Bella replied, "Bubblegum pink!" This was a new color, which was easy for Bella to remember because she knew the words "bubblegum" and "pink."

Creating the Unexpected

The strategy of creating the unexpected is commonly referred to by practitioners as *sabotage*. It's a magical strategy—one that really seems to get children using their spoken language and critical thinking skills.

To *create the unexpected*, the practitioner might bring out a "mystery" box that's never been seen before, full of trinkets that children don't typically see (e.g., an old-fashioned camera, kaleidoscope, an unwrapped present, clocks, calculators). *Magic tricks* are also a hit, and questions like "How did that happen?" "Where did it disappear?" "Can I try?" begin to flow. The unexpected is also created when adults pretend objects are something else. A banana becomes a telephone. A monkey can jump on a bed that's really a sandwich. This is a critical stage of development in play that children go through that *facilitates development of spoken language and cognition* (see Chapter 13). Finally, the unexpected can take a journey into the child's (and adult's) imagination, where *conversations with imaginary friends* or personified objects present limitless opportunities for development of Theory of Mind (ToM) (see Chapters 13 and 14) and role-play—key ingredients for social communication success.

Sabotage is created when something gets stuck or a bottle can't be opened. Parents learn to become "helpless" or "clueless" so that children are motivated to use their "spoken language savvy to save the day." It's important to ensure that any sabotaged situation can be easily rectified. Otherwise, unresolved conflicts or problems can create disappointment, frustration, and

Example
An AVT session appeared to be "falling apart" and 4-year-old Louis was quickly running out of patience. The practitioner brought out a large envelope that contained a map that leads to an old and forgotten treasure. Louis became interested when he heard the word "treasure." An unexpected departure from the AVT session plan brought the AVT session back on track. The practitioner was able to target all of the planned short-term objectives (and more) by the time the treasure was found.

distrust, especially for children who have sensory and/or emotional regulation challenges which hinder learning.

Emphasizing Actions, Relations, and Attributes

Babies and children learn to understand and use the language in which they are "bathed" by caregivers every day. While it is often easiest to talk about the objects in the child's environment (e.g., "Look! It's a bird!" or "Here are your hands."), children also need plenty of practice listening to and using other types of words. *Attributes*, like color and size, describe objects, while *relations* explain their relationships with one another. Objects and people can perform *actions* or have actions done to them. Emphasizing these words in everyday routines helps build larger, more flexible vocabularies and sets the stage for children to combine words into their first phrases and sentences

(Boehm, 1983). Attributes and relations, like position (*first/last*), location (*above/below*), and size (*long/short*), are part of a lexical category called basic concepts. Studies have shown that basic concepts, which are often unstressed in connected speech, can be difficult for children who are deaf or hard of hearing to acquire (Bracken & Cato, 1986; Rufsvold, Wang, Hartman, Arora, & Smolen, 2018).

Because children's early understanding of basic concepts has been shown to predict later academic success, practitioners and parents need to emphasize actions, attributes, and relations in their daily interactions with children. Narrating playtime or household routines is an excellent way to use this strategy. Instead of simply labeling an object of interest, such as a ball, adults can emphasize its attributes (e.g., "a big, squeaky ball") or actions the child takes with it (e.g., "You're bouncing the ball!"). They can also use relation words to describe its position, adding *acoustic highlighting* as appropriate (e.g., "The ball bounced *under* the table!").

Focusing on What the Child Knows

In AVT, the use of audition is the natural pathway to build fluent language skills, not to produce parrots who are able to produce speech (a physical skill) without the cognitive underpinnings of linguistic knowledge. As such, the focus in an AV session is on growing the child's receptive language skills (language understanding) before focusing on expressive language use. A child must *understand* a target (e.g., vocabulary word, grammatical morpheme, syntactic structure) before he is able to *use* it in his own conversational language.

For example, instead of asking a child to label pictures in a book by using questions such as "What's this?" and "What's that called?," the adult first bathes the child in language, providing abundant, context-bound models of the new vocabulary, and asks the child to participate in receptive tasks (e.g., "I want to play with the *elephant*, can you give it to me?") before expecting the child to use the target word ("elephant") expressively. While it can be tempting for parents to ask children to "Repeat after me" and produce desired words and phrases, a child's ability to imitate a phrase does not necessarily indicate that the child understands what he's saying or is able to use the words he's repeated in his own, novel linguistic combinations.

Example

Helga is a 3-year-old who was getting ready to give her older brother, Stefan, a birthday party. Stefan was in charge of blowing the balloons. Helga said, "I want a pink balloon!" Knowing that Helga was learning to understand and use combinations of attributes, Stefan replied, "You have so many pink balloons already! Look! You have a big, pink balloon, and a long, pink balloon, and a really short, pink balloon!" Helga pouted and said, "I want a small, round balloon!" Stefan replied, "Okay! How about a small, round balloon that's green!" Helga replied, "No, I want a small, round balloon that's pink!"

Example

Four-year-old Archie was playing with trains and his father was helping him build the track. When the track was constructed, it was time to put the trains together. Archie's father asked for the caboose. Archie looked puzzled because he had never heard the word before. Archie's father added, "The caboose is the very last train and it's red and has a deck." Archie quickly grabbed the caboose and put it in the last position of the line-up of trains.

Imitating Child's Vocalizations

When the adult imitates the child by repeating the child's vocalizations or utterances, the adult is facilitating several domains of development: auditory processing by strengthening auditory memory and increasing cognitive resources by accessing attentional reserves (AuBuchon, McGill, & Elliott, 2019) and spoken language by helping the child to learn to self-monitor and correct his/her own speech and expressive language—essential for the acquisition of fluent and intelligible speech (Perkell, 2008).

As children mature, their ability to remember information improves and this improvement has been linked to changes in verbal control processes such as auditory rehearsal (AuBuchon et al., 2019). There is evidence to suggest that children rely on "attentional resources" during auditory rehearsal and when there are irrelevant sounds (e.g., back-ground noise), or when children's attention is diverted, subsequently affecting their ability to remember what they heard (Elliott & Briganti, 2012). Verbal auditory rehearsal, therefore, is key to strengthening auditory memory. To raise the bar in listening, auditory rehearsal tasks can be made more difficult by introducing a variety of distractors such as engaging in a manual task (listening to multiple step directions while making a craft) or by introducing background noise. As the child grows older, he/she learns to use *internal auditory rehearsal* to aid the process of auditory closure when a spoken message was misheard. The child replays the "recording" of what was heard over and over in his/her mind, until the child figures out what the message likely was.

When facilitating the development of spoken language, parents are coached to imitate their child's utterances and add strategies such as *expansion, recasting*, or *expatiation*. In this way, children are able to learn from expanded models of their utterances. The "auditory feedback loop" also plays an important role in helping children learn to self-monitor and correct their own speech (output) by comparing their output with that of the adult model (Perkell, 2008). Mater-

---

Example

Jonah is a 7-month-old baby. He was in his daddy's arms, getting lots of cuddles and kisses. Jonah said, "Da, da, da, da!" and reached out his arms. Daddy replied, "Da, da, da, da? You want your daddy to give you another kiss?" and then he kissed Jonah's nose.

nal input influences children's language productivity; contingent language measures (e.g., imitations, interpretations, expansions) were related to high levels of productivity in children and such findings support the use of language intervention based on increasing maternal responsiveness for children at the one-word stage of language development (Girolametto et al., 2002).

Leaning Forward with an Expectant Look

Rather than constantly prompting children with "Say . . . " or "Repeat after me," practitioners make use of a more pragmatically appropriate prompt for conversational turn-taking: *the expectant look. By leaning in toward the child with eyebrows raised* (or any other appropriate cue of "your turn" in that child's particular language/culture), adults signal that a response is expected. The expectant look in AVT is perhaps just a slightly more exaggerated version of the nonverbal cueing used by all competent verbal communicators at the end of a conversational turn. Van den Dikkenberg-Pot and van der Stelt (2001) characterized *"a very expectant look"* (p. 4) as a strategy used by mothers of children who are deaf or hard of hearing to elicit conversational participation. The *expectant look* has also been identified as an elicitation strategy by researchers studying language of children with and without communication disorders (Strong & Shaver, 1991).

In an AVT session, if the practitioner asks a question and does not receive a response from the child, he/she may use one of several strategies discussed elsewhere in this chapter: *wait time, modeling,* or *giving the child an expectant look.* Likewise, parents may do the same at home during conversations when the child does not take his turn appropriately in the dialogue.

> **Example**
>
> Four-year-old Marisa, her older brother, and her grandmother were finishing their breakfast and making plans for the day ahead. Her grandmother asked, "I wonder what you guys would like to do today." Her brother replied, "Go to the library!" Marisa, not realizing that she was expected to take a turn, continued eating and did not respond. Her brother and grandmother waited a few moments and then leaned forward with their eyebrows raised. Marisa said, "Oh! I don't want to go the library. I want to play in the backyard."

Making Sound-Object Associations

Right from the beginning, practitioners use strategies that encourage children to attend to the sounds and speech of their daily environment. Once children spend time immersed in the sounds of their environment, they begin to attach meaning to what they hear. When children understand that sounds and spoken language have meaning, they are motivated to produce utterances to communicate their observations, wants, and needs.

Practitioners commonly use this strategy with the Learning to Listen Sounds (LTLS) that are used with beginning listeners, who need sounds and spoken language to be as acoustically salient as possible, and simple enough for the immature CANS to process. When sounds and spoken messages are easily processed, cognitive and sensory resources can be easily accessed that facilitate receptive and expressive language development.

LTLS (Estabrooks,1994, 2006) consist of a selection of onomatopoeic sounds, words, and/or phrases that imitate or resemble the source of the sound or are associated with their referent, such as "moo" for the cow and "choo choo" for the train. Representations of the LTLS vary among practitioners in different parts of the world because the LTLS need to match the linguistic and cultural system of the child and his/her family (Rhoades, Estabrooks, Lim, & MacIver-Lux, 2016).

The slower tempo of the LTLS (three sounds per second) facilitates the discrimination of sounds and words (auditory processing) (Goldstein & Schwade, 2008). Furthermore, changes in pitch and tone help gain and maintain the child's attention and facilitate auditory memory (Singh, Nestor, Parikh, & Yull, 2009) and understanding of the emotional content in language that promotes linguistic and social development (Kaplan et al., 1996).

Many LTLS consist of vowels and diphthongs that have first formants that are *audible* to most children with low-frequency hearing; other LTLS consist of consonant sounds that contain bursts of energy clustered in the mid- and high-frequency ranges (Estabrooks & Marlowe, 2000). When LTLS are presented, increased stress is placed on certain syllables or vowels; whispering is used, and the tempo (rate) varies from sound to sound; all are examples

> **Example**
>
> Two-year-old Shaneka was in an AVT session with her father where they were playing with a toy farm and farm animals. The practitioner had many farm animals that were waiting to join Old MacDonald. The practitioner sang, "Old MacDonald had a farm, ee-ii-ee-ii-oh! And on that farm, he had a cow, ee-ii-ee-oo. With a . . . " then *leaned in and looked expectantly.* Shaneka's father looked puzzled and looked at Shaneka for help. Shaneka sang, "moo, moo, here and moo-moo there!"

of strategies that provide acoustic highlighting. Thus, LTLS enhance auditory perception of speech.

Finally, LTLS are mostly vowels, diphthongs, and/or consonant sounds that children typically *begin producing* within the first two years of life. For example, infants pick up the vocal cues of infant/child directed speech and will often pattern their babbling after it (Goldstein & Schwade, 2008). From 12 months of age onward, children produce approximations of many of the LTLS and phrases heard throughout their daily routines and activities and begin to use novel combinations of *LTLS* followed by words and sentences to communicate their observations, wants, and needs, and thus these sounds help to facilitate spoken language and cognition.

Positioning Within Earshot

For children who are deaf or hard of hearing, seating is tremendously important, especially with today's hearing technologies that have directional microphone capabilities. When the speaker locates himself/herself in an ideal geographical manner (on the child's better ear if the hearing loss is asymmetric), the child has an easier time hearing spoken language, and perception of the speech signal will be clearer because of the higher integrity of cochlear and auditory-neural structures. Even the listener's head position (head up vs. head down vs. head positioned straight ahead) has an impact on the quality of the speech signal the listener receives due to directional/omnidirectional microphone capabilities. Finally, when the speaker *leans in close* (within 6 inches of the microphone) the integrity of the speech signal is at its best (Madell, Flexer, Wolfe, & Schafer, 2019). The adults can gradually introduce more challenging seating geography so that the child develops higher-level auditory processing skills that promote spatial hearing—key for listening success on the playground or in the preschool/nursery setting where children are constantly in motion. See Table 15–3 for ways that the AV practitioner and parent(s) can adapt speaker position in relation to the listener to fine-tune and develop higher-level auditory processing skills.

> **Example**
>
> During an AVT session, a parent asked the practitioner what could be done to make spoken language easier for her child to hear at a large family gathering. The parent explained that the table is rectangular and seats about 16 people. The practitioner suggested that the baby sit at the head of the table with his parents seated on either side. This way, the voices of multiple talkers at the table will not be directed toward the microphone of the hearing technology. Additionally, the parent was reminded to *lean in* so that speech becomes more acoustically salient against the background noise.

Table 15–3. Levels of Difficulty for Speaker Position in Relation to the Listener

Position of Speaker	Easier	More Difficult	Most Difficult
Distance Between Speaker and Listener	6–12 inches	3–6 feet	>6 feet
Speaker Position	In front of listener or beside listener on side of better ear/hearing technology.	Beside listener on opposite side of better ear/hearing technology.	Behind listener.

Presenting a Listening Look with a Verbal Prompt or an Auditory Hook

Children rely on auditory attention for both bottom-up and top-down processing, particularly when listening conditions are poor (Halliday, Moore, Taylor, & Amitay, 2011). When children demonstrate good auditory attention, they have developed a "listening attitude" (Holstrum et al., 2008).

Throughout the child's early stages of auditory development, there are four different components of attention. The first component is *arousal*—the ability to detect and respond to a sound (Gomes et al., 2000). Arousal appears to develop rapidly in the first two months of life (Leibold, 2012). The second component is *orienting*, which is an automatic behavioral response where the listener turns toward the sound (Gomes et al., 2000). The last two components are auditory *attentiveness* (or *sustained attention*) and *selective auditory attention*. Attentiveness is the listener's ability to maintain attention through hearing, while the sound is being presented and to remain "on task" at the same time (Leibold, 2012). Children rely on their attentiveness when they are listening to stories, songs, and spoken language. Selective auditory attention is the listener's ability to tune out unimportant sounds and focus on only the voice or sound that's desired (Leibold, 2012). It is helpful for children to be encouraged to listen to select auditory input of importance. Although practitioners observe all stages of development, attentiveness and selective attention are types of auditory attention in addition to auditory processing that are of particular interest.

When parents present a *listening look*, they are modeling positive listening behaviors that promote the development of auditory attentiveness and selective auditory attention. When the child observes the parents listening, he/she learns that there is something important to listen to.

If the child does not respond to the listening look, the practitioner or parent presents a *verbal prompt* or "*auditory hook*" to draw the child's auditory attention to the sound or spoken message. The practitioner and/or the parent will pair the listening look with a verbal prompt such as "Listen" or "I heard something" or "Did you hear that?" When the child is older, the person speaking may say the child's name to get attention or may use a variety of short phrases or expressions such as, "Hey! I got something to tell you!" or "Listen to this!" *These are auditory hooks.*

Verbal prompts/auditory hooks need to be used sparingly and only when necessary. Otherwise, the child will depend on verbal prompts/auditory hooks for auditory attention and speech

---

Two-year-old Hassan was enjoying a Learning to Listen Sounds Lesson with his practitioner and grandmother. As they played with the airplane, Hassan noticed that his grandmother became still and adopted a "listening look." Hassan became still and listened too. The faint sound of a plane flying overhead gradually became louder and louder. Hassan said, "I hear the airplane!"

perception. Children in AVT need to be in the "listening mode" at all times.

Prompting for Auditory Closure

It's not uncommon to hear practitioners say the beginning part of a sentence, phrase, or question only and then *lean in and look expectantly* at the child or parent, waiting for either one of them to say the rest. This is commonly referred to as promoting "auditory closure" and is used to facilitate auditory processing, promote knowledge of language, and facilitate spoken language and cognition.

Everyday environments force listeners to contend with background noise and conversational partners who speak with accents, dialects, quiet voices, etc. (Bellis, 2011). Children who are deaf or hard of hearing, despite the best hearing technology and AVT, are at an even greater disadvantage than their peers with typical hearing, in difficult listening scenarios (daycare, preschool classrooms, playgrounds), where a great deal of language is learned. Consequently, auditory closure skills are essential if children are to develop and experience conversational competence and social communication success in those important childhood places. Auditory closure refers to the listener's ability to fill in missing or distorted portions of the spoken message so that the whole message is understood. This is considered a component of a group of auditory processing skills (Bellis & Bellis, 2015). For example, if an older child who is a fluent communicator in English hears the message "Monday . . . Tuesday . . . Wednesday . . . Thursday . . . "

and then a fire engine drives by, sirens blaring, obscuring the next part of the message, the listener's command of the language and auditory processing abilities allows him/her to "fill in the blank."

Hassan, Eldin, and Al Kasaby (2014) noted significant differences in auditory working memory, including auditory closure abilities, in children with cochlear implants compared with typically hearing peers. Thus, practitioners and parents need to present many opportunities for children who are deaf or hard of hearing to develop strong auditory closure skills in a meaningful manner and to model appropriate communication repair strategies when required. At first, parents and practitioners may want to use the strategy of auditory closure only in phrases/sentences that are very familiar to the child. Leaving out the last few words of a familiar song ("The wheels on the bus go . . . ") or book ("Brown bear, brown bear . . . ") provides an easy and natural introduction to this task. Once a child has the ability to engage in conversation and with linguistic competence and some sophisticated top-down processing skills, the child will be able to figure out what the missing or misheard word/phrase is in the middle of a spoken message. For example, if a child says, "I'm hungry!" His father may respond, "Well, let's have ____ for a snack!" The child might reply, "Cookies!" Eventually, children learn to combine several other skills such as *internal auditory rehearsal* (repeating over and over in their mind what they did hear) and the ability to accurately judge the context of a situation and topic of conversation to make an educated guess as to what was said. They also learn to identify when conversational repair strategies need to be used.

Pausing, waiting, leaning in, and *looking expectantly* are strategies used to prompt auditory closure. Auditory closure strategies prompt the child to finish the sentence using his/her knowledge of language (semantic and syntactic context to provide cues as to what could be missing) (Gallun, Mason, & Kidd, 2007), enhance auditory memory (Hannemann, Obleser, & Eulitz, 2007), and express observations, wants, ideas, and other thoughts using expressive language skills (Cruz, Quittner, Marker, & DesJardin, 2013).

To get babies communicating, parents use strategies that promote auditory closure by singing songs or reciting rhymes that are accompanied by finger plays, hand actions, or facial expressions. After several repetitions of the song or rhyme, the practitioner stops and looks expectantly at the baby and waits for any facial expression, vocalization, and hand/body movement that might indicate comprehension and communicative intent. If the baby does not show any response, then the practitioner looks at the parents, and the appropriate response is modeled for the baby. It is during these playful activities that parents realize that they facilitate the development of their babies' linguistic and cognitive skills by:

- being warm, positive, attentive, and encouraging by using child-directed speech and smiling, leaning in, and looking expectantly;
- being excellent observers of their babies' subtle signs of receptive and expressive communication (e.g., the baby smiles and wriggles her body after the parent sings, "If you're happy and you know it, shout hooray!"); and
- immediately providing replies are dependent and directly related to their babies' communication attempts (e.g., "That was a hooray, wasn't it?") (Bornstein, Tamis-LeMonda, Hahn, & Haynes, 2008; Lloyd & Masur, 2014).

When babies approach their first birthday, they are encouraged to "fill in the blanks" with a vocalization or a word approximation. For example, the practitioner holds up a bubble wand, and the parent says, "One, two, three . . . " and then pauses and looks expectantly at the child, who eventually says a word approximation for "blow." In this instance, it is evident that the child has the linguistic and cognitive competence to realize that the phrase is incomplete and that they need to use their words to complete the message and make something happen (Gallun et al., 2007).

As children enter the toddlerhood years, they are encouraged to use words and phrases to finish songs and rhymes such as "Itsy bitsy spider went up the waterspout, down came the ____" or "Jack and Jill went up the ____." If the child has difficulty filling in the blank, then the practitioner redirects her/his attention to the parent so that the appropriate response can be modeled. After the parent provides the model, the practitioner looks back at the child, and the child imitates the parent's model, and then the rhyme continues.

Practitioners and parents facilitate the development of higher-level linguistic and cognitive skills (critical thinking skills) by presenting incomplete sentences about sequences of events (e.g., "First, we eat breakfast, and then we will . . . ") or cause and effect relationships (e.g., "Uh oh, I dropped the egg and now it's ____") that occur throughout the child's daily routines. As the child gains confidence and additional skills in listening and spoken language, adults may try more difficult or open-ended auditory closure tasks ("For my birthday, I think I'd like a ____") where there are many possible "right" answers, and the child must draw on his or her knowledge of language rather than memorization of familiar phrases.

The adult can vary the position of the missing word within the phrase or song and the amount of information omitted or distorted. The familiarity of the context can reduce or increase the demands of top-down processing and spoken language competence required for the listener to complete auditory-closure tasks. For example, it is easier for the child to verbally "fill in the blanks" when the missing/misheard word(s) is in the final position of the sentence than when the missing word is at the beginning of the phrase. Refer to Table 15–4 to see examples of auditory closure tasks that vary in levels of difficulty to scaffold learning for the development of higher-level auditory processing and spoken language skills.

Table 15–4. Levels of Difficulty for Auditory Closure that Facilitate Auditory Processing

Auditory Closure	Easy	More Difficult	Most Difficult
Position of omitted utterance	Brown bear, brown bear, what do you -----? Are you thirsty? Drink some ---. The car is dirty and needs to be --.	Brown bear, ----- -----, what do you see? Are you ----? Drink some water. The car is -- -- needs to be washed.	----- -----, ---- -------, what do you see? ---- ----- thirsty? Drink some water. ---- ---- is dirty and needs to be washed.
Length of omitted utterance	Brown bear, brown bear, what do you --? Are you thirsty? Drink some ---. The car is dirty and needs to be ---.	Brown bear, brown bear, ---- --- ----- ----? Are you thirsty? Drink --- -----. The car is dirty and ---- ---- ---- -----.	Brown ---, --- ----, ---- ---- ----- ------? Are you ----? ----- ----- ------. The car is --- ---- ------ ------ ----- -----.

continues

Table 15–4. *continued*

Auditory Closure	Easy	More Difficult	Most Difficult
Knowledge Context	Heard book read aloud many times and knows by heart. Speaker offers a water bottle. Standing beside a dirty car.	Heard book read aloud a few times and after re-introduction, recalls pattern. Water bottles nearby. Dirty car is far away but in sight.	Never heard book read aloud before. The phrase is used to abruptly change topic of conversation. The car is out of sight.

Example

Julius is a 14-month-old baby boy who wears hearing aids, and his mother loves to sing songs. Julius has had a lot of experience hearing his favorite songs, such as "Twinkle, Twinkle, Little Star" and "The Wheels on the Bus." The practitioner sang, "The horn on the bus goes . . . " then he stopped, leaned toward the child, and looked as if he were expecting Julius to say something. Julius babbled, "Ee, ee, ee" (beep, beep, beep) and punched his fists into the air. Julius' mom smiled and said, "Yeah, that's right, baby! The horn on the bus goes beep, beep, beep!"

Prompting for Listening First and Last

Sometimes children have difficulty hearing parts of a spoken message, particularly when auditory access is less than optimal or when the spoken message is presented in non-ideal listening conditions. Most daily communication takes place in noisy environments and speakers do not always use clear diction. Therefore, children who are deaf or hard of hearing need to develop strong auditory processing skills so they can experience lifelong listening and social communication success. Auditory processing skills are developed when listening is prioritized first and last; auditory pathways must receive auditory input in order for auditory processing (and development) to occur.

When it's clear that parts of a spoken message were misheard, the practitioner coaches the parents to use various forms of *acoustic highlighting* such as: using a slower rate of speech; putting additional stress on syllables, words, or phrases; and pausing to break longer messages into shorter chunks for easier processing. When these strategies are used, auditory input is prioritized and the central auditory neural system has the opportunity to fine-tune and develop new auditory processes and imprints (Bellis & Bellis, 2015; Madell, Flexer, Wolfe, & Schafer, 2019).

Once the previously misheard message is correctly perceived, the practitioner coaches the parents to repeat the spoken message again exactly as it was originally presented. For example, if the child requires additional cues to correctly perceive the spoken message (e.g., spoken message put into print/picture), then the spoken message is repeated as it was originally presented using natural spoken language with no additional acoustic highlighting or other cues.

Practitioners are often asked how many presentations of an acoustically highlighted message need to be presented before moving on to visual cues. The answer depends on a number of factors—an important one being the child's auditory attention. A general rule of thumb is that it's best to use

---

Example

Rosie is four and she loves to help her mother put freshly laundered and folded clothes away. Rosie grabbed some towels and raced to put them in the cupboard. Rosie's mother called out, "No, honey, those towels go in the bathroom!" Rosie replied, "Huh?" Rosie's mother waited and then decided to acoustically highlight the message by using a slightly louder voice. Rosie replied, "The bedroom?" Rosie's mother replied, "Nope! The bathroom!" Rosie said, "Oh, okay! The bathroom?" Rosie's mother confirmed, "Yes, honey, those towels go in the bathroom."

---

the "Three Strikes and Out" strategy (Estabrooks, 2006). This means that after three presentations of acoustically highlighted speech, with sufficient wait intervals between each one, other cues can be used to facilitate understanding; making sure to present the spoken message again into auditory-only condition using the originally presented delivery.

Recasting, Expanding, and Expatiating on the Child's Words and Utterances

Adults can help children grow their language skills through interactive conversations during which they model more mature, complex, and/or grammatically correct versions of child utterances. In their study of Facilitative Language Techniques (FLTs), Cruz, Quittner, Marker, and DesJardin (2013) used videotaped parent–child interactions and measures of child language development to identify what they categorized as "high level" and "low level" strategies, and identified *recasting, expansion*, and *extension* among those most effective at improving children's language skills. Extension may also be called "expatiation."

Recasting involves changing the child's utterance into a question. For example, if the child says, "Cookie?" with rising intonation to indicate a request, an adult might model, "Can I have a cookie?" *Expansion* takes the child's original utterance and reformulates it using adult syntax and semantics, but does not add new information, transforming the child's "He like cookie" to an adult model of "He like_s_ cookie_s_."

Extension adds new information to the child's utterance. If a child exclaims, "Cookie!" the adult would model, "A chocolate chip cookie!" These language facilitation strategies have been shown to significantly improve the expressive language skills of children who are deaf or hard of hearing (Cejas & Quittner, 2018). Duncan and Lederberg (2018) analyzed teacher talk in classrooms for children who are deaf or hard of hearing and in mainstream classrooms and found that *reformulations* (e.g., recasts, extensions, and expansions) along with explicit vocabulary instruction had the greatest effect on children's vocabulary growth. While child-directed talk is undoubtedly beneficial for children who are deaf or hard of hearing, incorporating these particular strategies into child-directed talk can further accelerate children's rate of language growth.

Example

Bai is a 16-month-old who was getting ready to welcome the practitioner into her home. Bai and her mother sat outside on the front steps. As Bai saw the practitioner, she yelled, "Hi!" Bai's mother yelled, "Hi, Sam!" Bai excitedly repeated, "Hi Sam!" After Sam greeted Bai with a hug, Bai said, "Dolly?" Sam replied, "I have the dolly right here!" Bai's mother gasped, "No way!" Sam nodded and said, "Yes, the dolly is in the bag." "Bag?" asked Bai. Bai's mother *asked*, "In the bag?" Bai shouted, "In da bag?"

Scaffolding for Language Production

When adults connect familiar vocabulary and concepts to the unfamiliar, they are scaffolding children's receptive and expressive language. Scaffolding also encompasses a variety of ways to help the child produce language that are slightly more complex than he/she could formulate without assistance. Like physical scaffolding on a building, this strategy builds a foundation of familiar, comfortable language and allows the child to stretch beyond this level with adult support (Vygotsky, 1978). Scaffolding has shown to promote faster vocabulary growth and the development of more complex language structures (Wood, Bruner, & Ross, 1976).

In AVT, *scaffolding* for language production might include a variety of other strategies, including *expansion, chunking*, or *the use of selected visual supports*. The adults might use expansion to scaffold expressive language when a child comments, "Doggie playing." The parent might expand, "Yes, the doggie *is* playing" and ask the child to repeat the expanded sentence. The adult may also *acoustically highlight* the word "is" to achieve the same goal. The parent might also use *chunking when modeling language* (e.g., "After we eat dinner [pause], we will get ice cream"), and then *pauses* to listen for the child to repeat each chunk separately and then produce the whole phrase. From time to time, the practitioner might have to use carefully selected visual supports, such as one block to represent each word in a target sentence, to help a child produce a new syntactic form. These visual supports

> **Example**
>
> Two-year-old Hako and his family were at the park, where they were enjoying a picnic lunch with a variety of foods. Hako took a bite of his cheese and declared, "Cheese!" with a smile. His father took the opportunity to scaffold Hako's production of a simple sentence using modeling. He took a bite of his noodles and said, "I love noodles!" Hako's mother took a bite of her pear and said, "I love pears!" Hako took another bite of cheese and said, "I love cheese!"

are used minimally and excluded as soon as the spoken information is modeled and understood in the auditory-only condition. This is also called "listen first and last" (see above).

Signaling with Objects

Children learn vocabulary, syntax, and cognitive skills through playful interaction with items in the real world. Signaling with objects occurs when the practitioner or parent points to or holds an object in order to gain the child's attention or prompt a verbal response. *Signaling with an object* has two major benefits for a child who is learning to listen and talk: it facilitates joint attention and initiates conversations about items of shared interest. Joint attention, also called shared attention, occurs when the adult and child look at the same object. Children learn vocabulary more quickly when adults establish joint attention before commenting, and the development of joint

attention facilitates more complex cognitive processing (Adamson, Bakeman, & Deckner, 2004; Brooks & Meltzoff, 2005). Picking up or gesturing toward an object while *displaying an expectant look* can also prompt children to verbalize, often by labeling or making a comment. This *joint engagement* has been shown to relate to higher expressive language skills in the future (Adamson, Bakeman, Suma, & Robins, 2019). By signaling with an object or with an expectant look, the child learns that it's his/her turn to contribute to the conversation.

Adults naturally signal with objects when playing with infants and young children. Parents pick up toys, shake rattles, and move colorful objects across the child's line of vision. Practitioners can encourage this behavior while coaching parents to pair this signaling with appropriate auditory input about the object and what it is doing. Seating the child and parent next to one another with the object of interest in front

> **Example**
>
> Eighteen-month-old Rolf was with his mother in an AVT session. Rolf suddenly demonstrated interest in his mother's mobile phone. The practitioner says, "Oh, do you want to call Daddy at work?" Rolf nodded his head. Rolf's mother picked up the phone and said, "Hi, Daddy!" and then passed the phone to Rolf. Rolf spoke into the phone and said, "Hi, Daddy!" and then he handed the phone back to his mother. Rolf's mother spoke into the phone and said, "It's me!" and then handed the phone back to Rolf, who said, "It me!"

of them encourages the child to look at the object while listening. Adults also signal with objects to promote expressive language when they pull a new toy from a bag or gesture toward an exciting item with an expectant look and then wait for a response.

Speaking the Language from the Child's Angle and View

This strategy is also referred to as parallel talk. Speaking language from the child's point of view provides rich language input about what a child sees or is doing. Just as adults are more engaged in a conversation when the topic interests them, children love to listen to language that connects to what they are doing. Research has shown that even though many strategies that "bathe" children in spoken language are very effective, parallel talk is particularly powerful (DesJardin, Ambrose, & Eisenberg, 2009; McNeil & Fowler, 1999). Talking about actions the child is making or objects he/she is noticing connects new vocabulary and syntax to items of direct visual interest to the child. In addition to building a significant repertoire of nouns (e.g., foods, toys, category names), *narrating from the child's point of view* enhances the child's understanding of verbs relevant to his/her stage of development (e.g., *holding, walking, jumping*) (Lund, 2018). Because parallel talk requires parents to attend to the child's communicative intent even before the child is able to verbalize feelings, the strategy also provides excellent opportunities to expose the child to "mental state" words related to emotions and likes/dislikes, which have been shown to develop Theory of Mind (Hofmann et al., 2016).

> ### Example
>
> Three-year-old Tunde was in the kitchen with her father and practitioner, making pancakes for lunch. Tunde's father said, "I need a bowl. A big bowl. Where is it?" He began to look for the bowl and Tunde shouted, "Up there, Daddy!" Tunde's father said, "Oh yes, that's right! It's up there in the cupboard. There it is!" As he reached up for the bowl, he said, "Oh, I'm stretching up, higher and higher! Oh, I can't reach it!" Tunde yelled in an encouraging tone, "Daddy go higher and higher! You can do it!"

Caregivers use parallel talk to narrate activities when they and the child are engaged together. Using parallel talk during playtime, parents can emphasize nouns (e.g., "You see the *kitten!*"), action verbs while *verbalizing in synchrony with movement* ("You are *rolling* the ball to Daddy"), or mental states (e.g., "You're crying because you're feeling *sad*"). Parallel talk involves simple sentences at the preverbal stage and moves on to more complex vocabulary language as the child grows.

Speaking Parentese (Infant-Directed Speech)

While many practitioners are familiar with the terms "motherese" or "parentese" (more formally and accurately called "infant-directed speech"), the speech register that includes greater pitch excursions, repetition, increased prosody, and other features designed

---

Example

A father and his 4-month-old, Haya, attend their first AVT session. The practitioner spent a few minutes observing Haya's father as he spoke to his daughter. He spoke loudly and slowly, using a tone of voice commonly used with adults. The practitioner encouraged the father when he verbalized in synchrony with his movement as he removed Haya from the car seat. As Haya's father removed his coat, the practitioner spoke using a melodic tone and had a rate of speech that flowed naturally as she narrated what the father was doing. Haya turned to looked at the practitioner. Haya's father noticed that the practitioner's voice was much quieter than his and Haya was completely engaged, listening attentively. The practitioner encouraged the father to quietly sing Haya's name, after which Haya immediately looked over to him and smiled.

---

to scaffold language learning in young children, fewer know of the term "motionese" or "infant-directed action." When comparing how adults interact with and demonstrate objects to other adults with how they talk and teach about objects with children, researchers note that infant/child-directed action is characterized by increased/exaggerated demonstrations of an object's features, demonstrations in closer proximity to the child, and performance of actions at a slower speed and with a greater number of repetitions (Brand, Baldwin, & Ashburn, 2002). This infant-directed action promotes children's attention (Koterba & Iverson, 2009), imitation (Williamson & Brand, 2014), and word learning (Brandone, Pence, Golinkoff, & Hirsh-Pasek, 2007; Matatyaho-Bullaro, Gogate, Mason, Cadavid, & Abdel-Mottaleb, 2014). Infant-directed action occurs across cultures (Gogate, Maganti, & Bahrick, 2015), and infants prefer this type of object interaction to adult-directed motion (Brand & Shallcross, 2008).

Use of infant-directed action is especially helpful to practitioners. Keeping an object of interest moving not only promotes word learning, but, when the object is held away from the talker's face, also serves as a *visual distractor* to promote listening. When playing with a toy, adults can sit beside children and hold the object of interest in front of them, moving it as they describe it and its features. Actions need to be slower and more repetitive than adult-directed action, just as infant-directed speech is slower and more repetitive than conversations between adults.

Taking Turns

Turn taking is the foundation of conversational competence. The term "a one-sided conversation" has negative connotations for a reason. While the initial research on parent–child talk focused on the quantity of words as a determining factor in child language and academic outcomes (Hart & Risley, 1995), later studies identified maternal responsivity and contingent responses to children's vocalizations as a determining factor in language growth for children both with and without hearing loss (Bloom, Russell, & Wassenberg, 1987; DesJardin & Eisenberg, 2007; Pressman, Pipp-Siegel, Yoshinaga-Itano, & Deas, 1999; Cruz, Quittner, Marker, & DesJardin, 2013; Smith & McMurray, 2018). This "serve and return" or "contingent reciprocity" has been acknowledged as a powerful tool to support the development of neural architecture in infants and young children, helping them build positive relationships with caregivers who can scaffold their language development. Zauche et al. (2017) call this interaction "language nutrition," describing it as "language exposure that is rich in quality and quantity and delivered in the context of social interactions" (p. 493).

New evidence using magnetic resonance imaging has shown what happens in the brain when children engage in more conversational turn taking with their parents and caregivers. Romeo and colleagues (2018) found that children who were exposed to more conversational turns throughout a typical day exhibited greater activation of Broca's area, the area of the brain associated with expressive language, while they listened to stories being read aloud. The children who participated in more conversational interactions had developed significantly greater expressive language through "serving up" language and having language "returned" to them by conversational partners, as well as returning the conversational attempts of others. The impact of turn taking on neural language processing and linguistic outcomes was above and beyond the effects of socioeconomic status and other factors, showing the importance of this "serve and return" strategy in children's daily lives!

It is often said that races are won in the turns, and the data teach us that language learning may be "won in the turns" as well. So how can practitioners support this rich, reciprocal, "serve and return" communication style in both AVT sessions and daily living? Harvard University's Center on the Developing Child (2019) has identified five steps for using the *serve and return* strategy; frequent practice should make these steps second nature for practitioners and parents. First, practitioners and parents need to be sensitive to early, non-verbal attempts at turn taking while sharing the child's focus of attention. A baby who repeats an action that gets a laugh or is able to push a ball back and forth with a caregiver is displaying early physical turn-taking skills. This is a foundational skill and predictor of later conversational turn-taking competence. Practitioners can help parents become attuned to their children's cues by encouraging time for observation of the child during the session and asking questions like, "What do you think interests him?" or "What do you think she is trying to tell you right now?" Second, the adult returns the child's serve by supporting and encouraging her/his curiosity and interest (e.g., by smiling or bringing an object of interest closer). Third, the adult responds in kind to the child's communicative attempts by naming or narrating the focus of their joint attention. Adults can use other strategies, such as *open-ended questions, self- and parallel talk*, and *modeling* of language to provide children with linguistic input that is responsive to their needs, interests, and desires. Fourth, the conversation continues by taking turns and waiting for responses (*wait time*). Fifth, the partners practice endings and beginnings, using pragmatically appropriate ways to initiate and end conversations.

Example

A practitioner goes to an apartment to visit a mother and her 3-month-old, Valeria, who was just fitted with hearing aids. Valeria was recently fed and was resting comfortably in her mother's arms. The practitioner watched as Valeria smiled upon seeing her mother's smile. The practitioner said, "Oh, that was lovely! Valeria is actually taking a turn in the conversation of smiles. Did you see that?" Valeria's mother smiled and said, "Are you a happy girl?" Vale-ria's eyes opened wider upon hearing her voice. The practitioner asked the mother to wait. After 5 to 6 seconds, Valeria smiled and gurgled. The mother immediately responded by saying, "You are? Yes, I think you are!" and then waited. Valeria smiled again and squirmed slightly in her mother's arm. Valeria's mother said, "Are you getting tired lying that way? How about we change positions?"

Talking Before, During, and After the Action or Object Is Presented

When the human brain experiences sensory deprivation—as is the case of children who are deaf or hard of hearing, auditory deprivation—neural "real estate" from one sensory modality can become re-purposed for other senses, in a process called "cross-modal reorganization." In children who are deaf or hard of hearing, the extent to which the auditory cortex has been reorganized to other sensory modalities (e.g., vision) is related to poorer speech perception skills (Campbell & Sharma, 2016; Glick & Sharma, 2017). Reliance on visual information for speech perception is notoriously unreliable. When the brain is "re-wired" to use vision, rather than audition, for the perception of spoken language, comprehension accuracy de-creases. Approximately 30% of the pho-nemes (speech sounds) in English are discriminable on the lips. The remaining 70% are what are called "viseme pairs"—sounds that are indistinguish-able on the lips (look in a mirror and mouth the words "pat, mat, bat" to your-self without voice—they look identical). Under the best circumstances (a clear, unaccented speaker without facial hair in a well-lit room, not chewing gum or eating food, etc.), the best lipreading is really 70% guessing—a difficult task even for an adult with a command of the language, and a nearly impossible feat for a child attempting to use this piecemeal information to *learn* a language system.

While all speech perception is an auditory and visual task (all of us—hearing and with hearing loss—use both eyes and ears to understand spoken language), children with prolonged periods of auditory deprivation may rely more heavily on visual information than auditory information, leading to decreased "bimodal fusion," the blend-ing of both visual and auditory signals for clear speech understanding (Schorr, Fox, van Wassenhove, & Knudsen, 2005). Children with cochlear implants, who rely more heavily on audition than on vision for speech understanding, display improved language abilities (Gori, Chilosi, Forli, & Burr, 2017). Thus, it is incumbent upon practitioners to help children with sensory deprivation due to hearing loss *first* overcome that deprivation with technology and *next* provide a rich, auditory-first environment to help promote appropriate neural organization of the auditory cortex for spoken language perception.

"Show and Tell" is a common feature of North American early childhood classrooms—children bring favorite items from home to show and describe to their classmates. In AVT, we flip that paradigm. Instead of "show and tell," to promote listening, AVT encourages, "tell and show." Just as it would be poor, for a physical therapist, when treating a patient with a sprained ankle to prescribe wrist exercises, it would also be poor for a practitioner to focus on *looking* when the mission is to build a child's brain architecture through listening, speech, language, and social and cognitive skills primarily through audition. Before presenting an object visually, adults need to talk about the object to help the children build their auditory-only language comprehension skills. For example, if a practitioner has planned a tea party for the AVT session, he/she needs to first introduce the activity and objects ("Let's have a tea party today! I brought a teapot, some cups and plates, and pretend cookies for us to share") before placing the items on the table. At home, parents can talk about daily routines ("Go get your shoes, it's time to go shopping") before providing visual cues (e.g., pointing to the shoes or the door, picking up the car keys or shopping bags). While this may seem like a small thing when

> **Example**
>
> Four-year-old Sitara and her aunt returned home from the nearby preschool. Sitara ran to get a coloring book and some crayons and sat down at the kitchen table. As she colored, Sitara exclaimed, "I'm hungry, Auntie!" As Sitara's aunt looked in the refrigerator, she talked about all the available snack options and Sitara listened as she colored. Auntie then closed the refrigerator door and waited for Sitara to respond. Sitara smiled and said, "Can I have a roti, Auntie?" (the third of six options presented).

a child is young, presenting auditory information first before visual confirmation at age 3 builds a brain that, in grade 3, can hear a complex auditory-only instruction (e.g., "Open your math workbook to page 15 and do all of the odd-numbered problems") without requiring visual cues. Children need to hear talk *before* an activity (to build that auditory cortex and build predictive skills), *during* the activity (to confirm what was heard, provide elaboration, and encourage conversation), and *after* the activity (to discuss the experience and cement new listening, speech, and language targets).

Transitioning Beyond the Comfort Zone

Like saplings, children may need to learn new skills in a controlled environment (think "greenhouse")—with minimal

---

Example

Five-year-old Devin is ready to order his first meal at McDonald's with his father standing beside him, ready to help or come to the rescue. Devin's father recalled the practitioner's words, "*Wait, smile, and . . . resist any urge to step in and repair conversational breakdowns.*" Devin is ready to take charge of ordering his meals!" When it is his turn, the employee says, "Hi there, how are you?" Devin looks surprised and doesn't know what to say at first. He is all ready to provide his order from the get-go. Devin's father smiles and waits. After a few seconds, Devin recovers by saying, "I'm good. How are you?" The employee replies, "I'm great! What can I get for you today?" Devin then proceeds with his order and has no difficulty answering questions.

---

noise, few cognitive demands beyond the linguistic task at hand, etc. However, listening, language, and speech do not always happen in such protected, facilitative environments—in fact, they rarely do. How then, do the practitioner and the parents help children transition from "greenhouse" to the "garden" of real-life communication?

Vygotsky (1978) proposed the concept of the "Zone of Proximal Development," focusing learning activities on the space between what the learner can do unaided (already learned tasks) and tasks far beyond the learner's current level. Tasks that the child can do with some adult support, scaffolding, and guidance provide a "just-right chal-

lenge" that pushes the child to new heights without introducing as-yet insurmountable challenges that may provoke feelings of failure or frustration. The objective is to set goals that are not so easy as to be unchallenging, but not so difficult as to be discouraging. If a child is currently producing one-word utterances spontaneously, modeling a complete, complex sentence and expecting the child to imitate it is unreasonable, but modeling a two-word phrase provides an appropriate level of challenge. Selecting tasks that are developmentally appropriate helps maximize the rate of progress while preventing or eliminating frustration (common in children with delayed language).

Transitioning beyond the comfort zone may also apply to parents, who often accept language from their child that is simpler than what the child is capable of using. Some parents avoid using language slightly higher in complexity than what the child currently understands and/or uses, thinking that it's what's required because of the hearing loss. Parents may also avoid certain situations or routines that they view as setting their child up for failure. The practitioner encourages parents to *transition beyond their comfort zone* so that children can expand their view and knowledge of the world and the spoken language that comes with it.

Waiting for the Child's Response

Practitioners and parents thoughtfully attend to what they say and how they say it, but *often not saying anything at all is surprisingly effective. Wait time,* or the *intentional use of silence* during an interaction with a child, signals to the child that a verbal or behavioral response is expected. Introducing an item or posing a question or comment and then *waiting quietly* cues the child that it is his/her turn to talk and prompts longer, more complex expressive language (Rowe, 1974). *Wait time* also allows the child to process what the adult has said and to formulate a response (Tobin, 1987). To use *wait time* effectively, *adults need to pause considerably longer than often feels natural.*

Wait time is a simple concept, but it can be very hard for adults, especially those who talk for a living! To implement this strategy effectively, the adult might ask a question or make a comment that requires a response (e.g., "What kind of cereal do you want?" or "I wonder how many trains you have"). If the child does not respond immediately, *the adult resists the urge to jump in and repeat or rephrase the message. Instead, the adult waits silently until he/she is uncomfortable and then waits some more.* This unexpected pause signals that the child is expected to say or do something. Then, the adult may *lean forward or use an expectant look.* Only after waiting at least 8 seconds does the adult ask another question. He/she needs to use more wait time before modeling appropriate language if the child still has not responded spontaneously. *Wait time* can also be implemented when the adult has not said anything at all, such as when a new object is introduced or when sabotage is used (e.g., a lid stuck on a jar).

One Strategy Can Address One Goal or Many Goals. Multiple Strategies Can Address One Goal or Many Goals

During any adult-child interaction, one strategy can address one or multiple goals of the AV Practitioner. Conversely, multiple strategies can be used to address one or multiple goals of the AV practitioner. AV practitioners observe parent-child interactions and identify the goal(s) and determine which strategy(ies) can most effectively accomplish the goal(s) given the listening, learning, and communication needs of the child and the communication style of the parent(s). Consider the following scenarios from an AVT session:

Scenario 1

A baby and his mother are playing in an early AVT session at home where there is hardwood flooring and the ceiling is high, causing speech to sound reverberant, and television is on. The practitioner addresses *Goal #1* by guiding the parents to turn off the television to reduce background noise and by introducing an area rug or blankets to reduce reverberation. Then he coaches mother to *stay within earshot* of the baby (be up close and personal) to ensure that the speech signal is louder than any background noise (*Goal #1*); capture and maintain the child's auditory attention with an acoustically salient speech signal (*Goal #2*); ensure that the integrity of the speech signal is at its best (*Goal #3*).

> ### Scenario 2
>
> A father says to his young child, "There's your chair, it's waiting for you. That's where you're going to sit." As he puts the child into the highchair, he says, "Into the highchair you go. We're going to buckle you in so that you're nice and safe! There you are. Now, you're sitting on the chair. Now you're ready to play!"

ADAPT STRATEGIES TO SCAFFOLD LEARNING

The practitioner understands that strategies can be adapted to scaffold learning. One strategy can be presented in varying ways that "raise the bar" in listening, spoken language, and cognitive development. The practitioner constantly evaluates the current functioning of the child and quickly adapts so the child becomes encouraged to develop new and more advanced skills and more listening and spoken communication success. Table 15–5 provides examples of how the practitioner might adapt a strategy to scaffold learning.

Today practitioners can rely on science, research, and cumulative practice to select strategies that work best to facilitate listening, talking, and thinking for any particular child and family (Rhoades, Estabrooks, Lim, & MacIver-Lux, 2016).

Table 15–5. Ways to Adapt Strategies to Scaffold Learning

Ways to Adapt Strategies to Scaffold Learning				
Strategy	**Easiest**	**Easy**	**Natural**	**Difficult**
Adjusting and Modifying the Listening Environment	The room is quiet.	The room is quiet with some noise outside.	The room has low level noise (e.g., fan, music).	The room is very noisy with multiple speakers.
Presenting a Listening Look with an Auditory Hook	*Sarah!* [*pause*] *Listen!* [*pause*] I hear a bird! It's in the tree!	*Listen* [*pause*] I hear a bird! It's in the tree!	I hear a bird. It's in the tree!	*Abrupt change in topic:* There's a bird's in the tree!
Acoustic Highlighting (AH) (*repetition,* singing, stress on syllable, pause)	Multiple forms of AH. *Brr, beep, beep!* I hear the [*pause*] <u>c</u>ar! Watch the <u>c</u>ar *go, go, go!* [*sing*] *Go,* <u>c</u>ar, *go!*	One form of AH. Brr, *beep, beep!* I hear the car! Watch the car *go, go, go! Go, car, go!*	No AH. Brr, beep, beep! I hear the car! Watch it go!	Fast/ mumbled/ distorted speech. Watch the car go! (spoken quickly)

TIPS FOR THE AV PRACTITIONER IN LEARNING AND USING THE STRATEGIES

AVT sessions sometimes look easy when delivered; however, they can be more difficult to plan, deliver, and evaluate than one thinks (see Chapter 18). Most new practitioners, using the strategies within interactions with the child while engaged in play, can be extremely challenged at first. Therefore, the aspiring practitioner and the parents may need to spend a lot of time learning the what, how, and why of these important strategies and then practice using them at the right time and in the right place. *Keeping It Simple and Specific* (KISS), the authors offer the *Top Five Tips* to help aspiring practitioners learn and practice these strategies.

Top Five Tips for Learning and Practicing the Strategies Used in AVT

1. Focus on practicing one new strategy each week.
2. Give yourself a short-term objective to raise the bar on your use of strategies.
3. Observe AVT sessions of highly experienced practitioners using the strategies.
4. Make a video of any AVT session and review it to evaluate your use of the strategies presented in this chapter.
5. Encourage parents to be your "armchair critic" by offering you feedback on your use of the strategies.

CONCLUSION

When parents learn how to effectively and efficiently use the strategies presented in this chapter to facilitate listening, talking, and thinking with their children in AVT sessions and in daily life, there can be considerable growth in the child's listening and spoken language outcomes and in the outcome of happy, productive parent–child interaction (Garcia, Bagner, Pruden, & Nicols-Lopez, 2015; Weitzman, 2017).

Rosenzweig and Smolen (2018) conducted an international survey on the use of strategies by practitioners who included speech-language pathologists, teachers of children with hearing loss, and audiologists, who served children with hearing loss and their families and were using listening and spoken language approaches. The results indicated that some strategies, such as *wait time*, are used by nearly all practitioners in the field. However, there were significant differences in the use of other strategies such as *whispering and asking "What did you hear?"* In these cases, practitioners who were certified Listening and Spoken Language Specialists were significantly more likely to use these evidence-informed strategies than their counterparts who were not certified.

Experienced practitioners combine observations of the child and child–family interactions with family preferences, and their cumulative experience and clinical intuition, to select and use the strategies that best serve a particular child and family at a particular time. Clinical intuition and hands-on experience analyses of child, family, and contextual factors developed through cumulative practice contribute significantly when making decisions about strategy use (Locke, 2015).

The evidence-based/evidence-informed strategies used in AVT to promote listening, talking, and thinking that are presented in this chapter can be found in best practices of typical child development. These strategies are also found in the toolboxes of most practitioners, who desire to *raise the bar* on their planning, delivery, and evaluation of the services they provide to families of children who are deaf or hard of hearing. Consequently, the authors of this chapter encourage more scientific research to verify the effectiveness of these strategies when used in the practice of AVT.

REFERENCES

Adamson, L. B., Bakeman, R., & Deckner, D. F. (2004). The development of symbol-infused joint engagement. *Child Development, 75,* 1171–1187.

Adamson, L. B., Bakeman, R., Suma, K., & Robins, D. L. (2019). An expanded view of joint attention: Skill, engagement, and language in typical development and autism. *Child Development, 90*(1), e1–e18.

Antia, S. D., Reed, S., & Shaw, L. (2011). Risk and resilience for social competence: Deaf students in general education classrooms. In D. H. Zand & K .J. Pierce (Eds.), *Resilience in deaf children: Adaptation through emerging adulthood.* (pp. 139–167). New York, NY: Springer.

AuBuchon, A., McGill, C., & Elliott, E. (2019). Auditory distraction does more than disrupt rehearsal process in children's serial recall. *Memory & Cognition, 47,* 738–748. Retrieved from https://doi.org/10.3758/s13421-018-0879-4

Bellis, T. J. (2011). *Assessment and management of central auditory processing disorders in the educational setting: From science to practice.* San Diego, CA: Plural Publishing.

Bellis, T. J., & Bellis, J. D. (2015). Central auditory processing disorders in children and adults. In G. G. Celesia & G. Hickock (Eds.), *Handbook of clinical neurology, 129,* (pp. 537–556). New York, NY: Elsevier.

Bloom, K., Russell, A., & Wassenberg, K. (1987). Turn taking affects the quality of infant vocalizations. *Journal of Child Language, 14*(2), 211–227.

Boehm, A. (1983). Assessment of basic concepts. In D. Paget & B. Bracken (Eds.), *The psychoeducational assessment of preschool children* (pp. 145–216). New York, NY: Grune & Stratton.

Bornstein, M. H., Tamis-LeMonda, C. S., Hahn, C. S., & Haynes, O. M. (2008). Maternal responsiveness to young children at three ages: Longitudinal analysis of a multidimensional, modular, and specific parenting construct. *Developmental Psychology, 44*(3), 867.

Bracken, B., & Cato, L. (1986). Rate of conceptual development among deaf preschool and primary children as compared to a matched group of non–hearing impaired children. *Psychology in the Schools, 23*(1), 95–99.

Brand, R. J., Baldwin, D. A., & Ashburn, L. A. (2002). Evidence for 'motionese': modifications in mothers' infant-directed action. *Developmental Science, 5*(1), 72–83.

Brand, R. J., & Shallcross, W. L. (2008). Infants prefer motionese to adult-directed action. *Developmental Science, 11*(6), 853–861.

Brandone, A. C., Pence, K. L., Golinkoff, R. M., & Hirsh-Pasek, K. (2007). Action speaks louder than words: Young children differentially weight perceptual, social, and linguistic cues to learn verbs. *Child Development, 78*(4), 1322–1342.

Brooks, R., & Meltzoff, A. (2005). The development of gaze following and its relation to language. *Developmental Science, 8*(6), 535–543.

Campbell, J., & Sharma, A. (2016). Visual cross-modal re-organization in children with cochlear implants. *PLoS One, 11*(1), e0147793.

Cejas, I., & Quittner, A. L. (2018). Effects of family variables on spoken language in children with cochlear implants. *Evidence-Based Practices in Deaf Education, 34*, 111.

Crandell, D., & Smaldino, J. (2001). An update on classroom acoustics. *The ASHA Leader, 6*(10), 5–20.

Cruz, I., Quittner, A. L., Marker, C., DesJardin, J. L., & CDaCI Investigative Team. (2013). Identification of effective strategies to promote language in deaf children with cochlear implants. *Child Development, 84*(2), 543–559.

DesJardin, J. L., Ambrose, S. E., & Eisenberg, L. S. (2009). Literacy skills in children with cochlear implants: The importance of early oral language and joint storybook reading. *Journal of Deaf Studies and Deaf Education, 14*(1), 22–43.

DesJardin, J. L., & Eisenberg, L. S. (2007). Maternal contributions: Supporting language development in young children with cochlear implants. *Ear and Hearing, 28*, 456–469.

Duncan, M. K., & Lederberg, A. R. (2018). Relations between teacher talk characteristics and child language in spoken-language deaf and hard-of-hearing classrooms. *Journal of Speech, Language, and Hearing Research, 61*(12), 2977–2995.

Elliott, E., & Briganti, A. (2012). Investigating the role of attentional resources in the irrelevant speech effect. *Acta Psychologica, 140*, 64–74.

Erber, N. P. (1981). Introduction to aural rehabilitation. *Ear and Hearing, 2*(5), 236.

Estabrooks, W. (1994). *Auditory-verbal therapy for parents and professionals.* Washington, DC: Alexander Graham Bell Association.

Estabrooks, W. (2006). *Auditory-verbal therapy and practice.* Washington, DC: Alexander Graham Bell Association.

Estabrooks, W., MacIver-Lux, K., & Rhoades, E. (2016). *Auditory-verbal therapy: For young children with hearing loss and their families, and the practitioners who guide them.* San Diego, CA: Plural Publishing.

Estabrooks, W., & Marlowe, J. (2000). *The baby is listening: An educational tool for professionals who work with children who are deaf or hard of hearing.* Washington, DC: Alexander Graham Bell Association.

Gallun, F. J., Mason, C. R., & Kidd, G. (2007). Task-dependent costs in processing two simultaneous auditory stimuli. *Perception & Psychophysics, 69*(5), 757–771.

Garcia, D., Bagner, D. M., Pruden, S. M., & Nichols-Lopez, K. (2015). Language production in children with and at risk for delay: Mediating role of parenting skills. *Journal of Clinical Child and Adolescent Psychology, 44*(5), 814–825.

Girolametto, L., Bonivacio, S., Visini, C., Weitzman, E., Zocconi, E., & Steig Pearce, P. (2002). Mother-child interactions in Canada and Italy: Linguistic responsiveness to late-talking toddlers. *International Journal of Language & Communication Disorders, 3*(2), 153–171.

Glick, H., & Sharma, A. (2017). Cross-modal plasticity in developmental and age-related hearing loss: clinical implications. *Hearing Research, 343*, 191–201.

Gogate, L., Maganti, M., & Bahrick, L. E. (2015). Cross-cultural evidence for multimodal motherese: Asian Indian mothers' adaptive use of synchronous words and gestures. *Journal of Experimental Child Psychology, 129*, 110–126.

Goldstein, M. H., & Schwade, J. A. (2008). Social feedback to infants' babbling facilitates rapid phonological learning. *Psychological Science, 19*(5), 515–523.

Gomes, H., Molholm, S., Christodoulou, C., Ritter, W., & Cowan, N. (2000). The development of auditory attention in children. *Frontiers in Bioscience, 5*(1), D108–D120.

Gori, M., Chilosi, A., Forli, F., & Burr, D. (2017). Audio-visual temporal perception in children with restored hearing. *Neuropsychologia, 99*, 350–359.

Halliday, L. F., Moore, D. R., Taylor, J. L., & Amitay, S. (2011). Dimension-specific attention directs learning and listening on auditory training tasks. *Attention, Perception, & Psychophysics, 73*(5), 1329–1335.

Hannemann, R., Obleser, J., & Eulitz, C. (2007). Top-down knowledge supports the retrieval of lexical information from degraded speech. *Brain Research, 1153*, 134–143.

Hart, B., & Risley, T. R. (1995). *Meaningful differences in the everyday experience of young American children*. Baltimore, MD: Paul H. Brookes Publishing.

Harvard University Center on the Developing Child. (2019). 5 steps for brain-building serve and return. Retrieved from https://developingchild.harvard.edu/resources/5-steps-for-brain-building-serve-and-return/

Hassan, H. E., Eldin, S. T. K., & Al Kasaby, R. M. (2014). Psycholinguistic abilities in cochlear implant and hearing-impaired children. *Egyptian Journal of Ear, Nose, Throat and Allied Sciences, 15*(1), 29–35.

Hofmann, S. G., Doan, S. N., Sprung, M., Wilson, A., Ebesutani, C., Andrews, L. A., . . . Harris, P. L. (2016). Training children's theory-of-mind: A meta-analysis of controlled studies. *Cognition, 150*, 200–212.

Holstrum, W. J., Gaffney, M., Gravel, J. S., Oyler, R. F., & Ross, D. S. (2008). Early intervention for children with unilateral and mild bilateral degrees of hearing loss. *Trends in Amplification, 12*(1), 35–41.

Huttenlocher, J., Vasilyeva, M., Cymerman, E., & Levine, S. (2002). Language input and child syntax. *Cognitive Psychology, 45*, 337–374.

Jones, G. (2012). Why chunking should be considered as an explanation for developmental change before short-term memory capacity and processing speed. *Frontiers in Psychology, 3*, 1–8.

Kaplan, P., Jung, P., Ryther, J., & Zarlengo-Strouse, P. (1996). Infant directed versus adult-directed speech as signals for face. *Developmental Psychology, 32*(5), 880–891.

Kornell, N., Hays, M., Jensen, M., & Bjork, R. A. (2009). Unsuccessful retrieval attempts enhance subsequent learning. *Journal of Experimental Psychology: Learning, Memory, and Cognition, 35*(4), 989–998.

Koterba, E. A., & Iverson, J. M. (2009). Investigating motionese: The effect of infant-directed action on infants' attention and object exploration. *Infant Behavior and Development, 32*(4), 437–444.

Kuchirko, Y., Tamis-LeMonda, C. S., Luo, R., & Liang, E. (2016). 'What happened next?': Developmental changes in mothers' questions to children. *Journal of Early Childhood Literacy, 16*(4), 498–521.

Leibold, L. J. (2012). Development of auditory scene analysis and auditory attention. In L. Werner, R. R. Fay, & A. N. Popper (Eds.), *Human auditory development* (pp. 137–161). New York, NY: Springer.

Lloyd, C. A., & Masur, E. F. (2014). Infant behaviors influence mothers' provision of responsive and directive behaviors. *Infant Behavior and Development, 37*(3), 276–285.

Locke, C. C. (2015). When it's safe to rely on intuition (and when it's not). *Harvard Business Review*. Retrieved from https://hbr.org/2015/04/when-its-safe-to-rely-on-intuition-and-when-its-not

Lund, E. (2018). The effects of parent training on vocabulary scores of young children with hearing loss. *American Journal of Speech-Language Pathology, 27*(2), 765–777.

Madell, J. R., Flexer, C. A., Wolfe, J., & Schafer, E. C. (2019). *Pediatric audiology: Diagnosis, technology, and management.* New York, NY: Thieme.

Matatyaho-Bullaro, D. J., Gogate, L., Mason, Z., Cadavid, S., & Abdel-Mottaleb, M. (2014). Type of object motion facilitates word mapping by preverbal infants. *Journal of Experimental Child Psychology, 118,* 27–40.

McNeil, J., & Fowler, S. (1999). Let's talk: Encouraging mother-child conversations during story reading. *Journal of Early Intervention, 22,* 51–69.

Nelson, P. B., & Soli, S. (2000). Acoustical barriers to learning: Children at risk in every classroom. *Language, Speech, and Hearing Services in Schools, 31*(4), 356–361.

Newman, R. S., Chatterjee, M., Morini, G. & Remez, R. E. (2015). Toddlers' comprehension of degraded signals: Noise-vocoded versus sine-wave analogs. *The Journal of the Acoustical Society of America, 138*(3), EL311–EL317.

Pepper, J., & Weitzman, E. (2004). *It takes two to talk: A practical guide for parents of children with language delays* (2nd ed.). Toronto, ON, Canada: The Hanen Centre.

Perkell, J. S. (2008). *Auditory feedback and speech production in cochlear implant users and speakers with typical hearing.* Paper presented at 2008 Research Symposium of the AG Bell Association International Convention; June 29, 2008; Milwaukee, WI.

Pressman, L., Pipp-Siegel, S., Yoshinaga-Itano, C., & Deas, A. (1999). The relation of sensitivity to child expressive language gain in deaf and hard-of-hearing children whose caregivers are hearing. *Journal of Deaf Studies and Deaf Education, 4*(4), 294–304.

Rhoades, E. Estabrooks, W., Lim, S., & MacIver-Lux, K. (2016). Strategies that facilitate listening, talking and thinking in auditory-verbal therapy. In W. Estabrooks, K. MacIver-Lux, & E. Rhoades (Eds.), *Auditory-verbal therapy: For young children with hearing loss and their families, and the practitioners who guide them,* (pp. 285–326). San Diego, CA: Plural Publishing.

Romeo, R. R., Leonard, J. A., Robinson, S. T., West, M. R., Mackey, A. P., Rowe, M. L., & Gabrieli, J. D. (2018). Beyond the 30-million-word gap: Children's conversational exposure is associated with language-related brain function. *Psychological Science, 29*(5), 700–710.

Rosenzweig, E. A., & Smolen, E. R. (2018, June). *Not just anyone will do: Trends in AV strategy utilization.* Presented to the Alexander Graham Bell Association for the Deaf and Hard of Hearing (AG Bell), Scottsdale, AZ.

Rowe, M. B. (1974). Wait-time and rewards as instructional variables, their influence on language, logic, and fate control: Part one-wait-time. *Journal of Research in Science Teaching, 11*(2), 81–94.

Rufsvold, R., Wang, Y., Hartman, M. C., Arora, S. B., & Smolen, E. R. (2018). The impact of language input on deaf and hard of hearing preschool children who use listening and spoken language. *American Annals of the Deaf, 163*(1), 35–60.

Schorr, E. A., Fox, N. A., van Wassenhove, V., & Knudsen, E. I. (2005). Auditory-visual fusion in speech perception in children with cochlear implants. *Proceedings of the National Academy of Sciences, 102*(51), 18748–18750.

Seep, B., Glosemeyer, R., Hulce, E., Linn, M., Aytar, P., & Coffeen, R. (2000). Classroom acoustics: A resource for creating learning environments with desirable listening conditions. *Acoustical Society of America Publications.* Melville, NY.

Shield, B. M., & Dockrell, J. E. (2003). The effects of noise on children at school: A review. *Building Acoustics, 10*(2), 97–116.

Singh, L., Nestor, S., Parikh, C., & Yull, A. (2009). Influences of infant-directed speech on early word recognition. *Infancy, 14*(6), 654–666.

Smaldino, J. J., & Flexer, C. (2012). *Handbook of acoustic accessibility: Best prac-*

tices for listening, learning, and literacy in the classroom. New York, NY: Thieme.

Smith, N. A., & McMurray, B. (2018). Temporal responsiveness in mother-child dialogue: A longitudinal analysis of children with normal hearing and hearing loss. *Infancy, 23*(3), 410–431.

Strong, C. J., & Shaver, J. P. (1991). Stability of cohesion in the spoken narratives of language-impaired and normally developing school-aged children. *Journal of Speech, Language, and Hearing Research, 34*(1), 95–111.

Suranata, K. S., Atmoko, A., Hidayah, N., Rangka, I. B., & Ifdil, I. (2017). Risk and resilience of students with hearing impairment in an inclusive school. *Baltic Journal of Special Education, 2*(37), 165–214.

Suskind, D., Suskind, B., & Lewinter-Suskind, L. (2015). *Building a child's brain: Tune in, talk more, take turns.* New York, NY: Dutton.

Tobin, K. (1987). The role of wait time in higher cognitive level learning. *Review of Educational Research, 57*(1), 69–95.

Tye-Murray, N. (2020). *Foundations of aural rehabilitation: Children, adults, and their family members.* San Diego, CA: Plural Publishing.

Van den Dikkenberg-Pot, I., & van der Stelt, J. M. (2001). Mother-child interaction in two year old deaf and hearing children. In *Proceedings of the Institute of Phonetic Sciences, University of Amsterdam, 24*, 1–13.

Vygotsky, L. V. (1978). Interaction between learning and development. In *Mind and society.* Cambridge, MA: Harvard University Press.

Weitzman, E. (2017). *It takes two to talk: A practical guide for parents of children with language delays* (5th ed.). Toronto, ON, Canada: The Hanen Centre.

Werner, L. A. (2002). Infant auditory capabilities. *Current Opinion in Otolaryngology & Head and Neck Surgery, 10*(5), 398–402.

Williamson, R. A., & Brand, R. J. (2014). Child-directed action promotes 2-year-olds' imitation. *Journal of Experimental Child Psychology, 118*, 119–126.

Wong, C., Ching, T., Leigh, G., Cupples, L., Button, L., Marnane, V., . . . Martin, L. (2018). Psychosocial development of 5-year-old children with hearing loss: Risks and protective factors. *International Journal of Audiology, 57*(suppl. 2), S81–S92.

Wood, D., Bruner, J. S., & Ross, G. (1976). The role of tutoring in problem solving. *Journal of Child Psychology and Psychiatry, 17*, 89–100.

Zauche, L. H., Mahoney, A. E. D., Thul, T. A., Zauche, M. S., Weldon, A. B., & Stapel-Wax, J. L. (2017). The power of language nutrition for children's brain development, health, and future academic achievement. *Journal of Pediatric Health Care, 31*(4), 493–503.

16

COACHING PARENTS AND CAREGIVERS IN AUDITORY-VERBAL THERAPY

Karen MacIver-Lux, Warren Estabrooks, and Joanna Smith

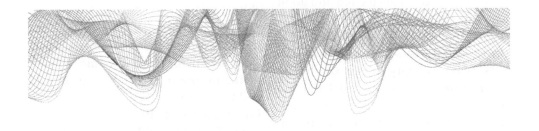

INTRODUCTION

Cultivated by its historical underpinnings and stated clearly in the Principles of LSLS Auditory-Verbal Therapy (AVT), *guiding and coaching parents* remain central to the current practice of AVT. Six of the principles begin with the words *guide and coach* and for the purpose of this chapter, the authors refer to the term as *coaching,* and to all caregivers as *parents*. The reader will find numerous examples of *coaching* parents throughout this book, and par-

ticularly in Chapters 15, 17, 21, and 22. The Auditory-Verbal practitioner (the practitioner) approaches coaching in synchrony with the planning, delivery, and evaluation of every AVT session (see Chapter 17) and the application of evidence-based/-informed strategies for listening, talking, and thinking (see Chapter 15). *Coaching parents is easier said than done* and since the concepts of coaching and adult learning do not appear in many curricula in audiology, speech-language pathology, or education of the deaf, most practitioners learn how to *coach parents on the job,* or in the processes of their own coaching and mentoring programs toward certification (see Chapter 26).

COACHING DEFINED

Coaching is an empirically based interactive process of reflection and feedback used to provide support and encouragement in refining existing practices, developing new skills, and promoting continuous self-assessment and learning (Rush, Shelden, & Hanft, 2003). The role of the *parent coach*, therefore, is to provide a supportive environment in which family members and the coach jointly reflect on current activities that encourage and enhance child and adult learning (Rush & Shelden, 2020). This definition applies very well to the practice of AVT and the development of parents as the primary agents of change in the listening and spoken language development of their children who are deaf or hard of hearing. The practitioner, as the coach, demonstrates for parents and gives them many opportunities to practice and then to evaluate by examining what they are doing in light of their intentions (Fenichel & Eggbeer, 1991).

PARENT COACHING IN AVT

Recognizing that *sound* education for the child who is deaf or hard of hearing is as much an attitude as it is an atmosphere (Silverman, 1963), Doreen Pollack, pioneer of AVT, urged practitioners to coach parents in creating the right learning environment, one in which their child who is deaf or hard of hearing could be bathed in sound, surrounded by people who believe he/she could hear, and expect the child to listen and respond in the relevant and meaningful context of daily experience (Pollack, Goldberg, & Caleffe-Schenck, 1997). In AVT, parents learn empirically based strategies that promote the child's development of listening, talking, and thinking skills that match the children's needs and real-life situations in an individualized manner (Estabrooks, MacIver-Lux, & Rhoades, 2016), and they also learn how to integrate listening into their child's entire being so that listening becomes a way of life (Estabrooks, 1994; Pollack et al., 1997). Parents develop confidence in the planning, delivery, and evaluation of strategies that promote learning in young children who are deaf or hard of hearing in AVT. This confidence has been identified as a significant variable that influences outcomes in listening, spoken communication, and cognitive skills of children who are deaf or hard of hearing (Estabrooks, 1994; Tomblin et al., 2015). Rhoades and MacIver-Lux (2016) delineated a list of the following top 5 parent coaching strategies for practitioners to use in AVT (see Figure 16–1) that mirror those used across a number of early intervention approaches in a variety of settings and include the following: (a) having conversations and sharing information, (b) collaborating in setting goals and planning activities, (c) demonstrating, (d) guided practice with feedback, and (e) providing video feedback. Parent coaching is primarily focused on promoting self-discovery that leads to greater levels of capacity and mastery of desired skills for both the child and the parents (Doyle, 1999; Dunst, Herter, & Shields, 2000; Rush & Shelden, 2020).

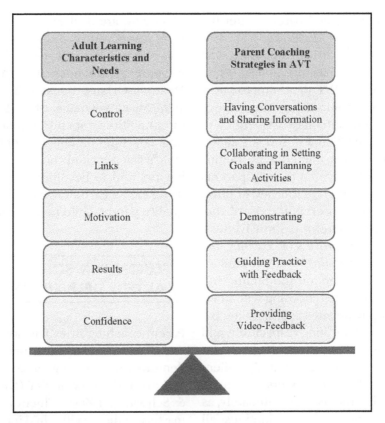

Figure 16-1. Adult learning characteristics and top five coaching strategies of AV practitioners.

Hanft and Pilkington (2000) describe a parent coach as a practitioner who has moved from being the lead player of direct intervention to one who sits alongside the parent. The concept of *coaching alongside* is also applicable to AVT. *Coaching alongside* provides more opportunities for promoting the development of listening, spoken language, and learning than practitioner-led intervention (Shelden & Rush, 2001). Even the strategic placement of the adults in an AVT session fosters the development of spoken language through listening rather than through visual stimulation. Successful parent coaching in AVT, however, is the work of the practitioner who knows how to use strategies described in detail in Chapter 15 and found throughout this book. The practitioner knows when these strategies are successful, when changes are required, and when and how to help parents generalize solutions to new and different circumstances and settings (Fenichel & Eggbeer, 1991; Flaherty, 2006; Kaiser & Hancock, 2003). Among many other responsibilities, the practitioner in AVT coaches the parents in ways to help them acquire competence and confidence in the independent application and generalization of strategies as they embrace their role as "agents of change." About 92% of children who are deaf or hard of hearing are born to parents with typical hearing (Mitchell &

Karchmer, 2004) and parents enter the world of childhood hearing loss with grief (Luterman, 2017) and a great deal to learn (Blum-Samson, 2006). When parents choose AVT, they want to know what to do to help their child achieve their desired outcomes (Alberg, Wilson, & Roush, 2006; Estabrooks, 2006). The practitioner immediately begins a process of coaching to help parents *chart a course* for the journey to those outcomes, by observing and enhancing positive parent responsiveness. Throughout the process of coaching, the practitioner remains ever mindful of the many stressors on the family, and always approaches coaching with kindness—by paying attention, showing patience, communicating respectfully, and expressing compassion and concern for others. To be an effective and resilient coach in AVT, practitioners also need to be kind to themselves. Ultimately, as the practitioner focuses on kindness all throughout the coaching process, the benefits of kindness will be transformative for the parents, the children, and the practitioner (Atkins & Salzhauer, 2018).

PARENT RESPONSIVENESS

Sensitive or responsive parenting refers to parent–child interactions in which parents are aware of their children's emotional and physical needs and respond appropriately and consistently (Safwat & Sheikhany, 2014). High parent responsiveness is what drives development in listening, spoken communication, and literacy development. Compared with the interactive behaviors of mothers and infants with typical hearing, mothers of infants and tod-

dlers who are deaf or hard of hearing were less sensitive and less responsive and showed less affect matching during parent–child interaction (MacTurk, Meadow-Orlans, Koester, & Spencer, 1993; Meadow-Orlans, 1997). Therefore, the practitioner spends a great deal of time coaching parents to identify their child's listening and communicative behaviors and to become responsive by using strategies that will facilitate high-quality parent–child interactions.

FLUENCY IN SCIENCE AND ARTFUL DELIVERY OF AVT

Parent coaching in AVT is holistic, and therefore it is critical that practitioners demonstrate *fluency* in the science and artful delivery of AVT (Estabrooks & Schwartz, 1995). "Fluency requires mastery of the specific child intervention procedures, understanding of the conceptual basis of the intervention and its core assumptions, and the ability to present information about the intervention in a way that is understood by the parents and is applicable to the individual children" (Kaiser & Hancock, 2003 p. 13). Fluency in the delivery of strategies that promote learning in young children who are deaf or hard of hearing is a significant variable that influences outcomes in listening, spoken communication and cognitive skills of children with hearing loss (Estabrooks, 1994; Moeller, Carr, Seaver, Stredler-Brown, & Holzinger, 2013).

The following represents the areas where *fluency of skills* is needed from the practitioners as coaches in AVT:

1. knowledge and expertise in planning and delivery of child interven-

tion and in coaching parents to do the intervention;

2. management of parent coaching (Kaiser & Hancock, 2003) and the referral process (Estabrooks, 1994; Estabrooks et al., 2016);

3. knowledge of typical childhood development in the domains of audition, speech, language, cognition, and communication (Estabrooks, 1994; Pollack et al., 1997); and

4. knowledge of hearing science and technology and expertise in interpretation of audiologic assessments and use of hearing technology (Estabrooks, 1994; Pollack et al., 1997).

COMPONENTS OF THE PARENT COACHING PROCESS IN AVT

Parent coaching in AVT is a dynamic process (Estabrooks, 2006). Rush and Shelden (2020) describe five components of effective parent coaching that are particularly applicable to the practice of AVT and match the Auditory-Verbal Therapy Session Cycle (AVTSC) described in Chapter 17: (1) initiation, (2) observation, (3) action, (4) reflection, and (5) evaluation. Each individual AVT session, situation, and/or family presents with a number of human variables that can determine how the coaching components occur, and the order of transition from one component to another will change depending on the parents' knowledge and competency.

Initiation

In general, the *initiation* component is described as the process of discovery in determining the parents' main reason for seeking out the intervention in the first place (Rush & Shelden, 2020). The initiation process typically occurs: (1) at the time of the initial interview with the practitioner and (2) at the time of every discussion that begins an AVT session.

The Initial Parent Discussion

At this time, the parents and/or extended family members learn about AVT. The practitioner gets to know the family and the child and begins a conversation to learn about the child and family's needs, their goals, and expected outcomes. The practitioner *listens to the parents* and responds to their questions and concerns.

The practitioner then provides information about the clearly stated policies and procedures of the AVT program and easy to understand documentation that outlines the Principles of AVT. Some practitioners recommend an agreement be reached and preferably signed by the parents and the practitioner, clearly stating the roles of both the parents and the practitioner.

In the AVT Session

The initiation begins the moment the practitioner meets and greets the family. They share anecdotes about the previous week and the practitioner *listens* as the parents offer pertinent information about the child's progress in listening, talking, and thinking as well as their own progress in the home and community in use of the strategies that were practiced since the previous session. The practitioner *listens to learn* of the family's culture, language, interests, routines, family members, friends, and what they might need then. They jointly develop a plan for the parent coaching process with clearly stated goals and desired outcomes (Kaiser & Hancock, 2003). The practitioner as coach may begin by:

1. *commenting on an observation of a new behavior/skill,*
2. *asking specific questions that require open ended answers.*

The subsequent conversation helps plan out the next steps and, not surprisingly, the practitioner may facilitate active parent engagement by using some of the same strategies used with the children to enhance listening, talking, and thinking.

Example

Adrianna is a 4-month-old girl who was diagnosed with a bilateral moderate sensorineural hearing loss when she was 3 months of age. She just received her first pair of hearing aids. As Mother takes Adrianna out of the car seat and lays her on a blanket, the practitioner observes the mother anxiously checking the hearing aids.

Practitioner: "Wow, I like those pink hearing aids! Perfectly sized and placed on her tiny delicate ears."

Mother: "You think so? I was worried. She cried a lot when the audiologist first put them on."

> The practitioner provides a *self-statement* to begin the initiation component of parent coaching, and to *provide support and encouragement.*

Practitioner: "Oh? [she smiles encouragingly at the Mother] It's tough to get the ear mold in . . . the sparkly part that goes in her ear . . . sticky isn't it?"

> The practitioner uses *plain language* to describe new hearing aid terminology.
>
> The *practitioner and parent jointly set a goal for the session*: to become familiar with a) hearing aid terminology (earmold) and b) demonstrate knowledge of what's to be expected when babies are adapting to new hearing aids.

Mother: "Yeah! Is that normal?"

Practitioner: "Well, they are new, and the silicone is sticky at first. It is really a lot like . . ." [She waits for about 4 seconds and Mother jumps in.]

Mother: "Getting new shoes?"

Practitioner (smiles and nods): "Yes, you got it! It won't take long for her to get used to her new molds."

> The practitioner *waits* and presents a thought for *auditory closure* to encourage the mother to come up with her own analogy. When parents think of their own analogy or comparisons, they are more likely to remember what they learn in the parent coaching session. *This promotes self-learning.*

Mother: "Oh, I hope so. Does it hurt her?"

Practitioner (looking carefully at the baby, who appears to be sitting happily in her mother's lap): "Well . . . I think she looks pretty comfortable right now . . . but you know her best of all. What's your impression?"

> The practitioner lets the mother know that she *recognizes the mother as the expert of her baby* and asks for her opinion to *provide encouragement and support* and to *help the mother gain confidence in her observation.*

Mother: "I think she's OK. Well, she cried for a bit when we put them in, but once they were in, she settled down after a minute or two."

Practitioner: "That must have been a relief for you to see that."

> The therapist attempts to *"put herself in the mother's shoes"* by demonstrating empathy.

Mother: "Yeah. It's just . . . [the tears start to flow] . . . *scary you know?"*

Practitioner (nods her head slowly, leans in, and keeps her arms open and relaxed. And brings a box of tissues closer. She looks attentively and smiles with understanding as the mother wipes her eyes).

Mother: "I'm sorry."

Practitioner: "It's OK. Most people have difficulty going through this period of change and adjustment. That's why I'm here, to provide you with support."

> The practitioner *demonstrates openness and acceptance.*

Mother: "I mean, will she hear with these hearing aids? Will she even talk?"

Practitioner: "Ah! most parents wonder the same."

> The practitioner demonstrates that *she heard and understood the question by rephrasing the mother's question as a statement.* This also encourages the mother to continue explaining her concerns.

Mother: "Yeah. The audiologist said she can hear some parts of my voice without hearing aids but not everything."

Practitioner: "But with hearing aids . . . ?" [She leans in and looks expectantly]

> *Leaning in and looking expectantly* prompts auditory closure and encourages the parent to continue sharing what she knows. This helps the practitioner to assess what the parents know so they can build upon the knowledge.

Mother: "Yeah, the hearing guy . . . oh gosh . . . can't remember what he's called."

Practitioner: "The audiologist?"

Mother: "Yeah, Nick said she would hear speech really well with hearing aids."

Practitioner: "That sounds right. What do you think she can hear with her hearing aids?"

The practitioner provides information to address gaps in the parent's knowledge by *answering questions in a conversational manner*. The parent tells what she was told, and the practitioner confirms it as correct (research shows that parents only retain half of the information provided within an appointment; half of the information that's recalled is incorrect).

Mother: "I'm not sure. I'm hoping you can tell me that."

Practitioner: "Well, we will find out together. Ready?"

The practitioner and the parent have jointly determined a learning goal for the AVT session.

Observation

In the observation component, the practitioner observes a parent–child interaction in which the parent uses an ex-isting strategy or practices a new skill that was discussed the previous week. On occasion, parents demonstrate their knowledge and understanding of a strategy or skill when they talk about an activity they did with their child during the week. An observation can help to support and build the competence and confidence of the parents so they will enjoy *engaging with the child for a purpose* until the next session. The observation component includes observing the practitioner as he/she demonstrates a particular skill or strategy prior to using it during the session. The Auditory-Verbal Therapy Session Cycle (AVTSC) is detailed in Chapter 17.

Example

Adrianna's mother and the practitioner proceed to the observation component of the AVT session. The practitioner gathers a few baby toys and a book of babies' faces and puts them nearby, between herself and the mother.

Practitioner: "OK" [She *adopts a listening look* and says] *"I'm listening here to make sure Adrianna's listening environment* [the practitioner spans the room with her hands] *is quiet and free of extraneous noise. It is important to see what Adrianna can actually hear—because we need to know she's responding to our voices. What do you think of this listening environment?"*

Mother (adopts a listening look)*: "I think it's pretty quiet, yeah."*

Practitioner: "OK . . . let's wait about ten seconds so there's nothing but silence. Then, I will make a sound and we will watch Adrianna's facial expression. We're looking for . . . " [the practitioner pauses and looks as if she's trying to find the right word].

Mother: "Any change in her facial expression . . . or?"

Practitioner: "Yes, exactly! OK, ready?"

Mother (smiles): "On your mark!"

The practitioner begins the observation component by *adopting a listening look*. This strategy helps parents learn to model positive listening behaviors that will facilitate the development of the child's auditory processing skills. She also effectively demonstrates what a positive listening environment is like and provides an explanation to go along with it. Finally, she uses *pausing* and the *natural facial expression for "searching for the right word" (auditory closure)* to encourage parents to *engage in self-learning*.

Practitioner: "Shhhhh"

Adrianna's eyes move to the side where the practitioner is sitting.

Mother: "Oh, my goodness. She heard that, right?"

Practitioner (nods and then raises her finger for silence): "Ssss" [Adrianna's eyes move to the side again.]

Mother (when she catches the practitioner's eyes): "Sssssooooo quiet in here, isn't Adrianna?"

Practitioner: "Why you don't you call her name, very softly" [practi-

tioner provides a model] *"On my signal. OK?"*

Mother nods quickly and waits.

Mother (using a sing song voice): "Adrianna"

Adrianna's eyes quickly move (followed by her head) to the other side where mother is sitting, and she sees her mother's smile. Adrianna's face erupts into a huge smile.

Mother: "Hi, Princess. Oh, I'm so happy for you."

Practitioner (quietly): "I'm so happy you heard me. Tell her that."

*Mother: "I'm **so** happy you heard me."*

Practitioner: "Wonderful! You want Adrianna hearing positive phrases that relate to listening and what she can hear. In AVT, create experiences that will help her love hearing and listening. I like how you put the stress and emphasis on the word 'so.' It's full of meaning and positivity—keys to listening and talking success!"

The practitioner first demonstrates *using talking before, and during and after the action and then coaches the mother* to call her daughter's name and then *models* exactly how she wants her to do it. The practitioner *provides in-session coaching by whispering from the side—the language to use*. The practitioner provides *immediate positive feedback on how the mother does* and explains *why the strategy she demonstrates was* so valuable for listening and spoken language development.

Action

Action is the component that involves events or experiences that occur in the context of a real-life activity and may take place when the coach is or is not present. The practitioner *retreats to the sidelines* and watches the parent practice newly learned skills without any in-person coaching. The practitioner's silence during this component is critical; parents must have the opportunity to independently practice newly learned skills from the start of the activity until the end. The practitioner then observes the parents' use of the new skills. This action component is a key characteristic of effective coaching for building the competency and fluency of the parent in AVT.

Example

As Adrianna and her mother exchange smiles, the practitioner sits quietly, smiling encouragingly, and observes the naturally occurring interaction as it unfolds. After about ten seconds, Adrianna's eye gaze moves midline, and she wiggles her body. Adrianna's mother waits for a few more seconds.

Mother: "Shhhh"

Adrianna smiles and moves her eyes toward her mother again. Mother looks thrilled.

Mother: "I'm so happy you heard me! You like it that you can hear now, don't you?"

The practitioner smiles, nods, and gives the thumbs up signal and the mother is happy.

When the practitioner sits quietly, smiles encouragingly, and nods, she encourages the mother to independently practice a newly learned skill. The practitioner observes and takes mental note of the strategies the mother uses and considers the next coaching steps.

Reflection Component in AVT

Reflection (Fenichel & Eggbeer, 1991; Gallacher, 1997) is a very important component that differentiates coaching from typical problem solving, consultation, and information sharing between the practitioner and the parents. The reflection component consists of the practitioner as coach, asking questions to give the parents cause to think about what is happening now, what they want to have happened, and what they can do to bridge the gap. Following reflection, the coach provides feedback and/or new information to promote continuous improvement by helping the parents to analyze their practices and behaviors through the use of a reflective discussion with the coach (Gallacher, 1997). During reflection, the parents come to recognize existing strategies and discover potential ideas to build upon current strengths to address identified questions, priorities, and interests.

Example

The practitioner and Adrianna's mother are finishing the last activity of the AVT session. Adrianna is sitting comfortably in her mother's arms and appears to enjoy listening to her mother's comments about the babies' expressions in a book. Mother tells Adrianna the next baby is going to be a hungry baby who's crying. The parent *learns to talk before, during, and after* each page she shows and the baby *listens attentively*, and at times looks up at her mother. The parent reports that she has never seen her daughter do that before hearing aids. When they finish the book, Mother puts the baby into the car seat and gives her a pacifier. She brings out her "parent book" at the practitioner's request.

Practitioner: "I enjoyed today with you and your baby!"

Mother: "Oh, thank you! We enjoyed our time with you too!"

Practitioner: "I'm also happy you remembered to bring your parent book. I usually forget to bring important items to my appointments. I once forgot my agenda on top of my car and drove down the street with it until it flew off."

Mother (laughing): *"Oh no!"*

Practitioner: "Yeah. Anyway, you have yours."

Mother: "I was surprised that I remembered. Sometimes things get so hectic at home with my boys. They're crazy about Adrianna and they play with her a lot."

Practitioner: "Oh, that's so great to hear. So much of what you did today, the boys can do too, right?"

Mother: "I think so. Yeah . . . well not as well as me. But . . ." (Laughs)

Practitioner: "I think they can learn a lot from you."

Mother: "I'll make sure that they talk to her even when she's not looking at them and she will hear what they're saying. And listen . . . " (She adopts the listening look).

Practitioner: "Great idea. So, what you just said there is what I will write down in my notes, and you can write down in your parent book. It will help you to remember those key strategies we use to help Adrianna learn to listen and talk."

Mother: "That's a good idea. OK."

Practitioner: "So . . . we will write that down . . . oh and what was the first thing we did? We . . ."

Mother: "We waited until the room got really quiet. Or we got quiet." (She laughs.).

Practitioner: "Perfect, yes. And just so I know I explained it right- why do we need to wait or . . . check to see that the room is . . ."

Mother: "Quiet . . . yeah . . . uhm . . . to make sure that we know that she is responding to our voices and not any background noise."

Practitioner: "Right. So, let's write that down together. We call that creating a listening environment."

Mother: "Got it."

Practitioner: "How do you think you can create a listening environment at home?"

Mother: "Well . . . I could make sure that we are in a room that doesn't have the TV blaring. Maybe turn off the television. Close the door. Um, make sure the boys are quiet . . .

which . . . I don't know if that will ever happen!"

Practitioner: "Well, let's talk about that for a minute. A house with two boys and a baby is not exactly quiet, but here's the thing . . . listening to the chattering is a great thing. Just make sure that it is talking that Adrianna . . . "

Mother: "hears . . . right. Got it. So, it doesn't matter that the boys are screaming . . . oh wait . . . will that bother her?"

Practitioner: "Maybe, but hearing aids make sure sounds and speech never get uncomfortably loud for her no matter how loud they are to you and me."

Mother: "Right. That's a relief."

Practitioner: "And something we can write down in the book!"

Mother (laughs): "Got it!"

Evaluation Component of Coaching in AVT

The purpose of the evaluation component is to review the effectiveness of the coaching process, rather than evaluating the parents who are being coached. The practitioner self-reflects during this personal evaluation after every AVT session. The practitioner decides whether to continue with coaching conversations (continuation) or if the intended outcomes of the coaching relationship have been achieved (resolution).

The practitioner uses a *self-statement that includes specific and encouraging feedback* about the AVT session. This is done to *create a safe and supportive environment for learning.* Then the practitioner asks for the *parent book.* She presents her "chart" as well and *they jointly reflect upon what happened* in the session within *an easy conversation. Together, they* record the strategies to be remembered throughout the week. The practitioner *listens carefully and responds in a sensitive manner* to the parent, *taking care to balance the turns in the conversation.* She does *not dominate the conversation or tell the parent what to do.* Through conversation, *new knowledge is presented.* The practitioner encourages the mother to *give clear examples of how she can create a listening environment at home,* and finally, they make *a plan for generalization of strategies.*

ADULT LEARNING CHARACTERISTICS AND AVT

The coach in AVT has acquired a specialized set of skills (Doyle, 1999) to help parents to purposefully, creatively, and skillfully influence their child's spoken language development, primarily though listening. In addition to demonstrating core competencies in the nine domains of AVT practice, the practitioner needs to demonstrate knowledge of the various characteristics of adult learners. Every family comes with a unique set of circumstances, including constellation, personality, culture, language, and needs, that impact the adult's ability to learn and generalize effectively. In early AVT sessions, the practitioner has to manage these circumstances, sometimes in addition to the shock that comes with the diagnosis of hearing loss and the uncertainty of what needs to be done. Consider the characteristics of adult learners (Figure 16–1) and how these apply to parent coaching in AVT in relation to the Top Five Coaching Strategies mentioned above.

Adults Want to Choose What They Need to Learn

Adults are accustomed to being in control of most aspects of their life. They make decisions about their occupation, purchases, life partner, etc. This control extends to their learning as well. When adults feel that they have control over *what* they learn, they are better able to adjust behaviors that create positive change. Control does not necessarily mean controlling what happens in the AVT session. Control means choosing the topic or concern they need to have addressed to help them to help their child.

Example

The practitioner was looking forward to seeing a mother and her 2-year-old son. She had planned an entire AVT session around *Thomas the Train*, the boy's current joy. Before the session, the practitioner asked, "What is one important thing you need to figure out or learn today?" The mother replied, "I'm actually wondering how I can go about convincing the CI [cochlear implant] surgeon that Harvey needs a CI. I'm nervous about the meeting tomor-

row and I'm convinced he's going to say 'no.' I'm losing sleep, I'm really distracted, and I'm constantly thinking about this, especially when I'm playing with Harvey." The practitioner quickly adapted the plan for the AVT session to focus first on the mother's main concern. Within 30 minutes, they jointly created a plan of action that included a script. The mother was visibly relieved, and the remainder of the session was spent in guided parent–child interactions that had the mother's full attention and capacity for new learning.

Adults Benefit from New Learning Linked to Life Experiences.

The adult's experience is a key resource in any learning and/or coaching effort. Adults tend to link any new learning (linking strategies that facilitate listening, talking, and thinking in AVT) to everyday adult experience. When the practitioner uses real-life examples and analogies when explaining complex information parents need to know, then the link is reinforced. For example, it takes time for the brain to learn what to do with new auditory input. The brain is like a factory that got a new machine for production. The employees need time to learn how to use it efficiently. When parents can link new information to what they already know, then there is a greater chance that the new information will be retained.

Example

Deema is a 1-year-old who has been listening for two weeks with her cochlear implant. The parents reported that it's really difficult to get her to put her CI on in the morning. In conversation, the practitioner learned that when they put the CI processor on the child, they immediately call her name and do a *listening check* using the Six Sound Test. The practitioner wondered aloud if Deema needed a period of quiet time to fully wake up. She asked the parents how they are feeling in the morning. Mother commented, "I get it now. Dad needs his mornings to be quiet until he has his first cup of coffee. He cringes when I talk to him first thing—so maybe that's what's happening with Deema." Father nodded and said, "Yeah, everything sounds loud to me in the morning. It takes my brain time to wake up and adjust to the sounds of the world. Makes sense!" The practitioner and parents jointly planned a new morning routine and a new and improved way of doing listening checks to ensure optimal CI functioning in a timely manner.

Adults Need to Know the What, How, and Why of Every Learning Experience and to See Results Quickly

Higher motivation is linked to the fact that most adult learning is voluntary (Kuhn, n.d.). When parents come to an AVT session, they identify their desired outcomes and are motivated to spend most of the session with the practitioner demonstrating the what, how, and why of strategies that promote listening, talking, and thinking. Then they need cumulative practice right on the spot. When parents see the positive ef-

fect resulting from using these strategies, they feel hopeful and motivated to continue at home. Therefore, the practitioner needs to create opportunities to: establish play activities that clearly demonstrate benefit of strategy use so that parents feel encouraged to use and practice them; coach parents through guided questions to become accurate reporters of response behaviors; and encourage parents to ask why this information is important to know.

Example

A practitioner is ready to begin the first session with an infant who was recently fitted with hearing aids. When the parent arrived, the hearing aids were not on. Instead of engaging in informational counseling about the importance of making sure the hearing aids are on during all waking hours, the practitioner just got started with the session instead. She observed Mother as she tried putting the hearing aids on with some difficulty. The practitioner coached her how to put on the hearing aids. Mother explained that she didn't think the hearing aids were providing any benefit, but through demonstration, the practitioner sets the baby up for listening success by starting with *sounds that are easy to hear* for babies with hearing loss (e.g. the sound–object associations [Learning to Listen Sounds]). She coached Mother to sit beside the child on the side of the *better ear*. The practitioner pointed out clear behavioral responses that suggested that the baby could, indeed, hear with the hearing aids. The practitioner used a number of strategies to engage the parent: using guided questions such as "Did you see that?" followed by

"What did you see?" so that Mother was focused on naming the child's response and providing evidence of why those responses were positive.

Lack of Confidence in Their Learning and Parenting Skills

Many adults have had somewhat negative learning experiences in their traditional schooling and may have preconceived notions about learning experiences in AVT sessions. Parents may also feel "tested" on what they know, "judged" on how they interact with their child, and may feel inadequately qualified to help their child learn to listen and talk. The practitioner must spend time building a positive and supportive relationship through formal and informal conversations.

Example

Bonnie is the mother of a 2-year-old girl who wears hearing aids. During their first session, Bonnie shared that she has anxiety that was identified when she was in school. The practitioner focuses on identifying Bonnie's strengths during parent–child interaction and builds upon them as she demonstrates a variety of strategies. Bonnie makes a video of the AVT session using her mobile phone. When something great happens in the session, the practitioner will immediately view the video playback to help Bonnie see the strategies put into action and their outcomes. Bonnie reports that watching video playback and engaging in self-analysis really helps to

boost her confidence. The practitioner also points out mistakes and missed opportunities she herself makes and asks Bonnie to be a help to her to "be the best practitioner she can be."

ELEVATING PARENT KNOWLEDGE

When coaching parents in AVT, it is very helpful for the practitioner to understand *health literacy*. Health literacy is commonly described as the degree to which individuals, and for the purposes of this chapter, the parents, have the capacity to obtain and understand basic health information and the services needed to make appropriate health decisions (Malloy-Weir, Charles, Gafni, & Entwistle, 2016). Low health literacy affects people of every age, race, socioeconomic status, and education level.

Some families of children in AVT are faced with a myriad of decisions regarding hearing technology, intervention approaches, education and life choices, etc. Information on topics related to hearing loss and care options may not only be difficult to obtain, but also to read and understand. In addition, approximately 40 to 80% of health information received by the patient/family member is forgotten immediately (Kessels, 2003) and nearly half of the information retained is incorrect (Anderson, Dodman, Kopelman, & Fleming, 1979; McGuire, 1996). Finally, some parents of children in AVT, especially those with low *health literacy*, have trouble providing information about medical history, auditory functioning, and listening and spoken language abilities/goals to the practitioner that may affect intervention and outcomes. When practitioners in AVT use health literacy–sensitive approaches, parent engagement, informed decision making, and desired outcomes will be enhanced. In coaching families, the following strategies are suggested for the practitioner to use in helping elevate parent understanding and recall.

1. Show what is meant by demonstrating instead of using long verbal or written statements and questions (Rush & Shelden, 2020).
2. Use the Teach-Back Method® (Farris, 2015) to assess what parents heard and understood ("I want to be sure that I explained everything correctly to you. Can you explain it back to me so I can be sure that I did?" or "We've reviewed the goals that we worked on today with your child. How do you think you can teach these at home during daily routines?").
3. Provide analogies (e.g., first MAP on a cochlear implant is like heavily tinted windows on a car—it will only let in an amount of sound).
4. Provide acronyms that are easy to remember (e.g., OWL = observe, wait, and listen) (Weitzman & Cupples, 2017).
5. Encourage parents to use ASK Me 3® (Institute for Health Care Improvement, 2019) questions such as: What is the main problem? What do I need to do? Why is it important for me to do this?
6. Ensure that materials and therapy sessions are provided in the parents' language of preference with interpreting services.

COACHING IN AVT—PUTTING IT ALL TOGETHER

In AVT, every family is respected as unique and each one may have different desired outcomes. Even in the same family, each member has a history different from the other, thus creating many challenges and many opportunities for the practitioner to consider as the coaching process begins. Often families of infants who are newly diagnosed with hearing loss, may be shocked, scared, anxious, angry, or frustrated. Family members may grieve differently and have different timetables for doing so. Practitioners know that every day counts for providing auditory access to a child and they are anxious to share their expertise along with the good news about hearing technology and what is possible through a family/professional partnership like AVT offers. However, training and expertise

1. Families are the only 24/7 experts.
2. Different strokes for different folks.
3. Influencer of change, not agent of change.
4. The Big Question: "What's in it for me?"
5. Listening, giving, getting: the first job.
6. Positive questions, rephrased responses, and reflections.
7. Proactive expectation management.
8. Challenging conversations.
9. Starting with *Why?*
10. Cultivating trust.

may also be roadblocks because it is the families who are the experts at living life 24/7 with their child.

The reader is invited to think about the following *10 Important Considerations* for the practitioner when coaching parents in AVT.

1. Families—the Only 24/7 Experts

Although practitioners develop close relationships with most families, they do not walk in a family's shoes, through their daily trials, tears, and joys. Consequently, families have much more knowledge about their needs and the needs of their child. Families are the experts at living their own lives and if practitioners understand this, it is the more likely there will be a positive and long-lasting influence on the decisions a family must make.

2. Different Strokes for Different Folks

Most families come to AVT with intrinsic motivation to do whatever it takes to ensure their child attains age-appropriate listening, speech, and language skills. They show up at every scheduled appointment. The data logging feature of their child's hearing technology indicates device use of 13 hours a day. On the other hand, some families don't arrive with the same level of internal motivation. This simply means that some families may have other needs that must be met before they can do what it takes to optimize the potential of their child.

A wise colleague once said, "Help is not help unless it's what you want, when you want it." For parents who are dealing with severe depression, grief, financial difficulties, unmanageable work schedules, transportation concerns, or a struggle to meet the most basic needs of life, it may simply be impossible to take on the stress and work associated with meeting the needs related to hearing loss. Practitioners are responsible for helping families identify those other needs before tackling listening, speech, and language development. Of course, some practitioners are not equipped to address the needs because they do not fit their scope of practice. Since interdisciplinary service provision is the best model of intervention for children who are deaf or hard of hearing, it is imperative that practitioners collaborate with social workers, psychologists, early interventionists, etc. as necessary to build a foundation that allows families to meet, head-on, the challenges that are specific to their family.

3. Influencer of Change

Once ready to tackle the needs specific to hearing loss, practitioners need to think of their role as effective influencers for good who, to serve well, can discover the best ways to meet the needs of families by uncovering and defining what motivates them. The word "influencer" is a concise definition of a leader. To clarify, an effective influencer gets others to do something they might not otherwise do on their own. For example, most families will be unaware of auditory brain development and plasticity and its relationship to the critical period of language development. When one is not equipped with that knowledge, then the importance of full-time hearing technology use during infancy and early childhood may not be obvious. A parent may feel like the importance of full-time hearing aid use is outweighed by the effort involved with facilitating that goal or the possibility that the child will lose or damage his/her hearing aids. Further, the parents might think that they can build up to full-time hearing technology use when the child is older, more cooperative, and is able to understand himself/herself. Family members might also think they can work extra hard when the child is 4 or 5 years old in order to catch up with speech and language development. These assumptions are all quite reasonable for someone who is unfamiliar with the speech and hearing literature and research showing the importance of early intervention. It is the practitioner's responsibility, as coach, to provide families with the resources they need to fully understand the implications of childhood hearing loss as well as the evidence-based interventions available to help the child reach his/her full potential. It must be remembered that families come with a wide variety of learning styles and communication dynamics. It is the responsibility of the practitioner to identify the most effective approach to connect with each family and provide them with the knowledge and skills they need. This is the job of the practitioner as coach—to serve their needs and support each family uniquely in their desired outcomes for their child.

4. The Big Question: "What's in it for me?"

Every moment of every day, each person is asking and answering one question unconsciously or occasionally consciously: "What's in it for me?" It's simply how humans are wired. One of the jobs of the practitioner as coach is to help families identify the fruits of the labor that need to be completed together. In other words, the practitioner can help a family realize what is in it for them when they are able to achieve their desired outcome by doing what it takes to get there. Families look for informa-

tion and advice, as well as ways to help them take care of needs that they may not even be able to articulate or have yet to even consider.

5. Listening, Getting, and Giving

To be a practitioner who is an effective influencer for good requires that the first job is not to give information, but to get information. As an effective influencer for good, the practitioner first helps families articulate what's in it for them. Paul Tillich quotes, "The first duty of love is to listen." Being in the business of coaching listening, the practitioner as coach needs to build a strong foundation for effective communication by giving families the opportunity to be heard. The practitioner needs to support each family in telling their own "story." What do they want to accomplish? What is their greatest fear? What are their dreams for their child? A question that is effective in supporting families as they tell their stories is, "What types of goals would you like to meet for your child in the next 1, 3, 5, and 18 years?" For a physical journey to be successful, it is important to know the desired destination. This is entirely true for the listening and spoken language journey with families. It is virtually impossible to meet families' needs and arrive at the coveted destination without first acquiring an understanding of each families' values, desires, and goals for their child.

6. Positive questions, Rephrased Responses, and Reflections

Asking positive questions, rephrasing the answers, and then giving the answers back to families in different words often helps identify what a family really wants for their child. By articulating what is motivating them to follow up, they are helping to establish what can and should happen. These conversations are often very similar, and many families share similar needs, wants, and desires. When families are offered the opportunity to tell their story without judgment or platitudes from the listener, there is power in the fact that they are important characters in their child's story, and they get to choose the outcome. For example, if a family is asked, "What are your goals for your child?" the answer may be, "I want my child to learn to listen, and talk, and when she is five years old, I want her to excel in our neighborhood kindergarten with other kids who are listening and talking." A follow-up response could be, "I hear you saying that you want your child to develop speech, language, and listening skills that are like her peers with normal hearing. That's great! We can do that if we consistently use the hearing technology that is most appropriate to meet your child's needs and we work together to create an auditory lifestyle that maximizes your child's development."

7. Proactive Expectation Management
Another important factor impacting the coaching partnership is that anger and frustration are nothing more than unfulfilled expectations. This principle is equally valuable when serving families, especially as practitioners listen to them share their stories and their expectations for what practitioners can provide. When practitioners listen well, expectations can be managed better. If anger and frustration are the result of unfulfilled expectations, it is critically important that families articulate their expectations, and practitioners inform families as to whether those expectations are realistic. If a family of a baby with a profound hearing loss expects their child will learn to listen and talk

while only wearing hearing aids for a couple of hours a day, then they are going to be disappointed and angry when the desired goal is not achieved. Families will be frustrated and angry if practitioners do not identify their desired outcome and then outline what is necessary for a child to achieve that outcome. Again, this responsibility does not reside with the family but rather with the practitioner, the coach.

8. Challenging Conversations
Focusing on the positive and promising outcomes for listening and spoken language in babies who are deaf or hard of hearing is at the forefront of communication with families. Yet it is important to not avoid ignoring the challenging aspects of the work accomplished with families. On the contrary, as in leadership, it is important to remember that success is directly proportional to the number of difficult conversations. Practitioners as coaches in AVT are educated, dedicated, and passionate, and have a fiduciary responsibility to families and colleagues to ensure that the information, advice, and therapy are provided. Sometimes, that means practitioners have to correct misinformation families may get from someone else or that they hold as truth. Sometimes it means gently and respectfully identifying the behavior or activity that a family holds sacrosanct that is inhibiting or getting in the way of the picture of success that has so inspirationally been painted. So, if difficult conversations are necessary, how do they happen?

9. Starting with *Why?*
Simon Sinek (2009) states that effective influencers for good always start with why they are doing what they do before proceeding on how to do it. This is an effective formula for any worthy

project, or a model for conducting a difficult conversation in most every setting. Start with *why*. Answer the question "What is it that you and the family or even perhaps a co-worker want to accomplish and why?" Getting the question answered clearly is often the hardest aspect to master in becoming an effective influencer for good. However, the "why" can serve as the force that drives families' motivation and the decisions that shape their children's intervention and outcome. For instance, a family may state that they want their child to learn to listen and talk (the what), because they want their child to have the best possible opportunity to be able to converse over the telephone, to be on their local high school's debate team, to pursue any occupation he or she chooses, etc. (the why). Once the why has been defined, then the how can be determined in order to make it happen. To achieve the "why goals," the child will need to have consistent access to intelligible speech. If the child has bilateral profound hearing loss, then the "how to" plan may include cochlear implantation at 8 months of age, use of digital remote microphone technology, consistent participation in AVT, etc. In the ideal world, practitioners and families can continually revisit the "why" when justifying and facilitating the motivation required to achieve the desired and optimal outcomes for the child.

10. Cultivating Trust

Key to long-lasting success as a practitioner and coach in AVT, an effective influencer for good, is **trust**. All satisfying, successful, and quality relationships are built on the foundation of trust. Families must trust their practitioner as coach, in order to partner effectively in the mutual goals of listening and spoken language acquisition for their child. Trust is one of those concepts that is highly valued but not understood well. There are many aspects to understanding trust and because it is foundational to an effective influencer for good. Trust comprises and is significantly affected by numerous components, including steadfastness, credibility, and time.

Steadfastness is all about being present when the chips are down. It means sacrificing something valuable to help another get something he or she wants. It implies devotion and loyalty, and it is built by ongoing contact, mutual interest, and pursuit of a common why. It can be nerve-wracking, difficult, and stressful to fit hearing aids on babies. Infants frequently cry and exhibit resistance when ear impressions for ear molds or real-ear-to-coupler differences for hearing aid verification are made. However, trust is built with families by remaining patient and positive and by serving as the stable beacon that ensures families that these types of services are innocuous and in the best interest of the child. In other words, they are an integral part of pursuing the "why."

Credibility may be the simplest and easiest term to define. Credibility means that individuals have the skills, knowledge, and experience to get something done. If one is a brain surgeon, she or he has both the scholastic training and the successful experience to perform surgery on peoples' brains. Although a carpenter uses basically the same tools as a surgeon, he does not have the credibility to do brain surgery (and vice versa). Credibility is earned by focusing on an area of expertise and obtaining the credentials necessary to convince others that an individual can do what he/she proclaims to be able to do. It can be very difficult to keep up with the rapidly evolving hearing technology and services that are imperative in the quest to optimize outcomes for children who are deaf or hard of hearing. However, practitioners who offer AVT remain current on the gold standard of AVT if trust is to be maintained with the families they serve.

Finally, trust is enhanced by time. Trust is something that is not immediately "there." Practitioners must capitalize on their credibility by providing the best they have to give, and they must remain steadfast to cultivate trust over time.

CONCLUSION

Coaching exists in business, education, and sports, among other domains, and it is considered foundational to current practice in AVT. The International Coach Federation (ICF), "the leading global organization dedicated to advancing the coaching profession by setting high standards and providing certification," presents core values of integrity, excellence, collaboration, and respect (2019). These are in harmony with the work of the AV practitioner in coaching parents to be the primary agents of change in the development of listening, talking, and thinking in their young children who are deaf or hard of hearing. In defining coaching as "partnering . . . in a thought-provoking and creative process that inspires them to maximize their . . . potential . . . " (http://www.coachfederation.org), the work of the

AV practitioner, who serves with kindness, compassion, respect, and gratitude, is once again in harmony with ICF. In addition to the educational credentials required to be an efficient AV practitioner, the authors forward the notion that coaching needs to be a required academic component of all academic preparation in speech-language pathology, audiology, and education of children who are deaf or hard of hearing.

REFERENCES

Alberg, J., Wilson, K., & Roush, J. (2006). Statewide collaboration in the delivery of EHDI services. *Volta Review, 106*, 259–274.

Anderson, J., Dodman, S., Kopelman, M., & Fleming, A. (1979). Patient information recall in a rheumatology clinic. *Rheumatology, 18*(1), 18–22.

Atkins, D., & Salzhauer, A. (2018). *The kindness advantage: Cultivating compassionate and connected children.* Deerfield Beach, FL: HCI Books.

Blum-Samson, A., (2006). The family-professional partnership: A parent's perspective. In W. Estabrooks (Ed.) *Auditory-verbal Therapy and practice.* Washington, DC: Alexander Graham Bell Association for the Deaf and Hard of Hearing.

Doyle, J. S. (1999). *The business coach: a game plan for the new work environment.* New York, NY: John Wiley.

Dunst, C. J., Herter, S., & Shield, H. (2000). Interest-based natural learning opportunities. In S. Sandall & M. Otrosky (Eds.), *Young Exceptional Children Monograph Series, (2),* 37–48.

Estabrooks, W. (1994). *Auditory-verbal therapy for parents and professionals.* Washington, DC: Alexander Graham Bell Association for the Deaf and Hard of Hearing.

Estabrooks, W. (2006). *Auditory-verbal therapy and practice.* Washington, DC: Alexander Graham Bell Association for the Deaf and Hard of Hearing.

Estabrooks, W., MacIver-Lux, K., & Rhoades, E. (2016). *Auditory-verbal therapy for young children with hearing loss and their families, and the practitioners who guide them.* San Diego, CA: Plural Publishing.

Estabrooks, W., & Schwartz, R. (1995). *The ABCs of AVT: Analyzing auditory-verbal therapy.* North York, ON: Arisa Publishing.

Farris, C. (2015). The teach back method. *Home Healthcare Now, 33*(6), 344–345.

Fenichel, E. S., & Eggbeer, L. (1991). Preparing practitioners to work with infants, toddlers, and their families: Four essential elements of training. *Infants & Young Children, 4*(2), 56–62.

Flaherty, J. (2006). Coaching: Evoking excellence in others (2nd ed.). *Development and Learning in Organizations: An International Journal, 20*(6). doi: 10.1108/dlo.2006.08120fae.002

Gallacher, K. K. (1997). Supervision, mentoring, and coaching. In P. Winton, J. A. McCollum, & C. Catlett (Eds.) *Reforming personnel preparation in early intervention: Issues, models, and practical strategies* (pp. 191–224). Baltimore, MD: Paul H. Brookes.

Hanft, B., & Pilkington, K. (2000). Therapy in natural environments: The means or end goal for early intervention? *Infants and Young Children, 12*(4), 1–13.

Institute for Health Care Improvement. (2019). *Ask me 3: Good questions for your health* Retrieved November 27, 2019 from http://www.ihi.org/resources/Pages/Tools/Ask-Me-3-Good-Questions-for-Your-Good-Health.aspx

International Coach Federation. (2019) Retrieved November 30, 2019 from http://www.internationalcoachfederation.org/core competencies

Kaiser, A. P., & Hancock, T. B. (2003). Teaching parents new skills to support their young children's development. *Infants & Young Children, 16*(1), 9–21.

Kessels, R. P. (2003). Patients' memory for medical information. *Journal of the Royal Society for Medicine, 96*(5), 219–222.

Kuhn, G. (n.d.). *ADTED 460 -Introduction to Adult Education-10 Characteristics of Adults as Learners.* Retrieved on September 12, 2019 from http://ctle.hccs.edu/facultyportal/tlp/seminars/tl1071SupportiveResources/Ten_Characteristics_Adults-Learners.pdf

Luterman, D. (2017). *Counseling persons with communication disorders and their families.* Austin, TX: Pro-Ed.

MacTurk, R. H., Meadow-Orlans, K. P., Koester, L. S., & Spencer, P. E. (1993). Social support, motivation, language, and interaction: A longitudinal study of mothers and deaf infants. *American Annals of the Deaf, 138*(1), 19–25.

Malloy-Weir, L. J., Charles, C., Gafni, A., & Entwistle, V. (2016). A review of health literacy: Definitions, interpretations, and implications for policy initiatives. *Journal of Public Health Policy, 37*(3), 334–352.

McGuire, L. C. (1996). Remembering what the doctor said: Organization and adults' memory for medical information. *Experimental Aging Research, 22*(4), 403–428.

Meadow-Orlans, K. P. (1997). Effects of mother and infant hearing status on interactions at twelve and eighteen months. *Journal of Deaf Studies and Deaf Education, 2*(1), 26–36.

Mitchell, R. E., & Karchmer, M. A. (2004). Chasing the mythical ten percent: Parental hearing status of deaf and hard of hearing students in the United States. *Sign Language Studies, 4*, 138–163.

Moeller, M. P., Carr, G., Seaver, L., Stredler-Brown, A., & Holzinger, D. (2013). Best practices in family-centered early intervention for children who are deaf or hard of hearing: An international consensus statement. *Journal of Deaf studies and Deaf Education, 18*(4), 429–445.

Pollack, D., Goldberg, D. M., & Caleffe-Schenck, N. (1997). *Educational audiology for the limited-hearing infant and preschooler.* Springfield, IL: C. C. Thomas.

Rhoades, E. A., & MacIver-Lux, K. (2016). Strategies that facilitate listening, talking and thinking in auditory-verbal therapy. In W. Estabrooks, K. MacIver-Lux, & E. Rhoades, (Eds.), *Auditory-verbal therapy for young children with hearing loss and their families, and the practitioners who guide them.* San Diego, CA: Plural Publishing.

Rush, D. D., Shelden, M. L. L., & Hanft, B. E. (2003). Coaching families and colleagues: A process for collaboration in natural settings. *Infants & Young Children, 16*(1), 33–47.

Rush, D. D., & Shelden, M. L. L. (2020). *The early childhood coaching handbook.* Baltimore, MD: Paul H. Brookes Publishing.

Safwat, R., & Sheikhany, A. (2014). Effect of parent interaction on language development in children. *The Egyptian Journal of Otolaryngology, 30*(3), 255.

Shelden, M. L., & Rush, D. D. (2001). The ten myths about providing early intervention services in natural environments. *Infants & Young Children, 14*(1), 1–13.

Silverman, S. R. (1963). The education of children with hearing impairments. *The Journal of Pediatrics, 62*(2), 254–260.

Sinek, S. (2009). How great leaders inspire action [Video file]. Retrieved on November 27, 2019 from https://www.ted.com/talks/simon_sinek_how_great_leaders_inspire_action?language=en

Tomblin, J. B., Walker, E. A., McCreery, R. W., Arenas, R. M., Harrison, M., & Moeller, M. P. (2015). Outcomes of children with hearing loss. *Ear and Hearing, 36*(suppl. 1), 14S–23S.

Weitzman, E., & Cupples, P. (2017). *It takes two to talk: A practical guide for parents of children with language delays.* Toronto, Ontario: The Hanen Centre.

What is coaching? (n.d.). Retrieved from https://internationalcoachingcommunity.com/what-is-coaching/

17

THE AUDITORY-VERBAL THERAPY SESSION: PLANNING, DELIVERY, AND EVALUATION

Warren Estabrooks, Louise Ashton,
Rosie Quayle, Frances Clark,
Karen MacIver-Lux, Sally Tannenbaum,
Lisa Katz, and Dave Sindrey

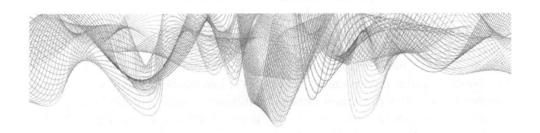

INTRODUCTION

Auditory-Verbal Therapy practitioners plan, deliver, and evaluate individualized AVT sessions reflecting the
interests of the child and the family,
their learning styles, the dynamic nature of daily life, the child's chronological
age, hearing age and stages of development, and the practitioners' own creative
processes and expertise. AVT sessions,
therefore, are as unique as the families
for whom they are created, and consequently there is no single and explicit
AVT session plan format suitable for all
practitioners, who themselves are unique
in their practical applications of AVT.

THE ART OF THE AUDITORY-VERBAL PRACTITIONER

Practitioners bring their personalities to the AVT session. Some practitioners are dramatic and outgoing, some are quiet and reserved, and some are somewhere in between. Some practitioners follow the child's lead most of the time (Bodrova & Leong, 2007; Girolametto, Pearce, & Weitzman, 1996a, 1996b; Pepper & Weitzman, 2004); some direct the child's attention to his or her own toys, books, props, and/or events in the environment or provide their own stimuli to help parents develop listening, talking, and thinking (Bergman Nutley et al., 2011; Eisenberg, 2004; Holmes et al., 2009; Lee & Van Patten, 2013); some do a combination of all of these (Snyder & Munakata, 2010, 2013). Some practitioners provide many activities during an AVT session; some provide a small number of activities capturing the child's interest and the parent's imagination; some follow themes and scenarios replicating real life and/or existing within the family's home environment. The number of activities presented during an AVT session can vary from week to week and can be difficult to predict, especially if the parent and the practitioner always follow the child's lead. Most children and their parents learn best when engaged in familiar routines (Kashinath, Woods, & Goldstein, 2006; Woods, Kashinath, & Goldstein, 2004); some, however, thrive on the excitement of evolving elements of surprise that also vary from session to session (Rush, Shelden, & Hanft, 2003). Some practitioners find that the best-planned sessions might not work, so flexibility is paramount to keep the AVT session focused on the short-term objectives regardless of the stimuli, taking care that it is meaningful to the child and parents (Fredricks, Blumenfeld, & Paris, 2004). Sometimes the best-planned AVT session might "fall apart." Practitioners are typically highly experienced in *expecting the unexpected* and can find ways to *save the session* and get back on course (Newbern & Lasker, 2012).

There are, however, common components and goals that act as compass, map, and chart rather than a global positioning system, to help the practitioner move the AVT session forward. These guiding components are driven by the principles of professional practice, by science, and by research. Consequently, there are many children who are deaf or hard of hearing in several countries in a variety of AVT programs who are learning to listen, to talk, to share in three-dimensional conversations (Chapter 10), to sing (Chapter 18), to read and write (Chapter 14), to go to school with typical hearing peers (Chapter 20), and to engage in all the activities of daily life (Latif Akbari, Khan, & Arshad, 2017; Percy-Smith et al., 2008; Torppa, Faulkner, Kujala, Huotilainen, & Lipsanen, 2018; Goldblat & Pinto, 2017).

CHARTING THE COURSE

Children born with typical hearing enter life with a system of dynamic interactive processes that occur automatically within the child and between the child and his or her significant others. They are equipped with perceptual, motor, cognitive, and linguistic abilities that develop in predictable sequences over time—along with the intrinsic motivation to communicate (Vanderwert et al., 2015). Consequently, when the family receives a diagnosis of hearing loss, and even before the child is fitted with hearing technology, the practitioner can begin right away to help parents *chart a course* toward the desired outcomes of listening and spoken communication (see Chapter 1).

Using a *sailing* analogy, the practitioner is primarily a *navigator*, especially during the early sessions of AVT, *where they help parents to chart a course for the future, to become captains of the ship,* and *to sail along with their child* from one port of call to another, discovering new destinations in audition, speech, expressive and receptive language, cognition, and communication. Subsequently, the parents take up sailing by themselves with the knowledge and skills acquired through coaching and guiding by the practitioner. Ultimately, the child takes up sailing by him/herself. By *charting the course* and *sailing together*, the adults who are part of the family's ongoing support team come to understand the following:

- It is only with parents that the course can be effectively charted.
- The parent is the captain.
- The practitioner is the navigator.
- The child is the precious passenger who is carried by the crew.
- They drop anchor at many ports along the way.
- At each port, they rest, study the maps, prepare new travel plans, and take on supplies

and additional crew when needed.
- Along the way, it will not always be clear sailing. The winds of hope and fear may collide and create storms.
- The weather will improve and there will be beacons along the shore to guide them.
- They all sail together.

Sometimes, however, the course may need to be changed. Maybe the chosen destinations really are impossible, and there need to be new ones. And sometimes those new choices involve principles of another kind of practice. Knowing when, where, why, and how to change course and chart a new direction so that the child reaches his/her highest communication potential is the AVT way.

BLUEPRINT: FROM AVT CARE PLAN TO AVT SESSION

Ernst (2012) states that "*treatment plans* are used throughout the medical community and in the social sciences whenever direct services are offered to an individual." In AVT, the treatment plan (AVT care plan) is seen in a broader context—one that includes the whole family and is typically revisited after each 3- to 6-month period. An AVT care plan contains various components such as name, chronological age, age at diagnosis, hearing age, auditory-verbal age, period of time covered by the AVT care plan, stated goals and objectives, some AVT session content, collateral concerns, and the support system and evaluation. This is very much in keeping with the individualized family service plan (IFSP), "a federally mandated plan of education for preschool children" (Tye-Murray, 2020) used in the US. The AVT care plan, therefore, is a blueprint used to:

- determine a trajectory of learning to listen and talk so that the child with hearing loss and the family move forward in a developmental manner to "close the gap" and reach the desired outcomes in a timely fashion.
- simplify and streamline the work of the practitioner.
- provide a template for charting diagnostic information and evaluating progress.

From time to time, sessions with only the parent may be requested and, in fact, required, based on the program's policies and procedures. These *consultations* or *counseling sessions* are part of the ongoing guidance and supportive services of the practitioner, and part of AVT practice.

COMPONENTS OF THE AUDITORY-VERBAL THERAPY SESSION

Based on numerous years of experience as practitioners, the authors suggest the following components to help in the

Six Goals of the Auditory-Verbal Practitioner

1. Create a listening environment.
2. Facilitate auditory processing.
3. Enhance auditory perception of speech.
4. Promote knowledge of language.
5. Facilitate spoken language and cognition.
6. Stimulate independent learning.

planning, delivery, and evaluation of an AVT session:

1. Pre-session
2. AVT session in action
3. Post-session

These components form a subset of the blueprint to assist the practitioner in planning and organizing the AVT session in ways that embrace the "Six Goals of the Auditory-Verbal practitioner" for every AVT session (Estabrooks, MacIver-Lux, & Rhoades, 2016).

These Six Goals ultimately become the goals of the parents during every interaction with their child (see Snapshots of AVT sessions below).

Pre-Session

1. Review the Child's Current Progress Summary and Long-Term Objectives (AVT care plan)

The practitioner will read the child's chart to review the following:

- the child's current skills as demonstrated in previous sessions.

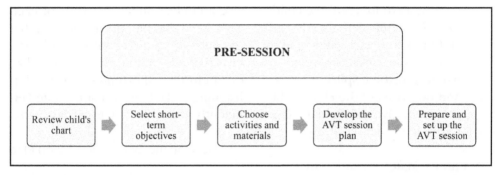

Figure 17-1. Pre-session.

▪ the *homework* or take-home messages generated by the discussion of carry-over from the previous sessions.

▪ the documented communication and current reports from professional partners (audiologist, occupational therapist, physiotherapist, psychologist, daycare/nursery/preschool teacher, etc.).

▪ the practitioner's additional notes on topics pertaining to the child and his or her family (e.g., child's current interests or upcoming events, any additional issues, strategies that the parent is currently using or needs to learn, new ideas for capturing the child's interests).

▪ the long-term goals to determine that the AVT session plan reflects practical steps to reach the long-term goals through short-term objectives.

2. Set Short-Term Objectives (STOs)

After reviewing the child's chart, the practitioner will:

▪ set short-term objectives (STOs) based on the child's hearing age, chronological age, stages of development in audition, speech, receptive and expressive language, cognition and communication and consider the child's *zone of proximal development* (Vygotsky, 1978). STOs can typically be accomplished in one to four sessions when the child is engaged with and helped by an engaging adult.

▪ consider parent suggestions about what they feel is important for the child to learn. For example, some families may have "behavior" objectives if they are helping the child to shape positive behaviors.

▪ set one or two goals to help the practitioner continually strive for optimal service provision to the child and parents (e.g., waiting longer for the child to respond, allowing more time to process the spoken message; using sabotage to demonstrate to the parents how to stimulate the child's thinking skills; finding ways to engage the parent more effectively).

▪ set one or two goals for the parent (e.g., observe the child closely; learn to "read" the child's *thought bubble* and give the child the language needed; allow problems and mistakes (e.g., when something spills or breaks) and not "rescue" the child right away, but give the child a chance to "fix it").

3. Choose Materials and Activities

Then the practitioner will create activities by choosing materials that:

- provide opportunities to facilitate achievement of all short-term objectives.
- capture and hold the child's interest without being too distracting.
- are culturally sensitive.
- can easily be carried over to the home, school, and community.
- contain intrinsic and extrinsic rewards—e.g., feeling excited about making cookies (intrinsic) and eating the cookies after baking them (extrinsic).
- are age and stage appropriate.
- are fun for the child, parent, and practitioner.

The practitioner encourages parents and their child to talk about things in their backpacks and welcomes toys and games, books, snacks, and traditions that reflect the family's interests and culture. For example: *a mother might offer freshly squeezed juice, a father may bring his prayer rug, or a parent may intentionally leave rollers in her hair.* The practitioner welcomes the unexpected and *knows how to chart the course.* The practitioner is always deci-

sive and clear about the STOs of each activity, so that parents understand that the outcome is not about a toy, objects, or activity, but about how to capitalize on multiple opportunities to develop listening and talking as naturally and efficiently as possible, in everyday living.

4. Develop the AVT Session Action Plan

The practitioner will then:

- document the short-term objectives and selected activities that will target them in the AVT session plan.
- plan how each one will be delivered.
- consider the transition from one activity to another.
- cite the planned strategies (Chapters 15).
- consider leading questions to ask the parents.
- collect resources (handouts, books, etc.).
- anticipate the "homework" or the possible take-home messages.

5. Set Up the AVT Session

An AVT session can take place almost anywhere and at any time: in the home, at the nearby park, an ice cream shop, a fire station, a grocery store, a laundromat, zoo, farm, restaurant, or in the garden. Where there is life, there is potential for auditory-verbal experiences. The child's natural play can be followed by the adults and subsequently, through coaching and guiding, parents learn how to adapt the strategies demonstrated in the AVT session (Chapter 15) and follow the child's play to enhance audition, facilitate language development, teach social skills, encourage speech development, and develop Theory of Mind (Chapter 13). Through play, the practitioner can address the Six Goals in each AVT session. Play, the Auditory-Verbal way, is discussed in detail in Chapter 12.

Prior to the AVT session, the practitioner:

▪ makes sure toys, books, and other materials are within reach and in good condition.
▪ selects appropriate seating for all participants.
▪ checks that the acoustic environment is as free from extraneous noise as possible.

Getting Started in the AVT Session (Figure 17-2)

1. Greeting and Setting the Stage

Practitioners work in a range of different settings (e.g., private practice, the family's home, a clinic, a cochlear implant (CI) program, daycare, nursery setup).

Regardless of the geography, the practitioner knows that an AVT session begins as soon as the practitioner greets the family. This demonstrates that right from the start, listening and spoken communication are always priorities.

When greeting the family, the practitioner:

▪ greets the family in a calm, friendly, and enthusiastic manner.
▪ invites the parents to join by getting down to the child's eye level to greet him or her, where they can respond if the child needs encouragement.
▪ recognizes that how one greets a child needs to be linked to his/her hearing age, chronological age, and stage of expressive language and the culture of the family.
▪ coaches the parents to help the child take a turn. The practitioner and the parents may model the greeting with one another as the child "listens" and observes. The child learns how interactions and conversations begin

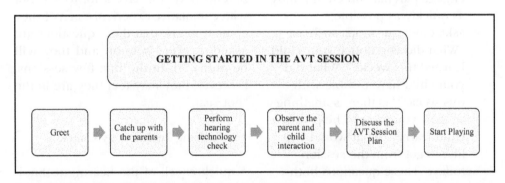

Figure 17-2. Getting started in the AVT session.

from the moment one meets another person. If the child is reluctant to take a turn, the practitioner coaches the parents to help the child to greet, even non-verbally, perhaps by giving the practitioner a smile or a "high-five."

2. Catching Up with the Parents

Following the greeting, the practitioner:

▪ asks the parents, "*How are things going?*"
▪ listens carefully to the parents' responses as they may change the direction, scope, and in particular, the STOs of the session. The child may simply observe the conversation, may play with a quiet activity or may join in depending on the age and stage of the child's development and on the child's temperament. The child really needs to be gainfully engaged in an activity and not left to sit too long. In fact, the "quiet" activity may stimulate the first joint activities of the AVT session. The adults help the child learn to wait but also engage parents and child jointly as quickly as possible.
▪ asks other questions such as: "What did you notice your child learned this week?" "What did your child have trouble with this week?" "Is there something specific you want to help your child learn?" "What would you like to get from the session today?" These questions both reinforce the parents' role as

their child's best expert and advocate and help them focus on being diagnostic themselves about what their child is doing and what they need to do next.
▪ considers the parents' responses to decide if the STOs, based on the child's current level of functioning, actually address the needs of the family. This might mean a quick change in the AVT session plan, or supporting the parents to understand the small steps required to achieve a specific objective (e.g., a parent wants to work on two-word phrases, but the child has just started producing Learning to Listen Sounds).
▪ responds in a way to demonstrate that the parents have been heard: "It sounds as if it might be useful to . . . ," "Based on what you have told me, it might be a good idea to . . . " or "Let's begin with the end in mind," or "Remember it's a process, not a performance."

The practitioner needs to establish realistic and measurable STOs in a discussion with the parents. Sometimes parents may not have a lot to say, but with cumulative experience in AVT they come to know that these questions are asked at every session and they will be prepared. In the first few sessions, however, they may feel they are in the "hot seat."

3. Hearing Technology Check

A quick check of the hearing technology is performed before the first activity begins to ensure that the child is able to optimally hear, so that spoken language is easy to hear, easy to say, and easy to learn (Estabrooks, MacIver-Lux, & Rhoades, 2016). Begin with a quick visual check of the hearing technology, being on the lookout for unexpected cracks in the casing, loose battery doors or compartments, microphone covers with debris, and ear hooks that are loosely fastened to the device. Loose connection of parts can cause intermittent sound or risk of hearing technology loss. Examine the tubing in the earmold to see that it is pliable and free of cracks or moisture build-up. Any problems with the above can cause a significant reduction in volume and sound quality and feedback often occurs. Batteries need to be fresh; and when in doubt, check the battery life with a battery tester. If a battery tester is not available, one can check that batteries are fresh by dropping the battery on the table. Dying or dead batteries when dropped on the table will bounce from one spot to another; conversely, fresh batteries will fall with a thud and bounce very little, if at all. When batteries are nearing the end of life, there can be a noticeable reduction in volume and sound quality. To check the sound quality of the hearing technology, couple the earmold tip (and hearing aid) to the hearing aid stethoscope and turn the aid on. The aid needs to sound clear and free of distortion and/or crackling/humming sounds. Many practitioners check the sound quality by producing the Ling Six Sounds and listening to ensure that there is sufficient gain and no distortion across the speech spectrum. If the hearing aid has multiple programs, check the sound quality in

each program. Finally, ensure that the volume is set at the correct level. For cochlear implants, sound quality checks are performed using monitor earphones that can be connected to the processor. Many cochlear implant processors have remote controls or mobile phone apps that will do a "systems check" of the CI processor. Again, one must ensure that the correct program has been selected and the volume and sensitivity levels are where they are recommended. In early AVT sessions, the practitioner will perform the visual and sound checks of the child's hearing technology but typically, after a few sessions, the parents know how to do this and often do it in advance of the session and report to the therapist.

4. Observation of Parent–Child Interaction

The practitioner and the parent know the child's current stage of development in listening, talking, thinking, and problem solving and move forward from one destination to another. By observing the parent and child engaged in doing a puzzle, blowing bubbles, reading a book, having a tea party, or playing with cars and trucks, farm animals, or a baby doll, the practitioner may discover:

- how the parent gets the child's attention.
- how the parent initiates interactions and conversations.
- if and when the parent "tunes in, talks more, and takes turns" (Suskind, Suskind, & Lewinter-Suskind, 2015).
- whether the parent requires a little or a lot of coaching in order

to adjust to the child's listening, language and social levels.

- the parent's ability to engage actively in play by modeling, narrating, and scaffolding.
- the parent's expectations that his/her child will be part of the conversation or whether the parent rescues the child when anticipating an error.
- the child's current skills, including those in play, gross and fine motor development, sensory skills, etc.
- how everyone is feeling in the session and if there are any obvious gaps that can be addressed immediately.

5. Discussion of the AVT Session Plan

Based on the above *observation of the parent–child interaction*, the practitioner subsequently shares the planned STOs and the parent restates them. The STOs may be changed or adjusted based on the parents' report or suggestions. For example, an STO might be to communicate using two-word utterances. The practitioner might have planned to target two-word utterances such as "want + object" during the session. Based on observation and discussion, however, the adults may decide it is better to target "no + object" because the child becomes upset and throws things when he does not want them and the child will benefit more from using "no + object" utterances to help other people to understand his desires and needs.

The practitioner discusses strategies the parent can use most effectively during the session (Chapter 15). Then the scene is set for the AVT session by discussing the session, the games and activities they will use and how they will provide multiple opportunities for practice.

6. Guiding and Coaching the Parents to Make a Plan with Their Child

The practitioner:

- guides the parents to explain the session to their child in language that is appropriate for the child. They will talk about the activity, what is going to happen, and how many steps it might involve. For a beginning listener, this might be: "We are going to say 'bye-bye' to the dolly and then we are going to get a car that goes 'brrm brmmm'." For a more sophisticated listener: "We are going to play with a dolly and then read a book. The dolly is very dirty! First, we will need to wash her, then feed her and then finally put her to bed."
- coaches parents of older children to negotiate the plan with their child by offering a choice of activities (e.g., "Shall we play board games or pretend to be pirates?" or "I would like to read a book and then play *Snakes and Ladders*. What are the two things you think you would like to do today?").
- demonstrates how short-term objectives are incorporated into each activity in a playful manner—from early sessions of detection and the Learning to Listen Sounds to sessions of higher-level auditory-cognitive skills.

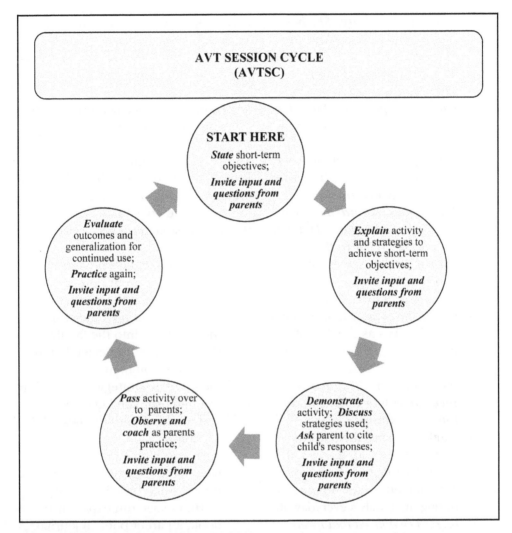

Figure 17-3. AVT Session Cycle (AVTSC).

7. The Auditory-Verbal Therapy Session Cycle

During each activity, the practitioner may follow the suggested steps of the Auditory-Verbal Therapy Session Cycle (AVTSC) (Figure 17–3) (Estabrooks, MacIver-Lux, & Rhoades, 2016). The practitioner:

1. states the short-term objectives for the parent (e.g., "*Today*

we're thinking about building Mary's repertoire of two-word sentences, and we're going to focus particularly on using 'No+' to reject and to mark absence").

2. explains exactly how the activity will work (e.g., "*As you said you love to cook at home, we're going to decorate cupcakes in a moment, but we'll forget to get a plate out for you. We can then*

go around and say, 'She has a plate, you have a plate, but Mummy has _____' and help Mary fill in the gap 'no plate.' Then have a laugh when the cup and a spoon are forgotten and see if she tells you there is 'no spoon' herself").

3. demonstrates the activity (one to three times) (e.g., *"Did you see how I leaned in closer when I said the /s/ sound? This will help Susie to hear it." "Did you see how she filled in the gap with 'no spoon' when you waited a bit longer and gave her a look of expectation?"*).

4. passes the activity to the parent and observes as the parent practices (e.g., *"Look how he is enjoying it! Why don't you try it now?"* or *"That was so nice Mary! Why don't you do this with Daddy?"*).

5. jointly evaluates the outcomes of the activity with the parent and talks about ways to generalize the outcomes at home during the family's everyday life (e.g., *"I've noticed that when you waited a little longer there, he vocalized! How do you think you can do this more at home?"*).

Practitioners may follow the AVTSC for some parts of the session and not for others; all steps may be followed in some activities and only a few in other activities. The AVTSC is a template that can be adjusted to the parent's level of comfort and skill. The practitioner may follow the AVT session plan exactly as planned in advance or may follow the lead of the child and the parents and may adapt the session as it happens. Sometimes all objectives can be addressed in one activity, one scenario, or one unexpected event.

8. Parent Guidance (End of AVT Session) and Farewell

The practitioner ensures that parents leave the session knowing what they are supposed to do during the following week. The final 10 to 15 minutes of the AVT session are reserved to:

- discuss the child's progress.
- discuss the parent's progress.
- jointly review the short-term objectives and how they can be incorporated into the family's daily routines and extended to life in the community.
- identify key strategies to develop listening, spoken language, and thinking until the next AVT session.
- encourage the parents to record take-home messages in an agreed upon format based on their learning style (an experience book, a parent book, a journal, a diary, a log, etc.).
- focus on two or three primary messages to follow before the next session. The practitioner informs the parents that the goals and the strategies used to accomplish them are most important. For example, the practitioner can help the parents in opening a conversation and keeping it going. *Statements such as "Look at my new shoes!" or "I went to the park"* or simple questions such as *"What did you*

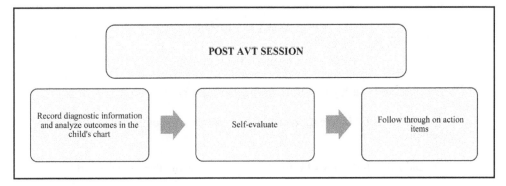

Figure 17–4. Post AVT session.

do at the park?" "Who did you go with?" can keep the conversation alive and outside of the "here and now."
■ review any parts of the video recording (e.g., with mobile phones/tablets) of the session to review key strategies and their outcomes that can be shared with other members of the family or intervention team.

9. Sample Questions for the Concluding Parent Guidance:

■ What happened during the AVT session that surprised you?
■ What happened that was new today?
■ Which short-term objective do you think was accomplished with ease or was challenging?
■ How do you think you will handle . . . during the next week at home?
■ What strategies might you use?
■ Did you see or hear how _____ did/said during . . . ?
■ Are you feeling encouraged by today's session?

■ Do you have any other concerns that I can help with at this time?

Post-Session

At the end of the session, the practitioner:

■ records the obtained diagnostic information in all the domains in the child's chart; evaluates and notes the strategies that did or did not promote success.
■ "raises the bar" by doing a quick analysis of personal performance and progress (service delivery) on the use of strategies for listening, talking, and thinking (Chapter 15), and strategies for parent coaching in AVT (Chapter 16) by responding to the questions such as those on WAVE Form I (see Figure 17–5) and/or makes a plan for continual improvement by using a form such as WAVE Form V (see Figure 17–6).
■ notes action items and follow through on any collaboration with other professionals.

WAVE FORM I ©

(WARREN'S AUDITORY- VERBAL EVALUATION I)

10 Questions to ask yourself, following the delivery of an AVT session:

1. Did I **EXPLAIN** the short-term objectives (STOs) before demonstrating the activity?

2. Did I **DEMONSTRATE** for the parents and invite them to take part?

3. Did I **PASS** the activity to the parents and observe them to do it?

4. Did I **STAY QUIET** while they did the activity?

5. Did I really **COACH AND ENCOURAGE** the parents?

6. Did I **DISCUSS** the outcome and really **LISTEN** to the questions and concerns of the parent?

7. Did I **USE** strategies that really encourage listening, talking and thinking?

8. Did I **ENCOURAGE** a conversation about carryover with leading questions?

9. Did I **MAKE** the session really **AUDITORY**?

10. Did I **HELP** the parents feel encouraged and hopeful?

© WE Listen International, 2020

Figure 17–5. WAVE Form I.

AVT SAMPLE SESSION PLANS, SNAPSHOTS OF AVT SESSIONS, AND ANALYSES

Rarely does a practitioner write such comprehensive AVT session plans as the reader can locate in other sources such as: *Auditory-Verbal Therapy for Parents and Professionals* (Estabrooks, 1994); *Cochlear Implants for Kids* (Estabrooks, 1998); *Songs for Listening! Songs for Life!* (Estabrooks & Birkenshaw-Fleming, 2003); *Auditory-Verbal Ther-* *apy and Practice,* (Estabrooks, 2006); or *Auditory-Verbal Therapy for Young Children with Hearing Loss and Their Families, and the Practitioners Who Guide Them* (Estabrooks, MacIver-Lux, & Rhoades, 2016). Many practitioners who train and mentor others may require the trainee/mentee to write detailed plans as an exercise in describing the step-by-step progression and transitions from one activity to another, and subsequently perform a diagnostic analysis of the AVT session. The AVT session plan and the snapshots of AVT sessions

WAVE FORM V©	
(WARREN'S AUDITORY-VERBAL EVALUATION FORM V)	
5 STRATEGIES **"TO RAISE THE BAR"** **STRATEGIES FOR LISTENING, TALKING AND** **THINKING AND/OR PARENT COACHING** **THAT I CAN IMPROVE**	**WHAT I CAN TRY OVER THE NEXT TWO** **WEEKS TO IMPROVE THESE STRATEGIES**
1	
2.	
3.	
4.	
5.	
© 2020 WE Listen International	

Figure 17-6. WAVE Form V.

presented here are for discussion and analysis, and not a prescription for all AVT practice.

In the following section the reader will find one complete step-by-step AVT session plan for an infant just starting in AVT, followed by a selected number of snapshots that have been taken from AVT sessions and analyzed based on strategies used in AVT to advance the SIX GOALS of the Auditory-Verbal practitioner (Estabrooks, MacIver-Lux,

& Rhoades, 2016). Following the previously discussed AVT session components, the practitioner can determine a personal template for the planning, delivery, and evaluation of the session and how to use the diagnostic information obtained to move forward *from one destination to another*.

User Guide for the Auditory-Verbal Practitioner during the Reading of the Following Section:

User Guide for the Auditory-Verbal Practitioner

1. Record each strategy used in the session or snapshot (strategies for listening, talking, and thinking and strategies for coaching and guiding parents).
2. Discuss the outcomes of each strategy.
3. List each goal of the Six Goals when they are presented in the session and cite an example of each one.
4. Discuss challenges one might find in the delivery of each strategy and give examples of how these strategies could be used in the child's daily life.

ENTIRE AVT SESSION PLAN

Pre-Session

Anna, an only child, is 3 months old. Following newborn hearing screening, she was diagnosed with a bilateral sensorineural hearing loss of unknown eti-

ology. She had repeated auditory brainstem responses (ABRs) that indicated a severe loss across all frequencies, absent otoacoustic emissions, and was fitted bilaterally with digital hearing aids at the age of 2 months. She and her family received counseling from the audiologist and the teacher of the deaf following diagnosis. This is Anna's first AVT session with her parents and it is planned, delivered, and evaluated in a clinic setting.

Current Progress Summary

Based on developmental norms, as reported by her parents, Anna's progress is as follows:

Audition

- Shows no responses to sounds with the hearing aids (parents are unsure if the hearing aids are working).

Speech

- Demonstrates no vocalization apart from crying.

Language/Communication

- Smiles (unclear if reflexive or communicative).
- Varies cries for different needs such as hunger and discomfort.

Cognition

- Fixes her gaze on mother's or father's face.
- Watches parents' faces when they talk to her (focuses for a few seconds, looks away, then looks back).

▨ Briefly explores objects with her hands.

Session Short-Term Objectives (STOs)

In one to four AVT sessions, Anna will demonstrate the following skills in each of four areas:

Audition

▨ Show consistent responses to some environmental sounds (start/stop moving, start/stop sucking, facial movement such as blinking).
▨ Demonstrate similar responses to some of the Ling Six Sounds and some Learning to Listen Sounds.
▨ Look in the direction of a sound source.
▨ Recognize singing as demonstrated by repeated change in behavior.

Speech

▨ Vocalize using gurgles and coos.

Language

▨ Watch faces of her parents when they talk to her (focus for a few seconds, look away, then look back).

Cognition

▨ Focus on pictures of faces in a book (e.g., *Baby Talk*).
▨ Anticipate daily events such as being fed when she hears "mmm mmm" and sees her bottle (demonstrable behavior such as beginning to move her lips).

Communication

▨ Use voice in vocal turn taking.
▨ Smile in response to parents' smiling.

Anna's AVT Session

Anna is sleeping in her pram when she arrives with her parents. They tell more about Anna, and the practitioner adds information to the case history.

Activity #1 Entering the Therapy Room

(Anna has awakened, and her eyes fix on her mother's face when her mother bends down to look at her in her pram.) The practitioner:

▨ coaches mother to lift Anna up while using a singsong voice and follow up with a natural gesture.
▨ says "*Make your voice melodic so that it sounds interesting to Anna and give her time to become aware of it. Say 'up, up, up,' then show Anna your hands.*"

(Mother seats Anna on a baby chair in the middle of the table and Anna closes her eyes again.)

Activity #2 Hearing Technology Check

Listening to the hearing aids.
The practitioner does the following:

▨ explains the Ling Six Sounds and why they are used every day.

- uses the stetoclip to demonstrate how to check the hearing aids using the Ling Six Sounds.
- demonstrates holding the hearing aid at the ideal distance from the adult's mouth to Anna's ear.
- says the Ling Six Sounds in this order ("m," "oo," "ah," "ee," "sh," and "s") and listens for clarity.
- observes the parents presenting the Ling Six Sounds following the model.
- explains that stimulation of her auditory cortex will develop Anna's auditory function.
- explains that detection of the Ling Six Sounds helps to identify what Anna can hear across the speech frequencies.
- moves within earshot of Anna's better ear and asks the parents to observe Anna's behavior when the practitioner voices a sound.
- makes sure her breath is not touching Anna's face, and explains why.
- says "aaaaaaaaah" at conversational level.
- points out a slight movement around Anna's eyebrows.
- repeats the sound again and both parents notice the same eyebrows movement.

(Anna begins to cry because she is hungry. Father leaves the room to heat a bottle. Mother tells the practitioner that Anna is unable to breastfeed because she has a tongue-tie. Father returns.)
The practitioner:

- coaches Father to "talk ahead" telling Anna that he has some milk for her and say "mmm mmm" before giving her the bottle.

- coaches him to use a louder voice. (Anna stops crying and Father is surprised as he has not observed this before. Father starts feeding Anna.)
- coaches the parents to observe changes in Anna's sucking behaviors during feeding.
- says "oooooo" close to Anna's right ear. (No response observed. Say "oooo" again, no reponse).
- says "oooo" a little louder using the pattern "ooooo oooo oooo." (Anna briefly stops sucking.)
- says "eeeeee" and "shhhhh" by using the same pattern and volume. (No response.)

(Anna starts to become unsettled.)

- asks Mother what she thinks Anna needs. (Mother says, "To be picked up.")
- coaches Mother to "talk ahead of the action." (Mother says "up, up, up," puts her hands out, and picks up Anna.)

Activity #3 Singing

The practitioner:

- asks Anna's parents if they sing. (Father becomes emotional. He is a musician and has not sung to Anna since the diagnosis of hearing loss.)
- explains that Anna has auditory access to the patterns and rhythms of singing that will stimulate her auditory brain.
- suggests Father begins singing *twinkle, twinkle, little star* as Anna's mother rocks her.

■ waits for a response before they begin rocking again.

■ coaches them to stop and wait for a vocalization from Anna before they continue.

■ explains that they are helping Anna understand that her voice can influence what happens around her.

Activity #4 Baby Faces *Book*

Anna calms from the singing and rocking. The practitioner coaches Mother to sit down and prop Anna up in her arms so she can see the book. (Mother says they have never shown her a book and is surprised that the practitioner is suggesting this since Anna is so young.)

The practitioner:

■ shows them the book of baby faces and explains that at 3 months of age, babies are very interested in faces.

■ coaches them to *talk ahead* using a mid-high frequency Learning to Listen Sound. (At this time, the practitioner and parents have not observed a response to "sh.")

Outcome Analysis

During the session, Anna did the following:

■ Detected "m," "ah," "oo" (Audition).
■ Vocalized in response to singing (could be incidental) (Speech).
■ Made eye contact with parents (Language).
■ Maintained attention to pictures in the book (Cognition).
■ Vocalized for singing (Communication).

Parent Guidance and Carryover

■ Check the hearing aids daily using the Ling Six Sounds.
■ Note any distortion or change in the quality of any of the sounds.
■ Review key reasons for the strategy of *planning and talking ahead (and especially when sharing books)*. Present the sound using acoustic highlighting. Follow up with action by presenting hands to lift her up, followed by the action.

■ Sing to provide Anna with lots of auditory information; then bring in movement.
■ Reinforce the value of *waiting* for Anna to make a vocalization and then carrying on with an action such as movement and singing.
■ Link the Ling Six Sounds and some Learning to Listen Sounds to daily life.

The practitioner asks, "*I wonder how you could use these sounds at home?*" The parents suggest they say:

■ "Mmm"—when she gets her bottle, "Ooo"—for her nappy "poooo,"
■ "Aaah"—for cuddling,
■ "Eee"—When they lift her ("wheeee!"),
■ "Sh"—when they put her down to sleep,
■ "S"—when they give her a kiss "kisssss!"

- demonstrates "splish splashhhhhhhh," and shows Anna a picture of the baby in the bath. Anna fixes her gaze on the picture. The adults wait while she looks at it.
- explains that this is really important for Anna to process what she is seeing. *Mother says the sound again but Anna does not react.*
- suggests trying a different picture (one of the baby eating). Father says "mmmmm," waits, and then shows the picture. Once again, Anna focuses on the baby's face. Everyone waits to give her time to process the information.
- coaches Father to do it again. (Anna raises her eyebrow.)

Post-Session

In Anna's chart, the practitioner records the diagnostic information obtained during the AVT session. This information will be used to plan, deliver, and evaluate subsequent AVT sessions.

SNAPSHOTS FROM AVT SESSION PLANS

In the following section, the reader will find a number of snapshots highlighting specific activities presented as part of the practitioner's entire AVT session. These snapshots have been analyzed to illustrate how the practitioner used particular strategies to achieve one or more of the Six Goals. The children have various hearing ages and chronological ages and varying AV ages, and come from a number of countries and cultures. The practitioners all have many years of experience in AVT.

SNAPSHOT #1: OMAR AT HOME (SALLY TANNENBAUM, PRACTITIONER)

Omar is 1 year, 2 months of age and has a bilateral profound sensorineural hearing loss due to bilateral cochlear nerve deficiency. He has been wearing his hearing aids for 10 months. This is Sally's second Auditory-Verbal Therapy session with Omar and his parents. In this session, Omar's mother learns how life in the home can create rich listening and language learning opportunities.

Changing Omar's Diaper

Activity Short-Term Objectives (STOs)

Audition

- Demonstrate detection and auditory attention to:
  - parent's voice (with varied intonation).
  - variety of vowels and pre-speech sounds.

Speech

- Produce pre-speech sounds (tongue click, raspberries).
- Make playful sounds (coos, yells, laughs).

Language

- Listen to someone talking and anticipate the next events.
- Share in vocal turn taking.

Communication

- Vocalize to indicate his needs.
- Make appropriate eye contact.
- Look at the person who is talking and engage in age-appropriate eye contact.

Cognition

- Sustain interest in desired object for two minutes or more.

Communication

- Attend to an object or person.
- Vocalize to make something happen, for attention and to have needs met.
- Request using vocalizations or gestures (puts hands up to be picked up).

Activity Description and Analysis

Omar begins to fuss and his mother determines he needs a diaper change. Omar's mother asks Sally if she and Omar can be excused for a few minutes. Sally tells Omar's mother that learning to listen and talk is a way of life and that the best activities are the ones that take place routinely. Sally offers to coach her with the activity, if she is comfortable.

> In coaching Omar's mother during the diaper change, Sally is *promoting knowledge of language* (Goal #4) by helping Omar's mother *transition beyond her comfort zone.*

Omar's mother looks at him and says, "Phew!" and waves her hand in front of her nose. Sally coaches the mother to kneel down next to her son and talk about what they are going to do. She says, "You have a dirty diaper. We need to change your diaper—phew. Let's change your diaper. Phew!"

> When Omar's mother kneels beside him, she *promotes knowledge of language* (Goal #4) by *speaking the language from the child's angle.* When she talks about what they are going to do, she *promotes knowledge of language* (Goal #4) by *talking before (during, and after) the action.*

Omar's mother encourages him to lie down and starts to take off his diaper. Sally coaches her to talk about what she is doing and mother says, "Phew— you have a very dirty diaper. I need to change your diaper!" To encourage Omar's mother, Sally explains she is using a lot of repetition, to help Omar hear words such as "diaper," "dirty," and "phew" over and over again.

> When Omar's mother repeats key words as she is changing his diaper, she promotes *knowledge of language* (Goal #4) by *emphasizing actions, relations, and attributes and by talking (before) during (and after) the action.*

Omar's mother says, "I am taking your dirty diaper off. Now, I have to wipe, wipe, wipe, and then put on a new diaper." Sally nods her head in encouragement and shares that by narrating what she's doing, Omar is hearing language that goes with the routine of diaper changing.

> Omar's mother narrates her actions and *promotes knowledge of language* (Goal #4) by *verbalizing in synchrony with movement.*

Omar begins making a few sounds. With Sally's guidance, Omar's mother imitates his sounds and then waits. Omar begins to babble again and Sally coaches Mother to smile and wait for him to finish before she takes a turn to "babble" back to him.

> By repeating his sounds, Omar's mother *facilitates auditory processing of speech* (Goal #2). *She helps to create an auditory-feedback loop* and *enhances auditory perception of speech* (Goal #3) by *engaging in vocal play.* She waits for Omar to finish babbling before she babbles back *and facilitates spoken language and cognition* by *waiting for his response.* She also *promotes knowledge of language* (Goal #4) by *taking turns* during the vocal play.

Omar vocalizes more frequently, and his vocalizations become more varied. Sally reminds Omar's mother to wait until Omar is finished before she talks back to him. Omar's mother waits a few seconds and Omar says, "Eh!" Mom says, "Eh!" and then waits. Omar then says, "Uh, uh!" and she repeats his new sounds and then waits. This very vocal interaction continues for several turns.

> By waiting a few seconds for his response, Omar's mother *facilitates spoken language and cognition* (Goal #5).

Omar's Calling Game

Activity Short-Term Objectives (STOs)

Audition

- Detect (respond to his name [by movement or smiling]).

Speech

- Make playful sounds (coos, yells, laughs).

Language

- Respond with appropriate actions when common words are used ("Omar!").

Communication

- Look at the person who is talking and engage in age-appropriate eye contact.

Cognition

- Sustain interest in desired object for two minutes or more.

Communication

- Respond to simple verbal requests when accompanied by gestures ("Bye-bye!" "Give it to Mama!").
- Vocalize when greeting a familiar adult.

Activity Description and Analysis

Everyone becomes quiet as Sally asks Omar's mother to hold him with his back on her chest, so they are both facing the same direction. Sally stands a short distance behind them and using a singsong voice calls, "Omar!" Omar's mother turns around to face Sally and points to his ear and says, "I hear that! Sally called you, Omar!"

> The family *creates a listening environment* (Goal #1) by becoming quiet. They control *the environment/ set the stage for what is coming next.* When Sally asks mother to hold him with his back to her chest, Mother controls the environment/setting by speaking within earshot. She *facilitates auditory attention* (Goal #2) *by pointing to her ear and saying, "I heard something!"*

Sally is very excited and says, "Hi! Omar!" and gives him a small toy to play with so that he learns that responding to his name has a payoff.

> These words and this action *stimulate independent learning* (Goal #6) *by creating the unexpected.*

After playing with the toy for a few minutes, Sally and Omar's siblings put the toy away by saying "bye-bye!" and waving.

> Sally and the family *promote knowledge of language* (Goal #4) by *verbalizing in synchrony with movement. Sally will coach the family to say "Bye-bye" before waving to see if Omar understands the concept.*

The siblings and Sally crawl behind Omar and his mother. Sally asks one of his siblings to call his name and explains that because Omar is very attached to his siblings, the activity will be more motivating and meaningful for Omar.

> By encouraging the siblings to play this calling game, Sally *promotes knowledge of language* (Goal #4) by *connecting the familiar to the unfamiliar.*

After the siblings call Omar, his mother waits a few seconds to see if he reacts. He moves in her arms, and she immediately turns around and everyone greets him enthusiastically.

> Mother *facilitates auditory processing* (Goal #2) by *waiting for her son to process what was heard.* By waiting for his response, she also *facilitates spoken language and cognition* (Goal #5).

Omar's Airplane
(Learning to Listen Sound)

Short-Term Objectives (STOs)

Audition

- Demonstrate detection and auditory attention to:
  - parent's voice (with varied intonation).
  - variety of vowels and pre-speech sounds.
  - his name (by movement or smiling).
  - the Learning to Listen Sounds.

Speech

- Imitate the following:
  - prosodic features of speech (duration, intensity, pitch).
  - make approximations of the Learning to Listen Sounds.
  - make playful sounds (coos, yells, laughs).

Language

- Listen to someone talking and anticipate the next events.
- Demonstrate association of the LTLS "ahh" and the word "airplane" with the object by using the gesture of flying airplane or searching for the object.
- Vocalize in response to talking.
- Share in vocal turn taking.
- Respond with appropriate actions when common words are used ("bye-bye," "all gone," "how big is the baby," "peek-a-boo," "where's mama").

Cognition

- Sustain interest in desired object for at least two minutes.

Communication

- Respond to simple verbal requests when accompanied by gestures ("bye-bye," "give it to Mama").
- Initiate interaction (point to something and then look at person, give something to person).
- Request or comment by using vocalizations or gestures: "I hear that!" (pointing to ear); or reaching out for a toy and vocalizing.

Activity Description and Analysis

Omar is lying on the rug. Sally puts a toy airplane in a brown paper bag and then says "Ahhh!" Sally coaches mother to point to her ear and says, "Listen, I hear an airplane. It says ahh." Sally explains that by keeping the airplane in the bag, she is helping Omar to focus on the sound and not the object.

> By keeping the airplane out of sight and saying, "Ahh!" Sally *facilitates auditory processing* (Goal #2) as she prepared Omar *to "listen first and last."*

Next, Sally holds the bag near Omar and waits for him to say a sound. He is quiet. She shakes the bag, points to her ear, and says, "Ahh! I hear the airplane!"

Then Sally brings the bag close to mother's ear and shakes it again. Mother points to her ear and says, "Ahhh. I hear the airplane!"

> Shaking the bag and pointing to the ear *facilitates auditory processing* (Goal #2) *and saying, "I heard something!" promotes knowledge of language.*

Sally gives the bag to the mother, who places it close to Omar's ear and then shakes it. Omar reaches for the bag, opens it, and finds the airplane.

> By opening the bag and finding the airplane after several repetitions of "I hear the airplane!" Sally *enhances auditory perception of speech* (Goal #3) by *associating sounds with objects and words* and *creates a listening environment* (Goal #1) by *speaking within earshot and leaning to the child's better hearing side.*

While Omar plays with the airplane, Omar's mother makes the same Learning to Listen Sound again. With Sally's coaching, she varies her pitch. When she flies the plane high, the pitch of "Ahhh" is high; when the airplane flies down, the pitch lowers.

> By varying the pitch of her voice in *stressing selected syllables, words, and phrases,* Mother *enhances auditory perception of speech* (Goal #3).

When it is time to put the airplane back in the bag, Sally asks mother to do it and she models it for everyone else and they say "Bye-bye," followed by a wave as they put it away.

> These words and actions *promote knowledge of language* (Goal #4) as they are *verbalizing in synchrony with movement.*

The family lives near an airport and often see airplanes. Sally encourages mother and the siblings to alert Omar to the sound of the airplane first, and then help him locate the airplane by searching for it and then pointing it out.

> This coaching and guidance help the family to *promote knowledge of language* (Goal #4) by *talking before, during and after the action.*

SNAPSHOT #2: DYLAN AND THE EXPERIENCE BOOK (DAVE SINDREY, PRACTITIONER)

Dylan is 3 years, and 4 months of age and he has been wearing bilateral cochlear implants for 2 years and 11 months. Dave has been providing Auditory-Verbal Therapy to Dylan and his parents for 3 years. Dylan went on a fishing trip with his grandfather and is excited to share with Dave what happened using his Experience book.

An Experience Book is a book the parent creates for his or her child that is "all about the child" (Sindrey, 2012). Listening to and talking about personal drawings of and/or collector's items from meaningful experiences will reinforce talking and listening the most. The Experience Books is one of the most powerful conversation starters. The book is also about what the child is most interested in hearing about or sharing, as he or she is often the hero/ine of the story. The book may contain mementos of a recent event like a bloody bandage from a bike fall or melted candles from the birthday party. The book may have flaps, envelopes with items, characters on strings, and other features that help the user of an Experience Book relive and retell a story that has, for that particular child, *the most bang for the buck* in terms of reinforcement and rich listening and language experience. It can be as creative as the parents desire— from the quiet to the ridiculous, but importantly, all bound to the family's interests and culture.

Activity Short-Term Objectives (STOs)

Audition

- Follow commands using two unrelated steps (e.g., "Take your plate to the kitchen and then find us a book to read").

Speech

- Produce /k/ in initial position of words (e.g., catch, cook).

Language

- Answer "How many?" questions.

Cognition

- Count out loud (up to 5 items).

Communication

- Respond to comments, negative assertions, sabotage, and pausing.

Activity Description and Analysis

As she enters, Mother scans the room and says, "Dylan! Can you close the door and then show Dave your *Experience Book?*"

Calling Dylan's name *facilitates his auditory attention* (Goal #2) as an *auditory hook*. The two-step unrelated direction *promotes his knowledge of language* (Goal #4) because it includes *language that he knows but does not yet use*.

Dylan follows her directions and then Dave praises Dylan and her. Dave points out that the more often Dylan demonstrates these types of directions, the greater his comprehension will become.

Guidance to provide additional practice will help *promote Dylan's knowledge of language* (Goal #4) when the mother uses *language that he knows but does not yet use*.

Then Dave asks, "Wow, Dylan! How many fish did you catch?" (Mother has drawn three fish to the left of the boat). Dylan begins to count "One, two, three! Three!" and Dave expands on his response by saying, "Three! Three fish. Three big fish!"

> "Three! Three fish. Three big fish!" promotes *Dylan's knowledge of language* (Goal #4) by *recasting, expanding and expatiating on his words.*

There is a bloody Band-Aid taped to the page and Dylan eagerly shows his finger and says "Ouch." Dave encourages Dylan to provide more information and Dylan's mother provides more too. Dave compliments them on the page as a great conversation starter.

> The Band-Aid is a great conversation starter and promotes *Dylan's independent learning* (Goal #6) by *creating the unexpected.*

Dave explained to Dylan's mother that photos of cleaning and cooking the fish could be a great addition to the Experience Book. The photos act as a simple three-step sequence story that Dylan's conversational partner can use to re-tell the story using new words such as "catch," "clean," and "cook."

> Dave's guidance helps *promote Dylan's knowledge of language* (Goal #4) by *connecting the familiar with the unfamiliar.*

Once Dylan's experience book is exhausted, Dave brings out a page from his own Experience Book (a traditional activity used at the start of AVT sessions). Dave models different ideas for displaying experiences within the file folder format. As the folder is retrieved from the shelf, Dave describes how he uses *wait time* and *expanded versions of Dylan's utterances* as ways to expand receptive and expressive language.

> Dave describes *how to facilitate spoken language and cognition* (Goal #5) by *waiting* for Dylan's response and by *recasting, expanding, and expatiating his words and/ or utterances.*

When Dave says, *"This is a sad story"* and then hands the folder to Mother, Mother opens it and says, *"What happened?"* in a concerned voice as she and Dylan look at the items. She gives Dylan lots of time to respond. Dave praises her and she continues to expand Dylan's language throughout the conversation about the demise of a pet turtle.

> Dave uses *a self-statement* that *facilitates spoken language and cognition* (Goal #5). When Dylan's mother *waits* after asking a question, she also *facilitates spoken language and cognition* (Goal #5). *Expansion of language promotes knowledge of language* (Goal #4).

SNAPSHOT #3: "I LIKE ICE CREAM" SONG (LISA KATZ (PRACTITIONER))

Emma is 4 years, and 6 months of age and she has been wearing bilateral cochlear implants for 1 year and 6 months. Lisa has been providing Auditory-Verbal Therapy to Emma and her parents for 2 years. In this session, Emma enjoys making ice cream desserts with Lisa and her mother and learns a new song about ice cream called "I Like Ice Cream" (Estabrooks & Birkenshaw-Fleming, 2003).

Activity Short-Term Objectives (STOs)

Audition

- Identify objects based on hearing their descriptions in a closed set with some open set ability.
- Demonstrate auditory sequential memory for four items.

Speech

- Enhance production of /s/ in final position of words.

Language

- Expand vocabulary (e.g., thunder, hail, bullies, liars, turnips).

Cognition

- Demonstrate ability to recall words in a new song.

- Demonstrate ease of identifying higher level auditory-cognitive concepts.

Communication

- Ask questions.

Activity Description and Analysis

Lisa begins singing the song "I Like Ice Cream" (Estabrooks & Birkenshaw-Fleming, 2003). After she sings the full song, she begins singing again and looks expectantly at Emma and her mother. Emma and her mother quickly join in.

> Lisa *facilitates Emma's spoken language and cognition* (Goal #5) when she *leans forward with an expectant look* and *waits for Emma's response.*

From time to time, Lisa sings "I like . . ." and then pauses and waits. Emma then sings, "Ice cream! All day long!"

> Lisa *facilitates auditory processing* (Goal #2) and *facilitates spoken language and cognition* (Goal #5) by *allowing time for auditory closure.*

Lisa then tells Emma that she has a tablet that can play the song as well. Emma responds, "Ablet?" Lisa says, "Yes, 'a,'" and then whispers the word "tablet."

Emma responds, "Oh! A tablet!" Lisa replies, "That's right, a tablet. Actually, mine is an iPad." Lisa, Emma, and her mother listen to the song again and sing along. This time, Emma demonstrates that she knows the song well.

> Emma's *auditory perception of speech is enhanced* (Goal #3) when *a word is whispered, and her auditory processing is facilitated* (Goal #3) *when she listens first and last*. Lisa *promotes knowledge of language* (Goal #4) by *recasting, expanding, and expatiating on Emma's words.*

Mother and Emma take turns singing the song and substituting the item in their box for the word "ice cream." After singing four times, Lisa asks Emma if she can remember what's in the boxes. Lisa and Mother verify the responses by indicating whether or not Emma is correct verbally, and then by revealing the item in the box.

> Lisa *promotes knowledge of language* (Goal #4) by *taking turns* singing the song and substituting the word ice cream for other items. She *facilitates spoken language and cognition* (Goal #5) by *scaffolding for language and asking age-appropriate questions* about what's in the boxes.

Emma has difficulty remembering one item. Emma's mother indicates that it's a fruit that monkeys like to eat. And

then she waits and looks expectantly. Emma finally remembers it's a banana.

> Emma's mother *promotes knowledge of language* (Goal #4) by *emphasizing actions, relations, and attributes* (e.g., a fruit that monkeys like to eat).

Lisa tells Emma's mother that the lyrics of the song can be changed to discuss things that children don't like (e.g., thunder, hail, bullies, liars, turnips).

> Lisa provides alternative ideas for Emma's mother to *stimulate independent learning* (Goal #6) by *creating the unexpected* (e.g., things that children don't like).

SNAPSHOT #4: GETTING READY TO BAKE (KAREN MACIVER-LUX (PRACTITIONER))

Michael is 5 years, and 10 months of age and has Auditory-Neuropathy Spectrum Disorder. He has been wearing his right CI for 4 months and has been wearing hearing aids since he was 2 years of age. Karen has been providing Auditory-Verbal Therapy to Michael and his parents for 5 months. In this session, Michael is preparing the oven to bake cookies with Karen and his mother.

Activity Short-Term Objectives (STOs)

Audition

■ Demonstrate auditory memory for three items in a closed set.
■ Maintain auditory attention when engaged in activities that involve multi-tasking (e.g., listening to directions while drawing a picture).

Speech

■ Produce word and phrase approximations.

Language/Communication

■ Ask questions.

Cognition

■ Demonstrate ability to identify letters in words.

Activity

Karen suggests to Michael's mother to go over to the oven and bring Michael along, saying "Michael, let's go and turn on the oven." When Mother arrives at the oven, Karen guides her to say, "Hm . . . how do we turn on this oven? Let's look together for the 'on' button. We're looking and looking . . . oh, here it is. Here is the 'on' button. Let's turn it on together. One, two, three, and we push the button!" Michael and his mother jointly push the "on" button as Mother says "push."

> When Michael's mother engages in self-talk as she figures out how to turn the oven on, she *promotes knowledge of language* (Goal #4) by *talking before, during, and after the action and by verbalizing in synchrony with movement.*

Mother says, "Okay, Michael, push 3, 7, and 5." He pushes numbers 3 and 5 but forgets to push the number 7. Michael's mother says, "Uh oh, we forgot to push the 7. Let's try again." She resets the oven, pretends that she forgot the numbers, and asks Michael, "What are the numbers again?" He shrugs and looks at Karen. Mom says, "Good idea, let's ask Karen." Michael's mother guides Michael word by word to ask Karen the question, by pausing between each of the words she says, and he repeats them.

> When Michael's mother pauses between each of the words she wants him to repeat, she *promotes knowledge of language* (Goal #4) by *pausing for grammatical spaces or emphasis.*

Karen responds by using a slightly louder volume, "Three, *seven,* five," putting stress on the word "seven." Michael turns to the oven and pushes the numbers 3, 7, and 5. Michael's mother gives him a thumbs-up signal. Karen says, "Yay, don't forget to say whatever it is that you say when you give a thumbs-up signal." Michael's mother says, "Yay! We did it!" and waits. He responds by providing an approximation of his mother's model.

When Karen emphasizes the word "seven," she enhances *auditory perception of speech* (Goal #3) by *stressing selected syllables, words, and phrases*. When she reminds Michael's mother to use a phrase with a gesture, she is helping her to *promote knowledge of language* (Goal #4) by *verbalizing in synchrony with movements*. Finally, after Michael's mother says, "Yay! We did it!" she *facilitates spoken language and cognition* (Goal #5) by *waiting for the child's response*.

Michael's mother says, "Okay, now we need to find a button that has the letter B on it." She waits. Michael looks for some time and finds the "bake" button. She says, "Yay, you did it!" without the thumbs-up gesture. She waits and then looks expectantly at Michael. Karen praises Mom and Michael grins and shows a thumbs-up gesture. Mom gasps with surprise and gives Michael a hug.

When Michael's mother gives the direction to find the bake button, she *facilitates auditory processing* (Goal #2) by waiting for the child to process what was heard. She *promotes knowledge of language* (Goal #4) by *talking before showing the action (talking before, during, and after the action)* and by *connecting the familiar with the unfamiliar* (by asking him to find the letter b in a word that he doesn't know. When she says, "Yay! You did it!" with the thumbs-up gesture, she *facilitates auditory processing* (Goal #2) by preparing the child to "listen first and last." She *facilitates spoken*

language and cognition (Goal #5) by *waiting for the child's response* and by *leaning forward with an expectant look*.

Karen tells Mother that Michael is able to follow single-step directions easily with numbers and letters, and asks what she thinks the next step might be to help increase his auditory memory. Mother replies, "Maybe I can ask him to push the 'bake' button and then push the 'start' button using the letters b and s."

When Karen asks the questions about how to stimulate his auditory memory, Mother's response helps *promote knowledge of language* (Goal #4) by *transitioning beyond Michael's comfort zone*.

CONCLUSION

In this chapter the authors proposed a framework or blueprint that can be generated when planning, delivering, and evaluating the AVT session. They suggested a number of components for the AVT session, provided a sample first session with a baby and additional snapshots from other sessions, complete with short analyses.

Through the planning, delivery, and evaluation of AVT sessions, practitioners carefully guide and coach parents of children who are deaf or hard of hearing in ways that will achieve the short-term objectives (STOs) of each session and the long-term goals (LTGs) in the AVT care plan. Practitioners *raise the bar* on their planning, delivery, and evaluation of AVT sessions by continuous quality improvement through self-evaluation and by engaging help from the family, the child, other partners on the family's team, and sometimes an extensive global network of colleagues.

Continuing the analogy of *charting the course* . . . to help children who are deaf or hard of hearing in AVT to reach the expected destinations that are shared by the family and the practitioner, *"all hands need to be on deck."*

REFERENCES

Bergman Nutley, S., Söderqvist, S., Bryde, S., Thorell, L. B., Humphreys, K., & Klingberg, T. (2011). Gains in fluid intelligence after training non-verbal reasoning in 4-year-old children: A controlled, randomized study. *Developmental Science, 14*, 591–601.

Bodrova, E., & Leong, D. J. (2007). *Tools of the mind*. Columbus, OH: Pearson.

Eisenberg, S. (2004). Structured communicative play therapy for targeting language in young children. *Communication Disorders Quarterly, 26*(1), 29–35.

Ernst, M. (2012). What is an auditory-verbal treatment plan? In *101 FAQs about auditory-verbal practice*, (pp. 334–337). Washington, DC: Alexander Graham Bell Association for the Deaf and Hard of Hearing.

Estabrooks, W. (1994). *Auditory-verbal therapy for parents and professionals*. Washington, DC: Alexander Graham Bell Association for the Deaf and Hard of Hearing.

Estabrooks, W. (1998). *Cochlear implants for kids*. Washington DC: Alexander Graham Bell Association for the Deaf and Hard of Hearing.

Estabrooks, W. (2006). *Auditory-verbal therapy and practice*. Washington, DC: AG Bell.

Estabrooks, W., & Birkenshaw-Fleming, (2003). *Hear & listen! Talk & sing!* Washington, DC: AG Bell.

Estabrooks, W., & Birkenshaw-Fleming, L. (2006). *Songs for listening! Songs for life!* Washington DC: Alexander Graham Bell Association for the Deaf and Hard of Hearing.

Estabrooks, W., MacIver-Lux, K., & Rhoades, E. (2016). *Auditory-verbal therapy for young children with hearing loss and their families and the practitioners who guide them*. San Diego, CA: Plural Publishing.

Fredricks, J. A., Blumenfeld, P. C., & Paris, A. H. (2004). School engagement: Potential of the concept, state of the evidence. *Review of Educational Research, 74*(1), 59–109.

Girolametto, L., Pearce, P., & Weitzman, E. (1996a). The effects of focused stimulation for promoting vocabulary in children with delays: A pilot study. *Journal of Childhood Communication Development, 17*, 39–49.

Girolametto, L., Pearce, P., & Weitzman, E. (1996b). Interactive focused stimulation for toddlers with expressive vocabulary delays. *Journal of Speech and Hearing Research, 39*, 1274–1283.

Goldblat, E., & Pinto, O. Y. (2017). Academic outcomes of adolescents and young adults with hearing loss who received auditory-verbal therapy. *Deafness & Education International, 19*(3–4), 126–133.

Holmes, J., Gathercole, S. E., & Dunning, D. L. (2009). Adaptive training leads to sustained enhancement of poor working memory in children. *Developmental Science, 12*, 9–15.

Kashinath, S., Woods, J. W., & Goldstein, H. (2006). Enhancing generalized teaching strategy use in daily routines by parents of children with autism. *Journal *of Speech, Language, and Hearing Research, 49,* 466–485.

Latif Akbari, R., Khan, M., & Arshad, H. (2017). Effectiveness of auditory verbal therapy in children with cochlear implantation and hearing aid users. *Journal of Riphah College of Rehabilitation Sciences, 5,* 8–11.

Lee, J., & Van Patten, B. (2003). *Making communicative language happen.* New York, NY: McGraw-Hill.

Newbern, K., & Lasker, L. (2012). What can the listening and spoken language professional do when the entire session seems to be "going down the drain"? In W. Estabrooks (Ed.), *101 FAQs about auditory-verbal practice.* Washington, DC: Alexander Graham Bell Association of the Deaf and Hard of Hearing.

Pepper, J., & Weitzman, E. (2004). *It takes two to talk®: A practical guide for parents of children with language delays* (2nd ed.). Toronto, ONT, Canada: The Hanen Centre.

Percy-Smith, L., Cayé-Thomasen, P., Gudman, M., Jensen, J. H., & Thomsen, J. (2008). Self-esteem and social well-being of children with cochlear implant compared to normal-hearing children. *International Journal of Pediatric Otorhinolaryngology, 72*(7), 1113–1120.

Rush, D., Shelden, M., & Hanft, S. (2003). Coaching families and colleagues: A process for collaboration in natural settings. *Infants and Young Children, 16,* 33–47.

Sindrey, D. (2012). What is an experience book and how is it used in auditory-verbal therapy and education? *101 FAQs about auditory-verbal practice* (pp. 142–145). Washington, DC: Alexander Graham Bell Association for the Deaf and Hard of Hearing.

Snyder, H. R., & Munakata, Y. (2010). Becoming self-directed: Abstract representations support endogenous flexibility in children. *Cognition, 116,* 155–167.

Snyder, H. R., & Munakata, Y. (2013). So many options, so little control: Abstract representations can reduce selection demands to increase children's self-directed flexibility. *Journal of Experimental Child Psychology, 116,* 659–673.

Suskind, D., Suskind, B., & Lewinter-Suskind, L. (2015). *Thirty million words.* New York, NY: Dutton.

Torppa, R., Faulkner, A., Kujala, T, Huotilainen, M., & Lipsanen, J. (2018). Developmental links between speech perception in noise, singing, and cortical processing of music in children with cochlear implants. *Music Perception, 36,* 156–174.

Tye-Murray, N. (2020). *Foundations of aural rehabilitation: Children, adults, and their family members* (5th ed., p. 374). San Diego, CA: Plural Publishing.

Vanderwert, R., Simpson, E., Paukner, A., Suomi S., Fox, N., & Ferrari, P. (2015). Early social experience affects neural activity to affiliative facial gestures in newborn nonhuman primates. *Developmental Neuroscience, 37*(3), 243–252.

Vygotsky, L. (1978). *Mind In society: Development of higher psychological processes.* Cambridge, MA: Harvard University Press.

Woods, J., Kashinath, S., & Goldstein, H. (2004). Effects of embedding caregiver-implemented teaching strategies in daily routines on children's communication outcomes. *Journal of Early Intervention, 26*(3), 175–193.

18

MUSIC AND SINGING IN AUDITORY-VERBAL THERAPY

Amy McConkey Robbins

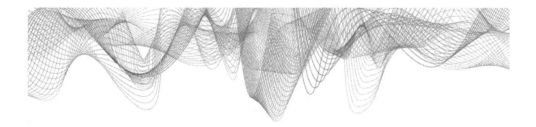

Historically, access to musical phenomena has eluded most children with severe-to-profound hearing loss. It is not just the music itself that is lost to these children, but the connection to others that music brings, the sense of community and the emotional outlet it makes possible. Musical experiences can and need to be part of the daily lives of all children who are deaf or hard of hearing. Given today's early identification of hearing loss, early fitting of hearing technology, early intervention, and habilitation, these children have unprecedented opportunities to experience and excel at music. Specifically, music experiences are well suited to be an integral part of Auditory-Verbal Therapy (AVT).

Throughout the evolution of AVT, many of the pioneers encouraged music, from Helen Beebe to Doreen Pollack and Daniel Ling. I first encountered the musical component of AVT at an Alexander Graham Bell convention in 1980, when I attended a short course given by an Auditory-Verbal practitioner (practitioner), who played the guitar and sang, "I'm Learning to Listen" (Estabrooks, 1994). He insisted that it was reasonable to expect children who are deaf or hard of hearing to participate in and enjoy music (see Figure 18–1). Leaders in the fields of music therapy and AVT combined efforts that same year when Carol and Clive Robbins published what they described as a "developmental music program" for children with severe

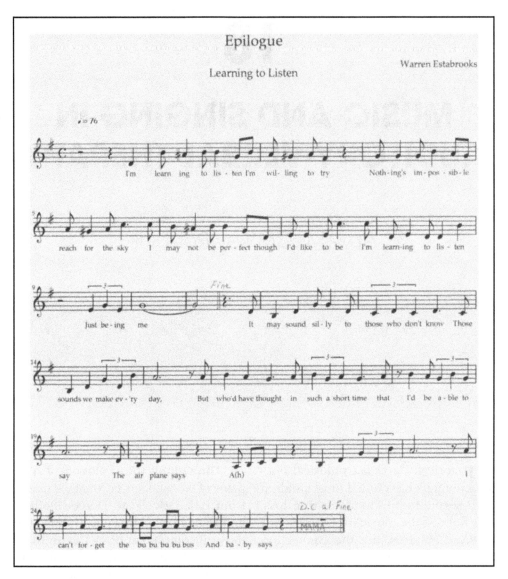

Figure 18–1. "Learning to Listen" music and lyric.

and profound hearing loss. Their book, *Music and the Hearing Impaired*, emphasized the importance of experiential music that was linked to emotion, rather than theoretical, rote music instruction. It included a chapter called "Audiological Considerations in Music with the Deaf" by Dr. Arthur Boothroyd.

Dr. Daniel Ling spoke and wrote often about the value of music for children who are deaf or hard of hearing. His forward to two volumes of music, singing and session plans for children in AVT (Estabrooks & Birkenshaw-Fleming, 1994, 2003) remains very relevant for today's children. In these two books, Ling listed reasons for practitioners to sing to children and to encourage them and their parents to sing (see Table 18–1 with some additions by this author). A review of the items in Table 18–1 introduces the reader to the timeless value of music for children who are deaf or hard of hearing and to many of the concepts reviewed in this chapter.

These leaders and many practitioners knew that music was a valuable component of AVT. They observed ways music supported a child's auditory and spoken language development. With advances in science, hearing technologies, and imaging techniques such as positron emission tomography (PET)

scanning and functional magnetic resonance imaging (fMRI) that allow viewing the brain in action, the reader can understand why this is true.

Why and How to Incorporate Music into AVT

This chapter is divided into two parts: Part 1, *Why include music in AVT?*, covers the rationale and research findings that support the integration of music

Table 18–1. The Value of Singing and Music for Children and Parents in AV Practice (Adapted from Ling, 2003[1])

Listening to singing gives pleasure.
Singing to children helps develop their listening skills.
Good listening skills enhance speech perception.
Putting words to music helps children remember them (music is a memory magnet[2]).
Singing songs focuses on voice pitch and rhythm.
Perception of pitch and rhythm is essential to understanding spoken language.
Singing tunes enhances a child's control of intonation in speech.
Rhythm in song helps to develop rhythm in speech.
Singing helps to develop breath flow and breath control.
Singing can help to avoid speech disorders such as weak breath flow, hypernasality, pharyngeal tension, and the prolongation and neutralization of vowels.
Singing can be used in the remediation of many speech problems.
Music offers repetition, repeated practice and rehearsal.[2]
Songs support executive functions, including planning, working memory and impulse control.[2]
Music enhances emotional discernment, including knowing the emotion of a speaker's voice.[2]
Singing or playing an instrument provides an outlet for feelings.[2]
Knowing the music of one's culture(s) allows for personal identity and group affiliation.[2]
Singing and musical experiences build children's confidence in listening.[2]

Source: [1]Ling, D. (2003). Introduction: Speech and song. In W. Estabrooks and L. Birkenshaw-Fleming (Eds.), *Songs for Listening! Songs for Life!* Washington, DC: Alexander Graham Bell Association for the Deaf and Hard of Hearing.

Note: [2]Added by the chapter author.

into AVT sessions. The author presents 10 underlying premises of the chapter, followed by the rationale for including music as an essential component for developing listening and spoken language in children with hearing loss, and the research demonstrating that children who are exposed to music, whether through didactic lessons or informal activities at home, are more proficient than their peers at developmentally important tasks, even non-musical ones. Part 2, *How to incorporate music into AVT,* describes activities that weave music into AVT with children at different ages and stages, including those with complex needs, and includes guidance for making music part of everyday living.

PART 1: WHY INCLUDE MUSIC IN AVT?

Ten Premises for Inclusion of Music in AVT

Ten premises form the foundation of this author's approach (see Table 18–2). These premises are convictions based on empirical evidence and personal experience, and the evidence-informed wisdom of mentors. In particular, board-certified music therapist Christine Barton offers hands-on demonstrations about the power music has to engage children who are deaf or hard of hearing (Barton & Robbins, 2018). The children are teachers too. By actively using music and singing in AVT sessions, one can observe what and how children can learn and the musical abilities they demonstrate. Some have asserted that these abilities are impossible for anyone wearing

hearing technology. Impossible? Not to the 4-year-old child with bilateral cochlear implants (CIs) who sings "Take Me Out to the Ballgame" mostly on pitch, with a tonal center that is like his peers with typical hearing. Not to the 12-year-old with complex needs and cognitive impairment who received bilateral CIs at an early age and loves classical music. While this child was attending a concert of Vivaldi music, the first piece was unfamiliar to him, but as it began, he immediately recognized it was different from "The Four Seasons" and exclaimed, "That's not MY Vivaldi!"

1. **Children are born with the ability to learn language and music; it defines us as human.** Every known culture possesses its own musical canon, and the instincts to sing and speak are universally human (Mithin, 2006).

2. **Music needs to be incorporated into a child's everyday life.** The most enjoyable and efficient way to provide musical experiences to children with hearing loss is to make music part of every AVT session and encourage families to infuse their home with musical opportunities. AVT is well suited to incorporating music, as it relies on the practitioner's ability to coach parents on how to integrate music experiences with listening and spoken language. In AVT we seek to foster development of a musical identity (Hargreaves, Miell, & MacDonald, 2002) in children, as we work to establish an "auditory personality" (Pollack, 1985). There may be a perception that to include music, one must provide formal instruction and use only published songs. In fact, studies show that, along with music training, informal musical experiences confer neurodevelopmental benefit and have the added advantage of encouraging

Table 18-2. Premises of this Chapter

1. Children are born with the ability to learn language and music; they define us as human.
2. Music should be integrated into Auditory-Verbal practice and incorporated into a child's everyday life.
3. Music must be experienced as active musicing. Children should "do" music.
4. Music and language have commonalities; developing one facilitates the other.
5. Music and spoken language also have important differences.
6. Research findings over the past decade are extremely encouraging regarding the benefits of music for those with typical hearing and hearing impairment.
7. Adult research findings underestimate the musical potential of children with hearing impairment.
8. Music is helpful for children with hearing impairment of all ages and stages.
9. Music holds promise for special populations.
10. The most valuable musical instrument we have is our voice.

Source: Adapted from "Language and Music and Ears, Oh My!" (Robbins & Barton, AG Bell, 2010)

emotional bonding between child and adult.

3. Music must be an active process that is experienced as "musicing." The term "musicing" implies human engagement and active involvement in musical experiences (Elliott, 1995). It is no coincidence that "musicing" is a verb, since music is something young children must "do" as part of an authentic musical experience.

4. Music and spoken language have commonalities; developing one facilitates the other. Speech and music share features such as rhythm, intensity, timbre (the unique quality distinguishing sounds, such as a trumpet versus a violin, or adult voice versus a child's voice) and pitch. However, the pitch spectrum in music is much greater than in speech. People can sing much higher and lower than they can talk, and many instruments can emit notes that one cannot sing. But access to these pitches helps us to hear birds, sirens, and other important sounds in the world. From a neurocognitive perspective, the human brain recruits similar cortical mechanisms for processing music and speech (Strait & Kraus, 2011). Patel's (2012) OPERA hypothesis posits that musical activities drive neural networks to function with higher precision than needed for ordinary spoken communication. Yet, since speech shares these networks with music, speech processing benefits.

5. Music and spoken language have important differences. Because it differs from language in some ways, music may be a bridge to spoken communication for children with a variety of learning profiles. For example, children with autism spectrum disorders (ASDs) may have difficulty with joint attention and eye contact and may not be responsive when spoken to. The author has observed that language seems confrontational to some of these children.

They may feel "on the spot" to make eye contact with the speaker, to reply verbally, and to take a conversational turn. In contrast, music can be invitational. When "invited" into a musical activity, a child may participate at his or her level of comfort. A child with ASD initially may just observe when the parent and the practitioner make music, then may pat his or her knees or tap out the beat with rhythm sticks but not sing along, and so on. Over time, the child becomes a full participant, having accepted the invitation to make music when ready to do so.

6. **Research findings over the past decade are extremely encouraging regarding the benefits of music for those with both typical hearing and hearing loss.** Musicians are better overall listeners than non-musicians on a variety of auditory tasks. One does not have to be a professional musician to experience this advantage, but simply must have musical experiences in life (Williams, Barrett, Welch, Abad, & Broughton, 2015). Everyday musical activities are a rich source of learning that has the potential to shape auditory skill development (Putkinen, Saarikivi, & Tervaniemi, 2013). The data show that music making contributes to "auditory fitness" (Kraus & Chandrasekaran, 2010) and has an age-decelerating effect on the brains of adult amateur musicians versus non-musicians (Rogenmoser. Kernbach, Schlaug, & Gaser, 2017). This phenomenon is described as "keeping the brain young by making music." Taken as a whole, the results of many studies indicate that music training can cause functional and structural changes to the brain across the lifespan. These changes have transfer ef-

fects that benefit speech and language tasks (Kraus & Chandrasekaran, 2010).

7. **Adult research findings underestimate the musical potential of children with hearing loss.** Until about the year 2000, the majority of music research with CIs had been done with adults, so expectations for children were extrapolated from adult research findings. This research, conducted with adults who were post-lingually deafened and had CIs, indicated that a substantial number were disappointed with their ability to appreciate music after receiving the CI. This remains true today. Many adults report music does not sound the way they remember it. In contrast, most children who are deaf or hard of hearing come to music experiences without any pre-conceived notions of "before" and "after" hearing. They seem to accept the musical input as something natural. Structural and functional MRIs of children with typical hearing who have received instrumental music training indicate that plasticity occurs in brain regions that either have control over primary musical functions or serve as multimodal integration regions for musical skills (Schlaug, Norton, Overy, & Winner, 2005). The higher potential for neuroplasticity in children versus adults allows for transfer effects (the impact of experience in one domain—music—on behavior in other domains) that benefit children who listen with CIs. Brain plasticity also might explain why children who receive CIs at very young ages show superior music processing and appreciation compared with most adults who were post-lingually deafened and have CIs. Putkinen, Saarikivi, et al. (2013) write: "the results of neural response studies are promising since

they give strong evidence against views that cochlear-implanted individuals are not able to perceive and appreciate music" (p. 4).

8. **Music is helpful for children of all ages and stages.** Even newborns benefit from music. Recent findings demonstrate that music is beneficial to children born prematurely and who are in the neonatal intensive care unit (NICU). On average, babies in the NICU who received specialized services from a music therapist were released from the hospital two weeks earlier than babies who did not (Colombini, 2019). Teens with CIs often indicate that music enjoyment is one of the strongest benefits they derive from hearing technology, as music connects them to others.

9. **Music holds promise for special populations.** Nowhere does one observe the value of auditory experiences more, and musical experiences, in particular, than in children with hearing loss who also have complex needs. This is especially relevant since about 40% of children who are deaf or hard of hearing also have other challenges (see Chapter 22). Access to music is often mentioned by parents of these children as one of the most important outcomes after the fitting of hearing aids or CIs. For some, music takes on the role that is usually played by spoken language as it can become the primary way they receive information and connect to others.

10. **The most valuable musical instrument is the voice.** Most people have a voice that can be accessed upon request or desire. The voice is the musical instrument most closely related to speech (Barton & Robbins, 2018). From a neurocognitive perspective the voice needs to be the first instrument

of choice, given that a baby's brain responds more robustly to tones produced by voices than by instruments and to a happy voice quality than voice that has neutral affect (Corbeil, Trehub & Peretz, 2013).

RATIONALES FOR EMBEDDING MUSIC INTO AVT

Spoken Language and Music Are Both *Auditory* Experiences

Music is a multisensory event—one experiences it through many sensory modalities, including audition, vision, and kinesthesis. It may be experienced without any visual cues, such as listening to music from a radio or a computer. However, without auditory access, music cannot be fully experienced. Thus, there is a recognized *primacy of audition* for music. The same is true of spoken language. Auditory input to the brain is the foundation upon which spoken language is built. Segal and Kishon-Rabin (2011) note that *auditory* exposure to linguistic input is critical for infants to develop an interest in spoken language.

There is a window for cortical development in auditory areas of the brain that is only open during the early years of a child's life and will effectively close if high-quality auditory stimulation is not available (Sharma & Nash, 2009). A young child's developing auditory neural structure is highly plastic during this early period but such plasticity deceases with age (Gordon et al., 2011.) Therefore, stimulating the auditory cortical centers early and consistently is imperative in order to influence the organization and maturation of these irreplaceable neural networks (see Chapter 1).

Spoken Language, a Major Focus of AVT, Inherently Contains Many Musical Elements

Music is considered by many to be a mode of communication (Trehub, 2013), one that has particular importance for pre-verbal infants. As a component of music, infant-directed (ID) singing is universal. Caregivers use ID singing when they sing songs, rock, pat, and soothe the infant in a responsive way. In addition, ID singing attracts the infants' attention and communicates the caregiver's emotional intent (Trainor et al., 1997; Trehub & Gudmundsdottir, 2015). The responsive nature of ID singing can be observed when mothers match their singing with the emotional state of the baby. If an infant is agitated, for example, mothers will rock, bounce, and sing to the child in a more intense way, using a louder singing voice if the child is crying. Fathers and older children make similar modifications to singing to babies, suggesting this is a universal response.

Caregivers unconsciously modify their speech when talking to infants using a universal behavior called child-directed (CD) speech (also known as infant-directed speech, motherese, or musical speech) (see Chapters 11, 12, and 15). CD speech occurs across all languages and is considered a "natural" first musical signal as it contains many features similar to music, such as melodic and exaggerated pitch contours, an overall higher pitch, a slow, deliberate tempo using short utterances, and use of repetition (Houston & Bergeson, 2014). Such input is acoustically salient because it captures and holds an infant's attention. The intrinsic acoustic patterns, grouping, rhythm, and phrasing found in CD speech are believed to prime the processing skills necessary to decode spoken language (Bergeson, Miller, & McCune, 2006). Infants with typical hearing detect rhythmic and melodic features in music and in the intonational contours of speech (Trehub, 2013) and they demonstrate a preference for listening to CD speech over other stimuli (Segal & Kishon-Rabin, 2011). As infants gain more auditory experience, mothers change the nature of their CD speech to complement the baby's new skills. For example, Bergeson et al. (2006) found when mothers of infants with CIs used CD speech, they adjusted their speech characteristics relative to the child's hearing age, not chronological age. This supports the notion that CD speech is naturally responsive and sensitive to a child's needs.

Coaching Parents Is Critical Both for Music and for Listening and Spoken Language Success

Home-based musical interactions between child and parent have wide-reaching benefits. Such interactions typically require that parents receive encouragement about how to utilize music in the home. Research suggests that informal musical activities such as singing and musical play, as part of daily routines, positively influence the maturation of auditory discrimination and attention in preschool-aged children with typical hearing (Putkinen, Saarikivi, et al., 2013). In AVT, carryover and extensions are suggested in every AVT session (see Chapter 17).

AVT Addresses Whole Child Learning and Development

What characteristics of music support whole child constructs? Shared music time engages the child and caregiver in joint attention—critical for social-linguistic development. Musical experiences often include dancing, marching, and other coordinated movements that benefit gross motor development. When one sings "Hokey Pokey" with words such as "You put your right foot in, you take your right foot out . . . you shake it all about" (Estabrooks & Birkenshaw-Fleming, 2003), one can stimulate motor planning in young children. Many action songs address executive functions as they require self-regulation, working memory, or impulse control (Chapter 13). Examples include songs such as "I Know an Old Woman Who Swallowed a Fly" (sequenced cumulative memory); "I Like to Eat Apples and Bananas" (working memory and phonological awareness); "Two Feet" (Barton, 2008), which contains a "freeze" moment in each verse (self-regulation); and the game "Musical Chairs" (impulse control). For children at the pre-verbal stage, finger plays or songs with gestures and cues pro-vide practice with coordination of fine motor skills and support overall meaning, even when linguistic competence is incomplete.

Music Aligns with AVT to Follow Typical Developmental Expectations

Central to AVT is guiding parents to help their children acquire developmental milestones in listening and spoken language as closely as possible to the time that they are biologically intended to do so (Robbins, Koch, Osberger, Phillips, & Kishon-Rabin, 2004). Practitioners seek to replicate the timeline and sequence of skill acquisition across a broad range of communication domains, taking into account the *whole child*, and synchrony across developmental areas (Robbins, 2016). The same is true of musical experiences in any AVT session. Practitioners need to be familiar with musical milestones for children with typical hearing and select goals and activities that are consistent with the age, stage, and listening experience of each child. Table 18–3 shows developmental milestones for children of increasing age, divided into those related to music and those related to language.

The Active Experience of "Musicing" Is Analogous to the Interactive, Reciprocal Nature of Spoken Communication

Much like spoken language, music is a dynamic process that occurs as part of social exchanges with other people.

Table 18–3. Music and Language Milestones in Typical Hearing Children with Associated Music Activities (Barton, 2010)

Age	Music Milestones	Language Milestones	Music Activities
Birth–3 months	Alerts and calms to music; prefers infant directed singing; coos/cries	Moves to the sound of a familiar voice; looks at speaker's mouth; coos/cries	Sing lullabies; gently rock and pat to music; narrate baby's day using "mama" interval
3–6 months	Musical babbling; repetitive movements in response to music; turns to the source of music; prefers higher pitched voices	Babbles; laughs; smiles; vocalizes pleasure and displeasure	Imitate baby's "musical" vocalizations; provide shakers, bells and simple rhythm toys, bounce gently to music
6–9 months	Occasionally matches pitch; larger repetitive movements; recognizes familiar melodies; uses descending vocalizations	Smiles at speaker; uses voice and gestures to show displeasure; responds to own name	Imitate spontaneous songs; play pitch matching games using "la-la" or "loo-loo"; easy finger play songs; nursery rhymes with movement
9–12 months	"Sings" spontaneously; recognizes and attempts to sing along with familiar songs;	Recognizes names of family members; waves bye-bye; says one-two words; responds to "no"; babbles with inflection	Provide songs for different activities like wake-up/bath time/bedtime; variety of recorded music; drums and xylophones;
12–18 months	Dances to music; pays attention to lyrics; sings snippets of learned songs; more pitch matching; starting to match movements to music	Jargon–like utterances with some words included; follows one step directions; 20–100 words	Dance baby on your feet; sing simple songs/chants/nursery rhymes; songs with repetitive chorus like E-I-E-I-O and B-I-N-G-O.

Table 18-3. *continued*

Age	Music Milestones	Language Milestones	Music Activities
18–24 months	Looks for dance partners; spins, marches to music; spontaneous songs have steady rhythm; able to imitate songs; lyrics more accurate than pitch	Two-word phrases; uses question intonation; repeats overheard words; starts using pronouns; understands "where?" and "what's that?"; >200 words	Experiment with different voices (big/little/high/low); Make sounds with voice to encourage vocal range (sirens, birds, animal noises)
2–3 years	Learns singing vs. speaking voices; sings in different keys and meters; matches pitch consistently; some instrument discrimination	Three-word phrases; refers to self as "me"; starts to use verb endings; answers questions with yes or no; follows two-step command; >900 words	Play guessing games with familiar songs and instruments; repetitive rhythmic accompaniment to singing; sequential songs like "If You're Happy and You Know it"
3–4 years	Begins to discriminate between familiar instruments; uses rhythm instruments to accompany their songs; melodic contour is intact; makes up songs	Uses many more pronouns; names colors; sentences of 5–6 words; tells stories; expresses feelings; enjoys poems; sense of humor starts to develop; >1500 words	Marching band with rhythm instruments; high/low up/down; play/stop; fast/slow; loud/soft; nonsense songs; read books based on familiar songs
4–5 years	Larger purposeful movements; imaginative songs and stories; beginning to recognize familiar melodies without lyrics; matches beat to others	Asks what, who, where, why questions; answers why and how questions; uses future tense; tells name and address; uses longer sentences; >2500 words	Rhythm stick games; movement songs using scarves, ribbons, etc.; story songs; group music experiences; xylophones, tone bars

continues

Table 18-3. *continued*

Age	Music Milestones	Language Milestones	Music Activities
5–6 years	Maintains steady beat while moving to music; sings melody with pitch accuracy; plays melodies on simple instruments; can remember songs in head; begins to read and write rhythmic notation	Uses past tense verbs, pronouns, prepositions correctly; sentences much longer; begins to read and write; knows time sequences; likes rhymes; >2800 words	Sing rounds like "Row your boat"; practice singing; provide diverse genres and styles of music recordings/ songs/games;
6–7 years	Develops tonal center;[1] starts to sing harmony and rounds; vocal range focused around 5–6 notes; expands rhythmic and melodic written notation	Uses many more verb tenses; can tell right from left; makes comparisons; tells well crafted, imaginative stories; > 13,000 words	Build a repertoire of familiar songs. Provide opportunities for music improvisation, reading and writing notation. Music lessons.
7–9 years	Vocal range expands; uses more complex meters and harmonies; demonstrates music preferences	Exaggerates; explains ideas in detail; likes vocabulary and word play; understands jokes, riddles and idioms; >20,000 words	Offer individual and group music experiences; provide music games (computer, board) that focus on music terminology, notation and discrimination

Note: [1]Tonal center is the "home key." When children have a sense of tonal center, they can sing a song all the way through in the same key.

The author is committed to "musicing," a term used since the seventeenth century. Elliott (1995) used musicing to highlight the human component essential to the process of making music—active participation rather than passive observation. It suggests the use of real music input, both through voice and instruments, rather than artificially generated stimuli that extract and isolate certain features from the musical gestalt. Recent shifts in the study of music posit that music is essentially a social activity—something people do in the company of others, either as co-creators or listeners, and that the social functions of music are extremely important (Hargreaves et al., 2002). Such a shift in focus from the individual to the relationship has also occurred in the field of communication science, as it is acknowledged that the connection to other human beings is the primary drive behind one's need and purpose to communicate. Pragmatics, conversational skills, and social thinking (Garcia-Winner, 2007) are all now subdomains of high interest in the communication sciences field.

Aigen (2005) wrote, "The judgment that musicing is occurring implies that there is intelligence, intention and consciousness present, although these qualities may not be verbally expressed." Active musicing happens during both music listening and music making, just as language learning occurs during both receptive and expressive tasks (Barton & Robbins, 2015). Musicing plays a part in the formation and refinement of the auditory feedback loop. The central elements in musicing are: a required understanding of silence; the necessity to actively listen; the incorporation of the individual within the group; the cultivation of respect for craft; and the

creation of connection. These all relate to the principles of AVT and the core work of the practitioner.

Evidence on the Beneficial Effects of Music for Neurocognitive Development

Research demonstrates the positive effects of musical experiences and training on a broad range of neurodevelopmental skills (Koelsch, 2009; Strait & Kraus, 2011). Kraus and Chandrasekaran (2010) write, "The effect of music training on brain plasticity is not just a 'volume-knob effect'; not every feature of the auditory signal improves to the same extent" (p. 601). Rather, music training and experience support fine-tuning of auditory signals that are salient with sound-to-meaning significance. Strait and Kraus (2011) put it this way, "In addition to great amusement and well-being, practicing music does, in fact, appear to make you smarter—at least smarter when it comes to how you hear" (p. 133). The evidence shows that music is an attention enhancer, a cognitive enricher, a behavior modulator, an emotional regulator, a communication facilitator, and a cultural connector.

Attention Enhancer

What a child understands through hearing is largely determined by how well he or she listens when attending to the input of highest interest, a concept known as the *attentional spotlight* (Strait & Kraus, 2011). Shared music activities in the home are associated with better attentional regulation (particularly persistence). Putkinen, Tervaniemi, and Huotilainen (2013) found that involvement in musical activities was linked to better attention in 2- and 3-year-olds with typical hearing. Torppa, Huotilainen, Leminen, Lipsanen, and Tervaniemi (2014) studied the auditory attention of a group of children with CIs, aged 4 to 13, and a control group of children with typical hearing. Children with CIs who regularly sang at home performed better than their non-singing counterparts with CIs on auditory attention tasks involving changes in timbre and pitch.

Cognitive Enricher

Participation in early music experiences has been linked with enhanced cognitive processing (Flohr, Miller, & deBeus, 2000) and with better numeric competency in children with typical hearing (Williams, Barrett, Welch, Abad, & Broughton, 2015). Hearing is a superior sensory modality for processing sequentially based material, such as music. Evidence from Conway, Pisoni, and Kronenberger (2009) suggests that experience with sound provides scaffolding for the development of general cognitive skills that depend on the representation of timing or sequential patterns. Speech and music share neurocognitive processing mechanisms and, compared with vision, sound and speech carry higher-level patterns of information related to timing and sequencing. Conway et al. (2009) assert that hearing is the primary gateway for perceiving sequential patterns of input that change over time rather than over space, as with vision. An assumption may be made that, because music is highly organized according to timing and sequencing, training and experience with music is a cognitive enhancer.

Behavior Modulator

Positive social behavior has been associated with music making in a number of studies. In children with typical hearing, the presence of shared music activities in the home (Williams et al., 2015) correlates with fewer behavioral outbursts (or "reactivity"). In addition, music can prompt and condition behavior without requiring conscious control. Rhythmic entrainment (synchronized movement), the body's ability to automatically synchronize to a steady beat, influences body movements. Preschool children who could entrain to an external beat scored higher on early language tests, likely due to their ability to encode speech syllables with precision (Woodruff Carr, White-Schwoch, Tierney, Strait, & Kraus, 2014).

Emotional Regulator

Better positive social skills (e.g., being considerate of others' feelings) have been documented in young children with typical hearing who participated in music compared with those who did not (Williams et al., 2015). Group music making has been shown to improve empathy in early (Kirschner & Tomasello, 2010) and middle childhood (Rabinowitch, Cross, & Burnard, 2012). Empathy in this context is the ability to experience another person's emotional state, a developmental construct that is often delayed in children who are deaf or hard of hearing. Those with CIs may struggle to extract the subtle emotional cues that are present in spoken language (Hopyan-Misakyan, Gordon, Dennis, & Papsin, 2009; Wang, Trehub, Volkova, & van Lieshout, 2013). Since music embodies a wide range of emotions and has the capacity to evoke moods and feelings, Hopyan, Gordon, and Papsin (2011) suggest that music be used with children with hearing loss as a way of providing more salient emotional cues than those available via spoken language. If empathy can be facilitated using music in addition to language, children in AVT could develop age-appropriate empathy skills—skills important for social learning, for literacy attainment, for narrative comprehension, and especially for understanding characters' actions and motives in literature. Since shared neural and acoustic mechanisms are active during the perception of both speech and music, it is known that music can enhance the ability to identify the emotional intent in spoken language (Strait, Kraus, Skoe, & Ashley, 2009).

Communication Facilitator

The effects of musical experience extend to language (Kraus, Skoe, & Parbery-Clark, 2008). Putkinen, Saarikivi, and Tervaniemi (2013) assert that musically rich environments promote general enhancement of auditory processing—favorable consequences for the development of language, especially for children with hearing loss. In a large-scale longitudinal study involving over 3,000 children with typical hearing, Williams et al. (2015) found that early music activities with children aged 2 to 3 years at home had a positive impact on the children's vocabulary age when they were 4 to 5 years old.

Perceptual Booster

Music training (Chen et al., 2010; Yucel, Sennaroglu, & Belgin, 2009) and home music activities (Torppa et al., 2014) can improve pitch perception in children with CIs for whom pitch discrimination is difficult, due to spectral limitations of the device (Hsiao & Gfeller, 2012). CIs primarily provide information that enhances speech recognition, while music requires more fine structure timing and pitch cues. Perception of speech in noise is better for children with CIs who have musical experiences than for peers with CIs who have little musical experience (Torppa, Faulkner, Kujala, Huotilainen, & Lipsanen, 2018; Welch, et al., 2015). This is noteworthy given that background noise is disruptive to language learning. Better speech-in-noise for these children is associated with faster attention shifting when listening for a change in musical instrument timbre, suggesting there is shared processing of timbre of musical instruments and speech in noise (Torppa et al., 2018).

Cultural Connector

Some of the most exciting events in AVT sessions involve music and a link between loved ones. This author has observed the following phenomena:

- A father sang a praise chant in the Navajo language for his young child with hearing loss. Jimmy learned it.
- Zeke's grandparents taught us (Zeke and the author) a Mexican finger play in Spanish from their childhood.
- Marcel, a bilingual French-English speaking child, learned to sing his national anthem and his father's alma mater song.

■ Adam learned to sing a song in Hebrew (written phonetically) for his bar mitzvah.

These evidence-informed findings indicate that music adds great benefit to the development of children with hearing loss in a variety of cultures and languages in AVT.

PART 2: HOW TO INCORPORATE MUSIC INTO AVT

Singing needs to be a priority in every AVT session because it is the musical activity most closely related to speech. The attitudes of the practitioner and the parents about singing and music are always conveyed to the child. So, adults are encouraged to be enthusiastic about musical activities and to sing joyfully. Babies adore the sound of their parents' singing and do not recognize a "good voice" or a "good song."

In the following section, the reader will find six types of songs used by the practitioner to enhance the development of listening and spoken language, and commentary regarding the importance of adults' attitudes toward music. Music activities are suggested for children in two age groups: (1) infants and (2) toddlers and preschoolers. Goals are established by the developmental expectations found in Table 18–3.

Singing Strategies: 6 Types of Songs to Use in AVT

When using a song with children, most adults think of a traditional, recognized piece of music with lyrics, such as, "Old MacDonald Had a Farm." But there are at least six types of songs the author uses regularly in AVT sessions—each with unique features—that serve useful purposes:

1. Traditional Songs
These belong to a collection or canon of children's music, widely recognized and associated with childhood experience and culture. The songs, usually listed as "traditional," evolved naturally and are passed down through generations. Table 18–4 contains a list of many popular North American children's songs, as examples. In AVT, the adults place great value on ensuring that children know these songs, as they provide familiarity with the culture. Lyrics to these songs are referenced in pop culture, poetry, and books, and the tunes are played on mobiles and wind-up toys found in a baby's nursery. Children with typical hearing are exposed to them from an early age, often through incidental listening, and consequently they are important for children in AVT programs to know.

2. Modern Children's Songs
Written, recorded, and copyrighted by children's songwriters and performers, these songs often come from movies or television and may be wildly popular (e.g., "Under the Sea" or "Let it Go").

3. Teaching Songs
Written with a specific learning goal in mind, using the vocabulary, concepts, and repetition that characterize spoken language input to children, these *teaching songs* have an express purpose in supporting a child's development. A number of such songs are presented

Table 18-4. Children's Tunes to Use with Traditional Lyrics or to Piggyback with New Lyrics

The Farmer in the Dell
Old McDonald
Ring Around the Rosie
Three Blind Mice
Row, Row, Row Your Boat
London Bridge Is Falling Down
Twinkle, Twinkle, Little Star/Baabaa Black Sheep/Alphabet song
Hokey Pokey
The Wheels on the Bus
If You're Happy and You Know It
Mary Had a Little Lamb
I Know an Old Woman Who Swallowed a Fly
Buffalo Gals, Won't You Come out Tonight?
The More we Get Together
Itsy Bitsy Spider
This Old Man
She'll be Comin' Round the Mountain
My Darlin' Clementine
Jack and Jill Went up the Hill
Three Sailors Went to Sea, Sea, Sea
On Top of Old Smokey
Are you Sleeping?/Frere Jacques/Where Is Thumbkin?
Scotland's Burning, Scotland's Burning
Good Night, Ladies
Round and Round the Garden
Hickory, Dickory Dock
It's Raining It's Pouring, the Old Man Is Snoring
I Had a Little Turtle, His Name Was Tiny Tim
Pop Goes the Weasel
Billy Boy
Doggie, Doggie, Where's Your Bone?
The Other Day I Met a Bear
Here We Go 'Round the Mulberry Bush
Heads, Shoulders, Knees and Toes
The Old Gray Mare
Rock-a-bye, Baby, on the Treetop
Do You Know the Muffin Man?
Where, Oh, Where Has My Little Dog Gone?
Oh, Dear! What Can the Matter Be?

here, including those of Estabrooks and Birkenshaw-Fleming (1994, 2003), Barton and Robbins (2008), and Chapin and Galdston (2013).

4. Piggyback Songs (Robbins, 2016)
Created by attaching new lyrics onto an existing, recognizable melody, *piggyback songs* change the words by "piggybacking" onto the melody of a familiar song and are customized to a child, a situation, or a theme. For example, one can use the melody to "If You're Happy and You Know It" and piggyback these words onto it: "If you're sitting quietly, nod your head [nod, nod]/If you're sitting quietly, nod your head [nod, nod]/ If you're sitting quietly, I'm as happy as can be/If you're sitting quietly, nod your head [nod, nod]." The adult uses the song as an auditory-only stimulus and starts singing it when a child has lost focus or is distracted. The music captures the child's attention so that the practitioner can guide the parent to engage the child to listen quietly and return to the task at hand. This song includes a motor response, nodding, which reinforces rhythm and helps the child focus. The traditional tunes in Table 18–4 are recommended by the author for piggybacking with new lyrics.

5. Practitioner-Composed (or Parent-Composed) Song
A practitioner or parent may compose non-rhyming simple tunes of just a few notes; they do this spontaneously on the spot to alleviate a tantrum, transition the child to another activity, or distract him or her from a toy or activity so that the next planned event can occur. One might call these "singing on your feet" songs, the musical equivalent to "thinking on your feet." Some adults

may sing the words using the "mama" interval as the tune (Barton, 2013). The simplest tune to sing, based on just two notes that are three half-steps apart, the *"mama" interval* is also called a minor third. This natural interval is heard in the voices of "nana, nana boo-boo" or "You can't catch me," sometimes adding one more musical note, the fourth tone in the scale. It's the back-and-forth interval one hears in "It's raining, it's pouring, the old man is snoring." Interestingly, the minor third is commonly used to express sadness in music, and research shows this mirrors its use in spoken language, as a tone similar to a minor third is produced during sad speech (Curtis & Bharucha, 2010).

6. Books Sung with the "Mama" Interval
This combines book reading and the "mama" interval to make a musical experience (C. Barton, personal communication). The text of the book provides the lyrics, and music is added easily by the adult singing the words on the back-and-forth "mama" interval (e.g., "Peek-a-Boo! I See You!", Phillips, 1990); "Blue Hat, Green Hat" (Boynton, 1995); and "Silly Sally" (Wood, 1992). These provide a host of musical experiences for adults who do not feel creative in making up their own songs. Parents name this strategy as a comfortable way to start singing to their child, noting that it builds their confidence to expand to other musical activities at home.

Music Activities for Infants with Hearing Loss in AVT

At this age, parents need to feel comfortable using music and especially singing. In AVT, parents will come to see music as

Table 18–5. Musical Activities for Infants in Auditory-Verbal Practice

1. Motherese
2. Swaying, rocking, patting the baby
3. Music is family heritage
4. First musical memory
5. "Put Your Ears On" Song
6. Use hand-to-ear cue at onset of music
7. Sing books using the "mama" interval
8. Encourage the Baby Bop: child's unique response to music
9. Start and stop to the music
10. Sensory songs with movement and actions (including parent choice)
11. Model the use of practitioner-composed songs
12. Associate routines and songs; credit comprehension and production
13. Learning to Listen Sounds and songs
14. Auditory-first with music to assess child's listening progress
15. "Up-Up-Up" song
16. "What's in the Bag?" song

a dynamic set of strategies that promote listening and talking, and emotional bonding. Parents are the "captains of the ship" for the journey of their child's progress and thus music and singing activities are included in every session and in interactions with the child, anywhere. (These activities will be reviewed in the following section and are listed in Table 18–5.) The effectiveness of these is highly dependent on the parent–practitioner level of confidence and the growing therapeutic alliance (Robbins & Caraway, 2010) established between parent and practitioner—an alliance based on mutual trust, respect, and authentic communication (Robbins, 2016). Through this communication, the practitioner helps the parents realize the benefits that music brings to the child's overall development. Estabrooks and Birkenshaw-Fleming (1994) guide practitioners when stating: "Share the child's

lead but provide direct instruction for the parents."

SNAPSHOTS OF MUSIC AND SINGING IN AVT SESSIONS—A PERSONAL EXPERIENCE

Motherese

Margot is a 5-week-old baby wearing hearing aids. Using *motherese* is a natural and musical way to encourage her interest in listening, talking, and singing. When I'm holding a baby during an AVT session, I often use *motherese* and coach the parent to follow the model with its musical quality. When the mother asks me if that is not just baby talk, I say, "Yes, and that kind of baby talk is very good for Margot to hear because it has a musical sound to it."

Swaying, Rocking, Patting the Baby

I show Margot's parents how to move in a rhythmic way when holding and singing to her. The parents report that this can quiet and calm her at home. I let them know that rhythm and movement are soothing to babies when they're trying to settle because these rhythms and movements mimic heartbeats and breathing rhythms. This lays the foundation for the steady beat that will be a later musical milestone for Margot. Her parents feel optimistic when they sense what they are doing in today's session contributes to future progress.

Music Is Family Heritage

I ask Margot's parents to make a list of songs, lullabies, chants, and finger plays they remember from their own childhoods, to use in subsequent AVT sessions. As they think back on their own musical histories, they may remember songs they haven't sung in years. I explain how it is vital to pass on their musical heritage so that Margot learns those songs, too. They had to think about them over the following week but finally retrieved some tunes. I assure the parents that music is a teaching tool, but also an emotional bonding agent. I share that some parents feel the bond with their newborn is compromised upon diagnosis of hearing loss and that music can help nurture the bond at this challenging time, bringing them closer together.

First Musical Memory

I encourage Margot's parents to "audiate," or play in their head, the song they associate with their first musical memory and invite them to sing it (Barton, personal communication). Margot's parents evoke a musical memory that involves a close family member such as their mother, father, or grandmother. I share that my own son described how I rocked him to sleep by singing "An Irish Lullaby" (Shannon, 1913). This was touching to Margot's parents and to me, as I recalled my own mother singing this to me and I heard her voice in my head. Reflecting on their past, Margot's parents realized that shared music could create an emotional bond between them and Margot.

"Put Your Ears On" Song

The amount of time a baby wears hearing aids or CIs is known to be a crucial factor in the development of listening and spoken language skills. Parents may struggle to keep the hearing technology on their babies and toddlers as indicated by recent research (Walker et al., 2015). The mother of Carly, age 6 months, tells me her daughter's fussiness keeps them from putting on her technology first thing in the morning. Hours may slip by without the child having auditory access, hours of bonding time with the parent during routines like diapering, feeding, dressing, and washing up that are prime for spoken language learning through listening, talking, and singing.

Singing offers a solution. I teach Mom the song "Put Your Ears On" (Figure 18–2) and encourage her to sing it

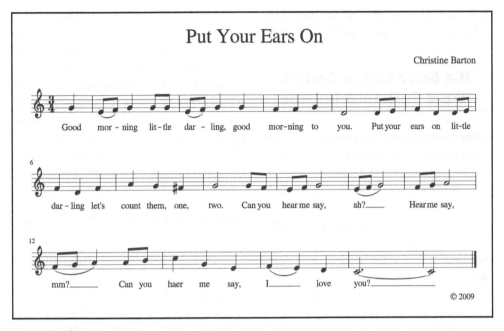

Figure 18–2. "Put Your Ears On" music and lyric.

every morning before she takes Carly out of her crib. We make a plan—the hearing aids will be close at hand as the parents approach the crib and begin slowly singing the song, with its lilting waltz tempo. Each line will prompt them to complete another step in the technology process. Subsequently as the song ends, both hearing aids will be on and working and Carly will be ready to start her day with optimal auditory access.

Hand-to-Ear Cue at the Onset of Singing (Pointing to the Ear)

This often-used strategy in AVT helps babies attend to meaningful sounds in the environment. But when the stimulus is singing, a follow-up feature is added. After pointing to my ear and using an excited expression, I rock or sway to the song, modeling the "baby bop" (see below). Sometimes I use a soft voice, hum, or sing "la" or "na" for each syllable. I explain to mother that an auditory stimulus is more salient when it first appears out of silence. So, we wait for silence before starting the music.

Sing Books, Using the "Mama" Interval

I sit Carly on my lap, so we are both looking at the pages of the book "Peek-a-Boo! I See You!" (Phillips, 1990). This posture facilitates joint attention and keeps my voice close to the Carly's hearing technology in a way that promotes listening first. I model how to sing the text on each page using the two- or three-note "mama" interval. Mother has a chance to practice and I am the "guide on her side." Then we talk about books they have at home that lend themselves to being sung on the "mama" interval.

The Baby Bop: A Child's Unique Response to Music

Babies with typical hearing learn early to recognize that the sounds of music are different than the sounds of speech. This is observed when the baby indicates his or her unique responses to music that are characterized by rhythmic movements (see Table 18–3). Depending on the infant's age, these may be kicking legs, waving, or thrusting arms and/or, as the child ages, swaying and rocking back and forth, even when no visual cues are present. One can refer to this as "the baby bop" (Barton, personal communication). Linking music with baby bop movements is important in AVT. Parents learn that when their baby shows this unique response to music, it confirms the effectiveness of hearing technology in replicating the auditory cues needed to form a perceptual category that is *music*.

Once the baby bop is modeled, I set up situations to assess whether Carly can demonstrate it. I ask Carly's mother to distract her while they're while seated on the floor playing with a toy. I start to sing a tune, out of Carly's line of vision, and Mom and I look to see whether Carly demonstrates a baby bop response by rocking back and forth (Barton & Robbins, 2018, Lesson 1). This response emerges by about six months in children with typical hearing, so we adjust this expectation according to the baby's developmental and hearing ages. As Carly does not do this spontaneously yet, we talk about

ways that mother can reinforce this more at home. We re-visit the discussion of full-time hearing aid use and note that Carly gets excellent benefit from her hearing technology, but only when she's wearing it during all waking hours. Mom asks if Carly's musical development will be delayed if she doesn't have full-time hearing aid use, then answers her own question.

Start and Stop to the Music

This activity extends the baby bop response. I model bopping with the onset of music then stopping when the music ends abruptly. Dane is a 9-month-old and wears hearing aids. His mother holds him in her lap, but sometimes he can sit for periods in a highchair. I explain that our objective is for Dane to link the presence of music with movement and the absence of music with cessation of movement. Mom previously told me that the song "Six Little Ducks" was an early musical memory for her, so we use it for this activity as it contains both sung lyrics and the Learning to Listen Sound "quack" throughout. Mom models starting and stopping with the music and Dane laughs and imitates her movements. However, we want to see a spontaneous response, so I encourage Mom to play this "game" often during the following week. I explain that over time, we generalize the baby bop to all musical stimuli, both sung live and recorded. For older children, I play this game to the song "I'm Going to Sing When I Hear the Music Play" (Estabrooks & Birkenshaw-Fleming, 2003) and substitute different actions (e.g., clap, skip, jump, tap) for the word "sing."

Sensory Songs with Movement and Actions (including parent choice)

Music is a multisensory experience, integrating kinesthetic, auditory and visual information. The strong kinesthetic cues draw and maintain the attention of babies, including 7-month old Wally who wears hearing aids. I sit him on my lap facing me, while I sing and bounce him on my knees to the beat of the song. This reinforces the first motor response that music elicits, and mother and I can experiment with different tempos (Barton & Robbins, 2018). I chant the traditional children's rhyme, "This is the way the _____ ride, bookity, booke, bookity, booke" (gentle tempo); "This is the way the _____ ride, bookity, bookity, bookity booke" (tempo quickening); "This is the way that Wally rides, bookity, bookity, bookity, boooooooke!" (fast tempo and lifting Wally into the air) When mom takes a turn, Wally begins to anticipate the rhythm changes, and the moment is playful for both of them.

Before babies talk, they often demonstrate comprehension of a song by using the motions they've learned with it. If the parent sings "Patty cake," "Itsy Bitsy Spider," or "I'm a Little Teapot" and the child begins to make the motions, he or she demonstrates auditory comprehension.

To strengthen the emotional bond, I ask parents about sensory songs, chants, and finger plays they knew as children. Wally's mother remembered a finger play, "Tabitha Cat" (Dowell, 1987) and taught it to us. The six lines are a rhythmic chant with a hand motion for each line: Tabitha Cat / Has a bell on her hat / The one she wears in the house / O listen! How nice! / How nice for the mice! / Said Ethyl, the old mother mouse/. His mother shares that, since the family focus is on Wally's auditory development, this finger play is more poignant now than when she was a child because of the line "O listen! How nice!" This is how music may stimulate parent engagement as they share suggestions, and music adds an emotional layer to the activity.

Model the Use of Practitioner-Composed Songs

In the AVT session if I'm looking for a toy for Wally, for example, I make up a little song on the "mama" interval: "Penguin toy, penguin toy, I can't find you" or "Fuzzy dog, fuzzy dog, where did you go-oh?" as I search. Wally's mother and I discuss how she narrates his life in song, as you would in a musical play or opera. I discuss again the "mama" interval. If I sit Wally on the floor, I describe what I'm doing by singing on the "mama" interval: "Down on the floor you go, Wally's on the floor." What one says one can also sing.

Associate Routines and Songs, Credit the Child's Comprehension and Production

I try to pair every activity with a particular song and help the parents to do so at home. We begin the AVT session

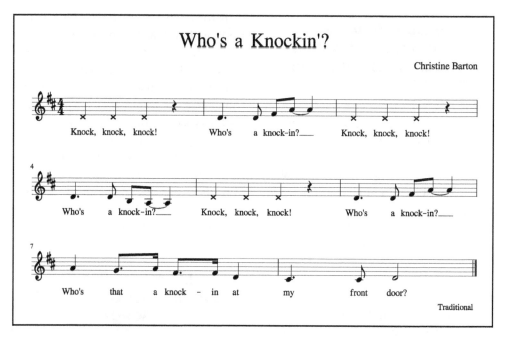

Figure 18–3. "Who's a Knockin'?" music and lyric.

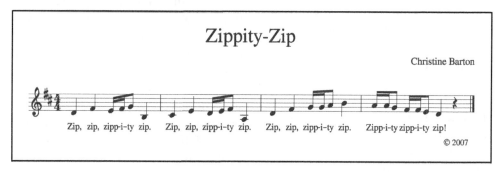

Figure 18–4. "Zippity-Zip" music and lyric.

with the song "Who's a-Knockin'?" (Figure 18–3). From outside, Wally's mother knocks on the door and sings the song. He joins in the knocking and I respond, encouraging them to use it when they greet someone into their own home.

Also recommended is the greeting song "Hi!" (Estabrooks & Birkenshaw-Fleming, 1994) set to the two-note "mama" interval. Once inside the room, we engage in some conversation, then sing a song as we remove Wally's coat: "Zip, zip, zippity zip" (Figure 18–4) or substitute another relevant verb, such as "Snap, snap, snappity snap." If the practitioner climbs a flight of steps to start the session, he or she can sing, "Up, up, up, up, up, up, up, up!" each time, in an ascending series of notes, or the reverse when going down the stairs. It is good to think of songs as units of comprehension and production for a baby. The parents credit Wally with understanding and producing a word but also with understanding and producing a song, or fragment of it, when he can demonstrate that it has meaning. The song is a unit of Auditory-Verbal communication, every bit as valid as a word, a phrase, or a sentence.

Learning to Listen Sounds and Songs

Learning to Listen Sounds (LTLS) are a hallmark of AVT (see Chapter 9, Appendix 9–1). LTLS are a set of acoustically salient onomatopoeic sounds and spoken words that children learn to associate with an object or an action through listening. From a linguistic perspective, LTLS are considered "proto-words" (Barton & Robbins, 2018, Lesson 4).

Auditory-First with Music to Assess Child's Listening Progress

An auditory-first presentation is familiar to practitioners and is used with music, too. I "announce" each activity by singing the song first. First, this captures the baby's attention by listening, and then I show the associated toy. The child demonstrates anticipatory comprehension (Barton & Robbins, 2018, Lesson 2). With repetition, Wally forms links between songs and activities. I have a toy with a ladybug floating in liquid that fascinates him. I start singing, on the "mama" interval, a self-created song, "Ladybug, ladybug, swimming in the wa-ter" and then pause expectantly. Because we've used the same song, each time we present the toy, I expect to

observe more progress. Wally shows he has linked the song and toy. Babies may do this by eye gaze and/or reaching toward the shelf where the ladybug toy is kept. I am planning, coaching, and evaluating in the AVT session (see Chapter 17). When I start to sing the Ladybug song, Wally turns to look at the ladybug toy and it is clear he has associated the song with it. His mother remarks, "That just made my day!"

"Up, Up, Up" Song

Infants such as Margot, Carly, and Wally may spend most of the AVT session playing on the floor, where it is easy to integrate fine and gross motor movements with listening, spoken language, and music. When possible, I also dedicate time during each session with the child in a highchair or booster seat: to help the baby adjust to a routine of being safely seated for short intervals; to allow the adults time to share information while the child is otherwise occupied; to assess the child's functional auditory responses in a semi-controlled way (see Chapter 17). I make a positive association between the highchair and music by singing "Up, up, up into your chair" (Figure 18–5). It's a moment to celebrate with the parents of 12-month-old Tucker, who has had bilateral CIs for 6 months. When I ask him, "Should we get you into your chair?" Tucker responds, "uh, uh, uh" and reaches upward.

"What's in the Bag?" Song

Children enjoy looking for objects hidden in bags, boxes, cans, gifts, or other

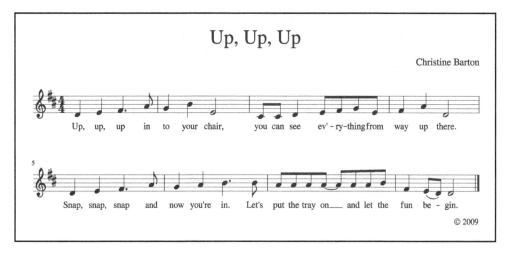

Figure 18–5. "Up, Up, Up" music and lyric.

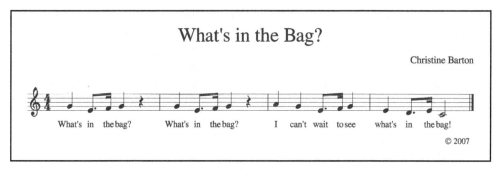

Figure 18–6. "What's in the Bag?" music and lyric.

containers (Estabrooks & Birkenshaw-Fleming, 1994). Two-year-old Blake (with bilateral CIs), his mom and I sing "What's in the Bag?" (Figure 18–6) together, emphasizing the lyrics of the first two lines as questions, before revealing the items hidden in a bag. The build-up of excitement increases Blake's anticipation and Mother and I weave appropriate Theory of Mind (ToM) concepts with the song, by using mental state words such as *think, guess, wonder*, and *believe*. As children are able, we use higher-level ToM mental state words, such as *suppose, predict*, and *hypothesize*.

MUSIC ACTIVITIES FOR TODDLERS AND PRESCHOOLERS

At this age, musical activities at the toddler/preschool stage typically shift because of rapid development and maturity. A child's increasing mobility and coordination allow more movement in musical activities. The child's attention span lengthens and he or she begins mapping symbolic language onto experiences, so the world is more predictable. The child seeks and is reinforced by patterns, too. A list of suggested

Table 18–6. Musical Activities for Toddlers and Preschoolers in Auditory-Verbal Practice

1. Presence versus absence of music
2. Expand the child's association of routines and songs
3. Build a musical word bank
4. Move like a slide whistle
5. Keeping steady beat
6. Rhythm instruments
7. Show me what I'm singing
8. I have different voices
9. Music guides motor actions
10. Acoustic highlighting with music
11. Be my echo
12. Early literacy songs
    Name songs
    Phonological awareness songs
13. Musical cousins
14. Doggie, doggie, where's your bone?
15. Our memory magnet
16. Executive functions (EFs) and music
17. Bossing your brain with music

musical activities for toddlers and preschoolers is shown in Table 18–6.

Presence Versus Absence of Music

Two-year-old Daisy, who wears bilateral CIs, is fascinated by monkeys, so she, her dad, and I make our toy monkeys dance together to the music, then stop when it stops. Next, Daisy demonstrates she can do this on her own, just by listening. We might choose the toy based on a current theme. Three-year-old Owen and I read a *Paddington Bear* book, play a Paddington Bear board game, and use small Paddington figures to move with the music.

As soon as children are successful, this activity may become more challenging in three ways: (1) I include a third stimulus, spoken language not music. This requires a child's perception of music versus non-music. (2) I start with moderately loud recorded music. As the game continues, the volume becomes progressively softer and I reinforce the child for listening carefully by saying, "You heard the very soft music, Owen. Way to go!" (3) We play the game in the presence of competing noise, such as recorded cafeteria noise or a podcast with a single speaker's voice, challenging Owen to attend to the musical signal. The game "Musical Chairs" focuses on the presence or absence of music with a gross motor component (e.g., sitting in a chair as soon as the music stops). As it is best played with four or more players, it can be recommended for family time at home.

Expanding the Child's Association of Routines and Songs

Whenever a new game or activity is introduced, it can be done with a song, as in the infancy period. When I sing the song to introduce an activity, I expect 2-year-old Daisy to provide some of the lyrics. I start by expecting her to supply just the last word of each line, which may be the same word for the entire song. As my AVT practice is in my home office, my dog joins us, and I sing a simple tune with only four words: "Oh my puppy, oh my puppy, oh my puppy (dog); Oh, my puppy, oh my puppy, oh my puppy (dog)" repeated, for a total of three or four lines. Daisy's father initially provides the missing word, "dog," and then Daisy has a turn at this early auditory closure task (Barton & Robbins, 2018, Lesson 2). Pause time and an expectant look cue her that it is her turn to sing (see Chapter 15). At the next stage, Daisy may be able to fill in several missing lyrics either alone or with Dad's help and, over time, may sing the whole song by herself. Eventually, I "raise the bar" by introducing songs that are longer and have multiple verses.

"Building a Child's Musical Word Bank"

Over time, children in AVT establish and expand their vocabulary to describe their musical percepts. The more capable that listeners are at describing the quality and nature of the sound heard, the better their listening, talking, and musical experiences become. For example, Tommy is 4 years old and wears a CI on one side and a hearing aid on the contralateral ear. First, I reflect on my own sound perceptions and use descriptors such as, "That drum I hear is very *low-pitched* and *booming*" or "I like the *fluttering* sound of the harmonica" and so on. Second, we play games to contrast the qualities of different sound makers and categorize them with words. Tommy, his mother, and I do some activities following a Peter Pan theme. I say, "Let's listen to each of these instruments put the 'tinkling' ones in this box for Tinker Bell." We play an instrument, describe it with words from our musical word bank, then decide if it goes in the "Tinkling" box. Tim decides that the bell, the xylophone, and the triangle belong in the box. The drum, kazoo, and maracas do not. Third, we find synonyms or words related to the target descriptor to expand Tim's word bank. "That bell *tinkles*, doesn't it? It *jingles*." Finally, we share books such as *Crash! Bang! Boom!* (Spier, 1972) that provide descriptors of sounds, including musical ones.

"Moving Like a Slide Whistle"

A slide whistle is excellent for reinforcing the concept of pitch change, as the instrument itself provides visual cues about whether the pitch is moving higher or lower (Barton & Robbins, 2018, Lesson 3). Also, children can play their own slide whistle, whereas many other instruments are inaccessible to them. For 3-year-old Joy who has hearing aids, I play a continuous sweep, gradually rise up on my tip toes as the pitch goes up, then slowly move to a seated or crouching position as the pitch lowers. After Mom models, Joy is ready to play. We may start with visual and auditory cues. Once Joy has this concept, I stand behind her so that she relies on audition alone to move in the correct direction. If she is adept at this, I speed up the game and make the slide whistle go up or down in pitch very slowly, moderately, quickly, or extremely fast. Like above, we encourage parents to build a word bank by using perceptual descriptors. For pitch, these might include "high pitch, low pitch, deep tone, shrill, and bass," depending on the instrument. Recommended preschool songs related to pitch change are "The Slide," "My Blue Yo-Yo," and "Small and Tall" (Estabrooks & Birkenshaw-Fleming, 1994).

When Joy is ready for a challenge, I'll use the slide whistle to help her differentiate melodic intervals of three varying notes. I play three tones following a pattern, such as: High-Low-Low or Low-High-Low or other combinations. Joy's task is to replicate the pattern of pitches by raising and lowering herself in the same pattern as the pitches. Some children sing the notes aloud as they imitate the pattern. Other children need to sing the words "high" and "low" as they move.

Keeping Steady Beat (Background)

The practitioner creates opportunities to keep a steady beat, using recorded music or live piano. Beat and rhythm are related but not synonymous: Beat is the steady pulse you feel in a tune, like a clock or heartbeat. It's what you clap along to or tap your foot to. Rhythm, on the other hand, is the actual spacing or timing of the notes that are the same as the words. As a newborn, a baby recognizes and is drawn to a beat because it is reminiscent of the mother's heartbeat. Within a few months, the baby will rock or kick to a steady beat (see Table 18–3) As motor skills improve, a preschool-age child will tap two toys or instruments together, tap a drum, and even run or jump to a steady pulse. Around the age of 4, a child begins to match an external steady beat. Practitioners and parents need to encourage children to keep a steady beat by rocking, patting knees or shoulders, tapping sticks together, or clapping during informal music enjoyment. This basic skill precedes keeping rhythm. Many young children, particularly those with motor delays, find that clapping is challenging because the hands must meet at midline. The difficulty of the motion might distract the child from the music task and that detracts from learning. A simpler way to keep steady beat is through bilateral, symmetrical movement such as tapping knees, shoulders, head, or feet with hands or rhythm sticks.

Using Rhythm Instruments

Every home, therapy room, studio, and early childhood center typically has a box of rhythm instruments for music making (http://www.westmusic.com). Rhythm instruments allow children to explore different timbres, loudness range, and even pitch. The practitioner might sing or play the piano while the child and parent keep steady beat on their instruments. Or, as they listen to a recorded song, they all play instruments together. Joy and I listen to a recording of the song "Tap Your Sticks" (Palmer, 1999) and explore the timbres of different objects when we use them as sticks, including pencils, carrots, plastic spoons, metal spoons, wooden spoons, dowels, pens, and bamboo sticks. Joy enjoys anticipating the points in the song where the lyrics instruct, "Tap your sticks in the air with a 1-2-3" or "Tap your sticks on the floor with a 1-2-3." Importantly, research has shown that a strong "beat sense" (ability to keep a beat) is critical for gross motor skills like crawling, walking, or clapping and cognitive skills involving language, speech, and reading. As a child gets older, a steady beat is found in activities such as using scissors, performing choreographed dances, and playing musical instruments.

Show Me What I'm Singing

The objective of this activity is for the child to demonstrate that he or she can choose from a limited set of objects that are associated with songs. I use only songs the child has heard in AVT sessions and at home. Two-and-a-half-year-old Roxy has CIs. I present a selection of toys, each of which corresponds to a familiar song. I start with three songs (and objects): "Baa Baa Black Sheep" (sheep), "Patty Cake, Patty Cake" (a rolling pin), and "The Itsy-Bitsy Spider" (spider). Roxy's mother sits slightly behind her and starts to sing a song. Roxy picks the correct object and spontaneously "sings" a fragment of each song. Since Roxy is successful, we increase the complexity of the activity by singing multiple lines, by mixing up the lyrics, or adding new words. I combine perception (listening) and production (talking) in the same game, to reinforce the auditory feedback loop, by switching the roles of "sender" and "receiver"—roles that

have different and equally important functions, each of great benefit to the child (Robbins, 2009). At this age, Roxy requires parent support when she is the leader or "sender."

With 4-year-old Gavon, the practitioner plays a variation of this game by singing one line of a multi-verse song such as, "She'll Be Coming Around the Mountain." I ask Gavon to pick out the key words (e.g., six white horses, old red rooster, chicken and dumplings), select the objects associated with them, and then sing the line himself. As an early-implanted child in AVT with excellent auditory discrimination, Gavon's rhythm on this song is excellent. The melodic contour of the tune is intact, although his tonal center may shift as he sings. The author recommends Laferriere (2003) for other engaging activities to use with this traditional song.

I Have Different Voices

Children who are deaf or hard of hearing need to know that people can have several different voices, an important auditory and vocal distinction (Barton & Robbins, 2018).

Singing Voice and Humming Voice

I show 3-year-old Josh, who has a CI and a hearing aid, a small wooden paddle that has a hand-drawn face with an open mouth on one side and a face with a closed mouth on the other. I sing "Lalalala, lalalala" while showing the open mouth, and label this my singing voice. I demonstrate humming, with a closed mouth and label it "my humming voice." Josh has many opportunities to produce the two voices while showing the correct side of the paddle. After this game, Josh sings to his teddy bear, "Lalalala" showing the singing side of the paddle and then we hum to him: "hmm, hmm, hmmm, hmmm" showing the humming side. I show Josh a side of the paddle to see if he can produce the corresponding voice on command. To check his ability to discriminate the two voices, I sing one or the other and Josh imitates what he hears and turns the paddle to the correct side.

Singing Voice, Speaking Voice, Whisper Voice, Shouting Voice

To address 4-year old Ella's ability to control vocal intensity, I work on levels of loudness: whisper, speaking, shouting. I use the song "Shout and whisper, that's our game. Shout and whisper, what's your name? Shout your name! (response). Whisper your name! (response)." Next, Ella is the leader and calls on mother to either shout or whisper our names. Once Ella can do this, we add the speaking voice. We combine it in the song with either shouting or whispering and do it in pairs, such as shouting and talking or talking and whispering. We may add an additional level, the quiet voice, which is fully vocalized at a very soft volume, depending on the child's ability to perceive and produce this. Ella's musical word bank increases with intensity descriptors such as *hushed, powerful, strong,* and *booming*.

Music Guides Motor Actions

When a child struggles repeatedly to carry out a task, I explore ways that music can help, including with motor planning. Ben, a 5-year-old preschooler, has

bilateral CIs, glasses, and visual-motor weakness. He crossed items off his printed schedule at our session every week, and yet seemed unable to find the starting point for his line, ending up with awkward scribbles across the paper. Since each item was numbered, I created a little song to the "mama" interval, "Start on the Number, start on the Number." I sang that whenever he prepared to cross something off the list. Mom did the same. Within a short time, Ben got his pencil ready and sang "Start on the Number" on his own. That prompted him to put his pencil down carefully and cross out the appropriate line.

Acoustic Highlighting with Music

Practitioners use acoustic highlighting in spoken language when a child omits grammatical morphemes or functor words such as "to, a, the, -ing." This draws auditory attention to the target by highlighting it (see Chapter 15). Singing can be considered a form of acoustic highlighting. Rhythm is advantageous as each word or syllable can be marked with a note in the music. Ben needs multisensory cues, so I add something tactile by singing and gently patting the rhythm on his arm as I highlight. If he omits a word, it will be clear that there is a missing syllable in the beat of the music.

Be My Echo

Echo songs can teach and evaluate a child's imitation of rhythm, pitch, and sung lyrics. The format is imitation or echo, where a line is sung by a leader and repeated by the follower(s). Some traditional children's echo songs are "The Other Day I Met a Bear" and "Down by the Bay." I also use the echo format with a "News of the Day" activity using a practitioner-created song. Six-year-old Elliott and I descend the stairs with Elliott one step behind, making this a listening-only activity. In the song, I review the date and say something noteworthy as Elliott echoes. Each line is sung one half-step lower than the previous line. We cover about one full octave of descending notes (Robbins, 2016). This allows me to hear Elliott's pitch matching and the accuracy of his open-set understanding. Elliott's "News of the Day" song goes like this: *"Today (Today) is (is) Wednesday (Wednesday) May First (May First) and this morning (and this morning) something happened (something happened) that made me (that made you) feel worried (feel worried)."* I added conversation to the song, and as we reach the bottom of the steps, Elliott asks, "What happened that worried you?" with genuine concern. Parents and children take their turns as leader and follower. Most early-implanted children who participate in this activity regularly show excellent pitch matching and open-set word repetition skills.

Sometimes echo songs are referred to as call-and-response songs, a category that includes question and answer songs—good for conversational turn taking. William, a 6-year-old with hearing aids, asks to sing, "Must Be Santa" at Christmas time. He wants to be the leader who sings each question, "Who's got a beard that's long and white?" while his mother and I sing the answer, "Santa's got a beard that's long and white!" There is cumulative working memory involved because after

every other verse, the list of features is repeated, and the list grows longer.

Early Literacy Songs

The foundations of music and singing begin in infancy like the foundations of literacy (see Chapter 14). Music and singing strongly support the development of reading, writing, and the use of electronic media across the life span. It is important then to indicate the relationship of music to literacy and vice versa. A few example activities are provided below, and others are found in Lesson 8 of Auditunes (Barton & Robbins, 2018).

1. Phonological awareness is a broad skill that includes manipulating units of spoken language such as sounds, syllables, onsets and rimes, and rhyming. The nature of many songs is prime learning material for children's phonological awareness and literacy, since it involves rhyming. I extend this by using a song Kevin knows well, "This Old Man." For each line, I stop short of the last word and find a different word that still rhymes. After Mom and I model a few, Kevin comes up with, "This old man / he played four / he played knick-knack on the floor," and he adds, "Or, in his store!" For 5-year-old Tate, I sing the song, "Apples and Bananas" to work on sound substitution as each verse requires the singer to replace the vowels in the title phrase with another vowel such as "ee" to become "I like to eat Ee-pples and Bee-nee-nees."

2. Name songs—Children love to hear their names mentioned in songs and enjoy having them spelled. Kevin is a 5-year-old with bone-anchored (os-

seo-integrated) devices. I use Barton's (2007) song with the lyrics "I know a boy and his name is Kevin, K-E-V-I-N." I contrast that with his mother's name, "P-A-M," and my name. I sing someone's spelled name in the song and Kevin identifies the person, then becomes the leader. The inviting name song "Welcome, Come On In" (Estabrooks & Birkenshaw-Fleming, 2003) is a recommended variation.

Musical Cousins

Since they can share features of rhythm, melodic intonation, and rhyming, poetry can strengthen a child's musical skills and vice versa. Poetry also brings light-heartedness and whimsy to an AVT session (Robbins, 2016). I read the poem "Happy New" (Silverstein, 2011) aloud with Abby, who is 6 and wears hearing aids as we target goals including: *Prediction*—What word do you suppose is missing from the title? *Phonological awareness*—What word substitutes for "new" in each iteration of "Happy New"? *Auditory closure*—how can we complete these silly greetings, so they make sense? *Rhyming*—Does my answer rhyme with the word it replaces? *Creativity*—Can we make up our own verses to extend the silliness? Parents are encouraged to read aloud poems that are meaningful to them—strengthening generational ties. Abby's mother brings her childhood poetry book, given to her by Abby's grandparents and suggests we read "The Swing" (Stevenson)—her favorite. Like a song, a poem may be associated with specific memories, eliciting emotion from its reader. Her mother tells Abby how much it means to her that they are sharing the experience.

"Doggie, Doggie, Where's Your Bone?"

Great auditory access includes the ability to recognize familiar people based on the sounds of their voices. This activity encourages the child to pay attention to indexical features of speech, the unique characteristics that give each speaker a *voice print*. It can be played with a minimum of three people, so we introduce it in the AVT session and then it can be played at home with a total of four or five people. This traditional song is sung on the "mama" interval. Mother, Gavon's sister, Anne, and I sit closely together. Gavon, age 4, is the *doggie*. He sits in front of us, facing backward. Mother, Anne, and I agree that Mother will hold the cardboard bone. All four of us sing together, *"Doggie, doggie, where's your bone? Somebody took it from your home."* Gavon sings, *"Who has my bone?"* Mom replies by singing, *"I have your bo-one."* Gavon recognizes his mother as the person who sang, so they trade places. To extend the game, I build Gavon's musical word bank by asking, "How are my voice, Anne's, and Mom's different?" He says Anne's voice is "littler" and we discuss whether he means "higher pitched," "softer," or "thinner."

Our Memory Magnet

Music is such an effective mnemonic device that I call it a "memory magnet" and recruit it for remembering facts, rules, or other rote information. I use piggyback tunes to help children learn their addresses and phone numbers as they are important for a child's safety. Several programs offer chants and songs to retain academic facts (see "Silly School Songs!" on YouTube). Tate, a 5-year-old with hearing aids, is fascinated by astronomy. He has learned facts about each planet by reciting a rap, *The Solar System Song* with a repeated chorus: *The sun, the moon and the stars* [Pause] / *Mercury, Venus, Earth and Mars.*

Executive Functions and Music

Executive functions (EFs) are a set of neurocognitive processes responsible for active management of cognitive resources, emotions, and behaviors in order to achieve a goal (see Chapter 13). Components include emotional regulation, controlled attention, planning, impulse control, and working memory. EFs are important in all the developmental areas needed for interpersonal, school, and life success. Children with CIs have been shown to have a two to five times greater risk of executive function (EF) deficits relative to hearing peers (Kronenberger, Beer, Castellanos, Pisoni, & Miyamoto, 2014), meaning this needs to be a focus for many children in AVT. The author has found music to be an effective way to improve EF deficits (Robbins & Kronenberger, 2019). Six-year-old Jay and I are using *Social Thinking* materials (Garcia Winner, 2007) including *the Social Explorers curriculum* (Hendrix, Palmer, Tarshis, & Garcia Winner, 2013), which has an accompanying music CD. Each EF concept is reinforced by a book, teaching activities, and a song (Chapin & Galdston, 2013). Jay sings "The Plan" song with the lyrics "*When it's you and only you/ you're alone, all on your own/But when it's you and me and we/*

There must be a plan." We have reviewed stories and songs about *"Show me what you're feeling," "Your Brain's where you think a thought"* and *"Size of the problem."* The automaticity of these songs reduces working memory load and allows Jay to internalize rules for how to accomplish important interpersonal and academic tasks.

Bossing Your Brain with Music

Meta-cognitive awareness allows us to think about how we think. Thinking is something children can get better at, but they have to practice it, to be the *"boss of their brain"* by using specific strategies that help them think smarter, not harder. Robbins (2005) described a set of strategies to help children *boss their brain.* The parent and I model the strategies frequently, even with preschoolers. I created piggyback songs for each strategy. These help Pete, age 6, to remember how to use them. Before we start an auditory memory game, Mom tells him, "You'd better boss your brain and re-auditorize what you hear." Pete sings to the tune of "My Bonnie Lies over the Ocean": *I ne-ed to sa-y things out loud /That's how I re-auditorize / I say it out loud and repeat it / My bra-ain can hear myself think!/* For the Finger Cues strategy, he sings (to the tune "I've Something in My Pocket"): *My fingers are like Post-its / they remind me what to do /I remember when my fingers help / how about you?* Singing each strategy to remember how he uses it helps Pete increase his meta-cognitive awareness and be a more active thinker and learner.

Musical Suggestions for Children with Complex Needs

Practitioners agree that music is one of the most effective tools for children who are deaf or hard of hearing who also have complex needs (see Chapter 22). Some suggestions for using music and singing with this population in AVT are as follows:

1. The developmental skills of children with complex needs in the "mild" range typically progress in the same sequence but at a slower rate than those of their peers with hearing loss alone. Though music itself may be delayed, music and singing in particular need to be considered to support other delayed skill areas.

2. The practitioner can use a progress-monitoring tool with individualized items designed for this population to chart musical and communication behaviors over time. Music is experienced globally, as a gestalt. For children with complex needs who cannot analyze or focus on parts, music provides a holistic way to be included in experiences.

3. Practitioners can learn from parents about the child's motivators and use songs and music based on these preferences.

4. Observe the child at home. Identify the communication targets of the highest functional value. Ask the question: *Can a song, a tune, or a rhythm be used to support or take the place of a word or phrase?*

5. Ask parents to identify the child's top hurdle. Explore how music can be a part of the solution. I worked with the family of Sam, a 6-year old with CIs and complex needs who used a wheelchair. He screamed when he wanted something. Responding to him, "We'll be there in a moment" was not effective, so I suggested we sing back to him instead. We composed a song, *"I will be there in a minute"* to the tune of "The More We Get Together." The parents were ecstatic to report that, for the first time, he was able to self-regulate and stay calm until they could attend to him.

6. Parents want their children to be a true part of their family and music can help. Families can assemble a band of rhythm instruments and find one their child with complex needs can play, either independently or with assistance. Sam's parents said that Sam's siblings felt he was a member of the team when he joined in their band by swiping at a hanging bell that was within his motor ability.

7. Share what we know with others and learn from them. *Listening connects a child to other people when the child can hear their voices and the music they make. If a child has limited independence, hearing and listening, talking, singing, and other musical activities can be a lifeline to the world.*

CONCLUSION

Of all musical experiences, the voice is the instrument that is most accessible and most related to talking. Singing therefore needs to receive top priority in AVT sessions and in all appropriate aspects of daily life. In this chapter, the author presented both the why and how of integrating music in AVT for children with hearing loss from birth to age 6, extensive activities in music and singing that may be integrated into AVT, and the generalization of music and singing far beyond the AVT session. The author also discussed abundant research to demonstrate the positive effects of music on various neurodevelopmental domains.

"My life flows on in endless song, above earth's lamentation . . . " so go the lyrics to the early American hymn "How Can I Keep from Singing?" Music and singing are integral to life and to our experiences as human beings. Music soothes, rejoices, grieves with us, and is associated with life's memorable moments. Music is with us when we gather as a family, as a faith community, as school friends, and at sporting events, birthday parties, and weddings. Music is one of the deepest expressions of feeling, often used when words are simply inadequate. Children with hearing loss are born with the ability to learn language and music and they deserve to have music and singing as part of their lives. Music aligns with AVT to enhance a child's cognitive, listening, spoken language, literacy, academic, and social outcomes. Music brings pleasure, provides an emotional outlet, and connects children to their family, their community, and the wider culture.

REFERENCES

Aigen, K. (2005). *Music-centered music therapy*. Gilsum, NH: Barcelona Publishers.

Barton, C. (2010). *Music, spoken language, and children with hearing loss: Definitions and development*. Course presented on http://www.SpeechPathology.com on 4/19/2010.

Barton, C. (2013). Children with hearing loss. In M. Hintz (Ed.), *Guidelines for music therapy practice in developmental health*, (pp. 233–269). Gilsum, NH: Barcelona Publishers.

Barton, C., & Robbins, A. M. (2008). *Tune-Ups: An integrated speech and music therapy approach*. Valencia, CA: Advanced Bionics.

Barton, C., & Robbins, A. M. (2015). Jump-starting auditory learning in children with cochlear implants through music experiences. *Cochlear Implants International, 16*(3), S51–S62.

Barton, C., & Robbins, A. M. (2018). Auditunes: A video resource of music activities to support listening and spoken language development. http://www.sjiresources.org

Beebe, H. (1985). *Educational audiology for the limited-hearing infant and preschooler*. Springfield, IL: Charles C. Thomas.

Bergeson, T. R., Miller, R. J., & McCune, K. (2006). Mothers' speech to hearing-impaired infants and children. *Infancy, 10*, 221–240.

Boynton, S. (1995). *Blue hat, green hat*. New York, NY: Little Simon.

Chapin, T., & Galdston, P. (2013). *The incredible flexible you*. Dobbs Ferry, NY: Sundance Music, Inc.

Chen, J., Chuang, A., McMahon, C., Hsieh J., Tung, T., & Po-Hunt, L. (2010). Music training improves pitch perception in prelingually deafened children with cochlear implants. *Pediatrics, 125*, e793–e800.

Colombini, S. (2019). Music therapy in NICUs can help babies get home sooner. Retrieved May 16, 2019 from https://wusfnews.wusf.usf.edu/post/music-therapy-nicus-can-help-babies-get-home-sooner

Conway, C., Pisoni, D., & Kronenberger, W. (2009). The importance of sound for cognitive sequencing abilities: The auditory scaffolding hypothesis. *Current Directions in Psychological Science, 18*(5), 275–279.

Corbeil, M., Trehub, S., & Peretz, I. (2013). Speech vs. singing: Infants choose happier sounds. *Frontiers in Psychology, 4,* 1–11.

Curtis, M., & Bharucha, J. (2010). The minor third communicates sadness in speech, mirroring its use in music. *Emotion, 10*(3), 335–348. doi: 10.1037/a0017928. PMID 20515223.

Dowell, R. I. (1987). *Move over, Mother Goose! Finger plays, action verses and funny rhymes.* Mt. Ranier, MD: Gryphon House.

Elliott, D. J. (1995). As cited in Nordoff, P., & Robbins, C. (2007). *Creative music therapy: A guide to fostering clinical musicianship* (2nd ed.). Gilsum, NH: Barcelona Publishers.

Estabrooks, W. (1994). Epilogue, learning to listen. In W. Estabrooks (Ed.), *Auditory-Verbal Therapy for parents and professionals* (pp. 292–293). Washington, DC: Alexander Graham Bell Association for the Deaf and Hard of Hearing.

Estabrooks, W. (2012). *101 frequently asked questions about auditory-verbal practice.* Washington DC: Alexander Graham Bell Association for the Deaf and Hard of Hearing.

Estabrooks, W, & Birkenshaw-Fleming, L. (1994). *Hear & listen! Talk & Sing!* Washington, DC: Alexander Graham Bell Association for the Deaf and Hard of Hearing.

Estabrooks, W., & Birkenshaw-Fleming, L. (2003). *Songs for listening, songs for life.* Washington DC: Alexander Graham Bell Association for the Deaf and Hard of Hearing.

Flohr, J. W., Miller, D., & DeBeus, R. (2000). EEG studies with young children. *Music Educators Journal, 87,* 28–32. doi: 10.2307 /3399645

Garcia-Winner, M. (2007). *Thinking of me thinking of you.* Santa Clara, CA: Think Social Publishing.

Gordon, K., Wong, D., Valero, J., Jewell, S., Yoo, P., & Papsin, B. (2011). Use it or lose it? Lessons learned from the developing brains of children who are deaf and use cochlear implants to hear. *Brain Topography, 24*(3-4), 204–219.

Hargreaves, D. J., Miell, D., & MacDonald, R. A. R. (2002). What are musical identities, and why are they important? In R. A. R. McDonald, D. J. Hargreaves, & D. Miell (Eds.), *Musical identities* (pp. 1–20). Oxford, UK: Oxford University Press.

Hendrix, R., Palmer, K., Tarshis, N., & Garcia Winner, M. (2013). *We thinkers!* Social Explorers (vol. 1). Santa Clara, CA: Think Social Publishing.

Holt, R., & Kirk, K. (2005). Speech and language development in cognitively delayed children with cochlear implants. *Ear and Hearing, 26,* 132–148.

Hopyan, T., Gordon, K. A., & Papsin, B. C. (2011). Identifying emotions in music through electrical hearing in deaf children using cochlear implants. *Cochlear Implants International, 12*(1), 21–26. doi: 10.1179/146701010X12677899497 399

Hopyan-Misakyan, T., Gordon, K. A., Dennis, M., & Papsin, B. (2009). Recognition of affective speech prosody and facial affect in deaf children with unilateral right cochlear implants. *Child Neuropsychology, 15,* 136–146.

Houston, D. M., & Bergeson, T. R. (2014). Hearing vs. listening: Attention to speech and its role in language acquisition in deaf infants with cochlear implants. *Lingua, 139,* 10–29.

Hsiao, F., & Gfeller, K. (2012). Music perception of cochlear implant recipients with implications for music instruction: A review of literature. *Update University S C Department Music, 31*(2), 5–10.

Kirschner, S., & Tomasello, M. (2010.) Joint music making promotes prosocial behavior in 4-year-old children. *Evolution and Human Behavior, 31*(2010), 354–364.

Koelsch, S. (2009). A neuroscientific perspective on music therapy. The neurosciences and music III—disorders and plasticity. *Annals of the New York Academy of Sciences, 1169*, 374–384.

Kraus, N., & Chandrasekaran, B. (2010) Music training for the development of auditory skills. *Nature Reviews Neuroscience, 11*, 599–605.

Kraus, N., Skoe, E., & Parbery-Clark, A. (2008). *Auditory processing of pitch, timber and time: Implications for language and music.* Paper presented at the Alexander Graham Bell Research Symposium, June 30, 2008, Washington, DC.

Kronenberger, W., Beer, J., Castellanos, I., Pisoni, D., & Miyamoto, R. (2014). Neurocognitive risk in children with cochlear implants. *JAMA Otolaryngology Head & Neck Surgery, 140*(7), 608–615.

Laferriere, J. (2003). Lesson plan. In W. Estabrooks & L. Birkenshaw-Fleming (Eds.), *Songs for listening! Songs for life!* Washington DC: Alexander Graham Bell Association for the Deaf and Hard of Hearing.

Mithin, S. (2006). *The singing Neanderthals: The origins of music, language, mind, and body.* Cambridge, MA: Harvard University Press.

Palmer, H. (1999). *Baby songs good night.* Racine, WI: Western Publishing.

Pasek, B., & Paul, J. (2017). *This is me.* New York, NY: Breathlike Music.

Patel, A. D. (2012). The OPERA hypothesis: Assumptions and clarifications. *Annals of the New York Academy of Sciences, 1252*, 124–128.

Phillips, J. (1990). *Peek-a-boo! I see you!* New York, NY: Grosset & Dunlap.

Pollack, D. (1985). *Educational audiology for the limited-hearing infant and preschooler.* Springfield, IL: Charles C. Thomas Publishing.

Putkinen, V, Saarikivi, K., & Tervaniemi, M. (2013). Do informal musical activities shape auditory skill development in preschool-age children? *Frontiers in Psychology, 4*, Article 572, 1–6.

Putkinen, V., Tervaniemi, M., & Huotilainen, M. (2013). Informal musical activities are linked to auditory discrimination and attention in 2–3-year-old children: An event-related potential study. *European Journal of Neurosciences, 37*, 654–661.

Rabinowitch, T., Cross, I., & Burnard, P. (2012). Long-term musical group interaction has a positive influence on empathy in children. *Psychology of Music.* https://doi.org/10.1177/0305735612440609

Robbins, A. M. (2005). Bossing your brain: A history lesson with a hard-of-hearing middle school student. *Volta Voices, 12*(4), 38–40.

Robbins, A. M. (2009). Rehabilitation after cochlear implantation. In Niparko (Ed.), *Cochlear implants principles and practices* (2nd ed., pp. 267–312). Philadelphia, PA: Lippincott Williams & Wilkins.

Robbins, A. M. (2016). Auditory-Verbal therapy: A conversational competence approach. In M. Moeller, D. J. Ertmer, & C. Stoel-Gammon (Eds.), *Promoting language and literacy in children who are deaf or hard of hearing.* Baltimore, MD: Paul H. Brookes Publishing.

Robbins, A. M., & Barton, C. G. (2010). *Language and music and ears, oh my!* Short course presented at the Alexander Graham Bell convention, June, Orlando, FL.

Robbins, A. M., & Caraway, T. (2010). Missing the mark in early intervention for babies who are hard of hearing or deaf learning spoken language. *Perspectives on Hearing and Hearing Disorders in Childhood, 20*(2), 41–47.

Robbins, A., Koch, D., Osberger, M., Phillips, S., & Kishon-Rabin, L. (2004). Effect of age at cochlear implantation on auditory skill development in infants and toddlers. *Archives of Otolaryngology, 130*, 570–574.

Robbins, A., & Kronenberger, W. (2019). *Principles of executive function intervention for children with cochlear implants.* Paper presented at American Cochlear Implant Alliance meeting, July 11, Hollywood, FL.

Robbins, C., & Robbins, C. (1980). *Music for the hearing impaired: A resource manual and curriculum guide.* New York, NY: MMB Music.

Rogenmoser, L., Kernbach, J., Schlaug, G., & Gaser, C. (2017). Keeping brains young by making music. *Brain Structure & Function*. Springer. doi: 10.1007/s00429-017-1491-2

Schlaug, G., Norton A., Overy, K., & Winner, E. (2005). Effects of music training on the child's brain and cognitive development. *Annals of the New York Academy of Sciences, 1060*, 219–230.

Segal, O., & Kishon-Rabin, L. (2011). Listening preference for child directed speech vs nonspeech stimuli in normal hearing and hearing impaired infants after cochlear implantation. *Ear and Hearing, 32*(3), 358–372.

Shannon, J. R. (1913). *That's an Irish lullaby*. M. Whitmark and Sons.

Sharma, A., & Nash, A. (2009, April 14). Brain maturation in children with CI. *Asha Leader*. Retrieved May 5, 2019 from https://leader.pubs.asha.org/doi/10.1044/leader.FTR3.14052009.14

Sherman, A., & Busch, L. (1963). *Hello Muddah hello Faddah*. Hendersonville, TN: WB Music and Burning Bush Music.

Silverstein, S. (2011). *Everthing on it*. New York, NY: Harper Collins.

Spier, P. (1972). *Crash! Bang! Boom!* New York, NY: Doubleday.

Strait, D., & Kraus, N. (2011). Playing music for a smarter ear: Cognitive, perceptual and neurobiological evidence. *Music Perception, 29*(2), 133–146.

Strait, D., Kraus, N., Skoe, E., & Ashley, R. (2009). Musical experience promotes subcortical efficiency in processing emotional vocal sounds. The Neurosciences and Music III—disorders and plasticity. *Annals of the New York Academy of Sciences, 1169*, 209–213.

Talbot P., & Estabrooks, W. (2012). What are the characteristics of an effective parent-practitioner relationship in auditory-verbal therapy and education? In W. Estabrooks (Ed.), *101 frequently asked questions about auditory-verbal practice* (pp. 23–26). Washington, DC: Alexander Graham Bell Association for the Deaf and Hard of Hearing.

Torppa, R., Huotilainen, M., Leminen, M., Lipsanen, J., & Teraniemi, T. (2014), Interplay between singing and cortical processing of music: A longitudinal study in children with cochlear implants. *Frontiers in Psychology, 5*, 1–16.

Torppa, R., Faulkner, A., Kujala, T., Huotilainen, M., & Lipsanen, J. (2018). Developmental links between speech perception in noise, singing and cortical processing of music in children with cochlear implants. *Music Perception, an Interdisciplinary Journal, 36*(2), 156.

Trainor, L. J., Clark, E. D., Huntley, A., & Adams, B. A. (1997). The acoustic benefits of musical training: Effects on oscillatory brain activity. *Annals of the New York Academy of Sciences, 1169*, 133–142.

Trehub, S. E. (2013). Communication, music, and language in infancy. In M. A. Arbib (Ed.), *Language, music, and the brain* (pp. 463–479). Strungmann Forum Reports, vol. 10. Cambridge, MA: MIT Press.

Trehub, S. E., & Gundmundsdottir, H. R. (2015). Mothers as singing mentors for infants. In: G. Welch, D. M. Howard, & J. Nix (Eds.), *The Oxford handbook of singing*. doi: 10.1093/oxfordhb/9780199660773.013.25.

Troxel, K. (1984). *Grammar songs*. http://www.kathytroxel.com

Walker, E., McCreery, R., Spratford, M., Oleson, J., Van Buren, J., Bentler, R., . . . Moeller, M. (2015). Trends and predictors of longitudinal hearing aid use for children who are hard of hearing. *Ear and Hearing, 36*(suppl 1.), 38S–47S.

Wang, D. J., Trehub, S. E., Volkova, A., & van Lieshout, P. (2013). Child implant users' imitation of happy- and sad-sounding speech. *Frontiers in Psychology, 4*(351), 1–8.

Welch, G., Saunders, J., Edwards, S., Palmer, Z., Himonides, E., Knight, J., . . . Vickers, D. (2015). Using singing to nurture children's hearing? A pilot study. *Otorhinolaryngology, 73*(7), 1043–1052.

Williams, K. E., Barrett, M. S., Welch, G. F., Abad, V., & Broughton, M. (2015).

Associations between early shared music activities in the home and later child outcomes: Findings from the longitudinal study of Australian children. *Early Childhood Research Quarterly, 31*, 113–124.

Wood, A. (1992). *Silly Sally*. Boston, MA: Houghton Mifflin Harcourt.

Woodruff Carr, K., White-Schwoch, T., Tierney, A., Strait, D. L., & Kraus, N. (2014). Beat synchronization predicts neural speech encoding and reading readiness in preschoolers. *Proceedings of the National Academy of Sciences, 111*(40), 14559–14564.

Yucel, E., Sennaroglu, G., & Belgin, E. (2009). The family oriented musical training for children with cochlear implants: Speech and musical perception results of two-year follow-up. *International Journal of Pediatric Otorhinolaryngology, 73*(7), 1043–1052.

19

ASSESSMENT AND AUDITORY-VERBAL THERAPY

Lindsay Zombek

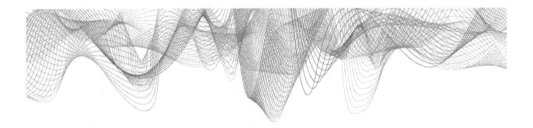

Assessment is an essential practice component of quality Auditory-Verbal Therapy (AVT) and appears in two of the Principles of AVT: (1) the use of natural developmental patterns of audition, speech, and language and cognition when teaching and communicating with the child, and (2) developing individualized plans, monitoring progress, and evaluating the effectiveness of the treatment plan. The impact of hearing loss on the multiple developmental domains of listening, speech, and language requires special considerations when assessing children who are deaf or hard of hearing in AVT.

Traditional assessments of communication skills in children may be limited to evaluation of speech articulation, receptive (comprehension), expressive (use) language, and pragmatic (social) language. Assessment in AVT includes all these *plus* formal and informal measures that evaluate and monitor a child's progress across the developmental domains of cognition, play, auditory function, speech development, language, literacy, along with other assessments as warranted, particularly when additional challenges are suspected. The AVT practitioner (the practitioner) goes even further and assesses family needs. The practitioner may not be able to complete some assessments related to personal or family matters if he/she has neither the necessary qualifications nor access to the required resources. It is then incumbent upon the practitioner to contact the appropriate professionals who can complete such assessments.

This chapter begins with a discussion of the purposes and timing of assessment in AVT, followed by descriptions of formal and informal testing, and scoring and interpretation considerations specific to AVT. From there, the reader will find the essential elements of assessment in AVT: (1) gathering case information, (2) ensuring auditory access, (3) assessing auditory function, speech, and language, and (4) assessing family needs. Special considerations for assessment of children who have unilateral hearing loss, complex hearing needs, and additional challenges will be suggested. The chapter concludes with two case histories that assimilate this information and serve to provide guidance for the practitioner.

INITIAL AND ONGOING ASSESSMENT IN AVT: PURPOSES, TIMING, AND CONTEXTS

Assessment of the child and family begins from the first meeting with the practitioner. The initial assessment provides the practitioner with information to (1) establish a child's developmental level with reference to typical listening, speech, and language milestones, (2) develop long-term goals in an individualized plan of care, and (3) provide a baseline for progress monitoring. Assessment beyond the baseline assessment in AVT is *ongoing*. *Ongoing assessment* is used to monitor a child's progress toward goal attainment and

can signal a need to change goals or conduct further assessment. When a child has met goals or is progressing adequately toward goal completion, ongoing assessment aids in the development of the next steps. If the ongoing assessment identifies lack of progress relative to the previously established goals, potential problem symptoms can be investigated and identified in a timely fashion. Possible problems that can be identified via continuous monitoring might be issues with hearing technology, changes in hearing, or undiagnosed concurrent disorders.

Ongoing assessment in AVT continues far beyond the initial assessment. In-depth assessment is conducted at regularly scheduled intervals of 6 or 12 months, typically using formal measures (see below) and frequently determined by insurance, school, or government requirements. Moreover, each AVT session is a *diagnostic* session during which the practitioner informally collects assessment and observation data during the course of an AVT session to monitor progress toward goals. The practitioner also monitors function and development in other domains throughout the family's journey in AVT. This is particularly helpful if a child is not making progress in established goals. For example, monitoring a child's behavior, attention, and cognitive development alerts the practitioner and parents to an underlying reason for inadequate progress and can prompt a referral for more specialized assessment. The practitioner might uncover a weakness in auditory skill development that affects a speech goal and can then develop a goal to help develop a fundamental auditory skill that supports the development of the speech target.

Ongoing assessment extends to environments beyond the AVT session. Parents are guided to observe and monitor a child's skills at home. Daycare providers and preschool classroom teachers provide information as well. These additional sources of information contribute to a more authentic and robust description of the child's ability and provide evidence for generalization of a skill from the clinical setting to the home or classroom. Information regarding how the child functions in environments outside the therapy setting helps determine a child's full range of service requirements and needs.

FORMAL AND INFORMAL ASSESSMENT IN AVT

Assessment in AVT is conducted both formally and informally. Formal assessment is conducted using standardized norm-referenced assessments. Norm-referenced assessments are standardized using a population of typically developing children who have taken the test; their scores serve as a reference, enabling the practitioner to compare a child's performance with that of the normative group of typically developing peers. Norm-referenced assessments enable the practitioner and families to determine whether the child is performing below, at, or above average. Many educational programs require these scores to make determinations about whether services are necessary, and the types of services required for a child to be successful in a particular program. A standard score also provides a consistent benchmark to assess

the progress of the child, as well as his/her current skill level. When possible, mastery of communication should be assessed using formal measures to allow for comparison to typically developing peers.

Informal assessments are indispensable to AVT and help provide a more authentic picture of a child's abilities. Informal testing uses criterion-referenced assessments and observations to identify mastered skills and functional performance. Criterion-referenced assessments use defined criteria that indicate mastery of a skill. A child's performance is compared with those criteria to determine whether a child's skills are approaching or have reached criteria for mastery. Many criterion-referenced assessments for children who are deaf or hard of hearing specify skills that children should achieve at a particular age. The practitioner uses this information to determine whether a child has developed age-appropriate skills or is lacking skills that should have been acquired.

Observations are especially valuable for getting information regarding how a child functions outside the AVT session. The practitioner can visit the home or child's classroom to conduct an observation. When a visit is not possible, regular communication and elicited input from parents, teachers, daycare providers, caretakers, and other important members of the child's team allows an evaluator to determine how the child is using his/her skill set in real-life settings.

Finally, informal assessment is an essential part of an overall assessment for children who have skill levels below what is captured by formal testing. Informal assessment of a child who has skills substantially below his or her age, whether due to a cognitive deficit, late identification, or other challenges, may provide more useful information about a child's true performance than a formal assessment.

Following assessment of a child who is deaf or hard of hearing in AVT, the interpretation of results is multi-dimensional. Interpretations take into consideration the results and observations from both formal and informal testing so that appropriate recommendations, goals, and an AVT plan of care can be developed. This requires that the practitioner understands how various scores are derived and knows what to do when a score may not give all the information needed. In addition, interpretation of the results of formal testing in AVT can proceed from several developmental perspectives, making it a bit more complex than traditional assessment.

Norm-Referenced Assessments and Standard Scores

Interpreting norm-referenced assessments requires an understanding of the kinds of scores that are obtained. The number of items that a child answers correctly is called the *raw score*. A *standard score* is derived from a child's raw score. Standard scores allow for comparison of a child's performance to typically developing peers, or the normative *mean*. Test developers assess a normative sample of typically developing children and then calculate the average raw scores that are attained by each age group within the normative group. This average score is the *mean*. On many standardized tests, the mean score is then translated into a standard score of 100. Typically developing 3-year-olds will perform on average differently than typically developing 4-year-olds. Accordingly, a mean raw score for 3-year-olds will be different than the mean raw score for 4-year-olds. When the raw scores for these two age groups are translated into standard scores, however, the mean raw score for each age group is given a standard mean score of 100. When a 3-year-old child in AVT completes a norm-referenced assessment and achieves a standard score of 100, it means that he/she is performing similarly to the average performance by 3-year-old typically developing children.

It is helpful for the practitioner and families to understand how far above or below the normative mean that a child is performing. *Standard deviations* give this information. When the standard mean is 100, each standard deviation is worth 15 points. For example, a standard score of 85 is 1 standard deviation below the mean. On a standardized test, 95% of the normative population performs within 2 standard deviations of the mean. In other words, if a child's standard score is greater than 2 standard deviations below the mean, he/she is performing below 95% of same-aged typically developing peers. The range of three standard deviations above and below the mean encompasses the performance of 99.7% of the normative population.

Table 19–1. Raw, Standard, and Age-Equivalency Scores of a Child Progressing from 12 Months to 24 Months on the *Preschool Language Scale–5th Edition* (Zimmerman et al., 2011)

	Chronological Age at Time of Testing	
	12 months	**24 months**
Raw Score	1	11
Standard Score	50	50
Age Equivalency	1 month	6 months

There are two issues of which the practitioner needs to be mindful when scoring and interpreting a standardized assessment. The first pertains to a child whose development is substantially below his/her same-aged typically developing peers. If a child's performance is so low that the standard score is greater than 3 standard deviations below the mean, the test may not be scored in a meaningful way. The practitioner finds another way to assess that child in order to obtain authentic information about a child's performance about the skills in question. Informal testing can be the solution in this case.

Another issue pertains to the range of raw scores that yield a single standard score. For example, raw scores on the *Preschool Language Scale: Fifth Edition* (*PLS-5*) (Zimmerman, Steiner, & Pond, 2011) obtained from a 12-month-old child that range from 0 to 8 will all yield the same standard score of 50. This is the case whether the child's raw score is closer to 0 or to 8. The range of raw scores that result in a single standard score makes it challenging to demonstrate progress from one test administration to the next. This is illustrated in Table 19–1. In this example, if a

12-month-old child attained a raw score of 1 on the Language Comprehension subtest, his/her standard score is 50, a concerning standard score because it is greater than 3 standard deviations below the mean. If the same child is retested at the age of 24 months, any score from 0 to 11 on the Language Comprehension subtest yields a standard score of 50, due to the higher number of items the average 24-month-old can respond to correctly. Consequently, a child who increases his/her raw score from 1 at age 12 months to a raw score of 11 at age 24 months would continue to achieve an alarmingly low standard score of 50 despite progress in the actual number of correct responses on the assessment. In this case, a notation of the change in the child's raw score may be an appropriate source of additional information in a conversation and in a report.

Age Equivalency Scores

Age-equivalency scores are an additional way to report progress and a child's current status of development. An age-equivalency score is the age at which at least 50% of children attain a specific raw score. For example, 50% of 2-year-olds in the normative group achieve a raw score of 27 on the Auditory Comprehension subtest of the *PLS-5* (Zimmerman et al., 2011). Age equivalency, like the standard score, is determined by the raw score achieved by the child. Age-equivalency conversions from raw scores for a particular assessment are often provided in the test manual. Calculation of equivalent age can be an effective approach to demonstrate progress, particularly for a child whose progress is not captured by a change in standard score. This is illustrated in Table 19–1, which shows the results from assessments of a child at ages 12 and 24 months. The child attained the same standard score for each assessment, scoring in the average range for the child's age at the time of testing. The unchanged standard score obscures what is revealed by the age equivalency, and indicates the child made 6 months of progress in a 12-month period. Although this child has made progress, the age-equivalency score informs the practitioner and family that the child is not moving forward at the rate, minimally, of 1 year's progress over 1 year of time. This alerts the practitioner et al. that further assessment of the child's needs is in order.

Age-equivalency scores can be unreliable, and use of these scores needs to be approached carefully. Maloney and Laravee (2007) reported that of 50 participants, 43 children who had normal, average standard scores demonstrated age-equivalency scores 2 or more years either above or below their chronological age. Age-equivalency scores indicate that a specific raw score was reached but do not indicate the specific questions a child correctly or incorrectly answered and are not sensitive enough to capture whether all age-appropriate targets were mastered. Furthermore, because the age equivalency is an average, half of the children in the normative sample group at that exact age scored above that score and half scored below. That is a wide variation and should be fully explained to parents when using age equivalency to track progress.

Hearing Age

Hearing age (HA), sometimes referred to as listening age, is an adjusted age that is used to account for the amount of time a child has had access to conversational speech using appropriate hearing technology. There is a similar model used for children born prematurely; for example, a child who is 6 months old born a month early may be more developmentally similar to a 5-month-old child. Age is adjusted for prematurity so that a child who is 6 months old but born one month prematurely may be given an adjusted age as 5 months old for developmental comparison.

In AVT, practitioners use the following formula to calculate HA: chronological age (CA) minus age at receiving appropriate hearing technology equals HA. Using this formula, a child who has a CA of 12 months who received hearing aids at age 2 months has an HA of 10 months. In the case of cochlear implantation, HA is slightly more complicated. An 18-month-old child with a profound hearing loss who was fit at age 2 months with hearing aids but did not have adequate aided auditory access to spoken language is considered to start listening at the time of cochlear implant activation. If that activation is at 12 months, the child has a hearing age of 6 months (CA18 months—12 months at implant activation—6 months HA).

Children who are deaf or hard of hearing in AVT tend to develop auditory, speech, and language skills developmentally; that is, skills develop in the same time frame as they do in typical development, based on the duration a child has had auditory access to conversational speech. Therefore, it is anticipated that a child with an HA of 12 months would demonstrate auditory, speech, and language skills of at least a typically developing 12-month-old child with no hearing loss, even if the child were chronologically older.

The use of HA assists the practitioner to determine if progress is being made developmentally in AVT. This is illustrated in Table 19–2, which shows a child's performance on the Auditory Comprehension subtest of the *PLS-5* (Zimmerman et al., 2011) in two administrations a year apart. The child in this illustration is 3 years old at the first test administration and has been listening with a cochlear implant for 1 year. That child's equivalent expressive language age of 1 year might be considered indicative of a severe language disorder according to an interpretation of test results that reference chronological age. If the practitioner uses the HA for analysis, however, a more optimistic picture of the child's developmental learning emerges. In this case, the age equivalency is appropriate for the child's HA. Looking at the second test administration 1 year later, the age equivalency has continued to match the child's HA, progressing the equivalent of 1 year over a 12-month period.

Ideally, a child needs to make more than a year of progress in a year's time to catch up to appropriate skills for his/her chronological age. If a child is not making sufficient progress, age-equivalency scores can reveal this, and the practitioner can determine if changes need to be made regarding the intensity and frequency of services or if additional evaluation of learning is needed.

Table 19-2. Comparison of Auditory Comprehension Subtest Scores on *Preschool Language Scale–5th Edition* by Chronological Age (CA) and Hearing Age (HA) with Two Administrations One Year Apart

	Test Administration Year 1		Test Administration Year 2	
Child "Age"	CA 3;0	HA 1;0	CA 4;0	HA 2;0
Raw Score	16	16	26	26
Standard Score	50	87	57	89
Percentile	1	19	1	23
Age Equivalency	1;0	1;0	1;11	1;11
Severity	SEVERE	WNL for LA	SEVERE	WNL for LA

Note: WNL = within normal limits; LA = language age.

Are Low-Average/Borderline Skills Acceptable?

Schools and private clinics may require that a child's skills need to be significantly below that of typically developing peers to qualify for services. The specific criterion deficit can vary with school or clinical program. For example, one program may require that a child's standard score on formal language testing be greater than 1 standard deviation below the mean to qualify for services; another may require a deficit of greater than 2 standard deviations below the mean. Using these criteria, a child with hearing loss in AVT whose standard scores on formal language testing fall within 1 standard deviation below average may be considered to be performing at an acceptable level and therefore ineligible for intervention services.

The practitioner takes a different perspective because he/she knows that children who are deaf or hard of hearing who are fit with hearing technology early in life have the potential to develop speech and language skills at a level commensurate with their peers. Consequently, a child with hearing loss who has average or above-average intelligence and low-borderline language scores may be demonstrating a deficit in language performance compared with his or her potential and is in need of intervention.

ESSENTIAL ELEMENTS OF AN ASSESSMENT PROTOCOL IN AVT

The essential elements of an assessment protocol in AVT include: (1) gathering case information, (2) ensuring auditory access, (3) assessing auditory function, speech, and language, and (4) assessing family needs.

Gathering Case Information

Case information is gathered for an initial assessment and updated throughout the duration of a child's journey in AVT. The case information includes the following:

1. Developmental history (e.g., global milestones in gross and fine motor skills and general communication), medical history (e.g., birth history, relevant diagnoses, hospitalizations), social history (e.g., how the child interacts with others, behavior), and presence of additional disability or other sensory deficits.

2. Hearing health: stability of hearing loss—congenital, progressive, or fluctuating—to understand a child's duration and stability of exposure to sound (includes history of recurrent otitis media); etiology to consider the possibility of concomitant disabilities that can affect learning or issues with fitting with hearing technology (e.g., cochlear malformation impacting implant effectiveness).

3. Audiological information and report of auditory access with hearing technology, including speech perception scores. Audiological and hearing technology information must be current and meet the guidelines in the *Recommended Protocol for Audiological Assessment, Hearing Aid and Cochlear Implant Evaluation, and Follow-Up* (A. G. Bell, 2019).

4. History of hearing technology use: date of initial hearing aid fitting or cochlear implant stimulation, hearing age, consistency of a child's use of his or her hearing technology.

Ensuring Auditory Access

It is essential to ensure that a child has auditory access with his/her hearing technology at the beginning of each session—including the initial evaluation, any reevaluations, and every therapy session. One way to do this is by using the Ling Six-Sound Test, explained in Chapter 8.

Assessment of Functional Listening

Assessment of functional listening is different from the audiological assessment described in Chapter 4. Functional listening assessment examines how a child uses his/her hearing to process information for meaning. The Erber model (1982), a hierarchy of auditory responses—detection, discrimination, identification, and comprehension, is useful for structuring auditory assessment (see also Chapter 9). This model, however, was created prior to the advancements in early identification of hearing loss and fitting with digital and implantable hearing technology. Today's young children who are deaf or hard of hearing in AVT are developing listening skills at similar ages to typically developing peers. Some response tasks associated with the Erber model are not developmentally appropriate, requiring adaptations appropriate for

today's young *developmental learners*. Erber's response stages are described below (see also Chapter 9).

A *detection* response indicates that a child is aware of the presence or absence of sound. The practitioner may observe an auditory detection response from an infant by raised eyebrows, cessation of sucking during feeding or when using a pacifier, becoming still, or head turning in search for a sound (once an infant has developed adequate neck muscle control). At around 18 months to 24 months, children may be able to participate in conditioned activities to demonstrate an awareness of presence of a sound, such as dropping a block or putting a ring on a stick, upon hearing a sound. Distance listening can be assessed by eliciting a detection response at 3, 6, 9, and 12 feet away from the child.

Discrimination is the ability to determine only if two sounds are the same or different. There is no implication that a child has associated meaning with the sounds. Examples of skills the practitioner can assess include differences between sort and long sounds, mono- and disyllabic words, high and low vowels, nasal and plosive consonants, etc. The practitioner may be able to observe a discrimination response by an infant if behavior changes when sound changes. An older child who understands the concept of "same" or "different" will be able to engage in a traditional assessment of discrimination and use the words same/different to describe the sounds (e.g., /ba/, /da/).

Toddlers and young preschoolers, however, are not developmentally ready to engage in a traditional same/different discrimination task and require developmentally appropriate adaptation. One adaptation is to elicit an imitation of the stimulus presented to the child.

If the child is able to imitate the model (e.g., /ba/, /da/), it can be assumed that the child recognized the difference. A failure to imitate correctly, however, may or may not be an indication of a failure at auditory discrimination. Full interpretation of the response requires understanding of the child's productive abilities and limitations.

The next step in Erber's hierarchy is *identification*, or the association of sound with meaning. A young child demonstrates auditory identification when he/she selects an object in response to hearing its label. Successful performance of this identification task requires that a child has a core receptive vocabulary. A young child who is not able to participate in formal discrimination tasks, for example, but has sufficient vocabulary to perform an identification task may require another developmentally appropriate adaptation. The identification and discrimination tasks can be combined, with a successful identification response indicating accurate discrimination. For example, if the child selects an object or picture from a group in which the labels differ only in one feature (e.g., pail, sail, whale, tail), the child demonstrates the ability to discriminate initial consonant manner when he/she selects the correct object/picture. This combined discrimination/identification task can be used to assess a child's ability with a full range of skills that are essential for processing the speech signal: suprasegmental features (duration, syllable number, stress patterns, pitch, intonational contour), vowels (height and front/back differentiation), and consonant manner (manner, place, and voicing). More in-depth descriptions are presented in Chapter 9.

The final stage in Erber's hierarchy is *comprehension*. Comprehension is the ability to fully understand the message and involves auditory processing of words, phrases, and sentences. Ultimately a child should be able to understand a message even if it is given out of context. Comprehension assessment of a young child can involve a child following directions. For example, "give mommy the ball" performed accurately indicates that the child understands the words "give, mommy, ball."

The related skills of auditory memory, sequencing, and processing of critical units each play a role in the comprehension of connected speech and can be assessed separately. Critical elements are the pieces of information in a message that need to be understood in order for the message to be understood. For example, identifying an object or a picture as described in the previous section is an example of processing one critical element. When a child follows directions, it generally involves processing and memory for more than one critical element. For example, the three-step direction "get out your pencil box, take out a pencil, and write your name on your paper" may be considered to contain the critical elements "box, pencil, write, name, and paper." It might be correct to say that "write your name on your paper" is a single element because writing one's name on paper on the school desk is a common classroom action. A more complex single step direction is, "Draw a green circle under the tall man wearing a purple hat who is standing next to the shortest animal." If the child has a paper featuring a lot of people wearing colored clothing items conducting various activities in the proximity of animals of variable heights, then "green, circle, under, tall, man, purple, hat, next to, shortest" may all be critical elements to process in order to follow the direction correctly. While the second direction, in theory, might appear to be easier to follow if comparing ability to follow one versus multistep directions, in reality there are potentially nine critical elements a child must detect, discriminate, identify, remember, and sequence in order to comprehend the second message and follow the direction correctly. The difference in these two directions is not the number of steps, rather the number of critical elements the child has to comprehend to follow the direction. When assessing the acquisition of critical elements, it is important that the practitioner select vocabulary the child knows so there is no question whether the child responded incorrectly due to vocabulary knowledge or issues with processing critical elements. At an even higher level, assessment of auditory comprehension could involve a story presented through the listening-only condition, followed by examining the details that a child remembers.

There are a number of assessments that can help determine a child's auditory skill level. The *Early Speech Perception Test* (ages 3 years and older) (Moog & Geers, 1990) and the *Contrasts for Auditory and Speech Training* (3 years to 12 years) (Ertmer, 2003) are criterion-referenced tests that assess the speech perception abilities of children. The *Cottage Acquisition Scales of Listening, Language, and Speech* (age birth to 8 years) (Wilkes, 1999) is also a criterion-referenced test that examines the child's ability to make meaning out of auditory signals and targets. Parent questionnaires such as *LittlEARS*

(Kuehn-Inacken, Weichboldt, Tsiakpini, Coninx, & D'Haese, 2003) and the *Infant Toddler Meaningful Auditory Integration Scale* (*IT-MAIS*) (Zimmerman-Phillips, Osberger, & Robbins, 2001) assist in determining if children are integrating meaning with what they hear.

When information is gathered from formal and informal assessments, and subsequently analyzed, deficit areas can be identified, and the practitioner and the parent can determine goals to target auditory skills.

To summarize, *auditory skills are the basis for listening and spoken language! Children's talking is listening translated into verbal motion.* By assessing speech perception skills through formal and informal assessment, a practitioner can get a full picture of the child's ability to process auditory information necessary for the development of talking.

Special Considerations

Infants and other new listeners. When children receive hearing technology for the first time, the initial experience with sounds is unfamiliar or new. Children respond to these in many ways. Some children respond by attending to the sound. An infant may become still (stop moving, cease sucking a bottle, pause during play), move his/her eyebrows, or exhibit movement of the eyes before the child is able to turn and look at sound. When assessing a new listener, one needs to notice any behavioral response to people talking or to environmental sounds. Some children may not respond at all. When children have not learned that things make sounds, there is no imperative to turn to a novel sound. No response in the early stages may indicate that the technology is not working, but may also indicate the child has not learned that sounds are created by something or someone and are meaningful. A child should begin responding to sound rapidly after initiation of hearing technology, and a lack of response or inconsistent reaction needs to be monitored as they can be interpreted as evidence of lack of auditory access.

The practitioner knows that *new listeners*, regardless of age, will usually follow the same auditory trajectory as a newborn with typical hearing. Following a developmental auditory hierarchy in assessment ensures children are meeting all auditory milestones. New listeners learn best in natural, meaningful interactions. Consequently, assessment needs to include informal assessment in the child's usual environments.

Advanced listeners. Advanced listeners require assessment to determine how well they can comprehend in a variety of noisy conditions at school and in the community. It is also useful to assess the benefit that FM or digital modulation (DM) systems provide (see Chapter 7).

The perceptions of important adults (parents, daycare attendants, teachers) help to determine how well the child is understanding spoken language in daily life. Checklists and assessments such as the *Functional Listening Evaluation* (ages grade 1 and higher) (Johnson & VonAlmen, 1993) and the *Screening Instrument for Targeting Education Risk* (*SIFTER*) (preschool: 3 to 5 years, elementary: first to sixth grade; secondary: middle school and high school grades) (Anderson, 1989) offers a formal assessment of the child's functional auditory performance. Finally, a child who can report information about his/her listening provides great information.

Children receiving a second implant. A child may receive a second implant in either a simultaneous or sequential fitting. Simultaneous cochlear implantation occurs when the child is provided with two cochlear implants at the same time (often same surgery, same initial stimulation activation date). Sequential cochlear implants occur when the child receives a second cochlear implant at a date after the first cochlear implant.

When a child receives cochlear implants sequentially, auditory function with the second cochlear implant should be assessed separately for each ear. The assessment may inform the practitioner that different auditory goals may be different for each ear. The brain must develop new neural pathways stimulated by information from the second implant. When the child listens only with the new cochlear implant, it may seem as though the child is starting over. The auditory learning process may also be different from the first implant but the child's success with this implant is independent of the first one (Smilsky et al., 2017). This process may occur faster or slower, and outcomes may be variable. Therefore, an assessment of a child who has just received a sequential cochlear implant is required to determine the auditory skills with the new implant in isolation, even though an assessment of the child's auditory skills with both cochlear implants represents auditory performance using all available technology. Auditory performance needs to be strong on both sides in case of technology failure (dead battery, broken cable, malfunctioning processor, change in a program, etc.) so the child could function in a unilateral condition.

Unilateral hearing loss. With unilateral hearing loss, it is not appropriate to assume the child will have sufficient auditory skills through the better hearing ear to develop speech and language optimally. There is a higher risk of poor academic achievement, speech and language deficits, reading difficulties, as well as auditory differences that could affect hearing in noise. (Krishnan & Van Hyfte, 2016). Auditory skills in the ear with hearing loss need to be assessed in isolation. Suggested strategies for this are presented in Table 19–3.

Speech Assessment

The ability to speak with the best intelligibility relies on hearing the characteristics of each sound and being able to monitor and match production of a sound with that of another person via the auditory feedback loop. Assessment for setting speech targets includes whether the child has auditory access to all the sounds and characteristics of speech.

Many children with typical hearing may receive intervention for articulation. They may have an underlying phonology but have difficulty with articulatory placement or coordination of the speech mechanisms, necessitating visual and tactile cues to help with production. Children who are deaf or hard of hearing, however, require help to develop that underlying phonology. Accordingly, an assessment of speech production begins with assessment of auditory function to determine which speech features a child is able to discriminate auditorily. If the child cannot identify one of these features, then an entire class of sounds may be misarticulated. Table 19–4 lists sounds that are

potentially misarticulated when each feature is not correctly identified by a child through listening. For example, if a child cannot recognize voicing, then the sounds /g d b z v ʒ ð/ are produced as their voiceless minimal contrast pairs /k t p s f ʃ θ/. Furthermore, if assessment revealed that the child was unable to produce /g k t d b p/, it would warrant assessment to determine if the child is able to recognize plosives auditorily using minimal pair contrasts before assuming that the child cannot produce plosives.

There are particular classes of consonants that are more challenging for children who are deaf or hard of hearing and therefore should be monitored:

1. *Fricatives* are challenging for many children because these sounds are more difficult to hear due to softer intensity and higher frequency.
2. *Velar stops /k, g/:* These sounds are not visual and the child must rely on audition. A child with typical hearing requires four years to complete the process of detecting, discriminating, and identifying the sound /g/ and how to coordinate the sound before being able to produce it (Smit, Hand, Freilinger, Bernthal, & Bird, 1990). While a child with hearing loss may have the coordination to produce the sound, he/she may require time learning how to identify manner, voicing, and place cues to hear the sound.
3. *Liquids*, /l, r/. These sounds are clearly challenging for all children, regardless of hearing status. It takes as long as six years for 90% of typically developing children to fully acquire these sounds (Smit et al., 1990). Liquids, like the velar stops,

Table 19–3. Strategies to Reduce Participation of the Unimpaired Ear When Assessing Auditory Skills in Children with Unilateral Hearing Loss

Method	Description	Pros	Cons
Earplug	Foam, putty, or energy absorbing resin material inserted into the ear Attenuates 35–48 dB[1]	Relatively low-cost and easy for home use for skill practice	Difficult to fit small ears
Earmuff	Fits over the ear, similar to a headphone Attenuates 40–55 dB[1]	Can offer greater volume reduction than earplugs depending on type	Relatively expensive Might not be available for home
Earplug and earmuff	Use of earplug and earmuff simultaneously Attenuates 44–66 dB[1]	Decreases intensity more than either strategy alone	Expensive, less practical for home
Masking	Sound directed into the unimpaired ear via earbuds or phones	Decreases the intensity of sound	Requires audiometer and masking level knowledge Not for home use Can interfere with comprehension in unmasked ear[2]
Direct Connect	Connection to the hearing aid or cochlear implant via FM or external microphone routed directly into the hearing aid (DM)	Child's hearing aid or implant may come with FM or DM systems Direct, clear signal to the amplification Can direct recorded material directly to impaired ear, enabling consistent signal from test to test	Expensive if the family does not own a system With live voice, requires signal attenuation in unimpaired ear Difficult for practitioner or parent to monitor signal presented to child

Sources: [1] Abel & Odell, 2006; [2] Corbin, Bonino, Buss, & Leibold, 2016.

Table 19–4. Phonemes Potentially Misarticulated When Consonant or Vowel Feature Misidentified

PHONEME FEATURE	PHONEMES IMPACTED BY FEATURE
TONGUE HEIGHT	
Low	æ ɑ a
Mid	ɛ e ɝ ɚ ʌ ə o ɔ
High	ɪ i ʊ u
VOWEL PLACE	
Front	ɪ i ɛ e æ
Central	ɝ ɚ ʌ ə a
Back	ʊ u o ɔ ɑ
CONSONANT MANNER	
Plosives	g k t d b p
Fricative	h s z v f ʒ ʃ θ ð
Affricate	dʒ tʃ
Nasal	ŋ m n
Liquid	l r
Approximants	j w
CONSONANT VOICING	
Voiceless	k t p h s f ʃ θ
Voiced	g d b z v ʒ ð
CONSONANT PLACE	
Velar/Glottal	g k h ŋ
Palate	ʒ ʃ r j
Alveolar	d t z s n l
Dental	θ ð
Labiodental	v f
Bilabial	b p n w

are not visually accessible unless exaggerated in production. Furthermore, they require precise placement of the articulators. If the placement is slightly incorrect, a distorted sound will be produced. For a child who is not hearing the sounds clearly or is unable to self-monitor, these sounds are very challenging to produce without distortion. Without the ability to hear a clear production and self-monitor, precision placement of the articulators is challenging for the child to achieve, and he/she is more likely to have a distorted production.

Assessment of speech for children who are deaf or hard of hearing should also include evaluation of *resonance and prosody*. Children with reduced access to sound at 500 to 1000 Hz are more likely to produce speech that is hyponasal (Ling, 1989). Children without consistently clear access to speech sounds in conversation are also more likely to have prosody irregularities such as staccato speech.

There are numerous assessments that the AV practitioner can administer to obtain a standardized articulation score. *The Goldman-Fristoe Test of Articulation* (ages 2;0–21;11) (Goldman & Fristoe, 2015), the *Khan-Lewis Phonological Analysis* (ages 2;0–21;11) (Kahn & Lewis, 2015), and the *Arizona Articulation and Phonology Scale* (ages 1;6–21;11) (Fudala & Stegall, 2017) are standardized assessments of phoneme production and phonological processes. These assessments require a child to label a picture with a word that contains a target phoneme or phonemes. The child's errors are recorded by the practitioner to yield a raw score

that is converted to a standard score to determine how far below or above average a child's skill falls.

The child's hearing age is considered when interpreting speech production assessments and can be used as a gauge to monitor whether the child is making adequate progress in speech development by comparing speech developmental milestones for typically developing children of the same chronological age with the child's hearing age. With this approach, a child with a hearing age of 3 years should be producing sounds similar to those produced by typically developing children with a chronological age of 3 years.

The tests listed above, along with informal assessments of conversation, can be used to determine goals. If articulation skills are below what would be expected for listening age, then the practitioner, with the parent's input, may choose to target improved articulation. Goals may include targeting a specific listening-age appropriate phoneme or discrimination and identification of minimal pair contrasts if auditory skills are also weak. Further assessment may be necessary if the child is not progressing with therapeutic intervention and/or motor speech involvement is suspected.

To summarize, speech articulation assessment is an important part of a comprehensive assessment in AVT. In addition to placement and coordination considerations, the practitioner must consider the child's ability to both detect and identify the phonemes in the child's language. For a child to develop speech skills through listening, the practitioner must determine that the child has clear, precise access to the sounds.

Language Assessment

A comprehensive language assessment examines the child's skills in semantics, syntax, morphology, pragmatics, and higher order language such as figurative language. Each of these linguistic aspects is impacted by hearing loss. Thorough language assessment includes the assessment of both receptive and expressive language. Receptive language is a child's understanding or comprehension of language. Expressive language is the child's use of language. Receptive and expressive language need to be treated as separate skills and assessed accordingly. This section will explore each of these areas as well as why children who are deaf or hard of hearing are at increased risk for deficits in each area.

Semantics pertains to the meaning aspect of language, including the child's lexicon, or receptive and expressive vocabulary. Children who are deaf or hard of hearing are at increased risk for reduced vocabulary, perhaps due to reduced language exposure prior to diagnosis and appropriate amplification as well as for reduced opportunities for incidental learning even while a child is using hearing technology (Davidson, Geers, & Nicholas, 2014). Incidental learning occurs when a child overhears language being used by others but is not directly taught that language. Children who are deaf or hard of hearing often easily learn concrete, basic vocabulary, and proper nouns, such as the names of objects that are frequently labeled (Houston et al., 2005).

These word types tend not to have multiple meanings, are easily represented by objects and actions, and are frequently used in basic conversation. Children who are deaf or hard of hearing may score well on receptive picture vocabulary where they are asked to identify these basic word types (Lund, 2016).

Children who are deaf or hard of hearing may have struggles, however, with vocabulary beyond basic labels, action words, and attributes. For example, children who are deaf or hard of hearing may have more difficulty with relational vocabulary such as category names and labels for function. Children may also struggle with synonyms, antonyms, and homonyms (multiple meanings of a word). By assessing multiple types of vocabulary, a practitioner may more roundly and completely determine whether the child has age-appropriate vocabulary skills and identify needs beyond the level of basic vocabulary. These skills serve a necessary foundation for later reading comprehension and writing.

Syntax comprises the rules that order the arrangement of words in a sentence. For example, a native English speaker would use a sentence form such as "Yesterday, the girl swam in the pool." If one were to translate the German form of this sentence into English, however, this sentence would result: "Yesterday has the girl into the pool jumped." This translated sentence would not be perceived as correct to a speaker of English. Each language has syntactic rules regarding word order and these need to be learned by the child. In spoken languages, word order is typically overheard and learned through incidental learning. Children who are deaf or hard of hearing may struggle to pick up these syntactic rules through incidental learning. Assessment of syntax will evaluate whether a child is able to comprehend and use the rules of order and grammar in the language. This is also a foundational skill for later literacy development.

Morphology pertains to the structure of words including the grammatical markers added to words such as (in English) plural /s, z/, possessive endings, past tense "-ed," and the present possessive "-ing" ending form. If a child does not comprehend these morphemes, then he/she may not recognize the difference in tense in a sentence, whether to pick one object versus multiple objects, possessive ownership of an object, and many other necessary parts of language. Morphological endings can be challenging to hear in a conversation. As a result, there is increased risk that a child will not hear the sound and will require direct instruction to learn the morphological rule. A thorough assessment should include examination of the child's receptive comprehension of age-appropriate morphemes as well as the child's expressive use of these morphemes.

Pragmatics of language refers to the manner in which language is used to interact with others. Pragmatic language rules include the choice of words in situations, whether that is through vocabulary choices, saying the correct response in a situation, or understanding the intent of others. Pragmatic language rules determine anticipated behaviors and responses in each interaction with a conversational partner. For example, the slang words and familiarity used with friends may not be appropriate in a formal encounter with a new person. A person using sarcasm anticipates the listener will comprehend the satire. A person talking about a tragic experience expects sympathetic responses from the listener. When pragmatic language rules are broken, the result can be awkward, frustrating for one or both partners, or humorous, depending on the situation. Pragmatic language may be more challenging for a child who has hearing loss. This is a combined result of reduced exposure to incidental learning along with possibly decreased abstract language and vocabulary comprehension and use. A deficit in pragmatic language may cause a child to misunderstand a social cue or unintentionally fail to use the correct language for a given situation. Assessment of pragmatic language will help identify children early who are struggling with these social language rules.

Figurative language is a higher order aspect of language that is useful to include in language assessment. Figurative language departs from the literal interpretation of the words or phrases. In short, figurative language comprises words and phrases that do not mean what they literally say but serve to provide comparisons or add effect to words or phrases. Examples of figurative language devices include similes, metaphors, hyperbole, idioms, and personification. Figurative language can pose a challenge to children who are deaf or hard of hearing. Children who have strong concrete vocabulary and poorer complex vocabulary and who process information literally often have greater challenges with figurative language (see also Chapter 15).

Figurative language plays an important role in pragmatic interaction. For example, children who are literal in their language comprehension may be disappointed when the friend who says he has "a million toy cars" at his house turns out to have only 10 cars. A child may wonder about the weather outside if a parent were to say, "it looks like a tornado went through the playroom." The ability to comprehend nonliteral meanings of words and phrases has a large social impact for children who are deaf or hard of hearing. Figurative language devices are routinely used by children and adults and successful communication relies on the ability to recognize when someone is being literal or deviating from the literal meaning. The comprehension of figurative language is also important to literacy development. Reading comprehension requires the ability to determine literal versus figurative meanings of words. Because figurative language is so important for social interactions and literacy, figurative language comprehension should be assessed informally in young children and formally when children are of age to participate in formal testing.

Standardized testing for language often requires a battery in order to assesses all aspects of language. The *Peabody Picture Vocabulary Test* (ages 2; 6–90+ years) (Dunn & Dunn, 2018) assesses receptive vocabulary, *the Structured Photographic Expressive Language Test* (ages 4;0–9;11) (Dawson, Stout, & Eyer, 2003) assesses expressive use of morphology and syntax. The *PLS-5* (Zimmerman et al., 2011) assesses overall receptive and expressive language. Other tests utilize a series of subtests that give information about specific domains and overall language ability when the full set of domains are considered. Examples include the *Clinical Evaluation of Language Fundamentals (CELF)* (age 5;0–21;11; preschool edition: age 3;0–6;11) (Semel, Wiig, Secord, 2013; Wiig, Secord, & Semel, 2004;), the *Comprehensive Assessment of Spoken Language* (ages 3;0–21;11) (Carrow-Woolfolk, 2017), and the *Test of Language Development* (primary: ages 4;0–8;11; intermediate: ages 8;0–17;11) (Hammill & Newcomer, 2008; Newcomer & Hammill, 2008).

Infant assessment of the precursors to language or the earliest language ability is predominantly conducted informally using criterion-referenced measures. Criterion-referenced assessments include *Rossetti Infant-Toddler Language Scale* (ages birth to 3;0) (Rossetti, 1990) and the *Cottage Acquisition Scales for Listening, Language, and Speech* (ages birth to 8;0) (Wilkes, 1999). These use observation and parent interview to determine whether the child has mastered age-appropriate skills in language.

When areas of language deficit are identified, the practitioner works with the parent to determine appropriate goals to target. It is common for children to have a variety of language goals simultaneously, e.g., increased vocabulary, the use of a specific morphological form, comprehension of figurative language.

To summarize, language assessment can be performed using a variety of commercially available and informal test measurers. A practitioner considers what parts of language are challenging. Language assessment should be thorough and cover a wide variety of language forms to ensure a child truly has age-appropriate receptive and expressive language.

Assessment of Family Needs

Six of the 10 Principles of AVT begin with the words "Guide and coach parents"

(Alexander Graham Bell Association Academy for Listening and Spoken Language, 2017). "Parent" is understood as primary caregiver or caregivers of the child as families are diverse. A fundamental idea of AVT is that the parent is the primary teacher of the child. Consequently, an assessment of family needs is an essential part of an AV assessment. Family needs assessment is handled with sensitivity and should be conducted regularly, to ensure the family's needs have been met. This section will discuss considerations regarding (1) the family system, dynamics, and daily life, (2) communication and language, (3) culture, and (4) access to support and resources.

The family system, dynamics, and daily life. The practitioner discovers who (a parent, a grandparent, a daycare worker) spends the majority of the day with the child so that each person in that child's day can receive support from the AV practitioner. Other critical questions include: Are there extended family members who should be included? Does the child reside in one home or in multiple homes? Are caregivers on the same page regarding hearing technology and the decision to pursue AVT? Do siblings have particular needs related to gaining parents' attention, communicating with a sibling with a hearing loss, or dealing with the social implications of having a sibling with a hearing loss? Does the family need support from professionals who can assist with such issues as family communication or conflict resolution? Are family members able to meet their physical and mental health needs and feel safe in the home without fear of domestic violence or threat from an external source?

The practitioner takes time to acquire an understanding about a family's daily life, so that he or she can guide parents and caregivers to target goals in functional ways that fit into the family's routines. For example, the practitioner may discover that grocery shopping is a time when siblings are not present, making that a good time for having language-building conversations with the child who is deaf or hard of hearing.

Communication and language. The AV practitioner determines the best way to communicate with a parent. Do parents like receiving written material, or do they prefer a verbal description or a demonstration, or more "hands-on" or "hands-off" instruction? The practitioner finds out the preferred *language* and determines whether a qualified interpreter is needed. It is helpful to also get a sense regarding the preferred language for written material because a family might be sufficiently fluent in the practitioner's language for AVT, but be more comfortable with written material that is in the home language.

Culture. Cultural considerations go to the heart of how the practitioner can become a partner with a family. Different cultures view disability differently and may have a culturally oriented perspective regarding how to best manage a child with a disability. This can influence the family's views of treatment approaches. Furthermore, some recommendations may unintentionally infringe upon a family's culture. It is important to know if a child's family will have support from their extended family or community if they were to decide to pursue treatment options or ways to help their child that might be antithetical to their culture. Cultural decisions can influence a family's decision about the use of hearing technology. For example, some sects within the Amish community may support cochlear implantation while others may not. Some Orthodox Jewish families may choose not to charge batteries on the Sabbath to adhere to Sabbath customs regarding the use electrical devices.

Access to support and resources. Does the family have emotional and social support from their community such as friends, religious or civic community, or parent groups? Family needs assessment includes determination of access to the resources required by the family to purchase hearing technology, batteries, and pay for repairs or other specialized equipment. The practitioner asks whether families require educational resources such as how to manage the behavior of children with communication challenges, appropriate disciplinary strategies, or even potty-training. Does the family have any transportation difficulties that would impact attendance at intervention, audiology, or otolaryngology appointments? Might the family need counseling support?

CONSIDERATIONS FOR ASSESSMENT OF CHILDREN WITH ADDITIONAL CHALLENGES

Children with additional challenges may require different means of assessment than other children who are deaf or hard of hearing. Children's unique individual needs will need to be taken into consideration during assessment. Assessment of children with concurrent disabilities is covered in deeper detail in Chapter 22.

Some children may require special accommodations. For example, a child with vision deficits may require special equipment to see pictures for a receptive language test or may not be able to access the pictures even with equipment, necessitating the use of objects. Children with cognitive or developmental deficits may require an assessment compatible with his/her developmental age rather than his/her chronological age. It may not be possible for a child with developmental delay to take a particular standardized assessment if his/her chronological age exceeds the normative range of the test, despite the format being appropriate for the child's developmental level. A child with attention deficit disorder in addition to hearing loss may be more likely to experience auditory fatigue and need more breaks during testing.

Interpretation of assessment results needs to incorporate the impact not only of hearing loss but also the additional disability. For example, a child with global coordination challenges may have difficulty in speech production due to motor issues as opposed to insufficient auditory access. Formal, standardized test results obtained from a child with a significant anxiety disorder may need to be compared with what is seen in an informal setting to be sure that the information is consistent.

CASE STUDIES

The following case studies synthesize the concepts presented in this chapter and demonstrate how these are applied to assessment in AVT.

Ella is 6 months old and arrives at the assessment with both parents. Prenatal and birth history was unremarkable with the exception of a 3-day neonatal intensive care unit stay for jaundice. She received a "refer" result on newborn hearing screening before leaving the hospital. Follow-up testing with an automated brainstem response (ABR) was completed at 3 months of age and waveforms were consistent with a severe hearing loss bilaterally. She was fit bilaterally with hearing aids at 5 months old. Genetic testing and imaging such as CT or MRI have not been completed. Developmental milestones are within functional limits for gross motor movements and cognitive development.

Auditory Access:

Ella wears bilateral hearing aids and her parents report that she wears her hearing aids approximately 4 hours a day. Results from the child's ABR were converted and used to predict thresholds through hearing aids. She is currently scheduled to return for aided testing. A Ling Six Sound Test was administered and Ella detected /a,u,m,i/ as evidenced by behavioral changes including raising eyebrows. There was no observed response to /s, ʃ/.

Assessment Results:

Ella's parents and the practitioner administered the Cottage Acquisition Scales for Listening, Language, and Speech Pre-verbal Level (Wilkes, 1999). Ella was determined to function as follows: Cognition/Play: 3 to 6 months; Listening: 0 to 3 months; Social Interaction: 0 to 3 months; Emerging Meaning: No behaviors to target prior to 6 months; Vocal Expression: 0 to 3 months. Ella fell in the "Below Average" range for applying meaning to sound on the LittlEars questionnaire

(Kuehn-Inacken et al., 2003). She was observed to startle to loud noises and quiet/excite to novel sounds, and responded when the mother and father used parentese. She did not turn to look for a speaker consistently. She did demonstrate joint attention, attended to a speaker's eyes and mouth, and had a social smile. She makes a reflexive vowel /a/ but is not yet imitating vowels and is not imitating suprasegmental features.

Family Needs Assessment:

Strengths identified: Ella's parents live together with the child and share a desire to work toward listening and spoken language. The family is fluent in speaking/reading/writing in the majority language in the community and deny any cultural or religious considerations. There are multiple family members locally who have been supportive with time and resources. A grandparent serves as a childcare provider on weekdays while both parents are at work. The family feels financially secure in regard to home and food.

Challenges identified: Ella's mother reports that she has been diagnosed with anxiety disorder and feels her anxiety has worsened since her child's hearing loss diagnosis, but has not seen her psychiatrist for assistance. Her parents acknowledge worry about recently buying expensive hearing aids and having to pay for ear molds and batteries regularly. Her parents have not seen major changes in listening with the hearing aids and are not feeling as motivated to keep putting them in as they were when they first got them. Ella's parents' concerns expressed in their own words are: "Are the hearing aids working?" "She only says /a/ and doesn't make other baby talk sounds." "How do we know if she hears us?"

Questions to Consider:

1. What details of the case history may impact therapy or outcomes?
2. What is the child's chronological age? What is the child's listening age?
3. Does the child have auditory access for listening and spoken language?
4. Are there any red flags in auditory access?
5. Does the child have chronological age-appropriate skills?
6. Does the child have listening age-appropriate skills?
7. What strengths can we use to help in therapy?
8. What support and/or resources can be offered to mitigate challenges?
9. What parent concerns overlap with challenges seen in the assessment section?
10. What goals address the family's concerns and help advance the child in auditory, speech, and/or language skills?

The AVT Plan of Care

The case history mentions that Ella has not had aided testing yet and the child is not showing much response to sound other than raising eyebrows to low and mid-frequency sounds. Also, she is not wearing the hearing aids for much time a day. In order to determine if Ella is appropriately aided and whether she is getting enough benefit from hearing aids, it is imperative to develop listening skills to see if Ella is capable of accessing enough spoken language through hearing aids. This also fits in with the parents' concerns that they are not sure if their child is hearing with the hearing aids and that they do not know how to tell if she is hearing. When looking at Ella's assessment testing, she demonstrated skills that were age appropriate for listening age (1 month listening age) but delayed when compared with her chronological age (6 months chronological age).

In the conversation with Ella's parents following assessment, the practitioner recommended enrollment in AVT. Ella's parents made a plan to alternate taking off of work so one parent could always be present. The grandmother who is providing care during the day is also able to be in attendance. To make this work, the parents will look into Family Medical Leave of Absence for their missed time at work. Ella's mother was encouraged to visit her psychiatrist to address her increased anxiety. The practitioner discussed state funding for medical supplies, including batteries. The family made a plan to reach out to Ella's otolaryngologist or pediatrician to start the paperwork to determine eligibility for this funding.

After collaboration with Ella's parents, the following goals were selected:

1. Wear hearing aids all waking hours 7 days a week with 90% accuracy in 1 month
2. Turn to sounds and voices in the environment on 70% of opportunities in 3 months
3. Imitate duration cues (long/short; continuous/broken), three of five attempts in 3 months

Parent goals include providing education and coaching for how to target each goal, strategies to support goals, and what to watch for in order to determine that their child is hearing them. The AV strategies that parents will learn are derived from Ella's goals and include wait time, expectant looks, talking to Ella from an optimal position, and the use of parentese.

Case Study #2

Carson is 3 years; 6 months old and arrives with his mother. Prenatal and birth history was normal. Carson failed newborn hearing screening at the birth hospital and his hearing loss was confirmed at 18 months via ABR. He has a profound hearing loss bilaterally. Genetic testing revealed a genetic cause for hearing loss, connexin-26. The MRI was normal. Carson was fit with hearing aids at 24 months. At the same time, he was enrolled in speech language pathology services and began wearing his hearing aids regularly but demonstrated minimal progress with hearing aids. At the age of 2 years; 6 months, Carson received bilateral cochlear implants that were activated at 2 years; 7 months old. Carson's family moved to this area a few months ago and would like to begin therapy services here. The previous therapist worked with Carson alone and his mother is not able to state the goals, though she thinks that he learned some sign language. Carson is in a local preschool program where he receives speech-language pathology services twice a week for a total of 40 minutes. His mother states she will bring the school Individual Education Plan to the next appointment and says that her child is receiving speech-language pathology services and accommodations including preferential seating and an FM system. She is not sure if Carson's school is using spoken or visual language modalities and cannot remember any of the goals on the plan. Carson has met development milestones appropriately with the exception of communication milestones.

Auditory Access:

Carson wears bilateral cochlear implants, and datalogging confirms that he wears his cochlear implants on average 8 hours a day. Conditioned Play Audiometry obtained hearing levels at 20 to 30dB HL across all frequencies when Carson was wearing his cochlear implants. A Ling Six Sound Test was administered, and Carson detected all sounds. After practice, he attempted to imitate /a,u,m/, produced /u/ for /i/, and blew air for both /s, ʃ/.

Assessment Results:

On the *Contrasts for Auditory and Speech Training* test (Ertmer, 2003) Carson scored 100% on Recognition of Suprasegmental Features, 100% on Recognition of Phonemically Dissimilar Words, 100% on Recognition of Vowels, 90% on Recognition of Consonant Manner Features, 70% on Recognition of Consonant Voicing Features, 40% accuracy on Recognition of Consonant Place Features, and 40% on Recognition of Final Consonant Differences.

On the *Goldman-Fristoe Test of Articulation–Third Edition* (Goldman & Fristoe, 2015), when compared with age-matched peers, Carson attained a Raw Score of 112, Standard Score of 51, percentile of 0.1, and test age equivalency of less than 2;0 years (on this test all scores 80 and above are considered to be less than 2;0). The *Goldman-Fristoe* could not be scored compared with Carson's listening age, as his listening age is below the norms provided by the test. Articulation errors included final consonant deletion with the exception of the ability to produce /t, n/ in final position, use and substitution of /h, m, n, b, p, t, d, w, j/ for all initial consonants, and use and substitutions of /m, n, b, p, t, d, w, j/ for all medial consonants. Carson did not use any fricative sounds or velar sounds, demonstrated occasional devoicing of voiced sounds, and did not use any consonant clusters.

On the *PLS-5* (Zimmerman et al., 2011), when comparing chronological age to age-matched peers, Carson scored a Total Language Raw Score of 137, Standard Score of 67, Percentile 1, and Age Equivalency of 2;1years. Carson scored as follows on the PLS sub-scores: (1) Auditory Comprehension: Raw Score 28 Standard Score 65, Percentile 1 Age Equivalency 2;1 and (2) Expressive Use: Raw Score 29; Standard Score 72, Percentile 3, Age Equivalency 2;1. When compared with his listening age in scoring and interpreting the PLS-5, Carson attained a Total Language Raw Score 300, Standard Score 150, Percentile 99, Age-Equivalency 2;1. On the subtests, still compared with listening age, Carson scored as follows: (1) Auditory Comprehension: Raw Score 28; Standard Score 150, Percentile 99, Age Equivalency 2;1; and (2) Expressive Use: Raw Score 29; Standard Score 150, Percentile 99, Age Equivalency 2;1.

During the evaluation, Carson demonstrated a reduced ability to request his wants and needs. When he needed help, he pulled an adult to the situation and pointed. He hid under the table when he desired to end an activity. He demonstrated reduced vocabulary including limited knowledge and use of verbs. Most utterances were one or two words in length. He is not using any grammatical forms.

Family Needs Assessment:

Strengths identified: Carson's mother is fluent in speaking/reading/writing in the majority language in the community and does not report any cultural considerations that require adaptations of treatment. She feels that she is financially secure with regard to her home and meeting food needs. She strongly believes that Carson should wear his cochlear implants all day long and says he does not resist the devices. She charges the batteries each night and is able to troubleshoot the cochlear implants when they do not work.

Challenges identified: Carson's mother has difficulties with transportation, reporting that her car breaks down frequently. She does not have a strong social support system because the family is new to the area. She has family and friends where she used to live, in another state. She is not sure what resources are available in the state where she currently resides. She is not familiar with AVT, but made the appointment with the practitioner upon recommendation by the local cochlear implant team. Carson's mother's concerns in her own words: "He yells a lot and won't tell me what he wants." "He's really smart but talks like a baby." "He can't answer my questions." "When he talks, it's not clear, like he can't say his r-sounds."

Questions to Consider:

1. What details of the case history may impact therapy or outcomes?
2. What is the child's chronological age? What is the child's listening age?
3. Does the child have auditory access for listening and spoken language?
4. Are there any red flags in auditory access?
5. Does the child have chronological age-appropriate skills?
6. Does the child have listening age-appropriate skills?
7. What strengths can we use to help in therapy?
8. What support and/or resources can be offered to mitigate challenges?

9. What parent concerns overlap with challenges seen in the assessment section?
10. What goals address the family's concerns and help advance the child in auditory, speech, and/or language skills?

The AVT Plan of Care

The case history indicates that Carson's hearing loss has a genetic basis that is not associated with deficits other than hearing loss. He did not receive hearing aids until he was 2 years old and then did not make sufficient progress using the hearing aids. His cochlear implants were activated at 2 years; 6 months, meaning that his listening age is of 0;11 months. His mother reports to have brought him to therapy, but because the mother is not sure of the therapy goals, it is likely she did not practice targeted goals at home as a component of the previous therapy program. Carson is in a school program so it will be important to be in communication with the school to ascertain the communication modality and goals targeted at school.

The family-needs assessment reveals that Carson's mother does not know what AVT is, nor is she sure what communication modality the previous speech-language pathologist used with her child. Carson's mother will be educated regarding communication options and given an opportunity to determine whether AVT is what she wants for her child. A period of diagnostic therapy with Carson and his mother can help them make an informed decision. Appropriate referrals will be made if the parents choose an alternative communication modality. Because Carson's mother is not familiar with the resources in her new locale, provision of information pertaining to financial, social, educational, or other resources and their connections is part of the plan.

When looking at auditory access, Carson should have access to all of the sounds across the speech frequencies. There are some concerns about high frequency access, and this should be monitored. Carson did appear to detect high frequency speech information by blowing air for /s, ʃ/, but he did not actually produce these sounds. In addition, Carson produces /u/ in imitation of /i/, an indication of errors in processing the high frequency second formant that characterizes /i/.

Auditory functional listening testing with the *Contrasts for Auditory and Speech Training* (CAST) demonstrated that Carson is not recognizing differences in consonant voice and place feature cues in initial position of words or final consonant differences.

The errors in speech articulation testing are consistent with Carson's CAST auditory scores. He deletes most final consonants, demonstrates inconsistent devoicing, and produces numerous substitutions. Furthermore, Carson is not producing any fricatives, consistent with performance on the Ling Six Sound Test. Carson demonstrated moderate deficits in speech production for his chronological age but is producing the sounds we expect from a 1 year old, consistent with his hearing age. The practitioner will monitor speech production and defer creating a specific articulation goal until Carson's delays in auditory development are addressed and he makes gains in the auditory domain.

Language testing with the *Preschool Language Scale–Fifth Edition* revealed chronological age performance consistent within the range of a severe deficit. When the raw score is examined with respect to hearing age, listening age skills are above hearing age expectations. His age-equivalency scores also give the practitioner similar information—although Carson performs better than his listening age, he is significantly delayed compared with his chronological peers.

In the conversation with Carson's mother following assessment, the practitioner recommended enrollment in AVT. The following goals were selected in collaboration with Carson's mother:

1. Use words to request objects, assistance, and end of activities with 90% accuracy in 4 months

2. Comprehend and use 10 verbs spontaneously in 3 months
3. Identify words with endings versus minimal pairs without endings with 90% accuracy in 3 months
4. Identify words with initial consonants varying in voicing cues with 90% accuracy in 3 months

Parent education will be provided regarding communication modalities. Parent use of AV strategies were selected based on Carson's goals—(1) Goal 1: expectant looks, wait time, repetition, and expand/extend, (2) Goal 2: auditory bombardment, self-talk/parallel talk, and acoustic highlighting, (3) Goals 3 and 4: acoustic highlighting and whispering.

CHAPTER SUMMARY

Assessment of auditory, speech, and language development for children who are deaf or hard of hearing is an integral component of AVT. Ongoing formal and informal assessment allows the practitioner to examine a child's success in all realms of communication. Children need to be successful in listening, talking, and thinking, at home, at school, and in their communities. Areas that challenge children and their families in AVT can be closely monitored through ongoing assessment and both prevention and timely intervention. Appropriate, comprehensive assessment of the auditory, speech, and language skills helps both parents and practitioners to chart the course in AVT so that families can reach their expected outcomes as efficiently and effectively as possible.

REFERENCES

Abel, S. M., & Odell, P. (2006). Sound attenuation from earmuffs and earplugs in combination: Maximum benefits vs. missed information. *Aviation, Space, and Environmental Medicine, 77*(9), 899–904.

A. G. Bell Academy for Listening and Spoken Language. (2017). *Listening and Spoken Language Specialist Certified Auditory-Verbal Therapist (LSLS Cert. AVT®) Application Packet.* Retrieved May 22, 2019 from https://agbellacademy.org/wp-content/uploads/2018/10/Certification-Handbook-1.pdf

A. G. Bell Association for the Deaf. (2019). *Recommended Protocol for Audiological Assessment, Hearing Aid and Cochlear Implant Evaluation, and Follow-up*. Retrieved July 6, 2019 from https://www.agbell.org/Advocacy/Alexander-Graham-Bell-Associations-Recommended-Protocol-for-Audiological-Assessment-Hearing-Aid-and-Cochlear-Implant-Evaluation-and-Follow-up

Anderson, K. (1989). *Screening Instrument for Targeting Educational Risk*. Retrieved from https://successforkidswithhearingloss.com/wp-content/uploads/2017/09/SIFTER.pdf

Carrow-Woolfolk, E. (2017). *Comprehensive Assessment of Spoken Language* (2nd ed.). Torrance, CA: Western Psychological Services.

Corbin, N. E., Bonino, A. Y., Buss, E., & Leibold, L. J. (2016). Development of open-set word recognition in children: Speech-shaped noise and two-talker speech maskers. *Ear and Hearing, 37*(1), 55.

Davidson, L. S., Geers, A. E., & Nicholas, J. G. (2014). The effects of audibility and novel word learning ability on vocabulary level in children with cochlear implants. *Cochlear Implants International, 15*(4): 211–221.

Dawson, J. I., Stout, C. E., & Eyer, J. A. (2003). *Structured Photographic Expressive Language Test–3rd Edition*. DeKalb, IL: Janelle Publications.

Dunn L., & Dunn D. (2018). *Peabody Picture Vocabulary Test–Fifth Edition*. Circle Pines, MN: American Guidance Service.

Erber, N. P. (1982). *Auditory training*. Washington, DC: Alexander Graham Bell Association for the Deaf and Hard of Hearing.

Ertmer, D. J. (2003). *Contrasts for auditory and speech training*. Austin, TX: Pro-Ed.

Fudala, J. B., & Stegall, S. (2017). *Arizona Test of Phonology Scale–Fourth Edition*. Los Angeles, CA: Western Psychological Services.

Goldman, R., & Fristoe, M. (2015). *Goldman-Fristoe Test of Articulation–Third Edition*. Shoreview, MN: American Guidance Service.

Hammill, D. D., & Newcomer, P. L. (2008). *Test of Language Development–Intermediate: Fifth Edition*. Austin, TX: Pro-Ed.

Houston, D. M., Carter, A. K., Pisoni, D. B., Iler Kirk, K., & Ying, E. A. (2005). Word learning in children following cochlear implantation. *The Volta Review, 105*(1), 41–72.

Johnson, C. D., & VonAlmen, P. (1993). The Functional Listening Evaluation. In C. D. Johnson, P. V. Benson, & J. Seaton (Eds.), *Educational audiology handbook* (pp. 336–339). San Diego, CA: Singular Publishing.

Khan, L. M. L., & Lewis, N. P. (2015). *Kahn-Lewis phonological analysis* (3rd ed.). Bloomington, MN: Pearson Education.

Krishnan, L., & Van Hyfte, S. (2016). Management of unilateral hearing loss. *International Journal of Pediatric Otolaryngology, 88*, 63–73.

Kuehn-Inacken, H., Weichboldt, V., Tsiakpini, L., Coninx, F., & D'Haese, P. (2003). *LittlEARS auditory questionnaire: Parents questionnaire to assess auditory behavior*. Innsbruck, Austria: Med-El.

Ling, D. (1989). *Foundations of spoken language for hearing-impaired children*. Washington, DC: Alexander Graham Bell Association for the Deaf and Hard of Hearing.

Lund, E. (2016). Vocabulary knowledge of children with cochlear implants: A meta-analysis. *Journal of Deaf Studies and Deaf Education, 21*(2): 107–121.

Maloney, E. S., & Laravee, L. S. (2007). Limitations of age-equivalency scores in reporting the results of norm-referenced tests. *Contemporary Issues in Communication Sciences and Disorders, 34*, 86–93.

Moog, J., & Geers, A. (1990). *Early speech perception test*. St. Louis, MO: Central Institute for the Deaf.

Newcomer, P. L. & Hammill, D. D. (2008). *Test of Language Development–Primary: Fourth Edition*. Austin, TX: Pro-Ed.

Rossetti, L. (1990). *The Rossetti Infant-Toddler Language Scale*. East Moline, IL: Linguisystems.

Semel, E., Wiig., E., & Secord, W. (2013). *Clinical Evaluation of Language Fundamentals* (5th ed.). Bloomington, MN: NCS Pearson.

Smilsky, K., Dixon, P. R., Smith, L., Shipp, D., Ng, A., Millman, T., . . . Chen, J. M. (2017). Isolated second implant adaptation period in sequential cochlear implantation in adults. *Otology and Neurotology, 38*, e274–e281.

Smit, A. B., Hand, L., Freilinger, J. J., Bernthal, J. E., & Bird, A. (1990). The Iowa Articulation Norms Project and its Nebraska replication. *Journal of Speech and Hearing Disorders, 55*(4), 779–798.

Wiig, E., Secord, W., & Semel, E. (2004). *Clinical Evaluation of Language Fundamentals—Preschool–Second Edition*. San Antonio, TX: NCS Pearson.

Wilkes, E. M. (1999). *Cottage Acquisition Scales for Listening, Language, and Speech*. San Antonio, TX: Sunshine Cottage School for the Deaf.

Zimmerman, I. L., Steiner, V. G., & Pond, R. E. (2011). *Preschool Language Scales* (5th ed.). Bloomington, IN: Pearson.

Zimmerman-Phillips, S., Osberger, M. J., & Robbins, A. M. (2001). *Infant-Toddler Meaningful Auditory Integration Scale*. Sylmar, CA: Advanced Bionics Corporation.

20

CHILDREN IN EARLY CHILDHOOD CLASSROOMS AND AUDITORY-VERBAL THERAPY

Helen McCaffrey Morrison, Karen MacIver-Lux, Stacey R. Lim, and Carrie Norman

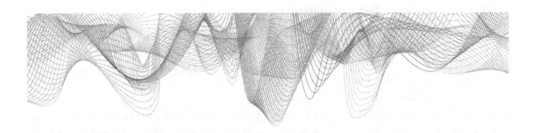

Auditory-Verbal Therapy (AVT) leads families to help their children who are deaf or hard of hearing to learn to listen, communicate, and participate in all of the ordinary, typical settings of child and family life (Caleffe-Schenck, 1992; Lim, Goldberg, & Flexer, 2018). AVT does not begin or stop at the AVT session—it travels with the family and child everywhere they go, including school. Participation in regular educational settings alongside typically developing children is one of the many ways

that children work toward a long-term goal of AVT—to help the child become a part of an inclusive society. Full inclusion is achieved when children who are deaf or hard of hearing become full and active participants, not only in regular classrooms and general school environments, but in the larger societal system as well.

Participation in regular education environments has been a hallmark of AVT since its inception (Pollack, 1970) and remains as the 10th Principle of

AVT—*Promote education in regular classrooms with typical hearing peers and with appropriate support services from early childhood onwards.* Surveys of AVT graduates consistently report that the majority of respondents enrolled in regular education from early childhood onward (Goldberg & Flexer, 1993, 2001; Lim, Goldberg, & Flexer, 2018).

Many children in AVT not only achieve high levels of positive outcomes across various domains, such as spoken language development and literacy skills (Kaipa & Danser, 2016; Percy-Smith et al., 2018), but they also achieve academic skills commensurate with typically developing peers and continue to do so well into adulthood (Goldblat & Pinto, 2017; Lim et al., 2018). Reports of outcomes regarding the efficacy of AVT (see Chapter 3) include this criterion for participants: children are enrolled in regular classrooms with typically developing peers from early childhood onward. If a practitioner is not guiding families toward inclusion as a first educational option, then the Principles of AVT are not being fully supported, and the practice is not truly AVT.

This chapter describes how practitioners and families in AVT carry out inclusion in early childhood settings. We define *inclusion* as placement in a classroom with typically developing children without hearing loss from the very beginning of a child's educational experience. *Early childhood settings* consist of preschool classrooms, pre-kindergarten classrooms (pre-K), and kindergarten. We define preschool as classrooms for 3-year-olds, pre-K as classrooms for 4-year olds and kindergarten as classrooms for 5-year-olds,

but acknowledge that there exists variability in the ages of children in each of these classroom types. The term *early childhood* is used in this chapter to refer to classrooms for 3 to 5-year-old children in general, otherwise the specific terms preschool, pre-K, or kindergarten are used to refer to these classrooms specifically. Children in AVT may begin school at 3 years or at later ages, depending upon the preference of the family and the child's needs.

The chapter begins by presenting the rationale for inclusion along with supporting evidence. This is followed by a "Game Plan" for inclusion—assessing readiness, program evaluation and classroom selection, implementing auditory access, collaborative support for child participation, and preparing the child, family, and school for inclusion.

RATIONALE AND EVIDENCE FOR EARLY CHILDHOOD INCLUSION IN AVT

Educational environments that are inclusive provide multiple and varied opportunities for interaction that foster and enhance a range of developmental skills, including play, language learning and conversation, socio-emotional development, and social well-being. Preschool children with special needs, in general, have been shown to perform as well in inclusion settings as in special education settings on both standardized developmental measures and on measures of participation (Odom, Parrish, & Hikado, 2001; Odom, Schwartz, & ECRII Investigators, 2002; Odom et al., 2004).

Children who are deaf or hard of hearing, in particular, benefit from the opportunity to listen and learn while listening to the speech and language models of their typically hearing peers (Pollack, Goldberg, & Caleffe-Schenck, 1997). Even if the language level of a peer model is higher than the child's own, the model is likely to be within the child's zone of proximal development and sufficiently accessible for learning to take place (Berk & Winsler, 1995). Classroom environments and peer interactions provide many opportunities for a child with hearing loss to overhear and develop rich language and communication/pragmatic skills (Akhtar, Jipson, & Callanan, 2001; Whorrall & Cabell, 2015). Inclusion in regular preschool settings is positively associated with auditory performance at school age (Wang, Liu, Liu, Huang, & Kuo, 2011).

High-quality interactions in non-teacher focused interactions (e.g., lunchtime, social activities) encourage children to answer and use open-ended questions, higher-level vocabulary, and pragmatic skills. Observation of preschoolers in regular classrooms reveals that children who are deaf or hard of hearing use strategies for initiating conversations similar to typically developing peers, including nonverbal entry, extending an invitation, offering an object, or producing a behavior similar to what the other children are doing (Weisel, Most, & Efron, 2005). Despite having lower language skills, children who are deaf or hard of hearing in early childhood inclusion settings have demonstrated levels similar to their typically developing peers for conversational initiation, topic maintenance, and contingent replies (Duncan, 1999; Duncan & Rochecouste, 1999). When educators provide guided opportunities for hearing peers

to be language models for the child with hearing loss in the classroom, the latter are more likely to use language and conversational rules that are accepted by that age group (Richels et al., 2016). Promotion of social skills has proven to be more effective when children who are deaf or hard of hearing practice these skills in an inclusion setting compared with practice in a classroom for children who are deaf or hard of hearing (Antia, Kreimeyer, & Eldredge, 1994).

A GAME PLAN FOR SUCCESSFUL INCLUSION

How does inclusion happen? Inclusion is not just the straightforward action of enrolling a child with hearing loss in a regular preschool, pre-K, or kindergarten class. Inclusion is a *process* that happens best when families have a sense of order and direction, or a Game Plan. The Game Plan for inclusion takes place in stages. The family and practitioner: (1) assess the readiness of the child, and the parents as well, for inclusion, (2) evaluate the program/classrooms that the family might select, (3) assess and plan for acoustic access in the selected classroom, (4) build the child's support team, (5) prepare the school, family, and child for inclusion, and (6) incorporate parts of the AVT session that fortify language development and participation in the classroom. The Game Plan for successful inclusion involves more players than just the AV practitioner and family. The child now has a *support team* that includes several members, and varies in membership with the specific needs of each child. Team building, collaboration, and clear communication are essential for support team function. The following describes each of these aspects of the Game Plan for successful inclusion.

READINESS FOR INCLUSION

AV practitioners and parents begin the conversation about early childhood inclusion early in participation in AVT. Parents are encouraged to give their child many experiences with typically developing peers, far before the time for preschool—in mothers and toddler programs in the community, play groups, children's hour at the library, family reunions, toddler gym classes, or even baby/toddler groups as part of attendance at services of faith. These early experiences give parents an opportunity to observe their child interacting with other children and to examine their own perspectives regarding these interactions. Successful inclusion calls for readiness on the part of the child *and* his/her parents.

Child Readiness Skills

Readiness is frequently thought of as a checklist of skills that a child must achieve in order to be *ready for school*. Another interpretation of readiness pertains to the process by which the practitioner and parents help a child *become ready* for school. In the latter, a checklist of skills is viewed as a guide for how the practitioner and parents prepare the child, rather than as a set of criteria that might prevent entry to the school experience.

A series of checklists that can help practitioners and parents apply either of these interpretations of readiness is the *PARC: Placement and Readiness Checklists for Students Who are Deaf and Hard of Hearing* (Johnson, Beams, & Stredler-Brown, 2011). These criterion-referenced checklists permit families and practitioners to consider both the child's skill levels and the learning environment when making educational placement decisions. The child readiness section guides the practitioner and parent to rate a child's skills in 13 areas. Among these, the following are pertinent to readiness for early childhood settings: knowledge of classroom routines and ability to handle transitions; following directions; attention to the teacher; comprehension of the teacher; behavior when the child does not understand; response to what is said; initiation of conversation; language skills; and self-advocacy.

Preschool

It is helpful to be mindful of the goal of preschool education when considering a child's "readiness." Preschool is a place where children develop a sense of belonging and membership, establish positive social relationships and friendships, make choices, and learn to be part of a group (DEC/NAEYC, 2009). They explore music, art, literacy, and take their first steps in science, math, and technology—all in a play-based environment. Most children enter preschool at 3 years of age. There exists a wide range of skill levels among typically developing 3-year-old children and a child with hearing loss in a regular classroom may find one or two classmates whose language and communication skills are close to his/her own.

It is helpful for a child entering preschool to have some independence in self-care. Some preschools require that a child be potty-trained prior to enrollment, but some do not. If a child is not potty-trained at the time that the family is considering preschool entry, they need to know the school's entry requirements. If the child is able to dress him/herself in a rudimentary fashion, particularly with regard to dressing as part of going to the bathroom, that is helpful. The preschool child needs to be able to separate from his/her parents without a tantrum and calm him/herself if upset.

Preschool activities tend to change every 10 to 20 minutes and a child should be able to participate in an activity close to that length of time; however, this is indeed one of the skills that children learn while in preschool. Much of what happens there is child directed, meaning that children often choose the activity or play center that they wish, so the ability to independently choose a preferred activity is helpful to successful participation. Book sharing, storytelling, and songs are prominent preschool activities. Children in AVT have abundant experience with these, which boosts a child's readiness for preschool. A preschooler also needs to be able to recognize his/her name when called, when the signal is audible. Entering preschoolers need to be able to share toys, sit and listen, and take turns in an age-appropriate manner.

Pre-K

Pre-K is a transition between preschool and kindergarten. The purpose and activities in pre-K are very similar to preschool, but there is an increase in the duration of activities and the number of structured activities that involve a full group of children. Literacy, phonological awareness, and early math concepts appear in pre-K curricula. Children entering pre-K need to be potty-trained and able to dress, play, share with others, and handle frustrations in an age-appropriate manner.

Kindergarten

Kindergarten introduces more structured organization and activities. The content becomes more academic, although kindergarten remains a place where experiential learning and social interaction are among the primary areas of focus. The child in AVT who is entering kindergarten needs to have behavioral, self-regulation, and self-help skills commensurate with his/her chronological age. The questions in the following text box can guide parents and practitioners regarding a child's readiness for kindergarten. Attainment of the skills addressed by these questions may help a child participate successfully in kindergarten, but a missing skill does not necessarily indicate that inclusion not be recommended. Rather, by discussing these questions the practitioner and parents can identify how a child needs to prepare for kindergarten.

Parent Readiness

Families also get ready for school. This can be an especially poignant time for families in AVT. Podvey, Mara, Hinojosa, and Koenig (2013) found that parents experience a shift in roles as their children transition from family-centered early intervention to the child-centered preschool setting. Parents who felt that they were integral members of their child's early intervention team experienced a feeling of being an "outsider" with regard to the school team. Many,

Auditory and Linguistic Competence:

- Can the child follow two- or three-step verbal directions?
- Does the child speak in complete sentences most of the time?
- Does the child understand vocabulary concepts such as direction, position, size, and comparison?
- Can the child make comments or simple predictions about a story being read aloud?

School Skills:

- Can the child classify objects by physical features (color, size, texture, etc.)?
- Does the child organize objects into groups?
- Can the child recognize, copy, or repeat patterns?
- Does the child have beginning-level print awareness (environmental print or logos, letter awareness)?
- Does the child recognize rhyme?
- Does the child attempt to make symbols or drawings to express ideas?

Social/Emotional Skills:

- Can the child follow social routines with guidance (line up, sit in a circle, dance to a song)?
- Does the child participate in group play?

- Does the child demonstrate the ability to use his/her language to make friends, keep them, and negotiate and solve conflicts?

Play:

- Does the child interact with other children?
- Can the child repeat or participate in songs, rhymes, and/or finger plays?
- Can the child ask for what he/she want or need using spoken words?
- Does the child allow other children to enter or change his/her play routine?

Social Intelligence:

- Does the child know his/her first and last name?
- Does the child know the names of family members?
- Can the child state his/her age?
- Can the child make his/her needs known using spoken words?

Self-Help/Advocacy Skills:

- Does the child demonstrate growing independence in personal care (washing hands, toileting, dressing)?
- Can the child indicate when the hearing device is working/not working?
- Can the child tell other children a little bit about the hearing device?

if not most, parents in AVT will retain their AV practitioner and participate in family-centered AVT when their child enters school. Nevertheless, parents in AVT also take on new roles. Although quality early childhood programs recognize that educating a child includes partnering with families (Keyser, 2006), the fact remains that parents are not in the classroom for the majority of the time and are not the child's primary teacher in the classroom. This is a shift from the parent's role in the AVT session and at home. The practitioner can guide parents in getting ready for this role change by helping them coordinate various tasks/meetings that facilitate successful inclusion (Constantinescu, Phillips, Davis, Dornan, & Hogan, 2015).

Parents can arrange for school personnel to attend an AVT session and/ or to visit their child in the home. This gives the school an opportunity to get to know the child and his/her needs. They can arrange for the child to visit the classroom and meet the teacher and the school principal. Parents are encouraged to take photos of the classroom and playground so that they can prepare the child for the start of school. These photos may also appear in the child's "experience book" (see Chapter 14).

FINDING A SCHOOL: PROGRAM AND CLASSROOM EVALUATION

Preschool is the first experience a family is likely to have with inclusion. Parents may visit several schools to determine the one that suits their needs best. Sometimes the selected preschool will be housed within their neighborhood school, but not all schools offer preschool services to typically developing children. Parents might also consider preschool settings in churches, synagogues, mosques, temples, community centers, co-ops, universities, daycare centers, or programs operated by for-profit corporations. Regardless of where the preschool is located, the Game Plan for inclusion proceeds in similar fashion, starting with a program and classroom evaluation.

Fortunately, today, more programs for typically developing children welcome inclusion for children who are deaf or hard of hearing in the preschool. In 2009, the U.S. Division of Early Childhood Education in the Council for Exceptional Children and the National Association for the Education of Young Children issued a joint position paper strongly supporting inclusion in early childhood settings (DEC/NAEYC, 2009). Classrooms that foster *successful* inclusion tend to have a lower student-to-teacher ratio and flexibility in class placement by age, so families can match a class to their child's developmental level. Successful programs have a specific curriculum and assessment protocols so families know what a child is learning and how well a child is learning. The curriculum does not necessarily need to be focused on pre-academic skills. A social skills curriculum is effective as long as it is clearly communicated and child progress is monitored and reported in a timely fashion to families. The degree to which children are actively engaged in learning supports successful inclusion, i.e., parents look for examples of guided and narrated discovery *vs* purely self-directed activity (Odom et al., 2001, 2002, 2004).

Evaluation of a school setting helps both practitioners and parents to identify the strengths of a program as well as areas where there might need to be extra support and accommodations. When information from the program and classroom evaluation are integrated with information about the child's readiness and level of function, practitioners and parents can further define the required accommodations. Ideally, evaluation of a school program and classroom is conducted by parents who are knowledgeable and effective advocates for their child. This takes time and practice, and it is part of AVT. From time to time the practitioner might join parents to observe programs and talk with the school team.

Table 20–1 lists questions that parents might ask when visiting and evaluating a school for their child (see also Johnson et al., 2011 and Sperandino, 2015 for additional examples of questions for preschool selection). Responses to the first set of questions could clarify the family's *purpose* for seeking inclusion in a regular early childhood setting. The information they seek from the subsequent program/school evaluation will vary depending upon answers to these questions. Parents evaluate the *program* or school as a *whole*, starting with the big picture, and then look at individual prospective classes. The overall characteristics of school programs tend to be more stable than individual classrooms that vary with the personality, interests, and skill level of the educator. *Classroom organization* refers to the makeup of the students, schedule, and transitions

Table 20-1. Questions that Parents Ask When Selecting a Preschool Classroom for Inclusion

Questions that Parents Ask when Selecting a Preschool Classroom
Clarifying my Purpose
What is my purpose for preschool inclusion?
What outcomes do I expect to achieve with my child's participation in the classroom?
What classroom characteristics do I think should be in place in order to meet my purposes?
The Program (or School) as a Whole
What are the entry criteria?
What is the curriculum?
What are the school's goals for their children?
What is the procedure for progress monitoring? How are children observed/assessed? How are parents informed of progress?
What is the length of the school day? Days per week?
What faculty teach the children in addition to classroom teachers (e.g., a music teacher, art teacher)?
What are the program's expectations for families?

Table 20-1. *continued*

Classroom Organization
What is the age range of the children?
What is the number of children/teachers/aides?
What is the daily schedule?
What are the various activities (play, reading, problem solving, music) that take place each day/week?
Is there daily reading to children?
Are there class songs?
Are there themes throughout the year?
Are there learning centers? How are they set up and how do children participate? How do teachers/aides participate in centers?
Are books displayed and available to children for looking at on their own?
How are transitions from one activity to the next handled?
What are the classroom teacher's expectations for entering children?
What are the classroom teacher's expectations for families?

Teacher and Child Talk (observed more than once, at different times of the day)
How would I describe the teacher's/aide's talk to children? Directive? Descriptive? Interactive?
How often does the teacher speak to individual children?
Does the teacher elicit conversation from individual children? Between children?
Are children encouraged to answer questions or to respond to the teacher?
How often does the teacher speak directly to the class other than to direct children to their places?
How often are the children left to their own devices while the teacher/aides tend to other things such as cleaning tables, setting out snacks, etc.?

Home and School Communication
How is school-to-home communication conducted? What are the expectations for family communication?
Are parents given copies of songs or themes or informed about weekly activities?
Is it possible for teacher to share lesson plans with the practitioner?
How open is the school/teacher to collaboration with parents and the AV practitioner?

Acoustic Environment
Describe the physical setting, including noise sources within and outside the classroom (e.g., heater or AC motors or fans).
What is the noise level when the classroom has children in it?
What is the noise level when there are no children?
How can the classroom be modified to reduce noise or reverberation?

continues

Table 20-1. *continued*

Acoustic Environment
How open is the school/teacher to FM use?
If the school/teacher have had experience with FM:
What did they feel helped them use the technology successfully?
What would they have wanted to happen differently?
How might FM use be organized (e.g., when does teacher talk to whole group, when does teacher talk to small groups)?

Inclusion
What are the school's and teacher's attitudes and experience with inclusion?
If the school/teacher have had experience with inclusion:
What do they feel has helped a child participate successfully?
What would they have wanted to happen differently in cases when it wasn't a successful experience?

in an individual class. These guiding questions help practitioners and parents identify the class content and evaluate how easily they might be able to help their child learn. Parents also observe *how teachers talk to the children* in their class. It is useful to observe more than once, and at different times of the day so that more than one activity is observed. Parents and practitioners look for indications that:

- the talking that teachers direct to children is learnable,
- teachers attend to what children say,
- teachers respond in ways are positive and constructive.

Communication between home and school is important to any family, but especially to a family with a child in AVT because parents and the practitioner will be helping the child learn the language of school routines and academic content. Families evaluate the *acoustic environment* and options for managing it. This is a crucial factor to successful inclusion; however, these questions are only the start of what families, the school, and the AV practitioner address when managing classroom acoustics (see below). Finally, program administrators and prospective teachers may have had some previous *experience with classroom inclusion*. Their experience and perspectives not only clue the family about any issues of concern, but importantly, these educators may have valuable suggestions that can support the family and child in this process.

MANAGING AUDITORY ACCESS IN THE CLASSROOM

Classrooms are noisy environments and present listening challenges for *all* children. Children who are deaf or hard of hearing, however, have more difficulty understanding speech in a noisy classroom than children with typical hearing (Lee, Ali, Ziaei, Hansen, & Tobey, 2017), especially if vocabulary and working memory are not fully developed. Children who are deaf or hard of hearing are obliged to use a greater share of cognitive resources than their typically hearing peers in order to process a message (McFadden & Pittman, 2008). This increases the likelihood that information will be misheard or missed entirely, particularly when the child is engaged in play or learning activities. Consequently, children who are deaf or hard of hearing benefit from a classroom that is acoustically friendly and there is consistent, appropriate use of hearing assistive technology (HAT). The following summarizes pertinent information from Chapter 7 as it relates to the preschool, pre-kindergarten, and kindergarten classroom. The reader is encouraged to go to Chapter 7 for more information about the HAT use in early childhood classrooms and steps teachers take to ensure that the child's HAT is functioning at all times.

Characteristics of an Acoustically Friendly Learning Environment

Classroom noise is generated by children's movements, traffic outside the room, other students' voices, and operational equipment. *Decreasing background noise* provides a more acoustically friendly classroom environment for the child with hearing loss. Some ways to achieve this include:

■ putting tennis balls on the chair and desk legs,
■ turning off background music or other media that is not use,
■ and closing windows and doors to prevent outside noise from entering the classroom.

Many early childhood classrooms adhere to a philosophy of child-directed learning. Children may be continuously moving from one learning center to another. With so much activity in the room, it can be very noisy. It may be necessary to help teachers design their classrooms so that learning centers that involve conversations between children and teachers (e.g., reading, story time, or even some of the science experiences) are positioned away from noisier self-exploration and play.

Some early childhood classrooms are large and open with high ceilings and hard surface areas that cause sound *reverberation*. Reverberation is the persistence of sound energy (similar to echo), even when the speaker has ceased speaking. The longer the reverberation time, the more likely the teacher's voice will be masked by reverberated speech. *Reducing reverberation time* is achieved by modifying the surfaces and layout of the room. An ideal early childhood classroom has lower ceilings with acoustic tiles, books on shelves, drapes over windows, and corkboards and posters on walls to absorb reverberation. Rugs that are strategically placed throughout the room in areas where teachers spend the majority of their time engaged in instruction, discussions, story time, and singing are especially helpful in creating a non-reverberant, acoustically friendly learning environment.

With a greater distance from speaker to listener, the intensity (loudness) of speech decreases, due to the loss of speech energy. As a result, some aspects of speech are lost, resulting in poorer speech understanding. *Reducing speaker-to-listener distance* often involves arranging classroom seating or child positioning so the child with is relatively close to the teacher. Reducing the speaker-to-listener distance also places the child within the teacher's line of vision so the teacher can monitor the child's listening behaviors and adapt or intervene when it appears that the child is not hearing optimally.

HATS in Early Childhood

None of the above solutions fully resolve the degradation of speech by noise, reverberation, or distance. It is critical, therefore, that children with hearing loss have access to remote microphone hearing assistive technology (RM-HAT) that is digitally modulated (DM) or frequency modulated (FM). RM-HAT helps children with hearing loss obtain *consistent and clear access* to spoken language even when the teacher is at a distance or listening conditions are poor. In AVT, RM-HAT is recommended as best practice for ensuring that a child has auditory access to classroom instruction. A comprehensive description of RM-HAT can be found in Chapter 7.

Listening conditions and communication demands vary throughout the child's day in early childhood settings and use of the RM-HAT will vary with these factors, as illustrated by Table 20–2. The table is a sample daily schedule for a preschool classroom and includes the communication demands for each activity. The child listens as a member of the whole class at the opening and closing of the day and as a member of a small group for phonological awareness activities. The teacher's RM-HAT needs to be turned on during these activities so that the child can more easily hear the teacher speaking. At other times in the schedule the child is likely in an activity/learning center where he/she is mostly exploring independently (e.g., art) or interacting with peers with minimal adult mediation. When the child is in a center/activity where the teacher is not present, the teacher's device should not be transmitting because that input is not relevant to what the child is experiencing. Instead, the child needs to be listening to peers through his/her personal hearing technology.

Orienting a classroom teacher to an RM-HAT must be done simply and carefully and scheduled at a time when the teacher has no other responsibilities. Device orientation is an ongoing process that takes place with each conversation about the equipment. Orientation needs to include listening check of the equipment on the child that is an easy to administer. It is beneficial to refrain from demonstrating all possible options at once to a teacher who has never used an RM-HAT device. The parent and practitioner can also describe the child's listening behaviors when the RM-HAT or the child's hearing technology may not be functioning properly. This can be provided as short description or even a short video for the teacher to watch so he or she can quickly identify when something is amiss.

Table 20-2. Communication Settings in a Day in the Life of a Preschooler

Time	Activity	Communication Setting		
		Teacher or Aide with Child	Child Alone	Child with Peers
9:15	Opening to whole group	Teacher		X
9:30	Phonological awareness in small groups	Teacher		X
9:45	Science/math center	Aide	X	
10:00	Art center		X	
10:15	Bathroom	Aide	X	
10:30	Snack with whole group	Both		X
10:45	Storytime to whole group	Teacher		X
11:00	Music to whole group	Both		X
11:15	Blocks center			X
11:30	Out of doors			X
11:45	Closing to whole group	Teacher		X

Many parents in AVT whose children are entering an early childhood classroom have been wearing RM-HATS at home since their children were infants. As a consequence, they already know how and when to use the RM-HAT, are adept at recognizing their child's listening behaviors when the RM-HAT is not working optimally and know how to trouble-shoot the device. The parents, therefore, can orient their child's teacher to device use and guide the teacher in checking and troubleshooting.

An ideal setup for equipment use is one that makes things "as easy as 1-2-3":

1. The teacher puts on the transmitter and turns it on,
2. the teacher mutes his/her microphone as necessary depending upon the child's listening environment, and
3. the teacher turns the microphone back on when it is needed again.

Making a 1-2-3 protocol possible requires consultation with the child's audiologist and highlights the necessity of including an educational audiologist on the child's inclusion support team, which is described in the next section.

BUILDING THE INCLUSION SUPPORT TEAM

The culture of inclusion consists of consultation, cooperation, and collaboration among parents, AV practitioners, regular education teachers, administrators, educational audiologists, and other school personnel. Innovation and flexibility among all involved adults are key to successful inclusion.

Parents

Parents are the key stakeholders in their child's future, and they are the most frequent liaison between the teacher and other members of the support team. They need to ensure that open communication is always available so they are able to monitor and manage their child's hearing and educational access in the classroom and address any questions from the teacher. Parents need to participate in the classroom as appropriate and get to know other families, and they need to carry over information learned in the classroom and communicate it regularly to the AV practitioner.

Classroom Teacher

The early childhood classroom is the domain of the early childhood educator. In general, teachers have favorable attitudes toward inclusion for children who are deaf or hard of hearing (Eriks-Brophy & Whitingham, 2013). If teachers are provided with practical information about children who are deaf or hard of hearing and their educational needs, their attitudes are more likely

to be positive regarding classroom management and knowledge about the education of children who are deaf or hard of hearing in inclusive settings (Sari, 2007). When a classroom teacher understands, respects, and welcomes the child with hearing loss into the classroom, this attitude permeates the classroom and is absorbed by the other children (Boothroyd-Turner & Sheppard, 2006).

AV Practitioner

The practitioner guides parents to be their child's advocate by helping with problem solving, rehearsing conversations with school personnel, and helping prepare orientation sessions with the classroom teacher and school. The practitioner collaborates with the classroom teacher—sharing lesson plans, adding goals to AVT based on the collaboration, inviting the teacher to observe an AVT session, or co-teaching in the classroom when invited to demonstrate strategies. The practitioner listens to teacher concerns and demonstrates respect for the teacher's expertise.

The practitioner may expand the content of AVT sessions to include aspects of the child's classroom experience—integrating classroom themes, songs, and books. The practitioner includes the language of classroom routines so that the child can participate at school more easily. For example, if phonological awareness is part of the child's school curriculum, activities about phonological awareness can be incorporated into any AVT session. The practitioner can help a child engage in social interactions with other children, and might encourage the parent to invite a classmate to join an AVT session so that the child and classmate can practice conversations. The practitioner also plans, delivers, and evaluates AVT sessions that preview language for upcoming classroom activities or field trips, and then reviews that language with the child and parents after the activity or field trip has taken place.

Finally, a child's entry into the school setting is a good time to begin practicing self-advocacy. The practitioner helps the child recognize when someone doesn't understand what he/she is saying and helps the child use strategies to address communication breakdowns. The child begins to learn to take responsibility for his/her hearing technology, beginning with letting adults know when something has gone wrong.

Educational Audiologist

The educational audiologist works to ensure that the child with hearing loss has optimal and consistent auditory access in the school environment. Aside from acoustic accommodations, the educational audiologist selects, fits, verifies, monitors, and maintains the child's hearing assistive technology (see Chapter 7). The educational audiologist may also monitor the child's hearing status through the academic year.

Collaborative Relationships

The best predictor of children's academic growth arises from the strength of collaboration and communication among members of the inclusion support team (Constantinescu-Sharpe et al., 2017). Collaboration takes many forms: the daily notes between teachers and

families, regular phone/text/emails among team members, scheduled meetings to review child progress and establish the next goals.

There are some practical strategies for building the support team, starting with helping team members recognize that they are indeed a team. The AV practitioner can team build by co-creating a team directory with the child's parents to be shared with each member. The directory includes contact information, preferred means of contact (e.g., phone, email, text, video chat), and preferred times for contact. Sometimes the practitioner and a team member may want to set up a standing date for contact—e.g., a phone call each 2 weeks or a weekly sharing of plans via email.

ORIENTING THE SCHOOL, THE FAMILY, AND THE CHILD

Once a family has selected a school program, the parents can begin to orient the school to their child, and the school can orient the family and the AV practitioner to that school's expectations and culture.

A first meeting with the family, child, and teacher is recommended. This is a getting-to-know-you session and may not necessarily include a lot of information about managing a child with a hearing loss. This is an opportunity for the teacher to meet the child just as he/she is—a young child. The child may bring a favorite toy or book to share, to help the child have a sense of security and to be a conversation starter. The child might share favorite photos on Mom or Dad's phone/tablet that can open a conversation. The teacher can show the child around the classroom—a special moment for making acquaintance with one another.

A more formal orientation may take longer and may involve many of the school staff, including the principal, school nurse, custodian, and even the crossing guard—all important people the child will come to know as a school family.

Orienting the teacher and school is most effective when the family and practitioner listen to questions and provide responses congruent with the type of questions that are asked—*information, insight,* or *implementation* (Norman, 2019).

1. *Information questions* are straightforward questions for information, usually "what" questions. Examples include:

   ■ "What is hearing loss?"
   ■ "What is that little microphone thing?"
   ■ "What is best practice?"
   ■ "What do you mean by accommodations?"
   ■ "What responsibilities does the student have?"
   ■ "What responsibilities does the teacher have?"

   Information questions are best answered with facts, data, or knowledge, using tools and resources such as a diagram of the ear, a familiar sounds audiogram, hearing assistive technology function, and general information about the child and his/her communication competence.

2. *Implementation questions* are questions about *how* to implement strategies in the classroom and are best answered with demonstration and practice. Examples might be:

   ■ *"How do I use the FM?"*
   ■ *"How does strategic seating work here?"*
   ■ *"How do I manage that behavior?"*

   The responses to these questions might be a straightforward demonstration or could be resolved by brainstorming together. A key factor to consider is that the classroom teacher will have the most success with implementation once they (a) *have sufficient background information about hearing loss* and (b) *have developed their own insight* about why the recommended strategies are effective for serving the child in that specific classroom.

3. *Insight questions* are "why" questions about the supports and strategies the family and practitioner are proposing. For example, a teacher might ask:

   ■ *"Why* do I need to wear that little microphone?"

   Insight questions are best addressed in conversations that bring about thought and problem solving that help a teacher develop insight. One way that parents or the practitioner can start the conversation with a classroom teacher is by asking their own *powerful questions* in response to the teacher's insight question. For example, the practitioner can respond to the insight question in the example above with:

   ■ "How close are you to the child when you are speaking to him during motor activities?"

This powerful question leads to discussion of distance and noise, the child's hearing levels while wearing his technology, etc. Table 20–3 outlines questions that will help teachers gain insight about strategies that can be used to support the child with hearing loss in the early childhood classroom.

Table 20–3. Examples of Powerful Questions for Developing Insight About Strategies for Support (Norman, 2019)

Examples of Powerful Questions for Developing Insight About Strategies for Support:	
"What do you hear?"	This helps teachers stop and listen to their own classroom and become aware of the sources of ambient noise. The AV practitioner can suggest strategies that maintain a listening environment: 1. identify sources of ambient noise 2. implement ways to reduce ambient noise 3. create learning environments that promote participation through listening
"How close is your voice?" "How close is the teacher's voice?"	This helps teachers and students think about how close or far away the sound seems to them. The AV practitioner can suggest strategies to help with distance listening: 1. strategic seating 2. use of an FM or other hearing assistive technology 3. verbally repeat other student's pertinent information
"Can they see your face?" "Can they see the words?"	This helps teachers think about how well the student can access the information being presented in the classroom. The AV practitioner can suggest strategies to help with communication access: 1. face the students when talking to them 2. be aware of lighting, glares and shadows 3. demonstration for assignments 4. visual reminder for behavior expectations 5. captions on all videos
"What is the need?"	This helps teachers remember that behavior is communication. The AV Practitioner can help the teacher figure out the child's underlying need and suggest strategies for managing classroom behaviors in a constructive way: 1. **Communication**—Can they understand you? Can you understand them? 2. **Academic**—Do they know the vocabulary? Do they understand what they read? 3. **Social**—Can they hear the group discussion? Do they feel included? 4. **Emotional**—Do they have a sensory need? Do they have listening fatigue?

PREPARING PEERS IN THE CLASS

Strategies that facilitate peer knowledge and acceptance of the child with hearing loss include:

- reading books about children who have hearing loss,
- implementing a buddy system to help peers improve their social skills,
- asking children to speak one at a time and to avoid interrupting each other,
- referring to visual information prior to having verbal discussions, and
- reminding children to avoid obstructing their lips or face when talking (Hughett, Kohler, & Raschke, 2013).

Peers can be taught to use a pass-around microphone that is coupled to the teacher's RM-HAT transmitter, not only for acoustic access for the child with hearing loss, but also for turn-taking skills. It's helpful if strategies the teacher uses for children who are deaf or hard of hearing are used with *all* children in the classroom. For example, if a buddy system is employed, everyone in the class needs to have a buddy, so the child with hearing loss is not singled out.

CHALLENGES FOR INCLUSION

Successful inclusion requires that a child have age-matched peers to model more advanced language and that the child possesses acoustic access to models, (Spencer, Koester, & Meadow-Orlans, 1994). Not all children are ready for preschool or kindergarten at the age most children might enter these classrooms. For example, a child might not have sufficient linguistic or social competence to participate in a school setting and need a bit more time learning the fundamental language of the home.

CONCLUSION

Entry into school is a milestone in any child's life, and a time for celebration in AVT. Children in AVT enter inclusive settings from their first enrollment in preschool. Evidence demonstrates that participation in inclusive classrooms results in gains in social skills and language competence and leads to participation in larger society over the lifespan. Children who are deaf or hard of hearing have the potential to achieve educational milestones on par with their hearing peers in an inclusive environment. This happens because parents and the practitioner jointly approach early childhood inclusion mindfully and systematically, beginning with an evaluation of the child's readiness and proceeding through the establishment of a collaborative team that supports the child and family. The ultimate goal is the child's participation in the world at large to the fullest extent possible. Graduates of AVT, historically and continually, show that this is possible. As teachers gain the knowledge they require and desire about children in AVT, they often want to learn more, and consequently teams of support come to share the same outcomes as those desired by the families of children in AVT. This sharing is paramount in supporting inclusion of children in AVT programs in regular education environments. Inclusion in early childhood classrooms is only the starting point.

REFERENCES

Akhtar, N., Jipson, J., & Callanan, M. A. (2001). Learning words through overhearing. *Child Development, 72*, 416–430.

Antia, S. D., Kreimeyer, K. H., & Eldredge, N. (1994). Promoting social interaction between young children with hearing impairments and their peers. *Exceptional Children, 60*, 262–275.

Berk, L. E., & Winsler, A. (1995). *Scaffolding Children's Learning: Vygotsky and Early Childhood Education. NAEYC Research into Practice Series* (vol. 7). Washington, DC: National Association for the Education of Young Children.

Boothroyd-Turner, D., & Sheppard, W. (2006). Auditory-Verbal therapy and school. In W. Estabrooks (Ed.), *Auditory-Verbal Therapy and practice* (pp. 191–200). Washington, DC: Alexander Graham Bell Association for the Deaf and Hard of Hearing.

Caleffe-Schenck, N. (1992). The Auditory-Verbal method: Description of a training program for audiologists, speech-language pathologists, and teachers of children with hearing loss. *The Volta Review, 94*, 65–68.

Constantinescu, G., Phillips, R. L., Davis, A., Dornan, D., & Hogan, A. (2015). Exploring the impact of spoken language on social inclusion for children with hearing loss in listening and spoken language early intervention. *The Volta Review, 115*(2), 153–181.

Constantinescu-Sharpe, G., Phillips, R. L., Davis, A., Dornan, D., & Hogan, A. (2017). Social inclusion for children with hearing loss in listening and spoken language early intervention: An exploratory study. *BMC Pediatrics, 17*(1).74.

DEC/NAEYC. (2009). *Early childhood inclusion: A joint position statement of the Division for Early Childhood (DEC) and the National Association for the Education of Young Children (NAEYC)*. Chapel Hill, NC: The University of North Carolina, FPG Child Development Institute.

Duncan, J. (1999). Conversational skills of children with hearing loss and children with normal hearing in an integrated setting. *The Volta Review, 101*(4), 193–211.

Duncan, J., & Rochecouste, J. (1999). Length and complexity of utterances produced by kindergarten children with impaired hearing and their hearing peers. *Australian Journal of Education of the Deaf, 5*, 63–69.

Eriks-Brophy, A., & Whittingham, J. (2013). Teachers' perceptions of the inclusion of children with hearing loss in general education settings. *American Annals of the Deaf, 158*(1), 63–97.

Goldberg, D. M., & Flexer, C. (1993). Outcome survey of Auditory-Verbal graduates: Study of clinical efficacy. *Journal of the American Academy of Audiology, 4*, 189–200.

Goldberg, D. M., & Flexer, C. (2001). Auditory-verbal graduates: Outcome survey of clinical efficacy. *Journal of the American Academy of Audiology, 12*, 406–414.

Goldblat, E., & Pinto, O. Y. (2017). Academic outcomes of adolescents and young adults with hearing loss who received auditory-verbal therapy. *Deafness & Education International, 19*(3–4), 126–133.

Hughett, K., Kohler, F. W., & Raschke, D. (2013). The effects of a buddy skills package on preschool children's social interactions and play. *Topics in Early Childhood Special Education, 32*(4), 246–254.

Johnson, C. D., Beams, D., & Stredler-Brown, A., (2011). *PARC: Placement and Readiness Checklist*, Retrieved October 15, 2019 from https://successforkids

withhearingloss.com/wp-content/up loads/2011/08/PARC_2011-Chap-7 .pdf

Kaipa, R., & Danser, M. L. (2016). Efficacy of auditory-verbal therapy in children with hearing impairment: A systematic review from 1993 to 2015. *International Journal of Pediatric Otorhinolaryngology, 86,* 124–134.

Keyser, J. (2006). *From parents to partners: Building a family-centered early childhood program.* St. Paul, MN: Redleaf Press.

Lee, J., Ali, H., Ziaei, A., Tobey, E. A., & Hansen, J. H. (2017). The Lombard effect observed in speech produced by cochlear implant users in noisy environments: A naturalistic study. *Journal of the Acoustical Society of America, 141*(4), 2788–2799.

Leigh, G., Ching, T. Y., Crowe, K., Cupples, L., Marnane, V., & Seeto, M. (2015). Factors affecting psychosocial and motor development in 3-year-old children who are deaf or hard of hearing. *Journal of Deaf Studies and Deaf Education, 20*(4), 331–342.

Lim, S. R., Goldberg, D. M., & Flexer, C. (2018). Auditory-Verbal graduates— 25 years later: Outcome survey of the clinical effectiveness of the listening and spoken language approach for young children with hearing loss. *The Volta Review, 118*(1–2), 5–40.

McFadden, B. & Pittman, A. (2008). Effect of minimal hearing loss on children's ability to multitask in quiet and in noise. *Language, Speech and Hearing Services in Schools, 39,* 1–10.

Norman, C. (2019). Children who are deaf or hard-of-hearing in the schools: Best practices and working interprofessionally. American Speech and Hearing Association. Retrieved October 17, 2019 from https://www.asha.org/Events/live/Chil dren-Who-are-Deaf-or-Hard-of-Hearing -in-the-Schools/

Odom, S. L., Parrish, T. B., & Hikado, C. (2001). The costs of inclusive and tra-ditional special education preschool services. *Journal of Special Education Leadership, 14,* 33–41.

Odom, S. L., Schwartz, I. S., & ECRII Investigators. (2002). So what do we know from all this? Synthesis points of research on preschool inclusion. In S. L. Odom (Ed.), *Widening the circle: Including children with disabilities in preschool programs* (pp. 154–174). New York, NY: Teachers College Press.

Odom, S. L., Vitztum, J., Wolery, R., Lieber, J., Sandall, S., Hanson, M. J., . . . Horn, E. (2004). Preschool inclusion: A review of research from an ecological systems perspective. *Journal of Research in Special Educational Needs, 4,* 17–49.

Percy-Smith, L., Tønning, T. L., Josvassen, J. L., Mikkelsen, J. H., Nissen, L., Dieleman, E., . . . Cayé-Thomasen, P. (2018). Auditory verbal habilitation is associated with improved outcome for children with cochlear implant. *Cochlear Implants International: An Interdisciplinary Journal, 19*(1), 38–45. doi: 10.1080/14670100.2017.1389020.

Podvey, Mara C., Hinojosa, J. & Koenig, K. P. (2013). Reconsidering insider status for families during the transition from early intervention to preschool special education. *Journal of Special Education, 46*(4), 211–222.

Pollack, D. (1970). *Educational audiology for the limited hearing infant.* Springfield, IL: Charles C. Thomas.

Pollack, D., Goldberg, D. M., & Caleffe-Schenck, N. (1997). *Educational audiology for the limited-hearing infant and preschooler: An auditory-verbal program.* Springfield, IL: Charles C. Thomas.

Richels, C. G., Bobzien, J. L., Schwartz, K. S., Raver, S. A., Browning, E. L., & Hester, P. P. (2016). Teachers and peers as communication models to teach grammatical forms to preschoolers with hearing loss. *Communication Disorders Quarterly, 37*(3), 131–140.

Sari, H. (2007). The influence of an in-service teacher training (INSET) programme on attitudes towards inclusion by regular classroom teachers who teach deaf students in primary schools in Turkey. *Deafness & Education International, 9*(3), 131–146. doi: 10.1002/dei .220

Spencer P. E., Koester L. S., & Meadow-Orlans K. (1994). Communicative interactions of deaf and hearing children in a day care center: An exploratory study. *American Annals of the Deaf, 139*, 512–518.

Sperandio, D. (2015). 29 Questions for how to choose a preschool. Retrieved from https://blog.medel.com/29-questions -how-to-choose-a-preschool

Wang, N.-M., Liu, C.-J., Liu, S.-Y., Huang, K.-Y., & Kuo, Y-C. (2011). Predicted factors related to auditory performance of school-aged children with cochlear implants. *Cochlear Implants International, 12*, S92–S95.

Weisel, A., Most, T., & Efron, C. (2005). Imitation of social interactions by young hearing impaired preschoolers. *Journal of Deaf Studies and Deaf Education, 10*, 161–170.

Whorrall, J., & Cabell, S. Q. (2016). Supporting children's oral language development in the preschool classroom. *Early Childhood Education Journal, 44*(4), 335–341.

Part V

EXTENDING AND EXPANDING THE PRACTICE OF AUDITORY-VERBAL THERAPY

Part V

EXTENDING AND EXPANDING THE PRACTICE OF AUDITORY-VERBAL THERAPY

21

CHILDREN WITH UNIQUE HEARING ISSUES AND AUDITORY-VERBAL THERAPY

Karen MacIver-Lux and Stacey R. Lim

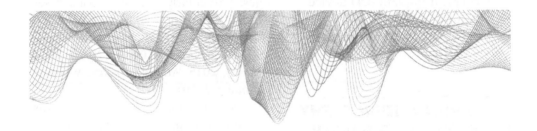

INTRODUCTION

Children who are deaf or hard of hearing can take excellent advantage of the critical period for listening and spoken communication learning if they are identified during the first few months of life and provided with consistent, binaural, auditory access to all sounds of the speech spectrum at soft and normal conversational loudness levels. Some children, however, have unique hearing needs that may require the Auditory-Verbal practitioner (practitioner) to modify the Auditory-Verbal Therapy (AVT) care plan or develop a transition plan to another communication approach. Therefore, the practitioner needs to understand the various unique hearing needs and the steps for management in AVT to help these children reach their highest listening and spoken communication potential.

If the child has a unique hearing issue requiring unique management, audiologists and practitioners rely on comprehensive information about the child's overall progress to distinguish delays and errors that are developmental and/or caused by additional issues unrelated to hearing loss, from those due to unique hearing issues such as abnormal temporal processing abilities, anatomical abnormalities, asymmetric hearing, and/or device malfunction. The audiologist, practitioner, and parents collaborate to determine the appropriateness of the current audiologic management and intervention and determine the next steps in AVT.

In relation to AVT, this chapter focuses on five unique hearing issues:

- auditory neuropathy spectrum disorder (ANSD);
- cochlear nerve deficiency/under-developed auditory nerve;
- unilateral hearing loss/single sided deafness (SSD);
- cochlear implant (CI) device failures; and
- congenital cytomegaolovirus (cCMV).

AUDITORY NEUROPATHY SPECTRUM DISORDER

ANSD occurs when there are disruptions in the neural synchrony of the inner hair cells or the auditory neural pathways, while outer hair cell function generally remains normal, primarily affecting perception of temporal aspects of speech (Rance & Starr, 2015; Roush, 2008). This dyssynchrony can affect speech understanding in the following ways:

- voiced and unvoiced consonants are difficult to distinguish because cues for voice onset time (Rance et al., 2007) and pitch discrimination (Rance & Starr, 2015) are poorly perceived;

- speech discrimination in general is more difficult (depending on the degree of dyssynchrony) because temporal resolution is poor especially in the low frequencies (Rance, et al. 2007; Wang, Wang, Psarros, & Da Cruz, 2014) particularly in noisy listening conditions (Rance & Starr, 2015); and
- localization of speech and environmental sound is difficult due to poor integrity of interaural timing cues (Rance & Starr, 2015).

If the degree of neural disruption is significant, the child's speech recognition abilities will be poorer than what results of behavioral audiometry would suggest, particularly in noise. In some cases, identification of ANSD can take longer due to the inconsistency of test results (Harrison, Gordon, Papsin, Negandhi, & James, 2015; Madell, Flexer, Wolfe, & Schafer, 2019).

ANSD is a disorder that causes distortion of temporal (timing) cues and altered discrimination of frequencies, as opposed to SNHL which affects perception of frequency or intensity (Berlin et al., 2010; Rance, 2005). Due to the variations of presentations of speech perception and listening and spoken language outcomes in children with ANSD (Berlin et al., 2010; Praveena, Prakash, & Rukmangathan, 2014; Rance et al., 2007), practitioners and parents are faced with challenges regarding audiologic management and intervention (Roush, Frymark, Veneditov, & Wang, 2011; Uus, Young, & Day, 2015), especially when the child is very young and has a mild to moderate hearing loss (Ching et al., 2013). The child's auditory abilities and progress in receptive and expressive language play a key role in determining audiologic management, in the selection, fitting, and management of hearing devices, and in the appropriateness of the early intervention model (Berlin et al., 2010). The general consensus is that after a determined period of AVT has yielded poor listening and spoken language progress, cochlear implantation be considered even if unaided or aided thresholds are in the mild hearing loss or normal hearing range (Berlin et al., 2010; Estabrooks, Houston, & MacIver-Lux, 2014; MacIver-Lux & Lim, 2016).

Auditory-Verbal Therapy and Auditory and Language Enrichment (ALE)

To meet the needs of children with ANSD who may or may not be fitted with hearing technology, some practitioners may offer two types of intervention, focusing on listening and spoken language development: AVT and *Auditory and Language Enrichment* (ALE) (Estabrooks, Houston, & MacIver-Lux, 2014; MacIver-Lux & Lim, 2016). AVT can be offered to children with ANSD who are fitted with hearing technology and follows the principles of practice outlined in Chapter 1. ALE follows nine of the same principles, and is for children who do not use hearing technology (Estabrooks, Houston, & MacIver-Lux, 2014). Both programs are diagnostic and use similar planning, delivery, and evaluation of short-term objectives, long-term goals, parent coaching, and strategies that facilitate listening, spoken language, and cognition (see Chapter 17), but ALE *is not* AVT because the children do not use hearing technology. ALE was specifically developed for

children with ANSD for whom hearing technology would be considered a contraindication. It is not uncommon for children with ANSD to begin intervention in ALE and subsequently transfer to AVT when and if it becomes clear the child would benefit from hearing technology. Conversely, a child may begin AVT and then transfer to ALE when it is clear that hearing technology is no longer required. In adherence to the A. G. Bell Academy Principles of Professional Behavior and Rules of Conduct (A. G. Bell Academy, 2007), it is important to clearly convey the distinction between ALE and AVT to parents and other members of their child's allied health team.

The reader may query why ALE is presented here as it is not AVT. The writers asked the same question by considering the history of the establishment of ALE. Some years ago, the practitioners at the Learning to Listen Foundation at North York General Hospital in Toronto were convinced by a parent of a child with ANSD who did not wear hearing technology that "they were the most qualified people" to manage his child diagnostically. The practitioners *bought into* his argument, because the parent indicated he had nowhere else go. Therefore, to remain ethical, the practitioners started ALE as an adjunct to the AVT program. They would be able to "do what they say and say what they do."

The practitioner monitors and records the child's progress and determines when: (1) hearing technology should be pursued if it has not been recommended (ALE), (2) whether hearing technology provides appropriate benefit or not (AVT), and (3) whether the child's intervention program (AVT or ALE) meets the child's overall listening and spoken language development needs.

In working with children with ANSD, the following steps are typically taken by the AV practitioner:

1. Observe the child's auditory functioning if the child is not wearing hearing technology.
2. Refer back to the audiologist immediately for consideration of hearing aid(s) if auditory functioning is poor and progress is limited (MacIver-Lux & Lim, 2016).
3. Observe auditory performance with and without hearing aids in the session. If the child performs better with hearing aid(s), then continued use of hearing aids can be monitored (MacIver-Lux & Lim, 2016).
4. Watch for behaviors such as removal of hearing aids and fluctuations in auditory performance, associated with body temperature sensitive ANSD (Varga et al., 2006; Zhang et al., 2016) and transient ANSD (Eom, Min, Lee, & Lee, 2013; Psarommatis et al., 2006).
5. Note listening conditions and/or child's health/activity level when fluctuations of auditory functioning are observed, to identify possibility of ANSD being temperature sensitive (Varga et al., 2006).
6. Consider cochlear implant candidacy evaluation if there is limited progress in listening, and spoken communication skills even if aids provide adequate audibility across the speech spectrum (Berlin et al., 2010).
7. Refer the child and his/her family to another intervention approach if CI(s) are not an option, or if the child who is implanted is making limited progress (Berlin et al., 2010; Esta-

brooks, Houston, & MacIver-Lux, 2014; MacIver-Lux & Lim, 2016).

As explained in Chapter 5, hearing aids provide benefit for only 30% (Berlin et al., 2010) to 50% (Rance & Starr, 2015) of children with ANSD. It is extremely difficult to obtain reliable behavioral measures of hearing thresholds from children with ANSD because of the unique nature of how sounds are perceived. It is not uncommon for an audiologist to have difficulty obtaining a reliable audiogram despite the child being able to reliably perform conditioned play audiometry tasks with the sounds of the Ling Six Sound Test in AVT sessions. This is why audiologists rely heavily on the practitioner and parents' reports of the child's auditory performance. Children with ANSD who demonstrate benefit from amplification usually meet milestones in language, articulation, and speech perception like their peers with sensorineural hearing loss (Walker, McCreery, Spratford, & Roush, 2016).

Cochlear implants need to be considered if children with ANSD do not receive adequate functional benefit from appropriately fitted hearing aids (Liu et al., 2014; Walker et al., 2016). The expected outcomes of early cochlear implantation (Cardon & Sharma, 2013; Liu et al., 2014) for children with ANSD, excluding children with cochlear nerve deficiency, are no different for children with non-ANSD sensorineural hearing loss (Breneman, Gifford, & Dejong, 2012; Daneshi et al., 2018; Rance & Barker, 2007). As a consequence, intervention should be auditory based (Praveena & et al., 2014) and accordingly, the value of AVT intervention for this population cannot be overstated.

Six Presentations of ANSD

Predictions cannot be made about the degree of disruption and speech understanding based on the pure tone audiogram because ANSD is primarily a timing disorder, not a frequency and intensity disorder (Berlin et al., 2010). As a consequence of the variable degrees of disruption, created by ANSD, a range of speech perception abilities and patterns of spoken language progress appears in children with this challenging auditory disorder. Six possible presentations of ANSD and their impact on the development of listening and spoken communication have been identified and are presented in Table 21–1.

Each of the six presentations of ANSD requires the AV practitioner's careful consideration and discussion with the parent(s) and audiologist. It is *critical* that practitioners are familiar with these presentations so that appropriate recommendations can be made to the audiologist and family regarding hearing technology management and intervention options in a timely and efficient manner.

ANSD Presentation #1

Children may have either normal hearing sensitivity or hearing thresholds in the hearing loss range. If hearing thresholds are in the hearing loss range, it's not uncommon to see a reverse slope configuration. Children usually demonstrate poorer than expected auditory functioning considering the child's audiogram or use of appropriately fitted hearing aids. Therefore, children make very limited gains in receptive and expressive language.

One very confusing aspect of this presentation is that when these children are in AVT or ALE, they learn to identify speech sounds, environmental sounds, or short phrases but there are limitations to their ability to attach meaning to what they hear. For example, these children may make progress in the initial stages of AVT repeating some of the Learning to Listen Sounds but have difficulty making the meaningful association between an object and its related sound. Eventually progress comes to a halt after 3 to 6 months of AVT. By this point, children demonstrate poor ability to hold and maintain eye contact and often repeat what they hear—almost sounding echolalic. Additionally, they often avoid or leave verbal parent–child interactions. This is why children with this presentation of ANSD are commonly misdiagnosed with autism spectrum disorder (ASD) (Berlin et al., 2010).

When it is known that the child has ANSD #1 and is not making progress with hearing aids, the practitioner will refer the child to a CI team to for investigation of CI candidacy. Imaging studies are ordered to ensure the cochlear nerve is intact—otherwise, the child will not benefit from a CI. Studies have shown that 80% of children with this presentation who are implanted demonstrate significant improvement in auditory development and in receptive and expressive communication growth (Breneman et al., 2012). Thus, timely referrals for CI investigations are essential during the early critical language learning years.

Case Study (ANSD Presentation #1)

▪ Antoine was a full-term baby, born without complications.

Table 21–1. Six Presentations of Auditory Neuropathy Spectrum Disorder (ANSD)

	Presentation 1	Presentation 2	Presentation 3	Presentation 4	Presentation 5	Presentation 6
Pure Tone Audiogram	Can vary from mild-profound or normal hearing sensitivity	Can vary from mild-profound or fluctuate or be progressive	Can vary from mild-profound or fluctuate or be progressive	Normal hearing sensitivity and may progress to hearing loss	Hearing levels "recover" or improve from previously obtained levels	Can vary from mild-profound or fluctuate or be progressive
Auditory Functioning in Quiet	Significantly poorer than audiogram would suggest	As expected given audiogram (similar to what's expected with SNHL)	Better than expected than what audiogram would suggest	As expected given normal hearing sensitivity	As expected given audiogram and then improves	As expected given audiogram or better, then declines with rise in core body temperature
Auditory Functioning in Noise	Significant difficulty	Mild to significant difficulty	Mild to significant difficulty	Mild to significant difficulty	Mild to significant difficulty; fluctuates	Mild to significant difficulty; fluctuates with core body temp
Speech and Language	Delayed; limited progress (Raveh et al, 2007; Praveena & Prakash, 2014)	At expected levels similar to those with SNHL (Raveh et al., 2007; Rance et al., 2007)	Better than expected (Estabrooks, Houston, & MacIver-Lux, 2014; Berlin et al., 2010)	At expected levels similar to those with typical hearing (Raveh et al., 2007; Berlin et al., 2010)	At expected levels similar to those with SNHL and then sudden growth (Psarommatis et. al., 2006; Eom et al., 2013)	Decline in auditory skills affects daily communication skills (Varga et al., 2006; Zhang et al., 2016;

- His hearing was screened three times and he passed on the third try.
- He met all milestones and his parents had no concerns about his hearing, speech, or language development.
- At 12 months, he could answer questions about what animals say, and he could say a few words like "more," "hi," and "bye-bye."
- At 14 months, he came down with a fever and was sick for a week.
- He recovered his health, but not his talking.
- At 24 months, he saw a speech-language pathologist.
- At 26 months, a moderate to severe sensorineural hearing loss was confirmed, and he was fitted with hearing aids.
- At 26 months, the family began AVT; Antoine and his parents and grandparents attended faithfully.
- Despite hearing aids meeting prescriptive targets (providing auditory access to all sounds of speech at conversational level speech), very little progress was made after one year of AVT. Data logging on hearing aids indicated the hearing aids were being worn all waking hours.
- Despite the parents' efforts, however, Antoine seemed to withdraw more and more from verbal interactions. His vocal productions and voice quality continued to decline and a cochlear implant investigation started.
- ANSD was identified bilaterally during the CI investigation.
- CI was received on the left side at 4 years of age.

- Immediately following activation of CI, his parents noticed a difference in his attention and level of engagement.
- Over the next three months, Antoine made significant progress in AVT and produced three- to four-word utterances to communicate his wants and needs.
- After four months of CI use, the hearing aid was re-introduced in the opposite ear. After three weeks, Antoine became quieter and his rate of progress regressed quickly.
- The hearing aid was removed.
- Antoine's listening, spoken language and speech production improved and he became interested again in engaging in conversation.
- He now is now fluent in English and French.

ANSD Presentation #2

Children typically have hearing thresholds in the hearing loss range. A hallmark characteristic is that auditory skills (and performance) and receptive and expressive language are observed to develop as expected given the child's hearing age (as children with sensorineural hearing loss who do not have ANSD do). Many children with presentation #2 benefit from hearing aid use and make steady progress in AVT.

Case Study (ANSD Presentation #2)

- Arif had a difficult birth.
- He received a diagnosis of ANSD at 6 months of age and

behavioral thresholds were reliably obtained.
- He was fitted hearing aids and enrolled in AVT.
- Over the next six months he made rapid progress.
- AVT progress reports (emails or telephone conversations) were provided to the audiologist and parents.
- At 2.5 years of age, Arif was discharged from AVT (assessment demonstrated he had reached age-appropriate stages of development across the domains).

ANSD Presentation #3

Children have hearing thresholds within hearing loss range. Based on test results, the audiologist confirms the need for amplification. However, parents often insist their child is hearing "normally." In fact, many parents report their child can *hear a pin drop*. Thus, audiologists may feel uncomfortable providing hearing technology and may not in most cases. In these cases, audiologists rely on the feedback of practitioners, as do the parents. If a child has not been fitted with hearing aids, the child and family will be enrolled in the ALE program. The practitioner usually sees better than expected auditory, speech, and language development, in some cases, matching typical development. It's not uncommon for there to be discrepancies in speech perception tests (child can repeat sounds of Six Sound Test and words), hearing thresholds obtained in the sound booth (results show evidence of hearing difficulties and thresholds in the hearing loss range), and observed excellent listening and spoken language performance in everyday life.

ANSD of this presentation type and others can be progressive. Meaning, in most cases, onset of auditory decline occurs during the teenage years. It's important to note that timing of auditory decline cannot be accurately predicted in this population, and may occur sooner or later than expected. Therefore, it is critical that practitioners help parents become astute observers and develop independent reporting abilities so that hearing technology can be provided when necessary.

Case Study (ANSD Presentation #3)

- Tameka was born at 32 weeks' gestation and spent some time in the NICU due to a variety of illnesses and complications.
- She did not pass the hearing screening in the NICU.
- Further testing at 6 months revealed bilateral ANSD.
- Parents were confused by the diagnosis; they indicated Tameka was responding appropriately to their voices and various environmental sounds at home.
- The audiologist, however, could not obtain behavioral thresholds. Although extremely concerned, she was not comfortable prescribing hearing aids because of the discrepancy between electrophysiological and behavioral audiometry results and the parents' report.
- Tameka and the family were referred to an AVT practitioner.
- ALE sessions commenced at 7 months of age.
- Tameka demonstrated excellent auditory access to all sounds of

the speech spectrum and excellent receptive and expressive language development followed.

▪ At 18 months of age, Tameka was speaking in four to six utterances and could answer a variety of age-appropriate questions.

▪ At 2 years, comprehensive speech and language tests were administered. Tameka scored in the 99th percentile.

▪ At 2.5 years of age, Tameka and her family were discharged from ALE.

▪ A reliable audiogram was obtained shortly before discharge from ALE. Results showed hearing levels at 10 dBHL across the speech spectrum except at 250 Hz which was at 20 dBHL.

▪ At 4 years during a recheck session the practitioner observed listening and spoken language skills that were ahead of her peers. The audiogram obtained one week prior, however, showed a moderate to moderately severe hearing loss.

▪ At 7 years, Tameka was asking for multiple repetitions during conversations in a very quiet environment.

▪ A visit to the audiologist showed that while hearing thresholds had not changed much, speech reception scores declined significantly in quiet and noisy listening conditions.

▪ Tameka was fitted with hearing aids.

ANSD Presentation #4

These children have hearing thresholds in the normal hearing range. The audiologist will only see evidence of ANSD on the ABR, but all other hearing assessments usually indicate results within normal limits. The parents report their child as hearing "normally" and developing listening and spoken language skills along normal trajectory. When families seek intervention, they are usually enrolled in ALE. Typically, auditory performance and listening and spoken language progress looks very similar to children with ANSD presentation #3, therefore, the authors do not provide a case study for this presentation type.

ANSD Presentation #5 (Transient ANSD)

Hearing thresholds are typically in the hearing loss range. The audiologist sees every indication for fitting of hearing aids. The AV practitioner will observe benefit with hearing aids and an obvious decline in auditory performance when the hearing aids are not worn. Receptive and expressive language development with hearing aids proceed at expected rates.

When the child turns 18 to 24 months of age, he/she begins taking off the hearing aids. The child demonstrates excellent auditory access all sounds of speech and excellent performance *without* the hearing aids. This is called *Transient ANSD*, and is observed in children who present recovery from ANSD in two ways: (1) when the ABR is performed, there is restoration of normal neural responses and it appears that the ANSD has disappeared along with hearing improved thresholds to normal or near-normal hearing sensitivity range or (2) the ABR continues to show presence of ANSD but hearing thresholds have improved to normal or near-normal hearing sensitivity range.

Transient ANSD is typically seen in children born prematurely, with low birth weight and severe hyperbilirubinemia. It is uncertain why the ANSD recovers or disappears. Therefore, it is important that the AV practitioner obtain a detailed birth history on every child with ANSD. Additionally, in every AVT session, short segments need to be conducted without the hearing aid technology to ensure that auditory performance does not indicate spontaneous recovery from ANSD.

Case Study (ANSD Presentation #5)

- Sameer was born at 24 weeks and spent several months in NICU.
- At 6 months, he was diagnosed with bilateral ANSD. Behavioral thresholds showed a severe hearing loss and he was promptly fitted with bilateral hearing aids.
- Enrolled in AVT at 7 months of age.
- Without his hearing aids, Sameer did not show any detection responses to speech or environmental sounds. There was a noticeable difference, however, when he was wearing the hearing aids.
- He demonstrated excellent progress in listening and spoken language development in both English and Arabic.
- At 21 months, he began pulling his hearing aids off abruptly and fussed whenever his parent(s) tried to put them on. Sameer's parents were surprised to

observe Sameer answer questions without the aids on.

- The audiologist tested Sameer several times and confirmed hearing thresholds at 25 dBHL across the speech spectrum. Speech awareness thresholds were obtained reliably at 15 dBHL, bilaterally.
- The audiologist asked the parents to keep the hearing aids off for the time being and to continue AVT.
- The practitioner provided functional verification of the audiologist's findings. Sameer identified all sounds of the Six Sound Test reliably, and he was even able to understand whispered speech without his hearing aids. He was transferred to the ALE program.
- Follow-up ABR confirmed continued presence of ANSD, yet behavioral audiometry and speech perception testing in the sound booth showed hearing thresholds across the speech spectrum at 15 dBHL and excellent speech perception in quiet listening conditions at soft conversational loudness levels. Hearing aid use was discontinued.

ANSD Presentation #6 (Temperature Sensitive ANSD)

Children have normal hearing or hearing thresholds in the hearing loss range. The hallmark characteristic is good auditory functioning and receptive and expressive language capabilities with (e.g., children who are fitted with hearing technology) or without (e.g., children who are not fitted with hearing technology) hearing technology at one time, and a significant decline in auditory functioning once there is a change in core body temperature (as little as one degree) (Berlin et al., 2010; Varga et al., 2006). The challenging aspect here is that these children often demonstrate fluctuations in overall progress and/or performance in listening and spoken communication. Therefore, it is recommended that the practitioner and parents plan for those situations when temperature sensitive ANSD is interfering with listening and talking so much that an intervention approach combining listening, talking, visual cues, and perhaps sign language is used instead of AVT or ALE.

Case Study (ANSD Presentation #6)

- Astrid was adopted shortly after birth.
- Her parents were assured that she passed all newborn screening tests, including hearing screening.
- Astrid experienced chronic middle ear infections during the first three years of life. Repeated visits to the local otolaryngologist's audiologist revealed presence of middle ear fluid, and as a result she had a conductive hearing loss.
- At 3 years of age, the audiologist referred Astrid to a speech-language pathologist for assessment.
- At 3.5 years, the audiologist discovered that Astrid's middle ear health improved but her hearing levels did not. Astrid was diagnosed with a moderate sensorineural hearing loss and was fitted with bilateral hearing

aids and referred to an AVT practitioner.
- Despite consistent use of hearing aids and AVT, Astrid continued to demonstrate slow progress in listening and spoken language development.
- Follow-up ABR showed presence of bilateral ANSD and a referral to the CI team was made.
- At 4.3 years, Astrid received a cochlear implant and immediately demonstrated open set speech understanding, and in the following months experienced rapid progress.
- One day, Astrid's mother called up the practitioner to report that Astrid could not hear at all with either of her hearing devices and that she was relying completely on lipreading and written communication to communicate.
- Her mother made a video using her mobile device and sent it to the practitioner, who clearly saw that Astrid could not detect any speech or environmental sounds, despite adequately functioning hearing technology.

  Astrid's mother updated the practitioner twice a day. On the second day, Astrid appeared to be hearing again, albeit not as well as usual. The following day, she was back "back to normal."
- The practitioner checked the weather on the days that Astrid had her episodes of hearing difficulty. The day of the first episode it was 102°F (39°C). Astrid's mother confirmed that episodes like these happened on hot and humid days or whenever Astrid was sick with a fever.

■ An ENT visit revealed that Astrid likely has temperature sensitive ANSD.

Cochlear Malformations

Cochlear malformations account for a significant number (20%) of sensorineural hearing loss (da Costa Monsanto et al., 2019; Dhanasingh, 2019). These can include, but are not limited to, enlarged vestibular aqueduct syndrome (EVAS), Mondini's malformation (incomplete cochlear partition), common cavity, or cochlear aplasia (Dhanasingh, 2019). Historically, cochlear malformations have been broadly classified as Mondini's malformation or Michel's aplasia. However, cochlear malformations can be categorized by embryologic development into five different types (Jackler, Luxford, & House, 1987), with later, further clarification between type 1 (Michel deformity) and type 2 (cochlear aplasia) (Sennarogalu & Saatci, 2002). Interruptions in earlier stages of cochlear development in utero are associated with more severe degrees of hearing loss (Farhood et al., 2017).

Differing degrees of hearing loss are associated with cochlear malformations. Imaging studies (Dhanasingh, 2019) and temporal bone studies (da Costa Monsanto et al., 2019) have shown a range of characteristics that have been present in different malformations. For instance, it is common for those with EVAS to have fluctuating or progressive hearing loss. Other characteristics of cochlear malformations include incomplete turns of the cochleae, abnormal mastoid bone structures abnormal facial nerve pathways, and abnormal round window (da Costa Monsanto et al., 2019). In approximately 71% of cochlear malformations, the auditory nerve has a normal structure (da Costa Monsanto et al., 2019). These factors can make it more challenging to approach cochlear implant surgery in a conventional manner and may require different surgical approaches (da Costa Monsanto et al., 2019). Approximately 80% of cochlear implant recipients with cochlear malformations have full insertion of the cochlear implant electrode array (Farhood et al., 2017).

Cochlear implantation has been an option for children who have cochlear malformations. There may be different considerations in selecting electrode arrays (e.g., short/compressed electrode array as opposed to a standard electrode array) in some cases. Considerations may also include preventing or minimizing the impact of gushers during the surgical procedure. Audiological considerations also include programming (e.g., incomplete cochlear implant insertion would necessitate different programming parameters, such as turning off electrodes or reallocating frequencies). Children with cochlear malformations may require higher T and C/M levels, or other changes in the programming parameters (Incerti et al., 2018). Pre-CI open set word and sentence recognition outcomes have been greater in children with Mondini's malformations (Farhood et al., 2017) and EVAS (Demir et al., 2019), and poorer word recognition has been exhibited by those with more severe malformations (Farhood et al., 2017). Post-CI open set sentence and word recognition performance has shown improvement across the group of those with cochlear malformations (Demir et al., 2019; Farhood et al., 2017). However, there is still a range of speech understanding performance and those who have more severe cochlear malformations may still have challenges with open-set recognition (Demir et al., 2019). Listening and spoken language outcomes, therefore, depend on the amount of neural stimulation the central auditory nervous system (CANS) ultimately receives. Some children with cochlear malformations demonstrate expected levels of listening and spoken language outcomes while other children will demonstrate poorer outcomes using an auditory-based approach like AVT. Thus, it is important that the AV practitioner refer children who make limited progress to early intervention programs/approaches that encourage lipreading, tactile, and/or signed communication as quickly as the differential diagnostic periods allows.

Case Study (Cochlear Nerve Deficiency)

- At 12 months of age, Anil was diagnosed with bilateral profound sensorineural hearing loss.
- He received powerful hearing aids shortly afterward and was enrolled in AVT.
- Despite consistent hearing aid use and the parents' efforts, Anil made very little progress.
- At 16 months, Anil and his family sought the assistance of a CI program.
- MRI showed he had a very narrow auditory nerve on the right side and a slightly larger auditory nerve on the left side.
- The CI surgeon agreed to proceed with cochlear implantation on the left ear but advised that the parents be guarded in

their expectations for improvement in auditory functioning.
- At 19 months, Anil was implanted. Following activation of the CI, he demonstrated detection responses to all sounds of the Six Sound Test.
- After 7 months of AVT and consistent use of the CI, however, he demonstrated few gains in the development of skills in audition, speech, language, communication, and verbal cognition.
- The practitioner and parents engaged in weekly discussions about Anil's current functioning and progress with the CI. Each week, Anil's parents reported that they did not see any meaningful auditory responses to environmental or speech sounds at home and that Anil was becoming increasingly frustrated.
- The practitioner indicated that she did not know what the future held for Anil in terms of listening and spoken language development, but what she did know for sure was that Anil needed an alternative way to communicate. Anil's parents agreed.
- It was agreed that the practitioner would refer the family to a program where Anil and his family would learn sign language.
- One month later, Anil was using two to four signs in combination to communicate his wants, needs, and observations. The parents and Anil were able to engage in a "conversation" that did not involve any misunderstandings or frustration.

Single-Sided Deafness

Unilateral hearing loss (UHL), or single-sided deafness (SSD), is present in 3.4% of infants identified with congenital hearing loss and affects up to 5% of school-aged children (Lieu, Tye-Murray, Karzon, & Piccirillo, 2010). Some of the known causes of UHL include bacterial meningitis, malformations of the ear canal, congenital cytomegalovirus (CMV), enlarged vestibular aqueduct syndrome (EVA), and premature birth (Prieve et al., 2000). Enlarged vestibular aqueduct (EVA) accounts for 23% of children with SSD (Clemmens et al., 2013). Although individuals with unilateral hearing loss have normal hearing function in one ear, they may still have compromised auditory ability, due to the lack of auditory information from the other ear. Unilateral hearing loss has been associated with differences in executive functioning and cognition (Lieu, 2013), poorer linguistic skills (Sangen et al., 2017), *worse* academic performance, and increased fatigue at the end of the day due to diminished access to auditory information (Lieu, Tye-Murray, Karzan, & Piccirillo, 2010).

A thorough review of the benefits of hearing technology for children with SSD has been provided in Chapters 5 and 6. The goal of bilateral input is to provide auditory support and stimulation so that the brain can develop auditory neural networks that will support strengthening of binaural/spatial hearing skills. When a hearing device is placed on the affected ear, the brain has to learn how to integrate two very different sounding auditory signals so that they sound as one (binaural integration). When both ears work together in an efficient manner, then binaural/spatial hearing can develop. Binaural/spatial hearing helps babies and young children to detect, localize, and perceive the spoken language of their peers and adults at a distance and/or in non-ideal listening conditions (e.g., home, daycare, playground, preschool), which is where the majority of spoken language is learned (Bodere & Jaspaert, 2017). The practitioner and parent(s) jointly work to help the child with SSD, and newly acquired hearing technologies *integrate* and process the two different auditory signals by creating meaningful experiences that facilitate binaural integration and the development of binaural/spatial hearing skills. There are several steps that the practitioner takes to help the child integrate two different auditory signals for these purposes:

1. The practitioner begins the session with a conversation or an activity and the child wears his or her hearing device (hearing aid [HA] and auditory osseointegrated implant system (AOIS) and leaves the ear with typical hearing unoccluded. The practitioner observes the child's hearing and listening behaviors and notes how the child engages in conversation to determine how the two auditory signals are being integrated.

2. Depending on the child's level of auditory functioning with the hearing device and the normal hearing ear, the practitioner presents a variety of activities that focus on auditory skill development *with the hearing device only*. The ear with typical hearing is either occluded with an earmold or an earplug so that the practitioner can gain infor-

mation about how the child is hearing with the hearing aid or cochlear implant only. The practitioner and parents create meaningful experiences to optimize auditory development. Therapy with the good ear occluded should be brief (no longer than 5 minutes) as the goal is to help the child integrate the two different auditory inputs.

3. For the remainder of the session, engage in activities that stimulate the development of auditory skills that are supported by binaural hearing/spatial hearing. When appropriate, a variety of tasks are then presented to facilitate refinement of binaural interaction skills (e.g., localization skills, understanding of speech-in-noise), speech sound discrimination skills (e.g., speech perception), and/or dichotic listening skills, e.g., ability to understand two competing messages presented at the same time (binaural integration) and ignore messages while concentrating on a message of importance (binaural separation).

It is important that bilateral auditory input is as symmetric and consistent as possible to provide the brain with ample opportunities to learn how to interpret two different auditory signals as one so that the world sounds balanced and natural. Therefore, the hearing device should be worn and the good ear unoccluded at all times to develop binaural/spatial hearing.

Children who wear an AOIS will receive auditory stimulation to both cochleae (via bone conduction). Thus, it is difficult for the practitioner to isolate the ear with AOIS to develop and/or enhance auditory skills. Therefore,

the majority of the AVT session is spent developing binaural auditory processing/spatial hearing skills which, again, should be a priority for all children with binaural input. A true measure of auditory functioning in the ear with the AOIS can only be obtained by the audiologist, who administers *speech perception tests with masking noise*. For these reasons, the practitioner plans, delivers, and evaluates AVT sessions for children with an AOIS similarly to those for children who wear bilateral hearing devices.

Case Study (Single-Sided Deafness)

- Andrina was diagnosed with a unilateral hearing loss during infancy.
- Shortly after diagnosis, she received a hearing aid and AVT sessions commenced. The family felt that bilateral hearing and early intervention was important for her overall development.
- The practitioner knew that many cases of unilateral hearing loss had genetic and/or imaging abnormalities, so the parents were supported in requesting a genetic workup and imaging studies.
- Follow-up imaging studies revealed that the unilateral hearing loss was caused by an enlarged vestibular aqueduct (EVA).
- Genetic testing and a series of other medical workups revealed that Andrina had Pendred syndrome, which affects the thyroid, inner ear, and kidney.
- At 3 years of age, Andrina's moderate sensorineural

hearing loss in her left ear had progressed to the severe to profound hearing loss levels.

- Despite steady progression of hearing loss, AVT and consistent audiologic management ensured that the hearing aid was continuously adjusted to provide sounds across the speech spectrum until it was no longer possible to do so.
- At 3.2 years of age, Andrina was approved for cochlear implant candidacy and received a cochlear implant.
- At a subsequent AVT session, Andrina greeted the practitioner, proudly showing off her "brand-new baby ear" and baby doll.
- The practitioner observed Andrina as she and her parents played with the baby doll and noticed her ability to hear, listen to, and process conversation. She sounded like she was her old self, which suggested that the auditory cortex of her brain was adjusting well to the electrical signal provided by the CI.
- Andrina allowed the practitioner to occlude her non-implanted ear with sparkly pink ear plugs and they continued to play with the doll, using conversation as the springboard for auditory skills development with the CI only.
- After several minutes, the practitioner decided it was appropriate to begin listening tasks and activities that encourage the development of auditory processing skills that support binaural hearing (e.g., distance hearing, localization of speakers,

understanding of two or more speakers who speak at the same time). The practitioner explained that strong binaural hearing skills would play a significant role in reducing Andrina's fatigue at the end of the day.

- The practitioner introduced "sabotage" into play with the doll, which got Mommy and Daddy "arguing" about who gets to hold/feed/change/bathe the baby first.
- Andrina enjoyed helping the practitioner "choose" who had the better argument by telling her who said what.
- Andrina's parents learned from the practitioner that playground play dates with multiple friends would provide meaningful and naturally occurring opportunities to develop binaural and spatial hearing skills.

Hard or Soft Failures in Cochlear Implant(s)

Over the course of a lifetime, a cochlear implant recipient may require one or more cochlear implant revision surgeries, due to device failure, suspected device malfunction, medical or surgical problems, and the desire for device upgrades (Wang et al, 2014). If a cochlear implant stops working entirely despite an adequately functioning processor, and results of integrity tests suggest a failed device, then it is considered to be a hard failure. When there is a suspicion that a cochlear implant is failing or has failed, yet results of integrity testing suggests otherwise (or repeated integrity tests over an extended period of time eventually shows malfunction), it is considered to be a soft failure. The practitioner and parents observe and document any changes in auditory functioning and report these to the audiologist.

Estimates of cochlear implant device failures in children have been cited anywhere from 9% (Parisier, Chute, & Popp, 1996) to 11.7% (Cullen, Fayad, Luxford, & Buchman, 2008). Hard failures make up 46% of the failures (Cullen et al., 2008), and are easier to recognize. In the case of hard failures, the child typically does not respond to auditory stimuli and may often refuse to wear the cochlear implant processor. Soft failures, on the other hand, are more difficult to recognize and may be confused with malfunctioning cochlear implant processors and/or changes in T and C levels.

Signs of Cochlear Implant Soft Failure

Typically, soft failures are suspected by the audiologist and/or practitioner when the child:

- refuses to wear the cochlear implant processor or inadvertently turns the cochlear implant processor off;
- has "good" hearing days and "bad" hearing days, with the "bad" hearing days outnumbering the "good" hearing days over time;
- displays auditory performance showing short term improvement programming of cochlear implant(s), followed by performance declines with subsequent programming sessions;
- makes consistent and unusual errors involving the omission

of previously produced speech sounds (e.g., "ka" for cats) or addition of sounds to words that were previously produced correctly (e.g., "airt" for air) which cannot be developmental according to the child's hearing age;

- becomes quieter, withdrawn, and/or more difficult to engage in conversation or becomes louder with displays of behavior suggesting frustration;
- demonstrates decrease in overall auditory functioning, particularly in areas of detection, discrimination, identification, and auditory attention;
- demonstrates eye twitching or complains of pain;
- reports funny sounds such as "popping," "buzzing," "static" and "whistles";
- experiences regression or lack of progress in receptive and expressive language skills/ development;
- has fluctuating hearing performance from day to day, or worsening of sound quality;
- experiences pain or physical sensation in the ear canal, middle ear, throat, forehead, eyebrows, area surrounding the coil, and/ or the mastoid in response to auditory stimulation (facial nerve stimulation), which are reliably reproduced when individual electrodes are stimulated during MAPping sessions. If five or more electrodes are deactivated, this may suggest an impending device failure (Zeitler et al., 2009);
- needs frequent programming/ MAPping sessions;

- experiences gradual changes in the primary goal of programming sessions that go from "improving speech reception/quality" to "finding a comfortable and stable listening program";
- experiences increased difficulty understanding speech in quiet and in noisy situations despite adjustments made in programming of the cochlear implant; and
- regresses steadily in overall auditory functioning and performance over time, especially with the phone, music, and other forms of telecommunications/media.

The decision for re-implantation is made in conjunction with the surgeon, audiologist, practitioner, parents, and/or other members of the cochlear implant team. Whenever appropriate, cochlear reimplantation surgery should take place as quickly as possible to avoid cross-modal reorganization (Peele, Troiani, Grossman, & Wingfield, 2011; Cardon & Sharma, 2019).

In most cases, revision cochlear implant surgeries are successful, and one can expect the child to return to or surpass the previous listening and spoken communication skills with the previously functioning cochlear implant (Gardner, Shanley, & Perry, 2018). The child and/or family need to be counseled that a return to previous functioning may take time and that failure to see any improvement with the new device may be a possibility.

Case Study (Cochlear Implant Soft Failure)

- Haakon received bilateral cochlear implants when he was 10 months of age.
- He had been attending AVT since he was 4 months of age and at 3.5 years of age, he was about to be discharged.
- Three weeks prior to discharge, Haakon's father emailed the practitioner about his concerns about his son's recent behavioral changes. Haakon was tugging on his left earlobe frequently and bringing the CI processor to his parents to "change the battery."
- Thorough troubleshooting and listening checks with the CI processor confirmed that all was functioning as usual. Haakon, however, kept insisting his CI processor needed a new battery.
- The practitioner suggested that a visit to the pediatrician was in order to rule out any ear infection. Haakon's pediatrician examined Haakon and pronounced his ears to be in excellent health. The next morning, Haakon resisted wearing the CI processor, proclaiming the CI ear sounded funny. Furthermore, the parents noticed that Haakon's speech clarity sounded poorer than usual and that he was asking for repetitions more frequently.
- MAPping parameters and impedances were checked by the audiologist and were outside normal limits.
- A week later, integrity testing of the internal part of cochlear implant was performed, and it was determined that the internal device was no longer functioning optimally.
- A month later, Haakon had surgery to replace the malfunctioning device. Two weeks later,

Haakon's new cochlear implant was activated he and his parents were thrilled to report that his "CI ear was back to its superhero ways."

Congenital Cytomegalovirus

Congenital cytomegalovirus (cCMV) is the most common cause of non-genetic hearing loss in children, with 6% to 30% of hearing loss associated with CMV (Diener, Zick, McVicar, Boettger, & Park, 2017). Congenital CMV is a viral infection in the same family as the herpes and chicken pox viruses. If a pregnant mother contracts CMV, the virus can pass through the placenta to the developing fetus. Depending on when the child was exposed to CMV (i.e., exposure to CMV in earlier stages of gestation, the birthing process, or post-natal exposure such as breastfeeding), the severity of different disorders can increase. These co-morbidities can include developmental delays, balance issues, neurodevelopmental disorders (e.g., autism spectrum disorder, pervasive developmental disorder, intellectual disability) and visual issues (Lee, Lustig, Sampson, Chinnici, & Niparko, 2005). Many children pass newborn hearing screenings and may not exhibit hearing loss until later in childhood (Kraaijenga et al., 2018) or even adolescence (Lanzieri et al., 2017). In fact, 90% of later identified cCMV-related hearing loss is asymptomatic at birth (Kraaijenga et al., 2018). Evidence suggests that medical treatment, as long as it is provided during the first months of life, can improve auditory outcomes (James & Kimberlin, 2016). If the child is older, hearing status needs to be carefully monitored. While most children in AVT have sensorineural hearing loss that was present

at birth, it is not uncommon for a child with cCMV exposure to later develop progressive hearing loss, fluctuating hearing loss, or late-onset hearing loss (Foulon et al., 2019). Additionally, vestibular loss can be progressive (Melo et al., 2019), which puts additional drain on the child's cognitive resources. Children with sensorineural hearing loss who demonstrate vestibular dysfunction have been shown to benefit from vestibular rehabilitation exercise programs (Melo et al., 2019).

In AVT, the writers note that depending on the degree of severity of neurological insults that often accompany cCMV, children demonstrate auditory functioning reflecting the presence of cognitive or auditory processing deficits such as a short auditory attention span, poor working memory, and word-finding difficulties, which could be confused with auditory comprehension deficits and vice versa. Language disorders and motor-speech difficulties related to the neurological issues from CMV may also be present.

It is recommended that the AV practitioner take the following steps for management of children who are deaf or hard of hearing secondary to cCMV:

1. If the child is younger than 3 months of age, encourage the parents to consult the ENT regarding ways to minimize future risks of progressive hearing loss.

2. Refer the child for a pediatric developmental assessment if a team is not already following the child.

3. Refer the child to the appropriate professionals (e.g., ENT or physiotherapist) to assess vestibular functioning.

4. Refer the child to an occupational therapist for assessment of sensory

(and emotional) integration and regulation abilities.

5. Monitor the child's auditory functioning and watch for any fluctuation or progressive decline.

6. If auditory functioning is poorer than expected, ensure that ANSD is ruled out.

Case Study (cCMV)

- Anna and her twin sister had a rough start in life. Complications at birth were managed in the NICU. The neonatal care physician was surprised that she tested positive for cCMV while her twin did not. After-effects of cCMV were quickly evident and imaging studies showed evidence of brain injury caused by cCMV.

- A bilateral moderate sensorineural hearing loss was identified, and hearing aids were fitted. The family received intervention from a speech-language pathologist who focused on feeding issues and communication skills development.

- Delays in a variety of developmental domains became evident over time, and a multidisciplinary team was assembled for monitoring, assessment, and intervention. Anna was considered medically fragile, and all efforts during the first half-year of her life were spent ensuring that she would thrive.

- At 10 months of age, Anna's left ear progressed to a severe-to-profound hearing loss and she received a cochlear implant in that ear at 12 months of age.

- At 2 years of age, the family sought the services of an AV practitioner who also provided intervention for children with auditory processing disorders (APDs). In the referral report, the speech-language pathologist expressed concerns about Anna's auditory processing abilities.

- During the session the practitioner noticed that Anna's auditory attention was poor. After observing Mother and Anna engaged in play, it was evident that Mother did not wait long enough for Anna to process spoken language and verbally respond.

- Mother appeared anxious, quickly repeated questions, and then provided the answer for Anna to repeat. The AV practitioner demonstrated the strategy of waiting and by the end of the session, Anna's mother could use the strategy well.

- Anna demonstrated vestibular functioning differences. She was unsteady on her feet while standing, and at times while walking. While Anna was receiving periodic support from a pediatric physiotherapist and occupational therapist, there was little knowledge among all the service providers of the impact that vestibular dysfunction had on listening and spoken language development. All service providers met to share goals.

- AVT continued and Anna made *slow but steady process*—encouraging, considering that Anna was receiving many other interventions.

▨ Weekly visits to a speech-language pathologist addressed her motor-speech issues.

▨ At 3.5 years of age, vestibular functioning declined, as did hearing in the left ear.

▨ At 4 years of age, Anna received a cochlear implant for her right ear.

▨ Close collaboration with members of the intervention team was maintained; Anna's mother kept everyone in the loop by sharing reports and conducting interdisciplinary team meetings to ensure that Anna received the care required.

CONCLUSION

Parents of children with unique hearing needs often build long-lasting partnerships with carefully selected teams of professionals who have the expertise to provide guidance and intervention that will meet their children's unique needs. AV practitioners are skilled at differential diagnosis and provide guidance to multidisciplinary team members about the impact of unique hearing needs on overall development, as indicated in this chapter regarding auditory neuropathy spectrum disorder (ANSD), cochlear nerve deficiency/underdeveloped auditory nerve, unilateral hearing loss/single sided deafness (SSD), and cochlear implant device failures. Parents learn to become accurate reporters of their child's auditory functioning and develop the skills to independently manage any auditory and/or non-auditory disruption as they materialize. When processes that support functioning in all

domains are nurtured and disruptions are kept to a minimum, children with complex hearing issues in AVT have the opportunity to experience listening and spoken language progress that's on a steady and upward trajectory.

REFERENCES

A. G. Bell Academy for Listening and Spoken Language. (2017). *Listening and Spoken Language Specialist Certified Auditory-Verbal Therapist (LSLS Cert. AVT®) application packet.* Retrieved September 23, 2019 from https://agbellacademy.org/wp-content/uploads/2018/12/AVT-Application-2017.pdf

Berlin, C. I., Hood, L. J., Morlet, T., Wilensky, D., Li, L., Mattingly, K. R., . . . Shallop, J. K. (2010). Multi-site diagnosis and management of 260 patients with auditory neuropathy/dys-synchrony (auditory neuropathy spectrum disorder). *International Journal of Audiology, 49*(1), 30–43.

Bodere, A., & Jaspaert, K. (2017). Six-year-olds' learning of novel words through addressed and overheard speech. *Journal of Child Language, 44*(5), 1163–1191.

Breneman, A. I., Gifford, R. H., & Dejong, M. D. (2012). Cochlear implantation in children with auditory neuropathy spectrum disorder: Long-term outcomes. *Journal of the American Academy of Audiology, 23*(1), 5–17.

Cardon, G., & Sharma, A. (2013). Central auditory maturation and behavioral outcome in children with auditory neuropathy spectrum disorder who use cochlear implants. *International Journal of Audiology, 52*(9), 577–586.

Cardon, G., & Sharma, A. (2019). Somatosensory cross-modal reorganization in children with cochlear implants. *Frontiers of Neurosciences, 13*(469), 1–14.

Ching, T. Y. C., Day, J., Dillon, H., Gardner-Berry, K., Hou, S., Seeto, M., . . . Zhang, V. (2013). Impact of the presence of auditory neuropathy spectrum disorder (ANSD) on outcomes of children at three years of age. *International Journal of Audiology, 52*(suppl. 2), S55–64.

Clemmens, C., Guidi, J., Caroff. A., Cohn, S., Brant J., Laury A., & Germiller J. (2013). Unilateral cochlear nerve deficiency in children. *Otolaryngology-Head and Neck Surgery, 149*(2), 318–325.

Cullen, R. D., Fayad, J. N., Luxford, W. M., & Buchman, C. A. (2008). Revision cochlear implant surgery in children. *Otology & Neurotology, 29*(2), 214–220.

da Costa Monsanto, R., Sennaroglu, L., Uchiyama, M., Sancak, I. G., Paparella, M. M., & Cureoglu, S. (2019). Histopathology of inner ear malformations: Potential pitfalls for cochlear implantation. *Otology & Neurotology, 40*(8), e839–e846.

Daneshi, A., Mirsalehi, M., Hashemi, S. B., Ajalloueyan, M., Rajati, M., Ghasemi, M. M., . . . Farhadi, M. (2018). Cochlear implantation in children with auditory neuropathy spectrum disorder: A multicenter study on auditory performance and speech production outcomes. *International Journal of Pediatric Otorhinolaryngology, 108*, 12–16. doi: 10.1016/j.ijporl.2018.02.004

Demir, B., Cesure, S., Sabin, A., Binnetoglu, A., Ciprut, A., & Batman, C. (2019). Outcomes of cochlear implantation in children with inner ear malformations. *European Archives in Otorhinolaryngology, 276*(9), 2397–2403.

Dhanasingh, A. (2019). Variations in the size and shape of human cochlear malformation types. *The Anatomical Record, 302*(10), 192–199.

Diener, M. L., Zick, C. D., McVicar, S. B., Boettger, J., & Park, A. H. (2017). Outcomes from a hearing-targeted cytomegalovirus screening program. *Pediatrics, 139*(2). pii: e20160789. doi: 10.1542/peds.2016-0789.

Eom, J. H., Min, H. J., Lee, S. H., & Lee, H. K. (2013). A case of auditory neuropathy with recovery of normal hearing. *Korean Journal of Audiology, 17*(3), 138–141.

Estabrooks, W., Houston, K. T., & MacIver-Lux, K. (2014). Therapeutic approaches following cochlear implantation in cochlear implants. In S. B. Waltzman & J. T. Roland (Eds.), *Cochlear implants*, (pp. 182–193) New York, NY: Thieme.

Farhood, Z., Nguyen, S. A., Miller, S. C., Holcomb, M. A., Meyer, T. A., & Rizk, A. H. G. (2017). Cochlear implantation in inner ear malformations: Systematic review of speech perception outcomes and intra-operative findings. *Otolaryngology–Head and Neck Surgery, 156*(5), 783–793.

Foulon, I., De Brucker, Y., Buyl, R., Lichtert, E., Verbruggen, K., Piérard, D., . . . Gordts, F. (2019). Hearing loss with congenital cytomegalovirus infection. *Pediatrics, 144*(2), 2018–3095.

Gardner, P. A., Shanley, R., & Perry, B. P. (2018). Failure rate in pediatric cochlear implantation and hearing results following revision surgery. *International Journal of Pediatric Otorhinolaryngology, 111*, 13–15.

Harrison, R. V., Gordon, K. A., Papsin, B. C., Negandhi, J., & James, A. L. (2015). Auditory neuropathy spectrum disorder (ANSD) and cochlear implantation. *International Journal of Pediatric Otorhinolaryngology, 79*(12), 1980–1989.

Incerti, P. V., Ching, T. Y., Hou, S., Van Buynder, P., Flynn, C., & Cowan, R. (2018). Programming characteristics of cochlear implants in children: Effects of aetiology and age at implantation. *International Journal of Audiology, 57*(suppl. 2), S27–S40.

Jackler, R. K., Luxford, W. M., & House, W. F. (1987). Congenital malformations of the inner ear: A classification based on embryogenesis. *The Laryngoscope, 97*(S40), 2–14.

James, S. H., & Kimberlin, D. W. (2016). Advances in the prevention and treatment of congenital cytomegalovirus infection. *Current Opinion in Pediatrics, 28*(1), 81–85.

Kraaijenga, V. J. C., Van Houwelingen, F., Van der Horst, S. F., Visscher, J., Huisman, J. M. L., Hollman, E. J., . . . Smit, A. L. (2018). Cochlear implant performance in children deafened by congenital cytomegalovirus—a systematic review. *Clinical Otolaryngology, 43*(5), 1283–1295.

Lanzieri, T. M., Chung, W., Flores, M., Blum, P., Caviness, A. C., Bialek, S. R., . . . Congenital Cytomegalovirus Longitudinal Study Group. (2017). Hearing loss in children with asymptomatic congenital cytomegalovirus infection. *Pediatrics, 139*(3), e20162610.

Lee, D. J., Lustig, L., Sampson, M., Chinnici, J., & Niparko, J. K. (2005). Effects of cytomegalovirus (CMV) related deafness on pediatric cochlear implant outcomes. *Otolaryngology–Head and Neck Surgery, 133*(6), 900–905.

Lieu, J. E. C. (2013). Unilateral hearing loss in children: Speech-language and school performance. *B-ENT* (suppl. 21), 107–115.

Lieu, J. E., Tye-Murray, N., Karzon, R. K., & Piccirillo, J. F. (2010). Unilateral hearing loss is associated with worse speech-language scores in children. *Pediatrics, 125*(6), e1348–e1355.

Liu, Y., Dong, R., Li, Y., Xu, T., Li, Y., Chen, X., & Gong, S. (2014). Effect of age at cochlear implantation on auditory and speech development of children with auditory neuropathy spectrum disorder. *Auris Nasus Larynx, 41*(6), 502–506.

MacIver-Lux, K. & Lim, S. (2016). Children with complex hearing issues and AVT. In W. Estabrooks, K. MacIver-Lux, & E. Rhoades (Eds.), *Auditory-verbal therapy for children with hearing loss and their families, and the practitioners who guide them,* (pp. 473–491). San Diego, CA: Plural Publishing.

Madell, J. R., Flexer, C. A., Wolfe, J., & Schafer, E. C. (2019). *Pediatric audiology: Diagnosis, technology, and management.* New York, NY: Thieme.

Melo, R. S., Lemos, A., Paiva, G. S., Ithamar, L., Lima, M. C., Eickmann, S. H., . . . Belian, R. B. (2019). Vestibular rehabilitation exercises programs to improve the postural control, balance and gait of children with sensorineural hearing loss: A systematic review. *International Journal of Pediatric Otorhinolaryngology, 127,* 109650.

Parisier, S., Chute, P., & Popp, A. (1996). Cochlear implant mechanical failures. *American Journal of Otolaryngology, 17*(5),730–734.

Peele, J., Troiani, V., Grossman, M., & Wingfield, A. (2011). Hearing loss in older adults affects neural systems supporting speech comprehension. *Journal of Neuroscience, 31*(35), 12638–12643.

Praveena, J., Prakash, H., & Rukmangathan, T. (2014). Auditory neuropathy: Better language outcomes in small study. *The Hearing Journal, 67*(11), 29–34.

Prieve, B., Dalzell, L., Berg, A., Bradley, M., Cacace, A., & Campbell, D. (2000). The New York State universal newborn hearing screening demonstration project: Outpatient outcome measures. *Ear and Hearing, 21*(2), 104–117.

Psarommatis, J., Riga, M., Douros, K., Koltsidopoulos, P., Douniadakis, D., Kapetanakis, J., & Apostolopoulos, N. (2006). Transient infantile auditory neuropathy and its clinical implications. *International Journal of Pediatric Otorhinolaryngology, 72,* 121–126.

Rance, G. (2005). Auditory neuropathy/dys-synchrony and its perceptual consequences. *Trends in Amplification, 9*(1), 1–43.

Rance, G., & Barker, E. (2007). Speech perception in children with auditory neuropathy/dys-synchrony managed with either hearing aids or cochlear implants. *Otology & Neurotology, 29*(2), 179–182.

Rance, G., Barker, E., Mok, M., Dowell, R., Rincon, A., & Garratt, R. (2007). Speech perception in noise for children with auditory neuropathy/dys-synchrony type hearing loss. *Ear and Hearing, 3*, 351–360.

Rance, G., & Starr, A. (2015). Pathophysiological mechanisms and functional hearing consequences of auditory neuropathy. *Brain, 138*(11), 3141–3158.

Raveh, E., Buller, N., Badrana, O., & Attias, J. (2007). Auditory neuropathy: Clinical characteristics and therapeutic approach. *American Journal of Otolaryngology, 28*(5), 302–308.

Roush, P. (2008). Auditory neuropathy spectrum disorder: Evaluation and management. *The Hearing Journal, 61*(11), 36–38.

Roush, P., Frymark, T., Venediktov, R., & Wang, B. (2011). Audiologic managements of auditory neuropathy spectrum disorder in children: A systematic review of the literature. *American Journal of Audiology, 20*(2), 159–170.

Sangen, A., Royackers, L., Desloovere, C., Wouters, J., & Wieringen, A. V. (2017). Single-sided deafness affects language and auditory development—a case-control study. *Clinical Otolaryngology, 42*(5), 979–987.

Sennaroglu, L., & Saatci, I. (2002). A new classification for cochleovestibular malformations. *The Laryngoscope, 112*(12), 2230–2241.

Uus, K., Young, A., & Day, M. (2015). Parents' perspectives on the dilemmas with intervention for infants with auditory neuropathy spectrum disorder: A qualitative study. *International Journal of Audiology, 54*(8), 552–558.

Varga, R. A., Kelley, M. R, Keats, B. J., Berlin, C. I., Hood, L. J, Morlet, T. G., . . . Kimberling, W. J. (2006). OTOF mutations revealed by genetic analysis of hearing loss families including a potential temperature sensitive auditory neuropathy allele. *Journal of Medical Genetics, 43*, 576–581.

Walker, E., McCreery, R., Spratford, M., & Roush, P. (2016). Children with auditory neuropathy spectrum disorders fitted with hearing aids applying the American Academy of Audiology pediatric amplification guideline: Current practice and outcomes. *Journal of the American Academy of Audiology, 27*(3), 204–218.

Wang, J. T., Wang, A. Y., Psarros, C., & Da Cruz, M. (2014). Rates of revision and device failure in cochlear implant surgery: A 30-year experience. *The Laryngoscope, 124*(10), 2393–2399.

Zeitler, D. M., Sladen, D. P., DeJong, M. D., Torres, J. H., Dorman, M. F., & Carlson, M. L. (2009). Cochlear implantation for single-sided deafness in children and adolescents. *International Journal of Pediatric Otorhinolaryngology, 118*, 128–133.

Zhang, Q., Lan, L., Shi, W., Yu, L., Xie, L., Xiong, F., . . . Wang, Q. (2016). Temperature sensitive auditory neuropathy. *Hearing Research, 335*, 53–63.

22

CHILDREN WITH ADDITIONAL CHALLENGES AND AUDITORY-VERBAL THERAPY

Kathryn Ritter, Denyse V. Hayward,
Warren Estabrooks, Noel Kenely,
and Sarah Hogan

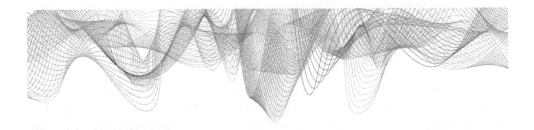

INTRODUCTION

Children with additional challenges, particularly those with *severe* additional challenges, have not, traditionally, been considered as candidates for Auditory-Verbal Therapy (AVT). This is due to a number of factors, including later prioritizing of audition in the child's development, a greater division of parental resources than that required by more typically developing children, and the reduced likelihood of spoken language as a primary outcome. However, with our current understanding of how audition contributes to overall brain and neurological development, as well as child and caregiver well-being (Flexer, 2016; Hayward, Ritter, Grueber, & Howarth, 2013; Hayward, Ritter, Mousavi, & Vatanapour, 2016), a greater number of children with mild to severe additional challenges are benefiting from AVT and are optimizing their use of audition for the purposes of neurological development, communication, connectivity, and inclusion (Perigoe & Perigoe, 2004). This chapter describes an expanded view of AVT that emphasizes the crucial connection that good access to sound provides, even when spoken language is likely to be limited, particularly for the 90% to 95% of children who are deaf or hard of hearing (including those with mild to severe additional challenges) who live with hearing and talking families (Cole & Flexer, 2015; Mitchell & Karchmer, 2004). We contend that audition is so important to these children and their families, that the Auditory-Verbal practitioner (practitioner) may be the best person to support the family in providing the needed advocacy for optimal audition in the context of other strongly competing developmental needs. Family and team support, assessment and intervention strategies are addressed. Our primary focus here is the infant-toddler and preschool years during which practitioners are usually most intensively involved with the child and family.

It is necessary to acknowledge at the outset that practitioners work in a wide variety of settings using a range of service delivery models, and various cultural and funding parameters. The writing cohort here share their own and sometimes differing perspectives of working in a large, publicly funded, interdisciplinary, rehabilitation hospital and a not-for-profit AV charity that works closely with parents and professionals outside of the UK's National Health and education services, respectively. Our goal is not to write a comprehensive review of AVT practice for children who are deaf or hard of hearing and additional challenges but to represent experiences that we have found most helpful in our own practices and that the global au-

dience of readers may find helpful in their own settings.

The population of children who are deaf or hard of hearing identified as having additional challenges is currently estimated at 40% to 45% (Ching & Wong, 2017; Holden-Pitt & Diaz, 1998). This is due to a number of factors including higher neonatal intensive care unit (NICU) survival rates and better diagnostic strategies combined with earlier intervention. Research is accumulating about the outcomes, particularly spoken language outcomes, of children who are deaf or hard of hearing and have additional challenges (Beer, Harris, Kronenberger, Frush-Holt, & Pisoni, 2012; Ching, Dillon, Leigh, & Cupples, 2018; Cruz et al., 2012; Olds et al., 2016). Additional challenges may be identified at birth or may emerge later. Increasingly, these children are being educated in inclusive placements, alongside peers with typical hearing. This alone suggests the need for optimal use of hearing, a primary goal of AVT.

Studies of AVT outcomes have rarely included children with additional challenges, as the heterogeneity of the impact of their additional challenges makes comparisons difficult both within a single population and when making comparisons with typically developing children (Hogan, Stokes, & Weller, 2010; Hogan, Stokes, White, Tyszkiewicz, & Woolgar, 2008). One of the ways of addressing the variability in this population is the use of an established classification system to help to organize variability in ways that more easily support systematic study. In 2017, the Royal College of Pediatrics and Child Health (RCPCH) and the British Academy of Childhood Disability (2017) endorsed an explanatory glossary of pediatric disability terms relating to the development of the Systemised Nomenclature of Medicine—Clinical Terms (SNOMED CT pediatric disability terminologies subset). The conceptual framework of disability was set upon the World Health Organization's International Classification of Functioning, Disability and Health (ICF). Utilizing this system, Hitchins and Hogan (2018) carried out an audit of preschool aged children participating in AVT programs that detailed the progress of children both with and without additional needs, whose abilities allowed them to participate in a formal standardized assessment of spoken language. The results indicated firstly that 40% of the cohort studied had at least one additional challenge; secondly, that one of every two children with additional challenges achieved age-appropriate spoken language while in the program; and thirdly, that on average, children with additional challenges doubled their rate of language development (RLD) while in the program compared with their RLD at the start of the AVT.

Other studies of outcomes of children with cochlear implants, closely allied with AVT research, have reported spoken language outcomes for children with additional challenges that are generally lower than those of typically developing peers with hearing loss (Cruz et al., 2012; Donaldson, Heavner, & Zwolan, 2004). Recent examinations have explored cochlear implantation benefit for children with more severe additional challenges, for whom spoken language may not be a possible primary outcome (Hayward, Ritter, Grueber, & Howarth, 2013; Hayward, Ritter, Mousavi, & Vata-

napour, 2016). Benefits cited by families and practitioners span a wide range of factors, including their child's enjoyment of music, improved quality of life for the child and the family, reductions in self-injurious behavior, increased verbal and non-verbal social interaction, improved behavior, and improvements in caregiver well-being. These point to the profound and pervasive influence of simple access to meaningful sounds in providing emotional as well as communicative connection to the world of sound and spoken language.

For children with additional challenges, management of hearing may be seen as a lower priority need by both parents and practitioners in light of other pressing physical and health demands. Indeed, families coping with the demands of their child's health and development are frequently overwhelmed physically, emotionally, and financially (McCracken & Turner, 2011). The role of the practitioner is enacted as one part of a complex care team that may involve dozens of professionals. How do we, as Auditory-Verbal practitioners, best support the child and family in this context? How do we make the case for optimizing the child's hearing in the midst of all the other strongly competing demands and priorities?

THOUGHTS ON FAMILY AND TEAM SUPPORT

At the outset, the reader is reminded of the work of David Luterman on counseling families of children with communication disorders (Luterman, 2016) and on living and coping with a loved one's chronic illness (Luterman, 1995). Luterman informs us that parents are often unable to absorb important information in the period following diagnosis and that period for a child with additional challenges can be quite drawn out. He reminds family members coping with a loved one's chronic illness that they are not responsible for what they think—only for what they do. He reminds caregivers to be compassionate with themselves. Support of families of children with additional challenges needs to be sensitive to the family's social-emotional process. Goals need to be realistic and achievable within the families' constraints.

Conceptually, Ritter and Hayward have found it helpful to first understand the process of adapting to a significant loss, such as a child's diagnosis, in terms of Martin and Elder's (1993) model. Most discussions of grieving follow the traditional Kubler-Ross (1969) model, which is based on those who are in the process of dying. It has become deeply embedded in our social and medical culture and suggests to parents that they should get to the point of acceptance, and that returning in a recursive way to the early experiences of grief is not normal. This is highly problematic for people who are living with grief as opposed to people who are dying. Martin and Elder (1993) challenge the Kubler-Ross model, with data based on parents who have lost their children to sudden infant death syndrome, and who are living with grief. The Martin and Elder model has since been validated with populations that have experienced a variety of life losses, including parents of children who are deaf or hard of hearing (Martin & Ritter, 2011).

Martin and Elder's model (as seen in Figure 22–1) places those experiencing a significant loss somewhere on a vertical, continuous figure 8, surrounded by external influences (extended family, friends, work situation, health and education systems, etc.). The upper portion of the figure 8 represents externally focused energies, such as hope and investment. In this part of the process, parents are better able to absorb information and ideas, to develop new skills (Luterman, 2016). The lower portion of the figure 8 represents internally focused energies such as despair and detachment. In this part of the process, parents may be less able to absorb new information and develop new skills. The affected person's location in the process is mediated by the meanings they assign to information and experiences.

From a clinical perspective, we suggest that part of the role of the practitioner is to assist parents and caregivers in constructing meanings that help them to move forward, often moving from the lower to the upper portion of the model. The process is continuous—there is no final resting spot called acceptance. On any given day and as a response to any given experience, parents may find themselves suddenly thrown into the inward, immobilizing phase of the process, or lifted into the outward, investing phase. Once parents understand that this is normal, it often becomes easier for them to accept their own process, as well as the process of a spouse or other family members. In accepting their own process, fear of being trapped in what some might characterize as unhealthy grief, something parents should "just get over," may be reduced, enabling parents to trust that they will move out of their inward phase in time. This ease

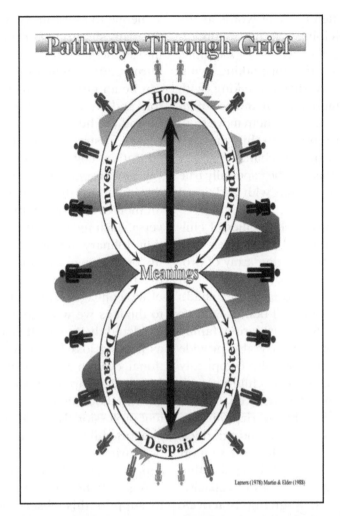

Figure 22-1. Pathways through grief model (Martin & Elder, 1993; Martin & Ritter, 2011).

may result in parents being more able to readily absorb coaching, guidance, and information for greater periods of time while also enhancing the practitioner's sensitivity to the timing and nature of support needed.

For children with additional challenges, helping parents assign meaning that allows them to invest actively in their child's intervention programs can often be a process of helping them recognize what Van Kaam and Muto (1993)

refer to as Just Noticeable Improvements or JNIs. The progress made by children with additional challenges may be in very tiny increments. Parents of a child with additional challenges may need to develop a deep and nuanced understanding of the many steps leading to children's understanding of what they hear and the ability to use it to support communication. For typically developing children, this complex process happens so quickly as to be unremarkable, so parents often think of words as the first step. Helping parents to understand the significance of, for example, eye gaze, nonverbal turn taking (without voice), pre-verbal turn taking (with voice), or comprehension and use of intonation can often help them move from despair to investment. In this sense, all of our therapy may be characterized as counselling. This may be especially true for parents of children with additional challenges.

At a systems level, families of children with additional challenges deal with an often bewildering array of professionals and the disparate information each offers, all of it crucial to their child's development and well-being. Dunst's (2017) model for considering family systems intervention may also provide insight into supporting the complexity with which families of children with additional challenges are faced. Dunst's model comprises the overlapping domains of family concerns and priorities, family member strengths, and support and resources. These are located within an overarching framework of capacity-building and help-giving practices. Within the capacity-building framework of the model lie the aspects of learning and development which are familiar territory for the practitioner. These are delineated as child learning opportunities, including everyday activity settings, parenting styles and instructional practices, parenting supports, and family and community supports. Any framework to model family systems intervention is always viewed against the backdrop of the demands of time, energy, financial resources, love, intellect and perseverance families, each of which is immense.

One of the things families report as most helpful to them is a case manager, someone to assist in weaving together the many strands of information offered into an integrated whole (McCracken & Turner, 2011). When this can occur, it can be an immense saving of time, effort, and even money for both the family and the health care system. Parents report frustration that their medical, education, cognitive, and physical development specialists don't understand the impact of the child's hearing loss on their overall development, and vice versa. Each member of the child's multidisciplinary support team will have his or her own area of expertise, and the practitioner will both learn from other colleagues and offer guidance to them as we work together with the child and the family. It is a reality that, as hearing loss in children with additional challenges is relatively low in prevalence (approximately one child per two thousand births), many competent professionals outside of services to support children who are deaf or hard of hearing may not be experienced in supporting the child's or family's needs in regard to hearing loss. The evidence to support this observation is starting to accrue: In a survey conducted with school-based psychologists and speech-language pathologists, Muncy, Yoho, and Brunson-McClain (2019) found that there was insufficient training or experience in the area of working with children who have hearing loss and other co-occurring disabilities.

The Auditory-Verbal practitioner may be in a position, at least in part, to fill the case manager role. Attending at least one of each specialist's appointments with the family, assisting other team members to understand, for instance, the need for special seating for the best use of hearing technology and the importance of hearing to the success of their own intervention can have big payoffs in terms of the relationship with the family and with the team. Since a positive relationship is the true fulcrum for change in our work, this can enhance our goal of optimal use of hearing technology. When this time is an early investment, the result can yield improved team function and family "buy in" into the therapeutic process.

McConkey-Robbins and McConkey (2008) and Palmer (1998) describe a critical concept: "standing in the gap." The gap that exists between what is possible, given resources and realities, and what would be ideal is ever present for all practitioners, and from our own experiences, most certainly for the practitioner. Palmer (1998) asserts that how well we occupy that gap greatly determines our effectiveness as practitioners. For example, leaning too far toward the restrictions of a child's situation can mean missing opportunities. Leaning too far toward the ideal may lead parents to be set up for dashed hopes—and damaged relationships with their practitioners. The Auditory-Verbal practitioner is not an exception, and, in fact, may be the person most frequently in contact with the family in the preschool years. Being conscious of helping the family (and the team) to "stand in the gap" productively provides a useful broad rubric for our practice.

INFORMAL AND FORMAL ASSESSMENTS

Children with additional challenges represent a very wide spectrum: from mild to severe, from a single additional chal-

lenge to several. Additional challenges may be sensory (e.g., vision, sensory integration), physical (e.g., cerebral palsy, oral-motor impairment), cognitive (e.g., learning disability, intellectual disability, autism), social (e.g., poverty, family dysfunction), or emotional (e.g., early trauma) (see Chapter 24). Additional challenges may be identifiable at birth or emerge later. The possibilities are essentially endless and present significant challenges to meaningful assessment that can point the way to effective intervention. The required assessment team often may need to include, in addition to the practitioner and audiologist, pediatric neurologists, ENT specialists, psychologists, speech-language pathologists, feeding specialists, physical therapists, occupational therapists, music therapists, social workers, early childhood educators, regular classroom educators, special educators, and assistive device and augmentative communication specialists, among others. As previously stated, the function of the team would benefit tremendously from a team coordinator or navigator to support the family (see Chapter 1).

All too often, the job of team coordination falls to the family. Some families excel at this, while others need more support to develop their skills in this role. Since access to all the sounds of life and the development of communication weave through every aspect of development, the practitioner may be the best family support for this role. In some practices, families are provided with a personal book at the outset of therapy, divided into sections for each of the specialists involved, to help parents organize documentation. Encourage the parents to take this book to all their appointments to reduce the number of times they may be required to "tell their story" by providing specialists with the documentation they need.

Assessment

We now turn to focus on assessments for which the practitioner may be responsible. The necessity of coordinating assessments with the interdisciplinary team cannot be overstated. Assessments can be very draining for children with additional challenges and for parents. Wherever possible, duplication needs to be avoided. Assessments of a child with additional challenges may begin best with observation of the child's interaction with family members, whenever possible in their most common environment, usually the home. Home environments tend to be complex (visually, experientially, and auditorily), making formal assessment in this setting challenging. Nevertheless, informal and specifically focused observation may yield the best idea of the child's real-life function in terms of listening and communication competence.

In a clinical environment, a formal assessment of the child's communication and functional listening administered by the practitioner needs to minimize external mitigating factors. Children deserve an optimized environment so that there is little strain on their attention and they are afforded the best opportunity to demonstrate their listening and spoken language capabilities. This should also be the case for children with additional challenges. Children who require a movement break every five minutes cannot be expected to sit still for 15, 30, or even 6 minutes in order to carry out a realistic assessment of their true communication skills.

Observation Protocols

Observation protocols and instruments administered by a practitioner and informed by parents (see Chapter 19) are helpful in the home environment to explore early communication behaviors in a systematic way for all children with additional challenges, but are especially important for very severely involved children. Scales of instruments for this group need to start at birth. Some of the tools that we have found helpful include: *It Takes Two to Talk* (Pepper & Weitzman, 2004); *The Production Infant Scale Evaluation* (PRISE; Kishon-Rabin et al., 2005); the *Rosetti Infant-Toddler Language Scale* (Rosetti, 2006); the *Champions Profile* (Herrmannova, Phillips, O'Donoghue, & Ramsden, 2009); and the *Six Sound Test* (Ling, 1976).

The *It Takes Two to Talk* materials are very helpful in pinpointing subtle preverbal behaviors that can be used as early building blocks for verbal behaviors. The *PRISE* can be helpful to the practitioner in documenting early vocal behavior. The *Rosetti Infant-Toddler Language Scale* can assist in documenting behaviors from birth to 36 months of age across the domains of interaction-attachment, pragmatics, gesture, play, language comprehension, and language expression. The *Champions Profile* provides a fairly extensive scaffold for both child observation and tracking of the team process, specifically related to cochlear implant candidacy. A video illustrating the use of the *Six Sound Test* for typically developing children as well as for those with severe additional challenges, developed by Ritter and Logan de Chavez (2011), can be instrumental in both identifying auditory behaviors and demonstrating to parents that their child actually *is* responding to sound.

Formal Assessment Tools

The *Sound Access Parent Outcome Instrument* (SAPOI) (Ritter & Hayward, 2016) was specifically designed to explore the impact of access to sound for children who have severe multiple challenges, and for whom severe to profound hearing loss might be considered a secondary driver of development. Grounded in parental reports of what matters most to them (Hayward et al., 2013, 2016), this criterion-referenced instrument was developed due to a strongly perceived need by professionals and parents to acknowledge and capture the more subtle communicative and quality of life improvements that were evident in children with additional challenges using hearing technologies. The call for this type of instrument has been virtually universal in the literature addressing this population (see, for example, Palmieri, Forli, & Berretini, 2014; Young, Weil, & Tournis, 2016). The SAPOI is designed to capture child and family changes resulting from use of hearing technology. Domains include the child's behavior and emotions, the child's interactions, parent-caregiver well-being, and the child's device use. It can be clinician administered or completed by parents independently. If administered by a clinician, it is also a useful counseling tool when hearing technology options, particularly cochlear implantation, are being considered. It is unique in including parent-caregiver well-being as a valid and important outcome.

Parent interview tools can provide more specific assessment information and can be done in the clinic or in the home. In many cases, the test norms and basal and ceiling rules will not be applicable to a child with additional challenges but may still provide important information to support counseling and intervention goals. Tools that the authors have found helpful for children with mild to moderate additional challenges include: the *Infant-Toddler Meaningful Auditory Integration Scale* (IT-MAIS: Koch, 2004; Zimmerman-Phillips et al., 2001); the *Little Ears Auditory Questionnaire* (Kuhn-Inacker, Weichbold, Tsiapini, Coninx, & D'Haese, 2003); the *Receptive-Expressive Emergent Language Scale* (REEL-3; Bzoch, League, & Brown, 2003).

The *IT-MAIS* and the *Little Ears* can provide insight into early auditory function as well as track progress. The *REEL-3* can be useful in pinpointing and tracking the levels of expressive and receptive communication development and can track progress. Additionally, the *REEL-3* serves as a good counseling and education tool as parents are learning about communication development. All of these tools are grounded in typical communication and listening development, starting at the very beginnings of development, and are consequently useful for children with additional challenges.

Literacy

For many children with moderate-severe additional challenges, access to literacy is often insufficiently explored because the child's education system may have a narrow definition of literacy.

Similar to our earlier discussion about communication, we believe it is important to broaden both the definition of literacy success for these children and the age range in which children acquire literacy skills. Framing literacy learning as a 50-year rather than a 13-year process frees educators and parents to support children in their progression along the literacy continuum rather than needing to or failing to meet specific grade level benchmarks (see Chapter 14). To support such an approach, Staugler (2007) developed a literacy rubric in which a child's behavior is observed during story reading or reading-related activities. The rubric is used to ascertain where a child falls along a continuum through early emergent literacy, transitional literacy, to early conventional literacy across five areas (phonemic awareness, concepts about print, word recognition, fluency, and comprehension). Once the child's skills are charted, the rubric can then be used to determine next steps and monitor a child's progress along the continuum over many years.

Practitioners and educators of children with additional challenges with mild-moderate diagnoses often focus primarily on language assessment and language interventions. The child's literacy skills, however, might be a relative strength and a means to enhance language development.

Additionally, focusing on language and literacy skills simultaneously allows for the identification of skill gaps that can be addressed earlier rather than later. Commonly used tests of language and literacy skills have inadvertently perpetuated the lack of simultaneous skill focus, since they are separate tests often administered by different clinicians, have strict age or grade testing criteria, and tend to offer limited information to support intervention. The *Test of Early Language and Literacy* (TELL; Phillips, Hayward, & Norris, 2016) was specifically designed to overcome these issues. The TELL evaluates language and literacy skills for children aged 3 to 8 years. The test format affords direct comparisons across language and literacy skills and provides insight into child strengths and difficulties, along with specific intervention goals and subsequent next steps. A major goal of the TELL is to establish what a child knows. While there are age-level basal and ceiling criteria, practitioners who give the TELL are encouraged to go backward or forward based on the child's ability to firmly establish what the child knows, irrespective of chronological age. Thus, the test can be used with much older children with additional challenges as a criterion rather than normative assessment tool.

GOAL SETTING AND THERAPY

The art of goal setting and therapy, guided by the science underpinning AVT, can take many forms. Dunst's work on family-centered intervention provides a good model for much of what practitioners deliver on a daily basis (see, for example, Dunst, 2018). At the family level, AVT is predicated on enabling a child's caregivers to be the best possible primary drivers of their child's development because we know that habit is far more powerful than isolated therapy as an influence on child development (Duhigg, 2012). Our therapy is aimed at helping parents and caregivers to develop habits of auditory living that are integrated into their family's daily routine. To do this well, a clear picture of what those routines entail is very helpful in developing goals that are a good fit for the family system. One of the most powerful ways to bring this about is to spend time in the family's home, if possible, particularly in the earliest years. While this is initially more time-consuming than seeing children and parents in a clinic, it offers a number of advantages, particularly for families of children with additional challenges. Transportation is often a challenge for parents of a child with additional challenges, especially when significant mobility issues exist. Furthermore, the home environment may be the place parents feel the safest and the surest of their ground, whereas within the clinic context, professionals may be seen as knowing more about their child than they do. The practitioner's willingness to work on the parents and child's home ground can provide a powerful shift in the balance of power from one of medical/professional expertise to one of honoring and inviting parental expertise and, thus, empowerment. It also makes it easier to include siblings and extended family members in goal setting and coaching. It may allow for more accurately set and collaboratively generated goals within the family's established routine, which are likely to have a higher chance of success than more decontextualized goals. If in-home contact is not possible, this potential perceived power differential

may be overcome through AVT as, over time, the parent comes to realize that he or she is the primary agent of change. Regardless of location of therapy, one of the most important questions to ask parents in the process of goal setting for a child with additional challenges is: "What would make the most difference to you in the short term/in the long term?"

The practitioner's first goal, always, is to establish consistent use of the hearing technology. This is often extremely challenging for a child with additional challenges. It requires as much certainty as possible about the correct fit of the amplification and real buy-in from the parents, and this requires the practitioner to educate the parents about the profound neurological and brain development advantages that access to good quality sound can provide. It can require tremendous creativity and persistence. Cochlear implant sites and Google and various agency websites provide a wealth of device retention suggestions. This is another instance where a strong understanding of the home environment is crucial.

▪ What does the child most enjoy?
▪ When are the child and parents most relaxed?
▪ Are the parents able to devote a full weekend, or even a week, to establishing consistent device use?

Concurrent with this first goal, and often most powerful, is to find ways for parents to enjoy interactions with their child with additional challenges. Parents of children with additional challenges can be so worried and overwhelmed by the routine demands of care for their child that simple joys become rare experiences.

For very young or severely involved children, *It Takes Two to Talk* (Pepper & Weitzman, 2004) can be extremely helpful in setting very early communication goals. This program offers a detailed breakdown of prelinguistic as well as early linguistic behavior and has excellent parent guidance material.

Augmentative Communication

Children whose motoric challenges make spoken language difficult or unlikely may benefit from augmentative communication strategies not typically within the Auditory-Verbal practitioner's scope. When it is clear that children will not be able to rely fully on speech for their expressive communication needs, referral should be made to an Augmentative Communication Specialist or team. It is important to note that what most augmentative communication strategies have in common is reliance on auditory comprehension of language. The Auditory-Verbal practitioner and the augmentative communication specialist can be a very powerful combination in optimizing communication access, even for "locked in" children.

Augmentative communication is an evolving area of research and practice (Romski & Sevcik, 2005; Wilkinson & Hennig, 2007) but beyond the scope of this chapter. It is an area that requires specific expertise both in terms of strategies and/or equipment and in terms of the best ways to approach language generation using augmentative communication (Tatenhove, 2007). The better the child is able to rely on audition for language comprehension, the more enhanced his or her ability will be to use augmentative communication as an expressive language mode. Augmentative communication strategies range from no-tech/low-tech strategies such as use of eye gaze in a variety of ways to the use of high-tech speech generating devices. Low-tech/no-tech strategies are easily used and cost-effective and open the door to expressive communication with what may be surprising breadth and specificity to those new to this arena. These include, but are not limited to, choice making with hand selection; eye pointing using an E-tran (eye transfer) board; laser pointing with partner confirmation; partner assisted auditory scrolling; sliding scale partner assisted scanning; and partner assisted row-column scanning (I Can Centre, n.d.). While this chapter's space limitations prevent detailed description of these strategies, simple Google searches will provide clarification.

CASE EXAMPLES

In the following section, the authors provide five case examples with explanations of the various goal setting and evaluation processes with a variety of children with additional challenges and their families. Examples are roughly organized from least to most complex.

Box 22–1. Harrison

CASE STUDY 1	
Name	Harrison
Chronological age	5 years, 5 months
Hearing age	2 years, 6 months (post CI initial activation)
Auditory-verbal age	4 years, 9 months
Type and degree of hearing loss	Bilateral, profound ANSD
Hearing technology	Bilateral cochlear implants (CIs): Fitted with hearing aids at 8 months of age but not implanted until 35 months: Delay attributed to complex needs.
Additional challenges	Born at 26 weeks' gestation with significant motor coordination difficulties—cerebellar insult from prematurity. Received support from a physiotherapist and occupational therapist.
	Difficulties with central visual processing—wore glasses and required materials to be of at least font size 24. Received support from a teacher of the visually impaired.
	Oral-motor difficulties—received support from a feeding specialist as he was just graduating to pureed food.
	Autism spectrum disorder (ASD).
	Sensory processing difficulties including poor sleep patterns.
	Attention deficit hyperactivity disorder (ADHD)—impulsivity and high level of activity.
	Increased processing time required for comprehension.

continues

Box 22-1. Harrison *continued*

Additional information	The diagnosis of ADHD and ASD were made at 5 years of age. Harrison attended a mainstream primary school and despite his many challenges, made progress in all areas. His auditory comprehension developed in advance of his expressive language with the rate of development of his expressive communication accelerating in the second year, post implantation. Although his expressive language improved, his speech was difficult for his peers to understand. In addition, Harrison had difficulty directing his message to conversational partners. Although his spoken language had developed rapidly over a short time, his slow process needed a supportive communication partner to know to wait for him to process the information and plan his reply—a skill to be developed among his teachers and his classmates.
Why Harrison and his family keep us "up at night"	Harrison's pragmatic skills had become a cause for concern. He made less direct eye contact and needed help providing information the listener needed to understand his behavior (a Theory of Mind skill).
The plan	Goal: Increase Harrison's effectiveness as a communication partner by encouraging him to make purposeful eye contact. Strategies: Previously, supportive adults got down to Harrison's level and being very close to him, pointed at the person to whom the message was directed; the next step was to encourage Harrison to do the same by using words: e.g., "I didn't know you were talking to me because you didn't look at me!" Goal: Help Harrison to provide the information that others needed to understand his behavior

	Strategy: Harrison needed to let others know his plan. He would often do things that were interpreted as "negative behaviors" as he would act on impulse. The practitioners and parents adopted a strategy for use at home and school: they would remind Harrison by saying "You didn't tell me your plan . . . So I didn't know what you were thinking!" or "What's your plan? You have to tell me because I don't know!"
Discussion	The strategy for increasing Harrison's eye contact paid off and was observable in his interactions with close family members. School staff continued to develop this skill and presented it as a goal in his IEP.
	Harrison gradually became accustomed to adults asking about his plan. Little by little, he started to tell them what he was about to do and subsequently there was greater understanding by adults about the behaviors he used for sensory well-being.
	In therapy sessions, it was difficult to determine which behaviors (a) reflected fatigue of being in a class for a whole day; (b) were due to being a relatively new listener to spoken language and with some atypical cognitive abilities, and (c) were indicators of a social communication disorder. A team of fourteen professionals attended his last IEP review meeting and included class teachers, educational psychologists, occupational and physiotherapists, teachers of children with visual and hearing impairments, speech-language pathologists, and auditory-verbal practitioners. The degree of overlap between his sensory needs and other challenges demanded a holistic and informed team approach.

Box 22-2. Maria

CASE STUDY 2	
Name	Maria
Chronological age Hearing age Auditory-verbal age	6 years 5 years, 10 months 4 years
Type and degree of hearing loss	Right severe mixed Left profound mixed (auditory nerve fused with facial nerve)
Hearing technology	Bone conduction hearing aid on soft band Behind the ear digital hearing aid (Rt. Ear) Bone conduction hearing aid (on abutment) (Left ear)
Additional challenges	CHARGE syndrome: a genetic disorder that occurs in approximately 1 in 10,000 live births (Blake, Trider, Hartshone, & Stratton, 2016). CHARGE syndrome is characterized by multiple congenital abnormalities that include a combination of major and minor features including: ocular coloboma (part of one or more structures inside an unborn baby's eye does not fully develop during pregnancy affecting the iris, retina and/or the optic disc), cleft palate, ear anomalies, developmental delay and cardiovascular malformations (Blake & Prasad, 2006). Maria had very little vision in her right eye and peripheral vision loss in her left. She was born with bilaterally absent semi-circular canals. In combination with reduced vision this created challenges with balance and proprioception. Maria had a complex audiological profile. She had a moderate sensorineural hearing loss in her right ear and a severe sensorineural loss in her left ear. Her hearing loss was further complicated because of a conductive element due to fusion of the auditory ossicles bilaterally.

	Furthermore, Maria had a submucous cleft palate that impacted her speech clarity.
	There have been a number of research studies linking CHARGE with difficulties in Executive Function (EF) (Figueras et al., 2008; Hall et al., 2018; Hartshorne, 2007). Maria had difficulties in all three areas affected by EF including working memory, inhibition, and flexibility of thought.
Why Maria and her family keep us "up at night"	Maria's parents chose listening and spoken language despite the different challenges. Although Maria's hearing loss was diagnosed early, the optimal arrangement for her hearing technology took time to be established. Her family began Auditory-Verbal Therapy (AVT) at the age of 2 years. Maria's spoken language plateaued from time to time and the clarity of her speech was severely compromised. She was a keen communicator and always wanted to be at the center of any conversation. However, the extra effort she used to control her vestibular and proprioceptive needs, and insufficient access to high frequency sounds meant that she often missed key parts of a conversation. Her limited language and speech intelligibility required her mother to often repeat what Maria was saying for the unfamiliar listener. Difficulties with EF often resulted in Maria pulling the listener by the hand away from a conversation or resorting to repeatedly asking the same questions to one person.
The Plan	Goal: Maria would try to verbally share a new piece of information with others about a recent personal experience.

continues

Box 22–2. Maria *continued*

	Strategies: Maria could initiate a conversation with peers and adults that were not family members. However, in a challenging environment such as a noisy party or when she was feeling tired, she often experienced a breakdown in communication that led to a repetitive, inflexible, verbal behavior of asking questions that were not pragmatically correct. With input from the occupational therapist (OT) to help manage self-regulation, the parents and her support person in school discussed topics to be used with others that were "news" and news was explained as information not known by another person. Maria would have an "Experience Book" to help her working memory. The parents and support person talked with Maria about the "news" for her experience book and decided what information needed to be shared verbally. The adult "rehearsed" a phrase that Maria could use to initiate the topic (e.g. "Yesterday I made pancakes").
Discussion	Maria used her Experience Book to initiate conversations in "challenging" situations with adults. This gave her a way to be involved socially in a context that would otherwise have led to a communication breakdown.
	As her working memory improved, Maria no longer needed the Experience Book to recall her "news." As she grew older, her ability to demonstrate more flexibility of thought improved and she was able to respond more appropriately to others, even in stressful situations.
	Maria transitioned from a special educational unit for children with hearing loss to her local mainstream primary school. A personal FM system was introduced to help her overcome background noise and she undertook a second assessment for a cochlear implant (CI).

The OT's involvement in collaboration with her specialist Multi-Sensory Impairment (MSI) teacher was very important in managing movement at school, as well as in using strategies to promote self-regulation and minimize stress.

Maria's language continued to progress, her auditory development was followed by her audiologist, and her educational environment was managed appropriately to ensure she could understand the information provided by the classroom teacher.

Following her second referral for a CI assessment, the parents decided on bilateral bone conduction hearing aids. These provided much better access to all the sounds of daily life, better speech intelligibility and eventually, age-appropriate spoken language.

Box 22–3. Elliott

CASE STUDY 3	
Name	Elliot
Chronological age	39 months
Hearing age	12 months
Auditory-verbal age	25.5 months
Type and degree of hearing loss	Bilateral profound auditory neuropathy spectrum disorder (ANSD)
Hearing technology	Bilateral cochlear implants at 23 months

continues

Box 22–3. Elliott *continued*

Additional challenges	Elliot was born at 26 weeks' gestation and started Auditory-Verbal Therapy (AVT) at 13.5 months of age. He was diagnosed with ANSD and at 23 months of age he underwent bilateral cochlear implant (CI) surgery. To this point his progress has been slow. Physiotherapy and occupational therapy helped in the development of motor skills. He started crawling at 14 months and walking at about 18 months. Progress in listening and spoken language was quite slow.
	The pediatrician diagnosed a global developmental delay and cognitive challenges that became even more evident as Elliot grew older. He spent a long period progressing from one cognitive level to the next and subsequently his language development was impacted.
Why Elliott and his family keep us "up at night"	By the time Elliot had completed six months of AVT with good auditory access, he was beginning to demonstrate understanding of familiar songs by his actions, and by using his voice to request that the singing continue. But, at the same time Elliot would often cry or scream to have his needs met. He needed a more appropriate way to communicate his wants and needs.
The plan	Goal: Elliot would point to what he wanted from a choice of items following the question, "What do you want?"
	Strategy: Elliot would often become frustrated at not being successfully understood by others. He had developed understanding of some familiar phrases such as "bye bye" and "Give it to Mommy," to which he would respond with a wave or by handing an object over to his mother. His understanding of everyday phrases would help ease the communication breakdowns. The auditory-verbal practitioner (practitioner) coached Elliot's parents in using the phrase "What do you want?" before they gave him options to choose from.

Discussion	This strategy developed into the use of the augmentative Picture Exchange Communication System (PECS) (Bondy & Frost, 1998). Upon the prompt "What do you want?" Elliot would find the picture that indicated his choice.

The practitioner suggested a parent consultation to discuss a plan going forward. Such consultations are held without the child in attendance, so the adults can concentrate fully on the needs, suggested solutions, and referrals.

They all looked at the "big picture." It was an occasion to celebrate Elliot's progress and, at the same time, review how the additional challenges required a change in programming. The option of a "signed language" was too challenging at that time. The parents eventually chose a Total Communication approach with the use of PECS and some Makaton signs, a communication system using signs and symbols developed specifically for children and adults with communication difficulties (Sheehy & Duffy, 2009). It was agreed that the family continue coming to the practitioner to support Elliot's auditory development. He was, however in a transition and using Auditory Skills Training (AST).

At the subsequent consultation 6 months later and one-year post CI activation, the parents decided to enrol Elliot in a full-time educational program that would better address his motor development, cognition, and communication. The program would focus on working with Elliot's new school and the family would no longer receive AVT.

A few months later the parents contacted the practitioner to say how well Elliot was doing at his new school and that having all the services available in one place made life much easier. He was always progressing in auditory development. |

Box 22–4. Ava

CASE STUDY 4	
Name	Ava
Chronological age	20 months
Hearing age	17 months, bilateral ear level hearing aids at 3 months
Auditory-verbal age	17 months
Type and degree of hearing loss	Progressive bilateral sensorineural, from mild-moderate at initial diagnosis at 3 months to moderate-to-severe at 12 months.
Hearing technology	Bilateral ear level hearing aids
Additional challenges	Ava had a progressive neurological disorder that affected hearing, vision, gross and fine motor control. Although she could hand feed herself, chew soft foods and swallow and occasionally babble isolated syllables /b/ plus neutral vowel, /d/ plus neutral vowel, her vocal behaviour had not progressed beyond that point. The primary evidence of her development of listening was her willingness to happily wear the hearing technology, her clear pleasure when hearing music, love of sound making toys and her parents' ability to soothe her verbally from a distance. Ava's disease meant that her life expectancy was 10 years or less; all vision was lost by 1 year of age, all motor milestones (head and neck control, sitting) were delayed. She was able to sit with support and had fairly good control of her arms and hands at that point.
Why Ava and her family keep us "up at night"	Ava's enjoyment of sound was the one constant in her life. She loved music, being sung to, being moved rhythmically to music, and loved noise making toys. Her quickly progressing hearing loss meant that she would likely require a cochlear implant to access sound—but would her overall health allow for the surgery? Would her brain be able to make the transfer from hearing aids to implant technology? It was critical to work with her parents to determine what was most important to them and to Ava on a day-to-day basis. What would make life easier? What would bring the most joy?

The plan	Goal: To help Ava's parents feel certain that she could identify her parents, and understand basic routines given her rapidly changing sensory status.
	Strategies: Ava could hear footsteps, voices, and environmental sounds, but she could no longer see to what these were attached. Ava's parents wanted to be certain that she recognized their voices and understood when basic routine actions were going to happen. Ava's quickly changing sensory and motor function made her parents unsure whether she understood verbal prompts alone. It is crucial to use anticipatory cues before touching a deaf-blind child to let him or her know something is about to happen. This can take the form of voiced cues alone or may be followed by a touch cue paired with a voiced label for what is about to happen to provide multiple sensory clues about the meaning. Failing to provide anticipatory cues means the child may repeatedly be startled, and may quickly become very passive (Chen, 1999). In order to systematize this way of communicating, a voice and touch dictionary was developed with the parents, the Auditory-Verbal practitioner (practitioner) and the vision consultant. Parents and practitioners found good information to support this process on both DB Link and on the California Deaf-Blind Services web site. Ava's first dictionary included (verbal cues always provided first, followed by brief pause before touch).
	1. *"Mom's here"* (voiced melodically); mom placed her hands UNDER Ava's (see Chen, Downing, & Rodriguez-Gil, 2016 for rationale for hand under hand) gently brought Ava's hands to Mom's hair, and stroked lightly.
	2. *"Dad's here,"* using shorter melodic pattern than Mom's. Dad placed his hands UNDER Ava's, gently brought them to his cheek, taps.

continues

Box 22–4. Ava *continued*

	3. *"come up,"* parent placed hands UNDER Ava's, and lifted them both up above her shoulders, before lifting her up. 4. *"diaper change,"* parent placed hands UNDER Ava's, gently brought them down to her diaper. 5. *"time to eat,"* parent placed one hand UNDER Ava's, and brought her hand to her mouth. 6. *"bath time,"* parent placed hands UNDER Ava's, brought them to her chest and gently rubbed up and down. 7. *"bed time,"* parent placed one hand UNDER Ava's, brought it up to lay her palm against her cheek.
Discussion	Ava's parents took about three weeks before they felt confident using this combination of strategies consistently. During that time, the practitioner, with consultation from the vision consultant, provided weekly coaching in the home. Once this strategy was consistently used, the parents reported that Ava seemed more settled, and less distressed. Importantly, Ava's parents felt more confident that they were communicating effectively with their child. Once the parents were confident that Ava knew what was about to happen in these routines, a reasonable goal was to reduce the use of the tactile prompts. However, given the swiftly changing nature of Ava's sensory-motor status, the parents chose to continue the tactile prompts, and to expand the dictionary to favorite toys, foods and activities.

Other important functions of the practitioner in this case were to assist in liaising with Ava's audiologists, make sure the parents were connected with support groups, had access to counselling, facilitated referrals to vision and deaf-blind consultants, early intervention programs and music therapists, and assisting in establishing the need for respite. The family's medical team facilitated access to physical and occupational therapy. Perhaps most importantly, the practitioner validated the parents' social-emotional process, allowing them to be open about how they were doing at each appointment.

Box 22–5. Remy

CASE STUDY 5	
Name	Remy
Chronological age	24 months
Hearing age	7 months
Auditory-verbal age	6 months
Type and degree of hearing loss	Profound bilateral sensorineural
Hearing technology	Cochlear Implant (CI), Left, at 18 months
Additional challenges	Remy had severe athetoid quadriplegic cerebral palsy (CP), etiology unknown. Athetoid CP is characterized by fluctuating hypo and hypertonia and involuntary movement in the face, torso, and limbs (http://www.cerebralpalsyguide.com). He was unable to control his swallow, so used a tube for feeding. He had limited and unpredictable control of his limbs and oral-motor musculature. Eye gaze was his most consistently available form of expressive communication (given a choice of two items he looked at the desired item), although vocalization with varying intonation pattern was present, and used to call attention, express discomfort or distress, and to express pleasure.

continues

Box 22-5. Remy *continued*

Why Remy and his family keep us "up at night"	Remy's overall engagement, responsiveness to the Six Sound test, environmental and voiced sounds (e.g., door opening, phone, Mom's voice from another room), speed in learning turn taking activities within his physical capability suggested no more than mild intellectual disability—average intelligence, but lack of control of oral motor and limb musculature made symbolic expressive communication extremely challenging. He seemed like a "locked in" child. We looked for ways to keep that spark of delight evident in his interactions alive. His access to good quality sound through his CI was an immensely important avenue for cognitive and linguistic stimulation but device retention was a challenge due to seating and head support requirements. Frequent hospitalizations interrupted device use as well. In studies of children with CP, severe CP usually co-occurs with severe intellectual disability and very poor listening, speech, language, and CI outcomes (Cejas, Hoffman, & Quittner, 2015). This level of intellectual disability did not appear to be the case with Remy, although spoken language beyond use of vocal intonation and possibly one syllable approximations may not have been possible for him. We had to wonder, given the difficulty in formally assessing a child such as Remy, about the means of accurately assessing intellectual function.
The plan	Goal: Explore enjoyable interactive turn taking possibilities (Precursors to conversation, Pepper & Weitzman, 2004); exposure to verbal prompt "push," maintain CI placement during activity.

	Strategy: Remy had somewhat more control of his legs than his arms and hands. In the home environment, reclining on the couch allowed Remy to be comfortable, his implant was unimpeded in this position, and the Auditory-Verbal practitioner (practitioner) could place his feet on her tummy and pair the verbal prompt "push" with his spontaneous (and possibly athetoid) push with his legs. The practitioner then pretended to fall backward, giving a big "pay off" to the child's action.
Discussion	Remy's quick grasp of turn taking provided evidence of his cognitive function. Specific assessment of comprehension is extremely difficult when only eye gaze is somewhat reliable. He expressed both pleasure and displeasure with appropriate vocal intonation but was unable to articulate differentiated speech sounds. This use of intonation was a starting point for spoken communication, but may have been all he was able to do given physical constraints.
	Remy (and his mother) enjoyed this activity a great deal as evidenced by Remy's smiles and squeals of pleasure. Furthermore, he was able to repeat the action several times.
	Remy's mother was happy to have found an activity that supported communication and listening development, was within her son's capabilities and was pleasurable.
	Referral to an Augmentative Communication team was a clear priority given evidence of cognitive function and pleasure in interaction but with very limited control of oral motor, arm and hand musculature. He was actively followed by physical and occupational therapists. Music therapy was also helpful given his evident pleasure when listening to music.
	Work was needed with his seating team to ensure that device retention was a priority.
	Ongoing strong advocacy was needed to keep continued CI use a priority in the midst of his other demanding physical needs.

CONCLUSION

The question may arise as to whether an Auditory-Verbal practitioner should be involved with children for whom spoken language may be an unlikely goal, as is the case with some children with additional challenges. Clearly, even for the child with the most severely involved additional challenges and their families, the Auditory-Verbal practitioner has a strong role to play on the interdisciplinary team supporting the family (Daniel & Ritter, 2012). Sound plays a crucial role in human connection in the vast majority of families of children with additional challenges. Furthermore, the emphasis on individualized coaching and guidance in AVT is uniquely suited to the highly varied and unique needs of parents of children with additional challenges.

Audition is the "way in" for many, even most, of these children, and language learning is most efficiently driven by auditory development when optimal access to the sounds of life is available. In fact, audition may be the primary avenue to the development of literacy for these children, and that in itself can act as a "bootstrap effect" for language. Furthermore, parents report that music is a source of great enjoyment for their child with additional challenges and for his or her parents too (see Chapter 18). The Auditory-Verbal practitioner may be even more needed as an advocate for audition for children with severely involved additional challenges than for more typically developing children who are deaf or hard of hearing because the impact of audition, access to sound, and the development of listening skills is often less immediately obvious for these children, particularly for those with significant intellectual disability.

Research cited in this chapter increasingly confirms that the emotional and linguistic benefits derived from the child's auditory access strongly affect the development of listening skills in the child with additional challenges and has a great impact on the family in many ways: the ability to comfort a child from a distance; the child's meaningful use of intonation to communicate emotional state even if words are not developed; the willingness of others to engage with the child because he or she responds to sound, even if only to tone of voice; a reduction in self injurious behaviors; reduction of inappropriate, persistent vocal behavior allowing parents to take their children out more often to public places without the inquisitive looks of strangers—these are profound impacts of access to sound. Children with hearing loss and additional challenges need strong advocates for the right to hear. The Auditory-Verbal practitioner is uniquely positioned to assist the parent in this advocacy.

Finally, we are all in this together and we believe that it is important to acknowledge that working with children with additional challenges and their families, particularly severely involved children, places extreme demands on the skills, resourcefulness, patience, and empathy of practitioners as well as caregivers. Being consciously aware of our own processes, taking care to pace and restore ourselves as we advise parents to do, will help us to be more effective in our work with children with additional challenges and their families. McConkey-Robbins and McConkey's (2008) *Whirlwinds and Small Voices: Sustaining Commitment to Work with Special*

Needs Children addresses practitioners' need for renewal and offers excellent resources to support that process.

REFERENCES

Beer, J., Harris, M., Kronenberger, W. G., Frush-Holt, R., & Pisoni, D. (2012). Auditory skills, language development and adaptive behavior of children with cochlear implants and additional disabilities. *International Journal of Audiology, 51*(6), 491–498.

Blake, K. D., & Prasad, C. (2006). CHARGE syndrome. *Orphanet Journal of Rare Diseases, 1*(1), 34.

Blake, K., Trider, C. L., Hartshorne, T. S., & Stratton, K. K. (2016). Correspondence to Hale et al.: Atypical phenotypes associated with pathogenic CHD7 variants and a proposal for broadening CHARGE syndrome clinical diagnostic criteria. *American Journal of Medical Genetics Part A, 170*(12), 3365–3366.

Bondy, A. S., & Frost, L. A. (1994). The picture exchange communication system. *Focus on Autistic Behavior, 9*(3), 1–19.

Bondy, A. S., & Frost, L. A. (1998). The picture exchange communication system. *Seminars in Speech and Language, 19*(4), 373–388.

British Academy of Childhood Disability. (2017). Explanatory glossary of paediatric disability terms to support data collection by paediatricians at the point of clinical care. Retrieved July 1, 2018 from http://www.bacdis.org.uk/policy/dataset.htm (accessed July 1, 2018).

Bzoch, K. R., League, R., & Brown, V. L. (2003). *The Receptive-Expressive Emergent Language Scale* (3rd ed.). Austin, TX: Pro-Ed.

Cejas, I., Hoffman, M. F., & Quittner, A. L. (2015). Outcomes and benefits of pediatric cochlear implantation with additional disabilities: A review and report on family influences on outcomes. *Pediatric Health Medicine and Therapeutics, 6*, 45–63.

Cerebral Palsy Guide. (n.d.). *Types of cerebral palsy: How CP affects your child.* http://www.cerebralpalsyguide.com

Chen, D. (1999). Learning to communicate: Strategies for developing communication in infants whose multiple disabilities include visual impairment and hearing loss. *reSources: California Deaf Blind Services, 10*(5), 1–9.

Chen, D., Downing, J., & Rodriguez-Gil, G. (2016). *Hand under hand.* Washington Sensory Disabilities Services. http://www.projectsalute.net

Ching, T. Y., Dillon, H., Leigh, G., & Cupples, L. (2018). Learning from the longitudinal outcomes of children with hearing impairment (LOCHI): Summary of five year findings and implications. *International Journal of Audiology, 57*(2), 105–111.

Ching, T. Y. C. & Wong, C. L. (2017). Factors influencing child development outcomes. In E. A. Rhoades & J. Duncan (Eds.), *Auditory-verbal practice: Family-centered early intervention* (pp. 103–117). Springfield, IL: Charles C. Thomas.

Cole, E., & Flexer, C. (2015). *Children with hearing loss: Developing listening and talking, birth to six years.* San Diego, CA: Plural Publishing.

Cruz, I., Vicaria, I, Wang, N. Y., Niparko, J., Quittner, A. L., & CDaCI Investigation Team. (2012). Language and behavioral outcomes in children with developmental disabilities using cochlear implants, *Society and European Academy of Otology and Neurotology, 33*(5), 751–760.

Daniel, L., & Ritter, K. (2012). What is the role of the auditory-verbal professional with children who have multiple challenges and their families? In W. Estabrooks (Ed.), *Frequently asked questions about auditory-verbal practice* (pp. 232–236). Washington, DC: Alexander

Graham Bell Association for the Deaf and Hard of Hearing.

Donaldson, A. I., Heavner, K. S., & Zwolan T. A. (2004). Measuring progress in children with Autism spectrum disorder who have cochlear implants. *Archives Otolaryngology Head Neck Surgery, (5)*, 666–671. https://doi.org/10.1001/archotol.130.5.666

Duhigg, C. (2012). *The power of habit.* Toronto, ON, Canada: Doubleday.

Dunst, C. J. (2017). Family systems early childhood intervention. In H. Sukkar, C. J. Dunst, & J. Kirby (Eds.), *Early childhood intervention. working with families of young children with special needs* (pp. 36–58). Abingdon, UK: Routledge.

Dunst, C. (2018). Family-centered practice: Collaboration, competency and evidence. *Research Gate.* https://www.research gate.net/publication/227665906_Family -centred_practice_Collaboration_compe tency_and_evidence >publication

Figueras, B., Edwards, L., & Langdon, D. (2008). Executive function and language in deaf children. *Journal of Deaf Studies and Deaf Education, 13*(3), 362–377.

Flexer, C. (2016). Maximising outcomes for children with auditory disorders: Auditory brain development-listening for learning. *Pediatrics, 16320.* https://www .audiologyonline.com/articles/Maximiz ing Outcomes for Children with Auditory Disorders: Auditory Brain Development—Listening for Learning

Hall, M. L., Eigsti, I. M., Bortfeld, H., & Lillo-Martin, D. (2018). Executive function in deaf children: Auditory access and language access. *Journal of Speech, Language, and Hearing Research, 61*(8), 1970–1988.

Hartshorne, T. S., Nicholas, J., Grialou, T. L., & Russ, J. M. (2007). Executive function in CHARGE syndrome. *Child Neuropsychology, 13*(4), 333–344.

Hayward, D. V., Ritter, K., Grueber, J., & Howarth, T. (2013). Outcomes that matter for children with multiple disabilities who use cochlear implants: The Cochlear Implant Parent Outcomes Instrument (CIPOI). *Journal of the Canadian Association of Speech Pathologists and Audiologists, 37*(1), 58–69.

Hayward, D. V., Ritter, K., Mousavi, A., & Vatanapour, S. (2016). The Sound Access Parent Outcomes Instrument (SAPOI): Construction of a new instrument for children with severe multiple disabilities who use cochlear implants or hearing aids. *Cochlear Implants International, 17*(2), 81–89.

Herrmannova, D., Phillips, R., O'Donoghue, G., & Ramsden, R. (2009). Advanced Bionics Europe, The Ear Foundation, UK. Manchester, UK: The Royal School for the Deaf and Communication Disorders. (Available through the EAR Foundation.)

Hitchins, A. R. C., & Hogan, S. C. (2018). Outcomes of early intervention for deaf children with additional needs following an auditory-verbal approach to communication. *International Journal of Pediatric Otorhinolaryngology, 115*, 125–132.

Hogan, S., Stokes, J., White, C., Tyszkiewicz, E., & Woolgar, A. (2008). An evaluation of auditory verbal therapy using the rate of early language development as an outcome measure. *Deafness and Education International, 10*(3), 143–167.

Hogan, S., Stokes, J., & Weller I. (2010). Language outcomes for children of low-income families enrolled in auditory-verbal therapy. *Deafness and Education International, 12*(4), 204–216.

Holden-Pitt, L., & Diaz, J. A. (1998). Thirty years of the annual survey of deaf and hard of hearing children and youth: A glance over the decades. *American Annals of the Deaf, 143*, 71–76. http://dx .doi.org/10.1353/aad.2012.0630

I Can Centre. (n.d.). *Partner-enhanced communication strategies.* Edmonton, AB, Canada: Glenrose Hospital.

Kishon-Rabin, L., Taitelbaum-Swead, R., Ezrati-Vinacour, J., Kronenberg, M., & Hildesheimer, M. (2005). Pre-lexical vocalizations in normal hearing and hearing impaired infants before and after cochlear implantation and its relationship to auditory skills. (Production Infant Scale Evaluation–PRISE). *Ear and Hearing, 26,* 17–29.

Koch, D. (2004). *Infant-Toddler Meaningful Auditory Integration Scale (IT-MAIS): Normal-hearing age equivalency.* Sylmar, CA: Advanced Bionics Corp.

Kubler-Ross, E. (1969). *On death and dying.* New York, NY: The Macmillan Company.

Kuhn-Inacker, H., Weichbold, V., Tsiapini, I., Coninx, F., & D'Haese, P. (2003). *Little Ears auditory questionnaire.* Innsbruck, Austria: MED-EL.

Ling, D. (1976). *Speech and the hearing impaired child: Theory and practice.* Washington, DC: Alexander Graham Bell Association for the Deaf and Hard of Hearing.

Luterman, D. (2016). *Counseling persons with communication disorders and their families* (3rd Ed.). Austin, TX: Pro-Ed.

Luterman, D. (1995). *In the shadows: Living and coping with a loved one's chronic illness.* Bedford, MA: Jade Press.

Martin, K., & Elder, S. (1993). Pathways through grief: A model of the process. In J. Morgan (Ed.), *Personal care in an impersonal world* (pp. 73–86). Amityville, NY: Baywood Publishing Company.

Martin, K., & Ritter, K. (2011). Navigating the emotional impact of diagnosis. *Volta Voices,* May/June, 14–16.

McConkey-Robbins, A., & McConkey, C. (2008). *Whirlwinds and small voices: Sustaining commitment to work with special needs children.* London, ON, Canada: Wordplay.

McCracken, W., & Turner, O. (2011). *Complex needs complex challenges: A report on research into the experiences of families with deaf children with additional complex needs.* London, UK: National Deaf Children's Society (NDCS).

Mitchell, R. E., & Karchmer, M. A. (2004). When parents are deaf versus hard of hearing: Patterns of sign use and school placement of deaf and hard-of-hearing children. *Journal of Deaf Studies and Deaf Education, 9*(2), 133–152.

Muncy, M., Yoho, S., & Brunson-McClain, M. (2019). Confidence of school-based speech language pathologists and psychologists in assessing students with hearing loss and co-occurring disabilities. *Language Speech and Hearing Services in the Schools.* https://doi.org/10.1044/2018_LSHSS-18-0091

Olds, J., Fitzpatrick, E., Steacie, P., Somerville, R., Neuss, D., Rabjohn, K., . . . Schramm, D. (2016, May). *Long term outcome after cochlear implantation in children with complex needs: Parents' perspectives.* Poster Presented at CI International, Toronto, ON.

Palmer, P. J. (1998). *The courage to teach: Exploring the inner landscape of a teacher's life.* San Francisco, CA: Jossey-Bass.

Palmieri, M., Forli, F., & Berrettini, S. (2014). Cochlear implant outcome for deaf children with additional disabilities: A systematic review. *Hearing, Balance and Communication, 12*(1), 6–19.

Pepper, J., & Weitzman, E. (2004). *It takes two to talk: A practical guide for parents of children with language delays.* Toronto, ON, Canada: The Hanen Centre.

Perigoe, C., & Perigoe, R. (2004). Multiple challenges—multiple solutions: Children with hearing loss and special needs. *Volta Review Monograph, 104*(4).

Phillips, L. M., Hayward, D. V., & Norris, S. P. (2016). *Test of early language and literacy.* Toronto, ON, Canada: Nelson Publishing.

Ritter, K., & Logan de Chavez, K. (2011). *The Ling Six Sound Test.* Produced and directed by the Northern Alberta Institute of Technology Digital Media Program, Justin Evans, director. Video available on AG Bell Pinterest page and the following YouTube web address: http://www.youtube.com/The Ling Six Sound Test

Ritter, K., & Hayward, D. V. (2016). *The Sound Access Parent Outcome Instrument (SAPOI)*. Retrieved from https://drive.google.com/file/d/1EvMlt06rcoAJoOGeornMRelS34P6gDRQ/view?usp=sharing

Rossetti, L. M. (2006). *The Rossetti infant-toddler language scale*. East Moline, IL: LinguiSystems.

Romski, M. A., & Sevcik, R. A. (2005). Augmentative communication and early intervention: Myths and realities. *Infants and Young Children, 18*(3), 174–184.

Sheehy, K., & Duffy, H. (2009). Attitudes to Makaton in the ages on integration and inclusion. *International Journal of Special Education, 24*(2), 91–102.

Staugler, K. (2007). Literacy rubric. Retrieved from https://wvde.state.wv.us/osp/supporting-literacy/assessment.html

Tatenhove, G. (2007). Normal language development, generative language and AAC. Retrieved from http://www.texasat.net/Assets/1--normal-language--aac.pdf.

Van Kaam, A., & Muto, S. (1993). *The power of appreciation: New approach to personal relational healing*. New York, NY: Crossroads Publishing.

Wilkinson, K., & Hennig, S. (2007). The state of research and practice in augmentative and alternative communication for children with developmental/intellectual disabilities. *Mental Retardation and Developmental Disabilities Research Reviews, 13*, 58–69.

World Health Organization's International Classification of Functioning, Disability and Health (ICF). Retrieved March 13, 2019 from https://www.who.int/classifications/icf/en/

Young, N., Weil, C., & Tournis, E. (2016). Redefining cochlear implant benefits to appropriately include children with additional disabilities. In N. Young & K. Iler-Kirk (Eds.), *Pediatric cochlear implantation*. New York, NY: Springer.

Zimmerman-Phillips, S., Osberger, M. J., & Robbins, A. M. (2001). *Infant-toddler meaningful auditory integration scale*. Sylmar, CA: Advanced Bionics Co.

Zimerman, I. L., Steiner, V. G., Evatt-Pond, R., Karas, G. B., & Marshal, J. (2011). *PLS-5: Preschool Language Scales*. Bloomington, MN: Pearson/PsychCorp.

23

MULTI-LINGUALISM AND AUDITORY-VERBAL THERAPY

Elizabeth M. Fitzpatrick and Suzanne P. Doucet

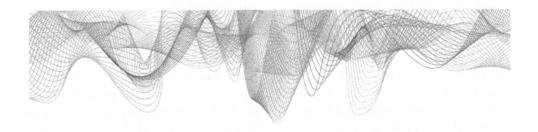

"If you talk to a man in a language he understands, that goes to his head. If you talk to him in his own language, that goes to his heart."
— Nelson Mandela

Multilingualism is a global reality. More than 7000 languages are used around the world and more than half of the world's population is multilingual (Grosjean, 2013). Even though multilingualism may also include the use of sign language with a spoken language (Grosjean, 2001), this chapter refers only to spoken language. Several definitions exist for multilingualism and common elements include the ability to use more than one language either actively (speaking and writing) or passively (listening and reading) (International Expert Panel on Multilingual Children's Speech, 2012; Li, 2008). Multilingualism involves linguistic competence in another language and also permits access to the social and philosophical dimensions of different cultures.

Multilingualism is acquired through a variety of contexts and circumstances. Children may grow up in families where parents or other family members speak more than one language. Parents, whether multilingual themselves or not, may choose to expose their children to more than one language. Many countries take pride in their bilingual or multilingual status. Switzerland, Belgium, and Canada, for example, are countries where many parents embrace multilingualism and create opportunities for their children to acquire more than one language. In some countries, minority groups of indigenous people such as those who speak Cree in Canada or Maori in New Zealand typically need to learn the dominant language for social and economic reasons. Similarly, immigrants usually learn the language of their new country in addition to their minority heritage language(s). In particular, many individuals choose to learn English as the international language that provides access to economic, educational, and social opportunities (Cenoz, 2013). Increasingly in a globally connected world, learning more than one language is viewed as an advantage for people of all ages. It is well documented that exposure to another language in early childhood has social and cognitive benefits (Bialystok, 2009; Genesee, 2015).

Historical Practices

It has been historically well established that a young child's brain is biologically ready to learn multiple languages with relative ease (Byers-Heinlein, Burns, & Werker, 2010; Werker, 2012). Most children with typical development can learn multiple languages fluently, especially when exposed to them at an early age (Byers-Heinlein et al., 2010; Genesee, 2015; Werker, 2012). Children who are deaf or hard of hearing and have identified communication disorders, however, have traditionally been thought to be at a disadvantage for learning more than one language. There is little or no published information on historical

practices with children who are deaf or hard of hearing and there has been considerable variation in delivery of services among practitioners. Auditory-Verbal practitioners frequently recommended that families of children with hearing loss choose one language, usually the language parents planned for their child's education (Fitzpatrick & Doucet, 2013; Levasseur & Rhoades, 2001). For the most part, practitioners believed that children needed to establish a dominant language first and only then be exposed to another language, most often at school age. These practices were likely influenced by the fact that children had limited auditory access, resulting in delayed speech and language (Karchmer & Mitchell, 2003; Marschark & Spencer, 2006). This applied particularly to children with severe and profound hearing loss primarily before cochlear implantation became a standard of care (Geers, Moog, Biedenstein, Brenner, & Hayes, 2009). These practices, however, tended to be applied to all children with hearing loss and Auditory-Verbal practitioners did not typically encourage parents to expose their children to multiple languages.

Essentially, past practices were based on beliefs that children with communication disorders had difficulty processing two languages (Grosjean & Byers-Heinlein, 2018). Sometimes called the *Cumulative Effects Hypothesis*, the theory that exposure to more than one language could have harmful effects on overall language acquisition was well accepted (Paradis & Govindarajan, 2018). Essentially, the belief was that a solid foundation in only one language optimized learning opportunities for the child and that it would facilitate development in that language, and in academics and literacy. This recommendation also applied to newly arrived families who were expected to use the language of the new country and essentially "drop" their native language in the home. In some jurisdictions, children with hearing loss were sometimes exempted from learning a second language in school and time at school was focused on speech-language development in the majority language and on academic subjects (Fitzpatrick & Doucet, 2013). These decisions were based on an understanding that learning more than one language was complex and would possibly confuse and/ or result in further vocabulary and language delay (Genesee, 2015; Ling & Ling, 1978).

EXAMPLE FROM A MINORITY LANGUAGE REGION

Despite the lack on emphasis on dual language learning, it is evident that some children developed bilingualism. For example, our recent research has shown that children with hearing loss, educated during the late 1990s, learned a second language, often as adolescents or young adults. We completed interviews with 12 young French-speaking adults and 9 parents who grew up in a minority French-speaking language context in the Canadian province of New Brunswick. Ten youth had bilateral severe or profound hearing loss and two had moderately-severe hearing loss. All had received Auditory-Verbal Therapy (AVT) shortly after the diagnosis. The primary objective of our study was to examine their outcomes in terms of overall social integration in post-secondary school or work life

and in their communities. Our findings provided interesting insights into their experiences growing up in a minority linguistic environment. Consistent with services at the time, they did not receive specific instruction in English during the preschool and elementary years and some were exempted from English courses throughout their school years. Others started attending English classes at school in their early adolescent years. Through interviews, we learned that the majority of these young people developed some level of proficiency in English. From the perspectives of some of the youth and young adults, not speaking English was a disadvantage as they entered adulthood. They informed us that learning to speak English was often motivated by a perceived need related to friendships, post-secondary study or work, and a sense of not belonging (see quotes below). Of the 12 young adults, 10 acquired a level of proficiency that permitted them to work in bilingual or English-only environments. While they were pleased with their progress in English, they also expressed their pride of continuing to communicate in French, their first language.

These young adults shared a variety of strategies they had used to learn their second language. These included listening to television with captioning, community-based extracurricular activities in English, and short-term immersion courses. The following quotes (translated from French) capture reflections of these francophone Canadian youth:

In school, I was afraid to speak in English because I had never heard the language, so I didn't know how to pronounce the words. As I was a perfectionist, I was afraid to say things because I feared that everybody would laugh at me since it wouldn't be the right way. (young adult, profound hearing loss; hearing aids)

I changed jobs and it was difficult to adapt because the team was more Anglophone and people spoke English together. So, when I went to lunch with them, there were one or two who spoke to me in French, but others just had their arms crossed because they didn't speak French, so that didn't make me feel that I was part of the team. (young adult, profound hearing loss; hearing aids)

I ended up working with a team of English-speaking guys and even though it was very difficult at first, they were very understanding. They even wrote out the technical terms and words to help me understand . . . Now I'm really happy that I forced myself to become bilingual because now when I travel, like I can speak French in Quebec or English in Ontario (young adult, profound hearing loss; cochlear implant)

I love watching Korean movies with English subtitles. I don't understand everything but reading the subtitles helps me learn English little by little. (young adult, profound hearing loss; cochlear implant)

BENEFITS OF MULTILINGUALISM

Typically Developing Children

Research has clearly shown benefits associated with multilingualism for typically developing children. Benefits in a range of linguistic and cognitive domains have been reported including: improved linguistic and literacy skills (Jasińska & Petitto, 2018; Kovelman & Petitto, 2008), attention, and executive functioning (Bialystok, 2009; Dong & Li, 2015). In addition to these behavioral results, there is emerging evidence from objective measures (e.g., event related potentials) that bilingual children outperform their monolingual peers on tasks related to executive functioning, referred to by the investigators as a type of "brain training" (Barac, Moreno, & Bialystok, 2016). Research using objective measures showed that in young 19- to 22-month-old English-Spanish bilingual children, even very brief exposure periods to a second language resulted in different patterns of neural activity (Conboy & Mills, 2006). This suggests that language experience influences language-relevant brain activity (Garcia-Sierra et al., 2011). Furthermore, these findings suggest that training changes the brain's responses to languages even with a brief period of exposure during childhood.

Benefits of Multilingualism for Children with Communication Disorders

Similar to our early beliefs for children with hearing loss, professionals working with children with other types of communication disorders adhered to the *Cumulative Effects Hypothesis*. Contrary to these early beliefs, several studies with children with communication disorders in multilingual environments have shown they are not at a disadvantage compared with their monolingual peers (Paradis & Govindarajan, 2018). Paradis and Govindarajan conclude that bilingual children with specific language impairment function similarly to monolingual peers in terms of grammatical structures and vocabulary and narrative abilities. However, as the authors point out, other studies have shown gaps between bilingual and monolingual children with specific language impairment in these areas. Similarly, for children with autism spectrum disorders (ASD), research with bilingual children has not shown important differences in their communication development compared with monolingual children with ASD (Paradis & Govindarajan, 2018). Based on a systematic review of the literature on multilingualism and neurodevelopmental disorders (Uljarević, Katsos, Hudry, & Gibson, 2016), the authors concluded that there are no negative effects on language and other developmental areas for children with these disorders. Our conclusion from this body of literature is that there is no convincing evidence that learning more than one language interferes with language acquisition for children with communication disorders.

Evidence Supporting Multilingualism in Children Who Are Deaf or Hard of Hearing

Our understanding for children who are deaf or hard of hearing has also shifted to recognizing the potential advantages of multilingualism. Combined with findings from neuroscience and clinical studies, a confluence of factors including greater acoustic accessibility through cochlear implantation and

other hearing technology, and early intervention, have influenced therapy practices. Consequently, multilingualism has become a possibility for more children and the need for culturally competent services has become a new reality (Bowen, 2016; McConkey Robbins, Green, & Waltzman, 2004; Rhoades, 2008; Rhoades, Price, & Perigoe, 2004) Various recommendations for models of practice have subsequently evolved; these will be elaborated in a subsequent section.

Despite this change in practice, there remains relatively little research on this new generation of children who are deaf and hard of hearing and who are bilingual and multilingual language learners. Reports suggest that there are increasing numbers of multilingual children who are deaf or hard of hearing in early intervention and educational programs. In an Australian population-based study of children with hearing loss, 25% of the children were from homes where parents spoke a language other than English (Crowe, McLeod, & Ching, 2012). In the United States, the Gallaudet Research Institute reported that almost 20% of children nationwide and up to 25% in some regions were English language learners from non-English speaking homes (Gallaudet Research Institute, 2013). At this time, in Canada, there is no specific information available related to those with hearing loss but in the most recent Canadian census, 20.6% reported using a home language other than English or French (Statistics Canada, 2016).

Much of what is known about outcomes in children with hearing loss and who are multilingual comes from the cochlear implant literature. There are many children from multilingual homes whose parents seek cochlear implants, and this has ignited an interest. Crowe and McLeod (2014) conducted a systematic review to investigate factors influencing linguistic outcomes in children who are deaf or hard of hearing who used languages other than English. The majority of the 117 studies retrieved were related to monolingual children and only 8 studies focused on multilingual children; 4 from children using cochlear implants, 2 with both children using implants or hearing aids, and 2 with children using only hearing aids. There is evidence that children who are deaf or hard of hearing can develop two or more languages, including their heritage language and the majority societal language. In 3 studies reported in the review, children with cochlear implants developed skills in their dominant language comparable to monolingual peers (McConkey Robbins et al., 2004; Thomas, El-Kashlan, & Zwolan, 2008; Waltzman, Robbins, Green, & Cohen, 2003). However, the same review also reported on studies of children with hearing aids or cochlear implants from multilingual homes who had more difficulty developing the dominant language than their monolingual peers (Kiese-Himmel, 2008; Teschendorf, Janeschik, Bagus, Lang, & Arweiler-Harbeck, 2011).

Recent studies have also reported better language outcomes in multilingual children who are deaf or hard of hearing compared with their monolingual peers (Bunta et al., 2016; Guiberson, 2014). Studies investigating the relationship between multilingualism and various linguistic outcomes (e.g., speech perception, speech production, language) have found that multilingualism does not have a negative effect on learning the community language (Bunta & Douglas, 2013; Lund, Werfel, & Schuele, 2015). Other recent studies on children with cochlear implants, however, have reported poorer outcomes in multilingual children (Deriaz, Pelizzone, & Perez Fornos, 2014; Forli et al., 2018). The authors do point out that these results may be related to the conditions for bilingual learning in particular study contexts (Forli et al., 2018). Like other areas of study in intervention outcomes, the small number of studies with mixed results limit the conclusions. The best available evidence seems to suggest that children who are deaf or hard of hearing can achieve multilingualism. The factors that lead to proficiency, however, are not yet well understood.

Similarly, there is also limited information on optimal interventions for children who are deaf or hard of hearing. In a scoping review, Guiberson and Crowe (2018) sought to retrieve studies related to appropriate interventions for multilingual children with hearing loss. Only two publications met the criteria (Cannon & Guardino, 2012; Guiberson, 2005) and described interventions with multilingual children with hearing loss. Guiberson and Crowe (2018) also reported on multiple interventions (e.g., enhanced vocabulary training, narrative or story grammar) that have been used with multilingual children without hearing loss, some of whom had special needs. Given the limited specific research on multilingual children who are deaf or hard of hearing, the authors concluded that little is known about the effectiveness of any particular intervention for this population.

Consistent with the literature on children who are deaf or hard of hearing more generally, and the heterogeneity in study populations, the problem of conducting large studies in low-incidence conditions such as childhood hearing loss, and the variability in study characteristics, and outcomes reported, make it difficult to draw good conclusions about the effects of multilingualism on spoken language outcomes, From the literature, it is evident that this is a developing field and more research is required before a clearer picture emerges. Taken together, the body of literature suggests that children can and do learn two languages and that exposure to another language in learning contexts that support multilingualism does not seem to have a negative impact on spoken language outcomes (Bunta et al., 2016; Crowe & McLeod, 2014; Guiberson & Crowe, 2018).

INTERVENTION PRACTICES

Multilingualism is valued in many different contexts in different countries. Embracing multilingualism involves much more than considering the linguistic needs of the child and family. It encompasses a multicultural approach to services that recognizes and respects the diversity of families (Bowen, 2016; Moeller, Carr, Seaver, Stredler-Brown, & Holzinger, 2013; Rhoades, 2008). Language is learned within a cultural context. Parent–child interactions and how children learn to communicate and socialize are anchored in their culture and beliefs. Rhoades (2008) emphasizes the importance of cultural awareness and sensitivity in providing services to families. A recent scoping review on culturally competent care in pediatric rehabilitation more generally showed

that parents from multicultural families experienced difficulty communicating their feelings and understanding treatment goals in therapy (Grandpierre et al., 2018). Interviews with Canadian parents from an AVT program who shared their perspectives indicated that important aspects of care included sensitivity around the notion of disability in some cultures, and clear and sensitive communication with practitioners (Grandpierre et al., in press). For example, these families viewed extensive use of written materials in English as a barrier. Parents also highlighted the need for practitioners to promote multilingualism, and to promote the parents' need to feel supported in their linguistic choices. Two main categories of children and families requiring multilingual support are serviced in the clinical context. The first consists of families who arrive in a new country and are required to learn the majority language to integrate into a new culture. Often referred to as culturally and linguistically diverse families, they are frequently adapting to both a new language and a new culture and lifestyle. The second large category consists of multilingual families who use the dominant language and choose bilingualism for their children. Although there are similarities in intervention approaches for these children and families, as discussed below, there are also differences that must be taken into account.

Much of what we know about multilanguage acquisition stems from an extensive body of research on children with typical hearing. This knowledge provides a useful foundation for intervention in young children with hearing loss who are using hearing to develop more than one spoken language, such as AVT. In other words, therapy and education programs have been influenced by best practices for children with typical development learning more than one language. A recent study suggests that providing dual language support that supports the development of both the heritage and majority languages is advantageous for children with hearing loss in AVT (Bunta et al., 2016). In this study, expressive language scores were better for children who received AVT in both languages compared with those with English-only AVT. Optimal intervention practices and recommendations for multilingual development in children with hearing loss are continuing to develop (Bunta et al., 2016; Douglas, 2014; Guiberson & Crowe, 2018).

Assessment of Multilingual Children

An assessment to determine the child's communication abilities and linguistic profile is an essential component of the initial encounter with the family in Auditory-Verbal Therapy. Early detection results in many young children entering intervention programs before they acquire spoken language, and therefore they will not receive an initial language assessment using standardized measures. Observation of the child's listening and communication skills, a parent report, and checklists and parent questionnaires are commonly used to assess the child's functioning in the early stages (Neuss et al., 2013). In addition, assessing and understanding the family's preferences and needs, as well as differences in parent–child interaction is a fundamental first step in planning an intervention program with multilingual families. For all children, regardless of age of intervention, early AVT sessions need to focus on coaching families with the practitioner's understanding of the language(s) in the home, school, and other learning and play environments (see Chapter 17). The assessment involves accounting for whether the child is learning multiple languages simultaneously or sequentially. Simultaneous acquisition generally refers to learning two or more languages at the same time by age 3 years, while sequential acquisition involves learning a second language after age 3 years (Genesee, Paradis, & Crago, 2004).

For older children who have some language ability, the Auditory-Verbal practitioner determines the language and nature of the assessment (e.g., measurement tools available). Douglas (2014) recommends when possible that an evaluation be carried out by a practitioner who speaks the family's heritage language, or with assistance from an examiner who speaks the language. If this is not possible, completing the assessment through an interpreter is the preferred option. However, these resources may not always be available, and practitioners may need to adapt assessments by working through a bilingual family, community member, or the parent.

It is well recognized that preferred assessment tools (e.g., standardized tests with good psychometric properties) may not be available in the heritage language and that results need to be interpreted and applied with caution (Douglas, 2014; Gaul Bouchard, Fitzpatrick, & Olds, 2009). Other tools such as criterion-referenced tools, parent questionnaires, and language samples may also constitute a core part of the assessment. For some children, a combined assessment using more than one language may be required to establish a comprehensive profile of the child's auditory and communication abilities. While children may appear to present delays or difficulties in one or more languages, the combined results may help to identify overall strengths and weaknesses in their communication skills. This can help focus intervention goals, such as those determined by the AV practitioner and the family in AVT. They can decide on the requirement for more emphasis on one language or the other, or both in therapy sessions and in the child's everyday environment. However, as noted by Paradis and Govindarajan (2018), differences in the rate of language acquisition in children with communication disorders can make it difficult to discern a true language delay in bilingual learners. For guidance and specific details on assessment and interpretation of various linguistic skills when working with multilingual children, the reader is referred to a useful published resource by Douglas (2014).

Early Intervention

In general, current practices in Auditory-Verbal Therapy support the provision of intervention based on the child's linguistic profile (Douglas, 2014). For early-identified children who are deaf or hard of hearing, the current tendency is to recommend using the home language as the primary language of intervention. This has been found to support healthy parent–child interaction and enhances language exposure because

parents are more comfortable and natural in their native language (Genesee et al., 2004; Kohnert, Yim, Nett, Kan, & Duran, 2005). Furthermore, children exposed to two languages at an early age are not disadvantaged compared with their monolingual peers and may even experience advantages in language and reading at school age (Petitto & Dunbar, 2009).

For families who choose multilingualism for their children, various options concerning their preferences and long-term goals can be discussed. It is often not feasible for the Auditory-Verbal practitioner to conduct therapy sessions in the child's heritage language. Possible options for service delivery, therefore, may include the following: (1) the AVT session takes place entirely or partially in the minority language of the family, but in the home language outside of the AVT session; and (2) the AVT session takes places in two languages, that is, the Auditory-Verbal practitioner uses the dominant language (family's minority language, e.g., English), and the parent stimulates the child in his or her own language. Douglas (2014) recommends that therapy be provided in the child's dominant language when children have already developed spoken language. However, when children do not show a clear language dominance (e.g., learning both languages simultaneously), the language of intervention is likely to be a joint decision between the parent and the AV practitioner. Furthermore, the emphasis placed on each language may vary depending on the child's development and exposure in different environments. In some cases, in order to strengthen the language parents have chosen for the child's education, the practitioner may opt to focus on the school language in AVT sessions, rather than the child's home language. What seems to be the most important is that, like typically developing children, the child with hearing loss be immersed in both languages. In summary, consistent with the principles of AVT (see Chapter 1), continuous monitoring of the child's auditory and communication competence in each language and consideration of parents' preferences help determine the needs for adjustment in the intervention program (Douglas, 2014.).

For children who are deaf or hard of hearing who have additional complex medical and developmental needs, decisions about multilingualism may involve other considerations, including the choice of educational facilities. There is very little in the literature that is related to multilingualism for these children. As discussed above, based on evidence from children with typical hearing and developmental challenges, there seems to be no disadvantage for these children to be exposed to more than one language (Genesee, 2015; Peña, 2016; Uljarević, Hudry, & Gibson, 2016). For some children with severe cognitive disabilities, spoken language may not be achievable. Qualitative interviews with parents of children with severe challenges and cochlear implants indicated that sound awareness, alone, and the child's connectedness with her environment were positive outcomes (Olds, Fitzpatrick, Steacie, McLean, & Schramm, 2007). Therefore, for these children, singing and exposure to rhythm and sounds in the parents' heritage language would not seem to interfere with the potential benefits from intervention (see Chapter 18).

Intervention Models

Various intervention models exist to accommodate a multitude of family situations seen in clinical and educational services. Douglas (2014) presents various simultaneous and sequential bilingual intervention models to guide practitioners. These models describe intervention practices that can support multilingual learning for children from different family profiles. For example, in a *monolingual minority language* speaking family, AVT can be offered in the minority language if possible or through an assistant or interpreter and the minority language is used at home. The child learns the majority language through exposure at preschool or daycare. In contrast, in a *bilingual-majority and minority language* speaking family, AVT is conducted in the majority language and parent uses the minority language at home. While these models may be effective and highly desirable, they may not necessarily represent what is offered, particularly in smaller regions and clinics where trained interpreters and assistants are not easily available. In these cases, parents and clinicians work together to find the best way to implement services that respect and promote the family's language and cultural values.

In many countries, *sequential* bilingual learning is a common practice, where children learn the majority language of the country or of the family and start acquiring another language in the early school years. Such is the situation in countries like Canada, where English-speaking families choose French immersion for their children or French-speaking children are exposed to English as a second language in school. Increasingly, children who are deaf or hard of hearing are expected to follow the same programs as their hearing peers with school support services when required.

Auditory-Verbal Therapy for Multilingual Learners

Auditory-Verbal therapy is based on typical developmental language learning sequences and involves facilitating language learning in as natural a way as possible. However, to enhance spoken language acquisition through auditory learning, numerous specific strategies have been developed and widely adopted over the years. Examples include selecting certain words or phrases that are acoustically salient and rich in suprasegmental information such as animal sounds (e.g., meow) and using acoustic highlighting to emphasize key words in a phrase (see Chapters 16 and 17).

To our knowledge, there has been no research on the use of specific strategies with children who have hearing loss who are learning more than one language. It appears reasonable to assume that the same strategies described in depth in Chapters 16 and 17 are applicable to multilingual children. For example, ensuring that the child is immersed in frequent, varied, and meaningful experiences in the languages the family has selected would seem most desirable. Douglas (2014) recommends that children spend at least 20% to 30% of their day immersed in their minority language, and also suggests that setting up clear linguistic boundaries may facilitate multilingual language learning. Families may wish to consider: (1) using the minority language at home, and children learn the majority language in their community (e.g., at daycare, preschool, playgroups); (2) using one parent-one language, where bilingual parents can decide that one parent speaks the minority language and the other speaks the majority language to the child; or (3) using language according to time and place, where the child is exposed to both minority and majority languages but in different environments; for example, the child is exposed to the minority language in the childcare setting (e.g., at a relative's home) and to the majority language at home; similar options may include different linguistic environments on different days, which might be achieved through a variety of childcare arrangements. These options likely reflect the diverse scenarios that naturally occur for typically developing children in multilingual environments. However, a fundamental difference is that for children who are deaf or hard of hearing, these situations may be more carefully planned and monitored than for children with typical hearing.

As noted previously, in multilinguistic contexts, the language of the AVT session is decided with the family depending on what is possible in the particular intervention program (e.g., availability of a bilingual practitioner or interpreter). The Auditory-Verbal practitioner supports the child and family by coaching them in the most effective ways to use the teaching strategies for listening, talking, and thinking that are outlined in Chapters 16 and 17. AV practitioners may need to adapt the flow of the session (see Chapter 17) to accommodate more repetition and to coach and guide in two languages to support families who are not comfortable in the majority language and/or who prefer to speak their home language during the AVT session. In addition, practitioners may enlist the assistance of social workers to engage support from members of the family or the family's linguistic community. Auditory-Verbal practitioners may be required to extend their coaching expertise well beyond the boundaries of the typical clinical or educational setting. This may involve teaching strategies to individuals who interact with the child in different linguistic settings (e.g., preschool) to maximize the opportunities for auditory and language exposure in all language learning environments.

In the school setting, Auditory-Verbal practitioners or specialized teachers often work with children at school age who are from bilingual families. Teachers stress the importance of understanding the family dynamic (e.g., cultural values, social environment) to better coach families about providing an optimal learning environment at home for the child's heritage language or second language depending on the child's linguistic strengths. Concrete examples include encouraging parents to expose their children to the weaker language through outside school activities such as friends, movies, books, and other family members. Since an important part of learning for the school-age child takes place in the classroom, adopting strategies that have been implemented to assist any child with multilingual needs would seem appropriate. Brice and Roseberry-McKibbin (2001) summarize several strategies for teachers working with bilingual children in classrooms such as: (1) reiteration for emphasis, (2) vocabulary expansion and vocabulary checking to ensure students have understood the information, (3) maintaining a flexible learning environment to encourage participation in any language, and (4) showing appreciation for the student's native language and culture.

For individual AVT sessions, the reader is directed to Chapter 17, which provides guidelines for a number of therapy session models that are applicable for the facilitatation of the development of two languages or more. In addition, examples of other recommendations and strategies used by Auditory-Verbal practitioners and specialized teachers, when working with multilingual children and families, are provided in Tables 23–1 and 23–2. Some of these are general parent coaching tips, while others are specific to an AVT session. The primary message from practitioners is that the goals, content, and strategies used in therapy sessions do not differ substantially when working with multilingual compared with monolingual children. Several practitioners indicated that the most striking difference in their sessions with multilingual children is related to how they coach parents about language stimulation at home. The reflections in Tables 23–1 and 23–2 highlight the diverse situations in which children who are deaf or hard of hearing are learning more than one language.

Table 23–1. Example of Recommendations for Bilingual Families (French and English) in a French Minority Context

- Understand the family dynamic (type of family, cultural values, social environment, etc.) to provide better coaching regarding language development for a child from a bilingual home by understanding which language is spoken in different situations.
- Provide information on the relationship between good language foundations and literacy acquisition and on social relationships and communication development.
- Talk about parents' attitude toward their second language and how to cultivate a positive attitude in themselves and their child toward the second language (e.g., for parents who say: "I'm awful at French." "I just can't learn the language").
- Encourage parents who speak French to use it on a daily basis with their child or to involve extended family members who speak French in the child's daily activities.
- Discuss with parents how to increase exposure to French as a second language (e.g., inviting friends from school to play at home, going to see a French movie, reading books, listening to audiobooks, singing together in French, spending time with a French babysitter).

Note: Information in this table is based on contributions from Auditory-Verbal practitioners: Jasmine Gallant, Mélissa Leblanc, and Deirdre Neuss.

Table 23–2. Examples of Recommendations and Strategies for Early Intervention Auditory-Verbal Therapy Sessions

- Encourage parents to use the language with which they are most comfortable; when parents are concerned about which language to use, remind them that early therapy is about stimulating the brain and the specific language is not important.
- Recognize that new immigrants are coping with new situations that require adaptation and this can affect interaction with their children. Cultural sensitivity and understanding parents' realities and barriers (e.g., cultural perspectives related to hearing aids, timing of appointments) are priorities.
- Use interpreters when necessary; however, it is important to recognize that interpreters can change the communication dynamic with parents during the therapy session.
- Include another family member when possible and when necessary to help with translation.
- Keep the focus on the parent during the session; continue to convey the message about auditory stimulation and ensure that parents are providing primary language input during the session.

continues

Table 23–2. *continued*

- Include some therapy sessions at home, when possible (if therapy is conducted provided in a clinic) to increase cultural sensitivity and to better understand the child's learning context.
- Use visual material extensively to assist with comprehension and use written or audio materials translated in the parents' language when possible.
- Conduct the therapy session in English and foster parent interaction in the home language.
- Provide appropriate vocabulary in the majority language when child uses vocabulary in the heritage language,
- Use a "sandwich" approach in therapy, teaching language through parents or siblings (when the therapist does not speak heritage language): heritage language first, then English, followed by heritage language or vice versa English first.
- Recommend that families use the sandwich approach at home, when one parent is fluent in English and the other not fluent.
- Recommend that families alternate language days at home, e.g., one day English, one day Chinese.
- Help parents to generate a list of learning to listen words in the heritage language and choose materials such as ethnic foods, animals, and toys to accompany these beginning words.
- Ensure that phonemes not used in the dominant language are practiced, if needed, through games and play activities.
- Use assessments including translated versions cautiously. The assessment tool can serve as a guide and parents can assist with conducting and interpreting the assessment.

Note: Information in this table is based on contributions from Auditory-Verbal practitioners: Jasmine Gallant, Mélissa Leblanc, Deirdre Neuss, Maha Shabana, and Rosemary Somerville.

CASE EXAMPLES

Tables 23–3 to 23–5 present case examples that capture practitioners' experiences with multilingual families in AVT sessions. These three scenarios illustrate how practitioners adapt their sessions to support multilingual development: (1) therapist uses majority language, parent uses heritage language, (2) therapist and parent use same majority language, (3) bilingual therapist uses school language in therapy; one parent is monolingual, and one is bilingual. These scenarios reflect the cultural and linguistic diversity as well as choices of families in today's Auditory-Verbal Therapy programs.

Table 23-3. Case Example 1

Name of child	Etiology
Yusuf	Unknown

Degree and type of hearing loss	
Severe bilateral sensorineural hearing loss	

Chronological age	Hearing age
18 months	2 months

Auditory-verbal age	Hearing technology history
2 months	Binaural hearing aids at 16 months

Developmental history

Full-term baby, no family history of hearing loss. Child has been seen by pediatrician. No other developmental concerns have been reported.

Case history/family context

The family arrived from Lebanon 10 months ago. Yusuf is an only child. The family speaks Arabic as their native language and Mother is proficient in French as a second language. Mom is a nurse but cannot yet practice in Canada. While taking courses, she has decided to provide daycare services in her home in French. The father, who is a teacher, is working as a youth support worker in a community center.

The family doctor referred Yusuf for an audiological assessment because the parents were concerned that he was not responding well to sounds. Since the hearing aid fitting, Yusuf attends weekly sessions with an Auditory-Verbal practitioner.

Auditory-Verbal Therapy

The Auditory-Verbal practitioner speaks English and French, but not Arabic. The Auditory-Verbal Therapy sessions take place in French, a decision that was made after discussion with both parents shortly after hearing aid fitting. This was decided because the child is exposed to French through the home daycare, and the parents indicated that they were likely to send him to school in French. Arabic is spoken in the home and parents were encouraged to continue to use Arabic in interacting with Yusuf.

Consistent with an Auditory-Verbal Therapy intervention plan for beginning listeners, the focus in therapy at this stage is on developing sound awareness, consistent response to sounds, early vocalizations and sound-word associations. In therapy, the auditory-verbal practitioner and Mother both interact with the child in French as the practitioner coaches Mother. Since Mother speaks French as a second language, the interactions take place as in any typical Auditory-Verbal Therapy session. Throughout the session and particularly in the wrap-up at the end, the practitioner encourages Mom to think of how she and Father can integrate the goals into their activities when speaking Arabic. For example, she prompts her to think of appropriate songs with lots of rhythm and repetition and she asks Mom to write out a short list of sound-word associations in their home language that can be shared with Father.

Note: Information in this table is based on discussions with Auditory-Verbal practitioners: Jasmine Gallant, Mélissa Leblanc, Deirdre Neuss, Maha Shabana, and Rosemary Somerville.

Table 23-4. Case Example 2

Name of child	Etiology
Tariqah	Meningitis

Degree and type of hearing loss	
Bilateral sensorineural hearing loss, profound in the right ear and sloping moderate to profound in the left ear.	

Chronological age	Hearing age
3 years, 2 months	14 months (hearing aids, both ears)
	11 months (cochlear implant right side)

Auditory-verbal age	Hearing technology history
14 months	Binaural hearing aids at 24 months; Cochlear implant in right ear at 27 months; Continues to wear hearing aid is left ear.

Developmental history
Full-term baby, no family history of hearing loss. Child has no known cognitive delay but has mild gross motor delays and is now followed in physiotherapy at the pediatric hospital where Auditory-Verbal therapy is provided.

Case history/family context
The family arrived in Canada from Somalia 16 months ago. Tariqah has three older brothers, age 5, 6, and 9 years. The family speaks Somali as their home language and they are now learning English to facilitate their integration into their new county. All three boys attend English-speaking schools and participate in neighborhood activities, such as Boy Scouts and soccer. Mother stays at home and Father drives a taxi. They live in a very multicultural neighborhood with many other families who have recently immigrated to Canada.
Tariqah contracted meningitis in her village in Somalia a few months before their departure, and the subsequent medical and audiologic care were rather limited based on family report. They were seen in the pediatric audiology clinic at the Children's Hospital within two months of their arrival at which time the hearing loss was confirmed. She was fitted with hearing aids and enrolled in the Auditory-Verbal Therapy program at the hospital. Through the local parents' group, the Auditory-Verbal practitioner arranged for them to meet another family from Somalia with a child with severe hearing loss, who has lived in Canada for several years.

Auditory-Verbal Therapy
An initial meeting was held with the Audiology clinic team (audiologist, Auditory-Verbal practitioner, social worker) to discuss the family service plan and a Somali interpreter was present for this session. The Auditory-Verbal practitioner is monolingual English speaking.

Table 23–4. *continued*

The Auditory-Verbal Therapy sessions take place in English, based on the parents' decision to educate their children in English and to integrate into their home country. Given that Taquira had access to her home language for the first two years of life and that parents use Somali at home, the Auditory-Verbal practitioner is fully supportive of the parents using their home language with her.

Given that the parents report that Tariqah continues to use some words in Somali, the practitioner arranges to have an interpreter for the first two sessions to better evaluate her level of competency in Somali through observation, play sessions and a language sample. In subsequent sessions, the practitioner speaks in English and the Mother interacts with the child in Somali. In the early sessions, the practitioner carefully selects beginning level words and phrases that she knows (from discussions with Mother) are familiar to the child in Somali. The program's social worker meets with a community worker and arranges that the child attend a play group in English three mornings a week. In addition, the practitioner arranges a home visit after school so that she can include the brothers and encourages them to speak English to their sister some of the time. At this point, after 14 months of intervention, they are working on auditory skills, enriching vocabulary, and Tariqah is beginning to combine words. The family is now considering a second implant and a meeting is arranged with the cochlear implant team, with the assistance of an interpreter, to further discussion this option.

Note: Information in this table is based on discussions with Auditory-Verbal practitioners: Jasmine Gallant, Mélissa Leblanc, Deirdre Neuss, Maha Shabana, and Rosemary Somerville.

Table 23–5. Case Example 3

Name of child	Etiology
Myriam	Genetic

Degree and type of hearing loss	
Bilateral moderate to severe sensorineural hearing loss	

Chronological age	Hearing age
3 years, 6 months (at start of Auditory-Verbal Therapy in French)	3 years, 2 months

Auditory-verbal age	Hearing technology history
3 years, 2 months (Auditory-Verbal Therapy in English start date)	Binaural hearing aids at age 4 months

Developmental history	
Full-term baby, maternal aunt with severe hearing loss. Child has no additional disabilities.	
Seen for diagnostic audiology assessment at age 1 month after being referred from the newborn screening program and diagnosed at age 3.5 months.	

continues

Table 23-5. *continued*

Case history/family context

This Canadian family lives in a typical village of about 3000 people in the province of New Brunswick, a bilingual province in eastern Canada. Mother is monolingual anglophone and Father is francophone and bilingual. Myriam has one older brother who attends grade 4 in the community French school. The family speaks primarily English at home. Mother is a computer programmer working with a private company and Father is an electrician working for extensive periods of several months in another province. The family's linguistic profile is quite typical for this region.

Early intervention services delivered through home visits are available through public education agencies in either French or English for children with hearing loss and bilingual audiological services are provided through regional hospitals. Shortly after receiving hearing aids, Myriam was referred to intervention services in English and received weekly home therapy visits from an auditory-verbal practitioner. Mother spoke English to the child who also attended daycare in English. Father spoke both languages to the children but was often absent for extended periods due to his work situation.

At approximately age 3 years, the parents indicated to their practitioner that they planned to enroll Myriam in the same French school as her brother. Since Myriam spoke only English, the practitioner transferred the child to the French intervention services.

Auditory-Verbal Therapy

Myriam's annual evaluation in English indicated that she was functioning at a level comparable to her peers with normal hearing in most language domains, with about a 6-month delay in expressive vocabulary. During the first sessions with the French-speaking Auditory-Verbal practitioner, an evaluation was completed in French. Myriam's receptive vocabulary was at an 18-month level and expressive vocabulary and language skills were limited to about a 12-month level with primarily single word utterances or French words inserted into English phrases. The practitioner interpreted the results as being typical of English-speaking children exposed to limited French.

Following the evaluation, the practitioner met with both parents to work in partnership with them to create an environment to expose Myriam to more French. One option explored was to transfer the child form English daycare to a French-speaking daycare program. However, Mother was very comfortable with the present child care situation and was reluctant to move Myriam at this stage, particularly because the brother attended the same daycare after school. Parents worked hard to find alternate solutions. They were able to involve the French-speaking grandmother who came occasionally to therapy and engaged in more play activities in French. They also enrolled Myriam in gymnastics at the local community center in French. In addition, they worked on a therapy schedule so that Myriam's brother could attend the session. Therapy sessions were increased to twice weekly. Finally, the practitioner arranged with the local library to have a selection of French books available for Father or Grandmother to read to the child.

Table 23–5. *continued*

Auditory-Verbal Therapy sessions continued in French; Mother understood some French but interacted with Myriam in English. By age 5 when Myriam started school, the evaluation showed that there was still a 12- to18-month delay in various language domains in French. The practitioner also carried out a mini-evaluation in English to ensure there were no language gaps. Myriam's school offered an enriched French program for all children as her situation was not unlike that of many children from bilingual families in this region where English was the majority language.

Note: Information in this table is based on discussions with Auditory-Verbal practitioners: Jasmine Gallant and Mélissa Leblanc.

SUMMARY

This chapter has presented an overview of multilingual learning in children who are deaf or hard of hearing. Practices have shifted tremendously in recent years, influenced by extensive research demonstrating the benefits of multilingualism in typically developing children and by increased auditory accessibility for children with hearing loss. In tandem with findings from neuroscience about the brain's capacity to process and transfer information between languages, substantive changes in approaches to early intervention with multilingual families have occurred. Current practices support and even promote multilingualism for the majority of children with hearing loss while respecting parents' preferences. Although high-quality evidence about the most effective interventions is limited for this population, there seems to be good reason to support multilingualism in children with hearing loss. The increasing numbers of multilingual children in Auditory-Verbal Therapy programs provide an opportunity to more systematically examine the effects of dual-language learning on multiple linguistic, social, and academic outcomes. Recommendations and best practices can be expected to continue to evolve to optimize interventions for today's children with hearing loss and their families.

REFERENCES

Barac, R., Moreno, S., & Bialystok, E. (2016). Behavioral and electrophysiological differences in executive control between monolingual and bilingual children. *Child Development, 87*(4), 1277–1290. doi: 10 .1111/cdev.12538.

Bialystok, E. (2009). Bilingualism: The good, the bad, and the indifferent. *Bilingualism: Language and Cognition, 12*(1), 3–11. doi: 10.1017/S1366728908003477

Bowen, S. K. (2016). Early intervention: A multicultural perspective on d/deaf and hard of hearing multilingual learners. *American Annals of the Deaf, 161*(1). doi: 10.2307/26235249

Brice, A., & Roseberry-McKibbin, C. (2001). Choice of languages in instruction: One language or two? *Teaching Exceptional Children, 33*(4), 10–16. doi: 10.1177/00 4005990103300402

Bunta, F., & Douglas, M. (2013). The effects of dual-language support on the language skills of bilingual children with hearing loss who use listening devices relative to their monolingual peers. *Language, Speech, and Hearing Services in Schools, 44*(3), 281–290. doi: 10.1044/0161-1461(2013/12-0073)

Bunta, F., Douglas, M., Dickson, H., Cantu, A., Wickesberg, J., & Gifford, R. H. (2016). Dual language versus English-only support for bilingual children with hearing loss who use cochlear implants and hearing aids. *International Journal of Language & Communication Disorders, 51*(4), 460–472. doi: 10.1111/1460-6984.12223

Byers-Heinlein, K., Burns, T. C., & Werker, J. F. (2010). The roots of bilingualism in newborns. *Psychologial Science, 21*(3), 343–348. doi: 10.1177%2F0956797609360758

Cannon, J. E., & Guardino, C. (2012). Literacy strategies for deaf/hard-of-hearing english language learners: Where do we begin? *Deafness & Education International, 14*(2), 78–99. doi: 10.1179/1557069X12Y.0000000006

Cenoz, J. (2013). Defining multilingualism. *Annual Review of Applied Linguistics, 33*(3–18). doi: 10.1017/S026719051300007X

Conboy, B. T., & Mills, D. L. (2006). Two languages, one developing brain: Event-related potentials to words in bilingual toddlers. *Developmental Science, 9*(1), F1–F12. doi: 10.1111/j.1467-7687.2005.00453.x

Crowe, K., & McLeod, S. (2014). A systematic review of cross-linguistic and multilingual speech and language outcomes for children with hearing loss. *International Journal of Bilingual Education and Bilingualism, 17*(3), 287–309. doi: 10.1080/13670050.2012.758686

Crowe, K., McLeod, S., & Ching, T. Y. (2012). The cultural and linguistic diversity of 3-year-old children with hearing loss. *Journal of Deaf Studies and Deaf Education, 17*(4), 421–438. doi: 10.1093/deafed/ens028

Deriaz, M., Pelizzone, M., & Perez Fornos, A. (2014). Simultaneous development of 2 oral languages by child cochlear implant recipients. *Otology & Neurotology, 35*(9), 1541–1544. doi: 10.1097/mao.0000000000000497

Dong, Y., & Li, P. (2015). The cognitive science of bilingualism. *Language and Linguistics Compass, 9*(1), 1–13. doi: 10.1111/lnc3.12099

Douglas, M. (2014). *Dual-language learning for children with hearing loss.* Durham, NC: Med-El Corporation.

Fitzpatrick, E. M., & Doucet, S. D. (2013). *Pediatric audiologic rehabilitation: From infancy to adolescence.* New York, NY: Thieme Medical Publishers.

Forli, F., Giuntini, G., Ciabotti, A., Bruschini, L., Lofkvist, U., & Berrettini, S. (2018). How does a bilingual environment affect the results in children with cochlear implants compared to monolingual-matched children? An Italian follow-up study. *International Journal of Pediatric Otorhinolaryngology, 105*, 56–62. doi: 10.1016/j.ijporl.2017.12.006

Gallaudet Research Institute. (2013). *Regional and national summary report of data from the 2011–12 annual survey of deaf and hard of hearing children and youth.* Washington, DC: GRI, Gallaudet University.

Garcia-Sierra, A., Rivera-Gaxiola, M., Percaccio, C. R., Conboy, B. T., Romo, H., Klarman, L., . . . Kuhl, P. K. (2011). Bilingual language learning: An ERP study relating early brain responses to speech, language input, and later word production *Journal of Phonetics, 39*(4), 546–557. doi: 10.1016/j.wocn.2011.07.002

Gaul Bouchard, M.-È., Fitzpatrick, E. M., & Olds, J. (2009). Analyse psychométrique d'outils d'évaluation utilisés auprès d'enfants francophones. *Canadian Journal of Speech Language Pathology and Audiology, 33*(3), 129–139.

Geers, A. E., Moog, J. S., Biedenstein, J., Brenner, C., & Hayes, H. (2009). Spoken language scores of children using cochlear implants compared to hearing age-mates at school entry. *Journal of Deaf Studies and Deaf Education, 14,* 371–385. doi: 10.1093/deafed/enn046

Genesee, F. (2015). Myths about early childhood bilingualism. *Canadian Psychology, 56*(1), 6–15. doi: 10.1037/a0038599

Genesee, F., Paradis, J., & Crago, M. B. (2004). *Dual language development & disorders: A handbook on bilingualism & second language learning* (vol. 11). Baltimore, MD: Paul H. Brookes Publishing.

Grandpierre, V., Fitzpatrick, E. M., Thomas, R., Potter, B., Sikora, K., & Thomas, O. (in press). Perspectives of parents of minority culture backgrounds on pediatric hearing loss services: A qualitative inquiry. *Canadian Journal of Speech Language Pathology and Audiology.*

Grandpierre, V., Milloy, V., Sikora, L., Fitzpatrick, E., Thomas, R., & Potter, B. (2018). Barriers and facilitators to cultural competence in rehabilitation services: A scoping review. *BMC Health Services Research, 18*(1), 23. doi: 10.1186/s12913-017-2811-1

Grosjean, F. (2001). The right of the deaf child to grow up bilingual. *Sign Language Studies, 1*(2), 110–114. doi: 10.1353/sls.2001.0003

Grosjean, F. (2013). Bilingualism: A short introduction. In F. Grosjean & L. Ping (Eds.), *The psycholinguistics of bilingualism* (pp. 5–25). Malden, MA: Wiley-Blackwell.

Grosjean, F., & Byers-Heinlein, K. (2018). *The listening bilingual: Speech perception, comprehension, and bilingualism* (F. Grosjean & K. Byers-Heinlein Eds.). Hoboken, NJ: John Wiley & Sons.

Guiberson, M. (2005). Children with cochlear implants from bilingual families: Considerations for interention and a case study. *The Volta Review, 105*(1), 29–39.

Guiberson, M. (2014). Bilingual skills of deaf/hard of hearing children from Spain. *Cochlear Implants International, 15*(2), 87–92. doi: 10.1179/1754762813y.0000000058

Guiberson, M., & Crowe, K. (2018). Interventions for multilingual children with hearing loss: A scoping review. *Topics in Language Disorders, 38*(3), 225–241. doi: 10.1097/TLD.0000000000000155

International Expert Panel on Multilingual Children's Speech. (2012). *Multilingual children with speech sound disorders: Position paper.* Bathurst, Australia: Research Institute for Professionnal practice. Learning & Education (RIPPLE). Charles Sturt University. Retrieved from https://www.csu.edu.au/research/multilingual-speech/position-paper

Jasińska, K. K., & Petitto, L. A. (2018). Age of bilingual exposure is related to the contribution of phonological and semantic knowledge to successful reading development *Child Development, 89*(1), 310–331. doi: 10.1111/cdev.12745

Karchmer, M. A., & Mitchell, R. E. (2003). Demographic and achievement characteristics of deaf and hard-of-hearing students. In M. Marschark & P. Spencer (Eds.), *Oxford handbook of deaf studies, language and education* (pp. 21–37). New York, NY: Oxford University Press.

Kiese-Himmel, C. (2008). Receptive (aural) vocabulary development in children with permanent bilateral sensorineural hearing impairment. *Journal of Laryngology and Otology, 122*(5), 458–465. doi: 10.1017/S0022215107000321

Kohnert, K., Yim, D., Nett, K., Kan, P. F., & Duran, L. (2005). Intervention with linguistically diverse preschool children: A focus on developing home language(s). *Language, Speech, and Hearing Services in Schools, 36,* 251–263. doi: 10.1044/0161-1461(2005/025)

Kovelman, I., & Petitto, L. A. (2008). Age of first bilingual language exposure as a new window into bilingual reading development. *Bilingualism (Cambridge, England), 11*(2), 203–223. doi: 10.1017/S1366728908003386

Levasseur, J., & Rhoades, E. A. (2001). If parents follow the auditory-verbal approach, can they talk to their child in their native language or must they speak English? In W. Estabrooks (Ed.), *50 FAQs about AVT*. Toronto, ON, Canada: Learning to Listen Foundation.

Li, W. (2008). Research perspectives on bilingualism and multilingualism. In W. Li & M. Moyer (Eds.), *The Blackwell handbook of research methods on bilingualism and multilingualism* (pp. 3–17). Oxford: Blackwell.

Ling, D., & Ling, A. H. (1978). *Aural habilitation: The foundations of verbal learning in hearing-impaired children*. Washington, DC: Alexander Graham Bell Association for the Deaf and Hard of Hearing.

Lund, E., Werfel, K. L., & Schuele, C. M. (2015). Phonological awareness and vocabulary performance of monolingual and bilingual preschool children with hearing loss. *Child Language Teaching and Therapy, 31*(1), 85–100. doi: 10.1177/0265659 014531261

Marschark, M., & Spencer, P. E. (2006). Spoken language development of deaf and hard-of-hearing children: Historical and theoretical perspectives. In M. Marschark & P. Spencer (Eds.), *Advances in the spoken language development of deaf and hard-of-hearing children* (pp. 3–21). New York, NY: Oxford University Press.

McConkey Robbins, A., Green, J. E., & Waltzman, S. B. (2004). Bilingual oral language proficiency in children with cochlear implants. *Archives of Otolaryngology: Head and Neck Surgery, 130*(5), 644–647. doi: 10.1001/archotol.130.5.644

Moeller, M. P., Carr, G., Seaver, L., Stredler-Brown, A., & Holzinger, D. (2013). Best practices in family-centered early intervention for children who are deaf of hard of hearing: An international consensus statement. *Journal of Deaf Studies and Deaf Education, 18*(4), 429–445. doi: 10.1093/deafed/ent034

Neuss, D., Fitzpatrick, E. M., Durieux-Smith, A., Olds, J., Moreau, K., Ufholz, L.-A., & Schramm, D. (2013). A survey of assessment tools used by LSLS Certified Auditory-Verbal Therapists for children ages birth to 3 years old. *The Volta Review, 113*, 43–56. doi: 10.17955/tvr.113 .1.696

Olds, J., Fitzpatrick, E. M., Steacie, J., McLean, J., & Schramm, D. (2007). *Parental perspectives of outcome after cochlear implantation in children with complex disabilities*. Paper presented at the 11th International Conference on Cochlear Implants in Children, Charlotte, NC.

Paradis, J., & Govindarajan, K. (2018). Bilingualism and children with developmental language and communication disorders. In D. Miller, F. Bayram, J. Rothman, & L. Serratrice (Eds.), *Bilingual cognition and language: The state of the science across its subfields* (vol. 54). Published online: John Benjamins Publishing Company.

Peña, E. D. (2016). Supporting the home language of bilingual children with developmental disabilities: From knowing to doing. *Journal of Communication Disorders, 63*, 85–92. doi: 10.1016/j.jcom dis.2016.08.001

Petitto, L. A., & Dunbar, K. N. (2009). Educational neuroscience: New discoveries from bilingual brains, scientific brains, and the educated mind. *Mind, Brain, and Education, 3*(4), 185–197. doi: 10.1111 /j.1751-228X.2009.01069.x

Rhoades, E. A. (2008). Working with multicultural and multilingual families of young children. In J. R. Madell & C. Flexer (Eds.), *Pediatric audiology: Diagnosis, technology, and management* (pp. 262–268). New York, NY: Thieme Medical Publishers.

Rhoades, E. A., Price, F., & Perigoe, C. B. (2004). The changing American family & ethnically diverse children with hearing loss and multiple needs *The Volta Review, 104*(4 monograph), 285–305.

Statistics Canada. (2016). Ethnic diversity and immigration 2016. Retrieved from http:// www.statcan.gc.ca/pub/11-402-x/2011 000/chap/imm/ imm-eng.htm

Teschendorf, M., Janeschik, S., Bagus, H., Lang, S., & Arweiler-Harbeck, D. (2011). Speech development after cochlear implantation in children from bilingual homes.

Otology & Neurotology, 32(2), 229–235. doi: 10.1097/MAO.0b013e318204ac1b

Thomas, E., El-Kashlan, H., & Zwolan, T. A. (2008). Children with cochlear implants who live in monolingual and bilingual homes. *Otology & Neurotology, 29*(2), 230–234. doi: 10.1097/mao.0b013e31815f668b

Uljarević, M., Hudry, K., & Gibson, J. L. (2016). Practitioner review: Multilingualism and neurodevelopmental disorders—an overview of recent research and discussion of clinical implications. *Journal of Child Psychology and Psychiatry, 57*(11), 1205–1217.

Uljarević, M., Katsos, N., Hudry, K., & Gibson, J. L. (2016). Practitioner review: Multilingualism and neurodevelopmental disorders—an overview of recent research and discussion of clinical implications. *Journal of Child Psychology and Psychiatry, 57*(11), 1205–1217. doi: 10.1111/jcpp.12596

Waltzman, S. B., Robbins, A. M., Green, J. E., & Cohen, N. L. (2003). Second oral language capabilities in children with cochlear implants. *Otology & Neurotology, 24*(5), 757–763.

Werker, J. (2012). Perceptual foundations of bilingual acquisition in infancy. *Annals of the New York Academy of Sciences, 1251*, 50–61. doi: 10.1111/j.1749-6632 .2012.06484.x

24

CHILDREN WHO ARE DEAF OR HARD OF HEARING AND FAMILIES EXPERIENCING ADVERSITY: THE ROLE OF THE AUDITORY-VERBAL PRACTITIONER

Jenna Voss and Susan Lenihan

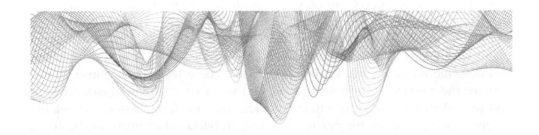

The experience of childhood adversity has a tremendous impact on the development and educational achievement of many of today's children (Bartlett, Smith, & Bringewatt, 2017; Harris, 2018). Sources of adversity such as poverty, violence, and family instability create trauma for young children and prevent healthy development. Recent evidence from pediatric neuroscience suggests that trauma creates changes in brain development and puts children at risk for delays in social, emotional, behavioral, and communicative development (Lipina & Posner, 2012; Noble et al., 2015; Shonkoff et al., 2012).

Children who are deaf or hard of hearing may also experience adversity and may be at even greater risk (Suskind et al., 2016). With a strong awareness regarding the negative impact associated with childhood adversity and a variety of effective practices and strategies that can be used to serve this population, Auditory-Verbal practitioners (practitioners) promote resilience and improve outcomes for young children who are deaf or hard of hearing and their families. Practitioners are not expected to solve, manage, or treat problems related to adversity, but they can assist families in accessing resources to reduce the harm caused by adverse childhood experiences. While professionals may feel that this is beyond the discipline's scope of practice, by encouraging, supporting, and facilitating relationships and attachment, practitioners can help caregivers buffer their children from the damaging effects of adversity. Because our work with young children and their families actively engages families and is often home based, these efforts can be embedded in our Auditory-Verbal practice and will enhance positive outcomes in multiple domains. In this chapter, we will describe adversity and resilience, explore the research on these topics, and provide a framework of effective practices and resources for practitioners to support children and families.

ADVERSITY AND RESILIENCE

In the last 20 years, much research has been done exploring the experiences of young children and how those experiences impact their development. Adverse childhood experiences are defined as traumatic events in a person's life before the age of 18. Approximately 35 million children—almost half of all children in the United States—have experienced one or more types of trauma. Trauma is defined as events that cause actual harm to the child's emotional or physical well-being causing a sense of intense fear. The most negative child outcomes occur when the trauma "begins early in life, takes multiple forms, is severe and pervasive and involves harmful behavior by primary caregivers" (Bartlett et al., 2017, p. 1).

ADVERSE CHILDHOOD EXPERIENCES STUDY AND RELATED RESEARCH

The term *adverse childhood experiences*, or ACEs, was first used by Felitti and Anda, who conducted a large public health study and found that individuals who were exposed to trauma such as physical abuse, neglect, or household dysfunction such as parental divorce or familial mental illness before the age of 18 were negatively impacted (Harris, 2018). These researchers chose 10 categories of trauma that impacted health outcomes and found a stunning link between childhood adversity and health as well as social and emotional problems (see Figure 24–1).

Although there are other forms of childhood trauma, these 10 were identified as most common and were extensively studied in the research literature. Data reported by the Health Resources and Services Administration (HRSA) in 2016 show that at least 48% of children in the United States have had at least one ACE and more than 20% have had at least two. In a study of childhood

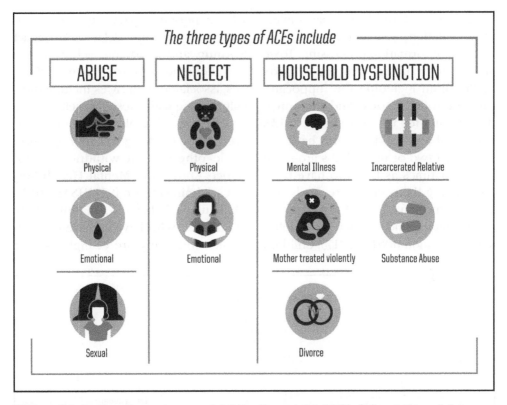

Figure 24-1. The three types of ACEs. Copyright 2013. Robert Wood Johnson Foundation. Used with permission from the Robert Wood Johnson Foundation.

trauma, Van der Kolk (2005) found that "eleven percent of the respondents reported having been emotionally abused as a child, 30.1% reported physical abuse, and 19.9% sexual abuse. In addition, 23.5% reported being exposed to family alcohol abuse, 18.8% were exposed to mental illness, 12.5% witnessed their mothers being battered, and 4.9% reported family drug abuse" (p. 402).

As researchers continued to explore the ways in which adversity impacted children, a dysregulated stress response emerged as a major factor. All individuals experience stress, and in some situations stress can be positive and tolerable, as opposed to the toxic or complex stress when a child experiences "strong, frequent, and/or prolonged adversity" (Harris, 2018, p 54). According to Harris, "This prolonged activation of the stress-response systems can disrupt the development of brain architecture and other organ systems" (p. 55).

Impact on Child and Family

Adversity can interfere with child development in several ways. Research has addressed the impact on brain development, cognitive development, and social development (Bartlett et al., 2017; Johnson, Riis, & Noble, 2016). Adversity limits brain volume and impacts executive function, self-regulation, attention, and information processing. Toxic stress can result in changes to parts of the brain including the hippocampus, prefrontal cortex, and the amygdala (Center for Youth Wellness, 2013). Preschool-age children who have experienced two or more ACEs are more than four times as likely to have trouble calming themselves, are easily distracted, and have a hard time making and keeping friends (Robert Wood Johnson Foundation [RWJF], 2017). Children who experience adversity show cognitive and language delays that impact learning and academic achievement. Social-emotional development difficulties associated with ACEs include difficulty coping with stress, low self-esteem, and feelings of helplessness. Some children have a tendency to hypervigilance, while others seem withdrawn (Substance Abuse and Mental Health Services Administration [SAMHSA], 2012). Challenging behaviors are more likely in children who have experienced adversity and many are at high risk for

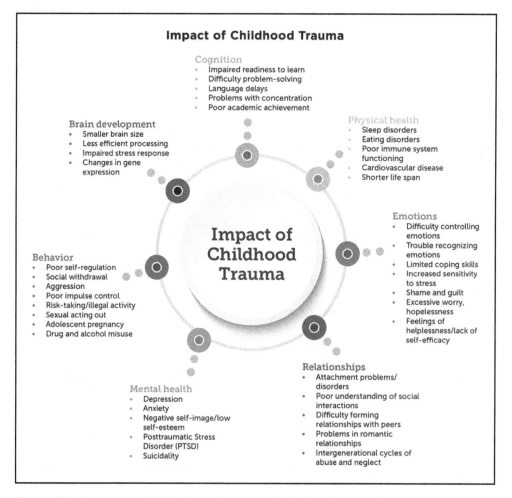

Figure 24–2. Impact of childhood trauma (Bartlett & Steber, 2019). Used with permission of *ChildTrends*.

anxiety and depression, and have difficulty forming and maintaining relationships. This is particularly problematic, since strong relationships have proven to be one of the most important factors in developing resilience in the face of adversity. In a study of children living in an urban setting, Burke, Hellman, Scott, Weems, and Carrion (2011) found that children who experienced four or more ACEs were 32 times more likely to have learning or behavior problems.

An excellent description of the impact of toxic stress on the brain and other systems can be found in Chapters 4 and 5 of Nadine Burke Harris' *The Deepest Well: Healing the Long-Term Effects of Childhood Adversity* (2018). The Center for the Developing Child at Harvard University (2017) provides videos, briefs, and resources on the impact of toxic stress.

In caring for a young child who has experienced adversity, the child's family can be greatly impacted (Bartlett et al., 2017). Parents may have difficulty responding in sensitive ways that are critical for the parent–child relationship and for communication development. For caregivers who are also experiencing adversity, the symptoms may be intensified and the child may be an emotional trigger for a parent who is overwhelmed and unable to respond in a caring way. Daily routines may become more difficult and conflicts between the parents may develop.

An additional important factor is the intergenerational nature of adverse childhood experiences. Research has shown a significant interaction between maternal childhood adversity and the experience of children. Bouvette-Turcot and colleagues (2017) noted the contribution of maternal history of early

adversity to other stressors and to the development of children.

SOURCES OF ADVERSITY AND TRAUMA

In addition to the ACE types, other sources of adversity have been shown to negatively impact child development and learning. Often an individual may experience a number of types of adversity and often sources of trauma are interrelated. For example, a mother who has untreated depression may be more likely to neglect her child and may have difficulty maintaining employment, thus impacting the economic status of the family. A family with limited financial means may be more likely to live in a community with high rates of violence.

Several sources of trauma can disrupt the development of children who are deaf or hard of hearing, including those whose families have chosen Auditory-Verbal services, and these can significantly reduce the positive impact of Auditory-Verbal strategies. Many such children may be experiencing the same negative conditions described above. With awareness and resources, practitioners may reduce the negative impact and enhance the child's and family's development and promote learning. Strategies and resources practitioners can use to buffer the detrimental impact of these sources of adversity will be addressed later.

Poverty

In the United States, 21% of young children under the age of 9 are living in poverty and 44% are living in low-income families (Koball & Jiang, 2018). For a family of four with two adults and two children, the federal poverty level threshold is $24,339 and the low income threshold is $48,678. Research suggests that families living below the low income level do not have sufficient resources to meet their most basic needs. Children are more likely to be living in poverty if they live in a single parent family, if their parents have a lower level of education, if their parents are immigrants, or if their parents are Hispanic or black (Koball & Jiang, 2018).

Johnson, Riis, and Noble (2016) summarized research on the impact of poverty on child development in this way: "As a group, children in poverty are more likely to experience developmental delay, perform worse on cognitive and achievement tests, and experience more behavioral and emotional problems than their more advantaged peers. In addition, child socioeconomic status (SES) is tied to educational attainment, health, and psychological well-being decades later. Increasingly, research is focused on understanding the extent to which these long-term outcomes are related to changes in the developing brain" (p. 1).

The primary issues for families living in poverty are housing, energy, health insurance, transportation, safety, and food security. Each of these issues may impact a child's success in general development and in education. Poverty impacts access to quality health and education services. Families who are striving to meet the basic needs of food, housing, and safety may have limited energy to bring to the important task of providing support for their develop-ing children. It is important to recognize that children living in poverty vary significantly with respect to adverse environments and that it would be unfair to stigmatize all impoverished families and communities when some children are thriving despite adverse living conditions. Practitioners who understand the impact of poverty on child development can emphasize the importance of communication between the child with a hearing loss and parents and can plan activities using readily available materials and routines that are appropriate for families with limited financial resources. Practitioners can also be knowledgeable regarding community resources for needs related to food, housing, transportation, and health care.

Child Maltreatment

Child maltreatment includes neglect, physical abuse, psychological maltreatment, and sexual abuse. Young children from birth to 8 years of age are the most frequent victims of maltreatment (Division of Early Childhood [DEC], 2016). Each year there are over 3 million children reported for abuse or neglect in the US and approximately 1 million of those cases are substantiated (Van der Kolk, 2005). The ACE study reported estimates of physical abuse at 28.3%, sexual abuse at 20.7% and emotional abuse at 10.6% (RWJF, 2017). In a study of individuals with hearing loss, participants reported significantly more instances of child maltreatment compared with hearing participants, with 76% of individuals with hearing loss reporting some type of childhood abuse or neglect (Schenkel, Rothman-Marschall, Schlehofer, Burnash, & Priddy, 2014).

The Council on Exceptional Children (2018) provides guidance for professionals in special education related to child maltreatment and the DEC position statement on child maltreatment reports that "despite being involved in multiple service systems, the health, developmental, educational, and social needs of young children with disabilities who have experienced maltreatment and their families often go unmet" (Corr & Danner, 2013).

In the US, professionals in education and health care, including Auditory-Verbal practitioners, are mandated reporters, required by law to report suspected cases of child maltreatment. The DEC position statement on maltreatment calls for practitioners to advocate for child safety and to assume responsibility for both prevention and intervention efforts. Johnson (2012) recommends that professionals in early intervention and early childhood education include protective factors in their practice such as nurturing and attachment, social connections, and social and emotional competence of children that prevent child maltreatment. An extensive collection of resources on child maltreatment is available at the OUR Children's Safety Project at the Hands and Voices website (Hands and Voices, 2019).

Caregiver Mental Health

It is estimated that approximately 20% of children have a parent with a mental illness such as depression, anxiety, schizophrenia, or bipolar disorder. Depending on the treatment and management of the illness, children may experience significant consequences such as impaired social functioning, poor academic performance, and feelings of anger, anxiety, and guilt (McCormack, White, & Cuenca, 2017). Depression, the most widely studied mental health condition, affects approximately 7.5 million parents in the US each year and may put at least 15 million children at risk for adverse health outcomes (National Research Council and Institute of Medicine, 2009). Extensive research has demonstrated the impact of maternal depression on child development (Shonkoff et al., 2012). Caregiver depression impacts the contingent reciprocity between mother and child that is essential for communication development at the core of Auditory-Verbal practice. Shonkoff calls for therapy focused on the dyadic relationship to provide care for both mother and developing child. Practitioners can support caregiver–child interaction and can refer families for therapeutic services as needed.

Family Instability

Approximately 25% of children experience parental separation or divorce that causes many children to be raised by a single parent, most often the mother (RWJF, 2017). Other situations of family instability include the death of a parent during childhood, a fragile family situation in which the child's parents are not married and may or may not be living together, or an incarcerated parent. Systems of immigration that separate children from caregivers and extended family, of course, result in family instability (Brabeck & Xu, 2010). While foster and adoptive placements may improve stability for children, the impact of early adversity remains (Forkey & Szilagyi, 2014).

These situations cause stress for the child and family and often result in economic hardship. Care for children may be compromised when family instability creates difficult living conditions. Parents may struggle to attend to their child's educational and developmental needs while trying to manage challenging family relations or early trauma. Typical routines such as meals, sleep, and positive parent–child interaction may be disrupted. Caregivers may struggle with missing appointments for audiology and for Auditory-Verbal sessions. Attendance at school may be more erratic. Housing may become an issue related to family instability and families may need to relocate. Parents experiencing grief related to the death or incarceration of a spouse may have less energy for supporting child development. In some situations, grandparents or other family members may become the primary caregivers for children. Each of these instances may impact the progress of a child who is deaf or hard of hearing. Practitioners who are aware of the family life of the children they serve can connect parents with needed resources and provide support through consistency of services and flexibility in scheduling.

Violence

Children may experience violence in a variety of ways. Domestic violence is defined as a pattern of physical, sexual, and psychological attacks against an intimate partner (UNICEF, 2006). In the ACEs Study, 12.7% of respondents reported witnessing domestic violence.

For example, a mother experiencing domestic violence must find ways to protect herself and her children and must also consider how she can provide for her children. Because Auditory-Verbal practitioners often work in families' homes, especially in early intervention, they may become aware of cases of domestic violence through the caregiver or child. Professionals must be aware of effective ways to respond to disclosures and be prepared with referrals to appropriate family support services. Practitioners can promote healthy social and emotional development for children by providing opportunities for children to express feelings and by ensuring that there are caring and stable adults in the child's life (Cohen & Knitzer, 2004).

Many children also experience violence in their communities related to crime (McGill et al., 2014). Research consistently shows that exposure to community violence impacts student learning. Another type of violence experienced by children is mistreatment or bullying due to race, sexual orientation, disability, or religion.

Substance Abuse

According to a 2016 Clinical Report from the American Academy of Pediatrics, one in five children grows up in a home in which someone uses drugs or misuses alcohol (Smith & Wilson, 2016). The impact of maternal drug and alcohol use on the developing fetus during pregnancy is well documented in the research, and professionals in education and child development often encounter learning and behavior challenges caused by drug or alcohol use during the pregnancy of the mothers of the children they serve (SAMHSA, 2012). When caregivers abuse alcohol or drugs, it is more likely that children in the family will experience toxic stress. Parenting skills may deteriorate, and caregivers may have difficulty interacting in warm and supportive ways, leading to feelings of insecurity and confusion in children. Substance abuse is often related to other sources of adversity such as child maltreatment, caregiver mental health, and domestic violence (SAMHSA, 2012). In situations of parental substance abuse, professional treatment is needed. Comprehensive programs that address addiction and parenting are vital, and consequently practitioners need to demonstrate awareness of possible substance abuse issues and the ability to make referrals to the appropriate community services.

RESILIENCE

Despite adversity, many children and families are able to flourish and many parents in some of these challenging situations do raise children who are socially and academically competent. These children and families demonstrate resilience, an important feature in successfully combating the negative effects of adversity. Resilience is defined as the ability to cope with the stress caused by challenging situations and can be understood at both the child and family level (Wilson-Simmons, Jiang, & Aratani, 2017). Children demonstrate resilience by engaging in age-appropriate activities, relating to others in positive ways, and understanding that they are not to blame for the adversity in their lives (Beardslee, Avery, Ayoub, Watts, & Lester, 2010). Many parents experiencing challenges remain deeply committed to their children and are able to provide competent, quality parenting (Wilson-Simmons et al., 2017) (see Figure 24–3). In the documentary *Resilience*, Jack Shonkoff describes resilience as being built over time and requiring learning how to deal with conflict, focusing on attention, controlling impulses, delaying gratification, and planning for the future.

Acknowledging families' strengths and achievements is a crucial first step. Implementing two-generation approaches that support both children and caregivers and providing evidence-based practices produce long-lasting positive outcomes (Wilson-Simmons et al., 2017). The best formula for success focuses on helping caregivers develop a parenting style that is both warm and nurturing, while providing consistent expectations and consequences. In this equation, children are able to develop social and emotional health that will support their continued development through adolescence and young adulthood.

Systems of service delivery may inadvertently add to barriers and burdens facing families. For example, fixed scheduling of session times may create hardship for working caregivers or those with limited access to transportation. With attention to both the individual qualities and the systemic factors, practitioners can provide substantial support to children and their families. Promoting resilience might involve bolstering individual interactions, and it might mean changing a rule, policy, or practice to be more inclusive, among other positive ways that practitioners and programs can support children and families in promoting resiliency.

Resilient Parents...

Can function well, even when faced with challenges, because they:

- Exhibit a positive outlook on life
- Communicate clearly and positively with all family members
- Establish and follow family routines and rituals
- Know how to seek help when needed
- Are flexible
- Promote family harmony, security, and unity
- Are able to manage their finances
- Have support networks
- Show appreciation and love for all family members
- Possess a strong sense of a greater good and purpose in life (e.g., spirituality)
- Have clear expectations of children's behavior
- Demonstrate consistency
- Make sure there is sufficient "family time"

Figure 24–3. Resilient parents (Wilson-Simmons, Jiang, & Aratani, 2017). Used with permission of the National Center for Children in Poverty.

ROLE OF THE AUDITORY-VERBAL PRACTITIONER

The Auditory-Verbal practitioner can take a primary role in promoting resilience for children and families experiencing adversity. The literature supports key features of interventions that serve to buffer children from the harmful impacts of early adversity. These include: the formation of positive relationships, feelings of safety and security, and opportunities to enjoy play and learn from both peers and caregivers (Bartlett et al., 2017). Practitioners can promote resilience through their implementation of the AG Bell Academy for Listening and Spoken Language (2019) LSLS Domains of Knowledge and Principles of LSL Specialists, which emphasize guidance and coaching of caregivers. However, a survey by Voss and Lenihan (2016) indi-

cates that professional preparation neglects to equip practitioners with the knowledge and skills needed to respond effectively and confidently to such adversity. Early Hearing Detection and Intervention (EHDI) practitioners were asked to rate the extent to which their professional preparation programs addressed challenges encountered by children and families living in poverty. The two highest rated challenges included access to hearing technologies (76.3%) and lack of enriching environments (59.7%). Further, more than 80% of the respondents indicated that the challenges associated with lack of transportation, housing insecurity, and food insecurity were infrequently or never addressed in their preparation programs. Few respondents indicated attendance at professional development activities that addressed challenges associated with increased risk of child maltreatment (51.4%), health disparities (47.7%), lack of transportation (27.1%), food insecurity (26.2%), and housing insecurity (25.2%).

A focus on resilience, in addition to identifying services that support individual children and families, also includes an opportunity to advocate for systems improvement and policy change. It is not a novel concept among Auditory-Verbal practitioners that children and families need support from the larger community. For those children and families who are most vulnerable, however, the supportive community has even greater significance. Responsive communities value individualized interventions that support families and build relationships grounded in respect (SAMHSA, 2012). This strengths-based approach prioritizes the provision of high quality information, in parent-friendly language, so caregivers learn to become consistently responsive to their children's needs. By working together as a community of learners who create interprofessional partnerships (Estabrooks, MacIver-Lux, & Rhoades, 2016), professionals can maximize their collective knowledge and skills to best support children and families experiencing adversity.

FRAMEWORK OF EFFECTIVE PRACTICES AND STRATEGIES TO PROMOTE RESILIENCE

An Auditory-Verbal practitioner may want to promote resilience but may not know how to do it. Over the years, study of this topic has resulted in the development of the *Framework of Effective*

Practices practitioners can use to foster resilience for children and families experiencing adversity. The Framework continues to provide a structure by which practitioners can organize those strategies, interventions, and activities that are utilized to meet the needs of families experiencing adversity while promoting positive outcomes. By considering the categories of adversity presented earlier as well as their own professional experience serving children and families, Auditory-Verbal practitioners can categorize the strategies used in practice.

1. Identify personal bias.

The first practice is to recognize one's implicit bias and become aware of the experiences, values, and attitudes that lead to an individual's unconscious prejudices. Individuals have varying degrees of self-awareness relative to their own biases as a result of varied motivation, desires, interests, and experiences. According to Cohn-Vargas (2015), "One of the challenges of changing implicit bias is that, because we are often not conscious of our beliefs, we can take actions based on them without realizing it." In addition to individual practitioners working to recognize the implicit bias they hold, recognition of how one's personal bias influences service delivery can also be prioritized institutionally. By prioritizing this at a systems level, it becomes possible to recognize the ways service delivery systems that are built on the personal/professional interactions with others might fail to support all clients and families to the same extent. It becomes important to recognize that every conclusion one makes about a family's circumstances such as how they choose to spend their money, time, and energy, are all judgments made through one's own lens of experience. Resisting the tendency to assume that one's own decision making is the only, or most correct, decision to be made is challenging. The truth remains that there are many ways to do things, many paths to success, and many opportunities to achieve one's preferred outcomes. There are many ways to communicate, many ways to raise children into healthy, productive adults, and many ways to interact with family members, neighbors, and community members. The families we serve have the right to make their own choices. We can help them evaluate the anticipated outcomes of the choices they make, but in the end, it is their right to make a choice. Ultimately, when we ensure that the power to make decisions for their children remains with caregivers, we allow them to own the *wins* and *losses* of parenting. As Auditory-Verbal practitioners, we can walk alongside them to celebrate the successes they accomplish and scoop them up in supportive arms when they stumble. As we examine circumstances of great adversity, we are challenged to set aside our own judgments, because for many of us, we have not, or are not, experiencing the same adversity. Further, for those of us who do have personal experience with great adversity, we must acknowledge that our own lived experience is not necessarily reflective of others' lived experience. The decisions we may have made for our own families need not be the same decisions others make for their families.

David Luterman, audiologist turned counselor, has provided our field with much wise guidance on serving families of children who are deaf or hard of hearing (Luterman, 2004, 2015). His simple "PNS" reminds us to be *present* in every conversation, session, or home visit, to be *non-judgmental*, and to understand that our work is *selfless*. The purpose of the professional–caregiver relationship is about supporting caregiver capacity. Practitioners work to put their own agendas aside in order to meet the families wherever they are on their own journeys.

Finally, Auditory-Verbal practitioners need to model high expectations, so the caregivers and families come to know it is possible to hold high expectations for their children. In contrast, low expectations are as detrimental to a family's success as if the family itself had low expectations.

Questions for Reflection:

- *How did I engage with medical professionals and educators?*
- *How have my own experiences in educational and medical intervention influenced my career choice?*
- *Have I ever thought. . . ?*
  - *If I wouldn't do it that way, it must not be the right way to do it.*
  - *If other people in my circle of friends wouldn't do it that way, it must not be the right way to do it.*
  - *If my own parents didn't do it that way, then it must not be the right way to do it.*

2. Build relationships.

The next practice is to build relationships including both parent–

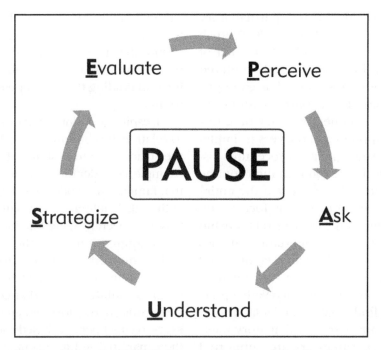

Figure 24-4. The PAUSE framework. From A. M. Tomlin and S. A. Viehweg (2016). *Tackling the tough stuff: A home visitor's guide to supporting families at risk.* Baltimore, MD: Paul H. Brookes Publishing, Co., Inc. Reprinted with permission.

practitioner relationships as well as the parent–child relationships. Tomlin and Viehweg (2016), in *Tackling the Tough Stuff: A Home Visitor's Guide to Supporting Families At Risk*, present a problem-solving framework grounded in family relationships that encourages both practitioner and caregiver reflection (see Figure 24–4). The acronym PAUSE indicates a five-step cycle: *Perceive, Ask, Understand, Strategize*, and *Evaluate*. Step one, *perceive*, calls for practitioners' full attention to observe and listen to the caregivers. Next, practitioners *ask* a variety of open-ended and more specific questions as a means of information gathering. Considering varied viewpoints, including those of the child and the caregivers, encourages practitioners

to better *understand* the family's experience, further bolstering the relationships. Step four, *strategize*, indicates a shift from information gathering to action. During this phase the practitioner and caregiver identify potential action steps. Finally, in the *evaluate* phase, caregiver and practitioner reflect on the action taken to determine effectiveness. This PAUSE cycle is a combination of both relational and reflective approaches to intervention and may be useful for Auditory-Verbal practitioners who seek to improve their family-centered practice that is grounded in strong professional–caregiver relationships.

Professionals, including Auditory-Verbal practitioners, are encouraged to provide intervention that is grounded in both relational and participatory practice (Dunst & Trivette, 2009; Rush & Shelden, 2011). Without one-half of this critical equation, family-centered intervention falls short. For example, without strong relationships, Auditory-Verbal practitioners will not be effective in supporting caregivers to implement the strategies and procedures discussed during sessions in their routine interactions. Alternatively, if the entire Auditory-Verbal session is focused on practitioner and caregiver relationship building, then the important strategies used to develop listening, talking, and thinking in our children will remain a mystery. Effective Auditory-Verbal practitioners find a balance of relationship building and active participatory intervention, so caregivers are supported and empowered to promote their child's listening, spoken language, and cognitive development.

Wilson-Simmons and colleagues (2017) describe resilient parenting styles of lower-income parents as those that provide a balance of warmth and nurturance with consistent rules and consequences. Children of caregivers with these parenting styles experience competent functioning through young adulthood, further affirming the value of healthy early attachment between caregivers and their children.

Adapted from work by Seibel, Britt, Gillespie, and Parlakian (2006), the SAMHSA Community Action Guide outlines five R's that all children need (2012). Children need safe, loving **relationships** that include **respectful, responsive** interactions with adults. Children also need **routines** that allow for the necessary **repetition** that promotes development of memory and organizational skills. Auditory-Verbal practitioners can support the caregiver–child relationship, focused on responsive communicative interactions through coaching and guiding them in repeated daily routines.

Despite good intentions, challenges to relationship building are inherent in the structures and systems of care. For example, consider the micro-aggressions that families and colleagues experience in their daily interactions. Columbia professor Dr. Derald Wing Sue has defined micro-aggressions as "the everyday verbal, nonverbal, and environmental slights, snubs, or insults, whether intentional or unintentional, that communicate hostile, derogatory, or negative messages to target persons based solely upon their marginalized group membership" (2010). The impact of these covert messages on the recipient scrvc to intimidate, threaten, and relegate them to an unwelcome, inferior position. If Auditory-Verbal practitioners are unaware of their implicit bias, they may harm the very relationships they are working to build. Therefore, effective strategies to lessen the negative impact of micro-aggressions include noticing when they occur in routine meetings or daily interactions, owning the impact instead of doubling down on the intent, and apologizing to the harmed individual.

Questions for Reflection:

- *How does the structure of my clinic, practice, or school facilitate or limit relationship building?*
- *How are families and children scheduled?*
- *Do families meet with consistent service providers, including*

audiologists or physicians, at each visit?

▪ *When are families assigned to a consistent Auditory-Verbal practitioner?*

3. Assess family needs.

Assessment of family needs, through a strengths-based model—examining what the family is doing well, what supports and resources they have—and then looking at what areas are remaining needs is an effective practice. For some family systems experiencing a great deal of adversity, or even generational trauma, this needs assessment can be overwhelming for both the Auditory-Verbal practitioner and for the family. Only when needs are named or identified can the practitioners efficiently and effectively position the appropriate resources and supports to address those needs. It is important for the family to identify and prioritize its own needs, with professional guidance. The Auditory-Verbal practitioner does not choose or identify the needs on the family's behalf. The work on Routines Based Interviews (RBI) by Robin McWilliam (2010) provides examples of an honest family-centered needs assessment. Even if a program is not able to utilize the RBI in its original form, the model of questioning and active listening before prioritization of intervention may be useful.

As noted previously, within the five-step PAUSE cycle, three steps are dedicated to practitioners understanding family needs, and the fourth step is focused on implementation of strategies to meet those stated and unstated needs (Tomlin & Viehweg, 2016). After a family prioritizes its needs, Auditory-Verbal practitioners are challenged to

probe a bit further to understand what has caused this to become a need. Just because a need has been identified doesn't mean the practitioner understands the source. For interventions to be successful over the long term, the strategy provided by the practitioner must match the source of the need. For example, if families are working to achieve all-waking-hours hearing device use, the Auditory-Verbal practitioner needs to figure out the actual roadblock to achieving this goal. If the roadblock is characterized by the Auditory-Verbal practitioner as a problem of caregiver buy-in, then the practitioner needs to find a strategy to help the family understand the importance of hearing device use during all-waking hours. But, for a family who lacks financial resources, the true roadblock to full-time device use may be an inability to afford the cost of batteries. Knowing the true roadblock to achieving this goal, the Auditory-Verbal practitioner can spend time and energy finding an appropriate strategy that might include seeking out funding sources or discount programs for batteries or assistive technology.

Questions for Reflection:

▪ *What resources are available within my own intervention system to assist with family-needs assessment?*

▪ *Do I have access to data analysis to track documentation, appointment no-shows, or patterns of caregiver behavior?*

▪ *How can I assess family priorities and needs within the forms, interview scripts, and curricula I currently utilize?*

4. Provide resources and support.

Provision of resources and support for basic needs such as food, clothing, shelter, and transportation encompass both tangible resources and information that can increase caregiver knowledge and confidence. Certain needs are most easily met by providing a specific resource or short-term gift. However, these temporary, or get-by, resources may be insufficient, and a family may require more long-term supports. The Auditory-Verbal practitioner's collaborative partnerships with other social service professionals and agencies can support families with both short- and long-term needs.

The Auditory-Verbal practitioners and other practice partners need to know area food banks and shelters, and be prepared to make referrals for families. For families who need more sustained support, the child's educational planning team may offer the most help. Early intervention programs can add a social worker to a family's team, especially when basic family needs overshadow individual child developmental needs. Maslow's Hierarchy of Needs reminds us that if the most basic needs are not met, families will be unable to focus on higher-level priorities such as responsive communicative interactions. The resources and supports described below are organized into four categories: listening technology; access to services; food, housing, and health; and keeping everyone safe.

Listening Technology

- Seek funding to provide free hearing screenings to childcare programs in neighborhoods with limited resources.

- Find pediatric audiology programs that provide services at low or no cost.
- Seek funding to provide hearing aid batteries at low or no cost.

Access to Services

- Obtain gas cards or bus passes to support transportation needs.
- Assist in arranging transportation for audiology services.
- Host an open house for community agencies that provide services for families.
- Meet with the family at the local public library where the Auditory-Verbal session can take place while encouraging literacy activities.

Food, Housing, Health

- Identify community resources for food assistance such as the "backpack snack," food pantries, or community garden programs. In the US and Canada, the United Way offers the 211 hotline and associated websites (http://www.211.org/) to efficiently connect individuals with available community resources. Religious organizations often provide support related to food, housing, and health.
- Explore governmental agencies that may provide support. For US based practitioners, consider Supplemental Security Income and Departments of Health and Human Services/Regional Centers. Homeless youth are afforded special protections under federal law, the McKinney-

Vento Homeless Education Assistance Improvements Act of 2001.

■ Develop collaborative relationships with social workers and social service programs in the community; use the Individual Family Service Plan (IFSP) team to engage a social worker to assist with goals related to food, housing, and health.

■ Encourage healthy eating by using appropriate snack activities during sessions.

Keeping Everyone Safe

■ Discuss safety concerns related to scheduling of time and place of family sessions, lead paint poisoning, and access to outdoor play.

■ Protect children from child abuse and neglect by providing resources and support and by using the OUR Children's Safety Project from Hands and Voices.

Questions for Reflection

■ *Listening Technology—Where might interprofessional partnerships aid in the provision of resources and supports related to hearing and assistive technology?*

■ *Access to Services—Are families able to access the resources and supports? Is transportation to and from clinics, appointments, and school a challenge? Are necessary referrals, insurance approvals, and permissions in place to connect families to needed resources and supports?*

■ *Food, Housing, Health—Do I think focusing on a family's*

basic needs is beyond the Auditory-Verbal practitioner's scope of practice? Who might I partner with to support families' basic needs? How might I share this information between systems?

■ *Keeping Everyone Safe—As mandated reporters of child maltreatment, how often do I observe, understand, and respond to concerns related to child well-being? What prevents me from making reports? Who or what resources can support us in helping to keep children safe?*

5. Increase awareness and advocate.

An effective practice is to increase awareness and advocate, on both the personal and individual levels as well as for community-wide policy and systems change. Clinics, programs, and schools whose outcomes are challenged by the adverse experiences facing families may choose to prioritize professional development to better understand the impact of adversity. Auditory-verbal practitioners who provide home visits may notice the family's adversity first-hand. However, all practitioners who interact with families will find benefit in participating in this focused professional development.

The National Center for Children in Poverty (2019; http://www.nccp.org) at Columbia University has a plethora of resources. One particular resource simulates a family budget based on national poverty levels. By changing the number of dependents and the percentage of income, viewers can contemplate the real challenges associated with limited money. To extend organizational awareness and empathy, one might consider participation in a community-based poverty simulation to help face the systemic injustices at play and to debunk myths about people who live in poverty.

Questions for Reflection

- *What systems changes across medical and hearing technology, therapy and educational services, policy, and research domains might allow the community of Auditory-Verbal practitioners to function as a responsive community?*
- *What professional development opportunities have I participated in relative to increasing awareness and advocating for families experiencing adversity?*

6. Educate families on quality instruction.

Finally, educating families on quality instruction is an effective practice to promote resilience. One primary recommendation from *Helping Young Children Who Have Experienced Trauma: Policies and Strategies for Early Care and Education* (Bartlett et al., 2017) is to ensure children who have experienced trauma receive high-quality, stable early childhood education. In order for this to be possible, the report acknowledges a need for a strengthened workforce of professionals who have the necessary knowledge and skills to provide such support. Early childhood settings can provide nurturing caregivers who facilitate the child's ability in coping with trauma in addition to supporting caregiver well-being. These supportive early care settings promote safety and trust, self-regulation, and the development of social-emotional skills.

By facilitating partnerships with other agencies and organizations, Auditory-Verbal practitioners can support families and potentially enhance their own outcome measures. For example, if an Auditory-Verbal practitioner is able to spend time assisting a family in seeking a quality educational setting for their child who is deaf or hard of hearing, it is likely that the child's outcomes will improve more efficiently than if the child remained in an unsupportive educational setting. Families from poverty may have difficulty selecting quality childcare centers and early education programs. If the only programs in their neighborhoods are not high quality, they may believe those are their only options.

Auditory-Verbal practitioners can spend time during sessions talking with families about the characteristics to consider when selecting childcare. While Auditory-Verbal practitioners may be quite used to talking about topics related to listening, spoken language development, and thinking skills, it is also important that they have engaging conversations with parents that include a variety of characteristics that make for quality instruction.

Questions for Reflection

- *How much do I know about the quality of the educational and childcare settings of the children on my caseload?*
- *How often do I initiate conversations with families about their child's educational setting and supports?*
- *What about these conversations do I find challenging?*

OPPORTUNITIES FOR AUDITORY-VERBAL PRACTITIONERS TO INFLUENCE FAMILY RESILIENCE

The Creating Nurturing Environments framework (http://promiseneighbor hoods.org), from the Promise Neighborhoods Research Consortium (2010), articulates the outcomes and influences through a model of development that encompasses cognitive, social-emotional, behavioral, and health outcomes across the lifespan. A review of empirical evidence identified primary influencers of outcomes at each phase of development. These influencers were categorized as immediate (those relating to quality of parenting, school, and peer relationships, etc.) and background (physical environment, availability of financial resources, social cohesion in the community, etc.). Of the immediate and background influences that have significant effects on child development outcome, interventions related to social cohesion, caring parents, effective schools, and peer influences are worthy of the attention of Auditory-Verbal practitioners. The influences listed in Table 24–1 identify areas where Auditory-Verbal practitioners are well suited to provide resources and engage caregivers in activities that will promote positive family outcomes, while limiting the cumulative family risk.

CONCLUSION

"With policies that help families to raise healthy children, and the consis-tent presence of caring adults in their lives, the impact of trauma on children's health can be significantly reduced and the children and families can thrive in the face of adversity" (RWJF, 2017). This is of monumental importance to Auditory-Verbal practitioners everywhere who have caseloads that involve many such children, who deserve the right to learn to listen and talk in loving, nurturing environments.

Reflect

Calling to mind a family with whom I have worked, I consider the challenges the family faced during our time together, the strategies and activities I utilized as their Auditory-Verbal practitioner, and the successes and barriers that impacted our relationship and the family's participation in the session. Then I can ask myself further questions such as:

- *What programs or approaches might have benefitted this family? What strategies might I have used from the Framework of Effective Practices to increase the chance of success for this child? How might I have included these strategies in my interactions with the child and caregiver? What influences, from Table 24–1, might have been malleable through Auditory-Verbal practice?*
- *Where might I find collaborations and accountability partners in my own professional community? What Effective Practices can I implement with the support of my professional community?*
- *How can I engage others in a conversation about my opportunity to promote resilience?*

Table 24–1. Ways to Promote Positive Family Outcomes

Background and Immediate Influences		What Does this Influence Mean?	How Might an Auditory-Verbal (AV) Practitioner Address this Influence during Intervention? AV Practitioners Can . . .
Caring Parents		*Parents Are Teachers*: Since babies are active learners from birth, their caregivers are teachers from the start too! Caregivers can create responsive, interactive environments and opportunities for play and communication across daily routines and experiences. When caregivers provide enriched experiences, share books, and seek opportunities to help their children develop conceptual knowledge in addition to language, they set their children up for success.	• Utilize books and songs in sessions helping caregivers identify ways to read and sing during daily routines. • Focus on making cognitive links—pointing out the language that must be readily accessible to allow for the acquisition of concepts—to assist caregivers in recognizing their role in helping children grow critical background knowledge. • Identify ways to learn about family routines so they can connect the LSL strategies during an AV session to a family's lived experience.
		Reinforcing Interactions: When parents engage in consistent, contingent verbal interactions, they build a trusting relationship with their young children. Parents utilizing proactive parenting, give positive reinforcement for desirable child behavior, and set clear consequences for non-desirable behaviors.	• Notice when a parent recognizes and responds to a child's communication attempt, providing specific feedback so the parent is encouraged to continue the facilitative behavior. • Encourage parents to provide contingent responses to their children and avoid pitfalls for incessant self-talk, naming, or labeling without first obtaining the child's attention. • Support parents in utilizing language just beyond a child's current level of functioning to continue to extend and challenge the child's language development without going so far beyond that the child is no longer able to make sense of the caregiver's message.

Non-harsh Limit Setting: Parenting practices that provide consistent limits and are responsive to children's needs are the most effective in promoting adolescent social advantages, school performance, and maturity. Related to the reinforcement of interactions, this type of warm, positive behavior support is indicative of mutual respect between parent and child.	• Discuss the intersection of language and behavior management during sessions. Help caregivers identify the way ineffective behavior management may be related to inappropriately high levels of language or vocabulary. • Model practices of positive parenting, for example *Love and Logic*, making note of any language-related modifications to support child's ability to access the message. • Connect caregivers with other parents who have faced periods of challenging child behavior, even when the behaviors may not relate to the impact of the child's hearing loss. • Provide parents with web resources related to behavior, discussing the language and behavior link, or handouts such as "What to do when your two-year-old bites?" or "Ways to help your preschooler self-regulate"
Positive Role Modeling: Parents themselves are role-models for their children. By setting high expectations, expressing positive beliefs, attitudes, and behaviors, parents model desirable behaviors and beliefs. Alternatively, when parents model substance use, such as smoking or alcohol use, youth are more likely to engage in these behaviors.	• Use language such as, "When you go to college . . ." or "When you're working as a 'desired professional' . . ." to model high expectations. • Disclose their own challenges in implementing specific strategies or techniques to acknowledge that with practice and appropriate support, these challenges can be overcome. Sometimes if the practitioner makes it look easy, without revealing the years of practice, caregivers and children can feel less self-efficacious.

continues

Table 24–1. *continued*

Background and Immediate Influences	What Does this Influence Mean?	How Might an Auditory-Verbal (AV) Practitioner Address this Influence during Intervention? AV Practitioners Can . . .
Caring Parents		• Start working on self-advocacy early and often. In early intervention and early childhood, caregivers take on the advocacy role for their children. AV practitioners can encourage parents to transfer the advocacy role to their children early and often, at developmentally appropriate levels. This may look like helping a young child put their hearing devices back on when they slip off, or move closer to the speaker to improve the signal to noise ratio.
	Involved Monitoring: Monitoring refers to the way caregivers engage in supervising their children's behavior. While monitoring activities may evolve as a child ages, some examples include, parents who: know what is happening in the child's school, attend open houses, limit independent use of TV/technology, know their child's friends and their parents, and setting and naming clear rules.	• Encourage parents to monitor across all areas of development, social included, not just the auditory and language domains. • Inquire with parents about what they've observed or learned at school open house or parent-teacher conferences. • Assess family needs relative to monitoring behaviors and connect caregivers with other families or professionals who might be able to offer tangible supports relative to monitoring. • Make sure the way screens are used to motivate in the AV session, nor the recommendations for strategies and activities to promote LSL development outside of the session, do not violate the parent's preferences related to quantity of screen-time or technology use.

Health Maintenance, Hygiene, and Provision of Healthy Food: Parents serve as the gatekeeper for a child's access to medical services, even as young children grow into adolescents. Parents can encourage healthy nutrition and sleep habits.	• Check in often regarding a child's hearing health, making sure caregivers share a commitment to ensuring proactive hearing health by aggressively managing otitis media, visiting otologists and audiologists for routine check-ups, and keeping hearing technology in good working order. • Offer healthy snacks instead of sugary reinforcers during intervention. • Address safe boundaries and healthy relationships with peers and other adults to ensure children's safety is protected. Consider use of safety objectives in IFSP/IEP documents. • Connect caregivers with resources about healthy sleep habits, making referrals when appropriate. • Check in about caregiver mental health, facilitate caregiver support groups, and make referrals when appropriate.
Effective Schools — *Importance of Early Childhood Education*: Children benefit from enrollment in high-quality early educational settings which provide skilled educators, low adult to child ratios, safe facilities, well-planned curricula, exposure to early literacy, and toys/materials for play.	• Seek opportunities for engaging caregivers in conversations about ideal/supportive inclusive educational settings. • Offer to tour or visit potential programs with caregivers. • Share parent checklists for school placements, like that available from *Hands & Voices* or *Supporting Success for Children with Hearing Loss*. • Communicate child's strengths, goals, and suggested strategies to support development of listening and spoken language with child's early childhood practitioners. Inquire about child's performance in those settings to inform priorities being addressed in Auditory-Verbal sessions.

Table 24–1. *continued*

Background and Immediate Influences	What Does this Influence Mean?	How Might an Auditory-Verbal (AV) Practitioner Address this Influence during Intervention? AV Practitioners Can . . .
	Effective Reading Instruction: Participation in schools with school-wide reading practices which are designed, implemented, and sustained through community support ensures that all students can become readers by third grade. School-wide reading instruction should focus on prevention of reading difficulties. Further, the curriculum should be guided by scientific evidence and monitored and evaluated objectively.	• Find out how literacy is being implemented and monitored in the child's classroom environment. • Discuss, with caregivers and the child's educational team, the impact of receptive, expressive, auditory skills on the child's ability to access curriculum • Pre-teach and reinforce relevant vocabulary and concepts being taught in the school setting. • Coordinate with child's team of educators, the assessments being given to ensure no unnecessary reduplication of assessment or gaps in the assessment. Make recommendations for accommodations and modifications to the school-based assessment and intervention.
	Afterschool Education and Activities: Participation in physical activities, music, art, and literacy experiences help children develop both academic and interpersonal skills. Participation in afterschool programming Is associated with decreased health-risk behaviors including substance use, violence and criminal activity, risky sexual behavior, and obesity.	• Start early conversations about what children can do, so parents are encouraged to envision their child participating in sports, theater, music, or other extracurriculars. • Identify role models, adolescents and young adults who have hearing loss, who are engaged in extracurricular activities.

	• Work with the child and caregiver to identify the accommodations that will support the child's participation in afterschool activities. Will the child have auditory access? Will CART services be available? Will a coach/director wear the child's DM/remote microphone? Discuss specific adaptations to equipment (i.e., helmets) that will allow children to safely participate with their hearing technology.
	• Debunk the myth that learners who are successful do not need ongoing support through the school age years. Even the most successful youth with hearing loss benefit from supportive peer and adult relationships as they grow and develop across inclusive settings. • Facilitate peer to peer support groups, among children with hearing loss who may have shared experiences relative to identity development. • Make recommendations of literature and media that center characters with hearing loss. • Provide families and youth with lists of enrichment opportunities to connect with peers and role models. Examples include: AG Bell's LOFT program or summer camps for youth who are deaf or hard of hearing. • Arrange pen-pal or distance technology meet-ups to connect youth who have hearing loss with one another, even if there are limited opportunities for face-to-face meetings within a community or school setting.
Peer Influences	*Prosocial Peers, Role Models:* Positive role models, or people that youth look up to, are influential on youth behavior. Youth benefit from pro-social relationships with peers and adults they admire. Benefits of these healthy peer and role-model relationships include: enhanced feelings of self-worth, increased grades, and decreased substance use.

Who do I work with, or who do I influence, that might also benefit from this information?

■ *What can I alter or implement in my next interaction with a child and family? What practices might I implement that will enable a caregiver to make actionable change in his or her own life? What systems-level changes can I advocate for in order to better promote resiliency?*

"Every child deserves a healthy start. A loving home, a good school, a safe neighborhood—these things are the foundations for a long and happy life, yet far too many children don't have them," said Richard Besser, president and CEO of the Robert Wood Johnson Foundation. "Too often children experience trauma that can be devastating. But trauma doesn't have to define a child's life trajectory. They can be incredibly resilient" (RWJF, 2017).

SELECTED RESOURCES

Books

The Deepest Well: Healing the Long-Term Effects of Childhood Adversity by Nadine Burke Harris, 2018, Houghton Mifflin Harcourt.

Helping Children Succeed: What Works and Why by Paul Tough, 2016, Houghton Mifflin Harcourt.

Reaching and Teaching Students in Poverty: Strategies for Erasing the Opportunity Gap by Paul Gorski, 2013, Teachers College Press.

Tackling the Tough Stuff: A Home Visitor's Guide to Supporting Families At Risk by Angela Tomlin and Stephan Viehweg, 2016, Brookes Publishing.

Websites

These websites provide resources on adversity and resilience:

Center for Parent Information and Resources, https://www.parent centerhub.org/ and https://www .parentcenterhub.org/trauma-basics/

Center for Youth Wellness, https:// centerforyouthwellness.org/

Center on the Developing Child, https://developingchild.harvard.edu/

Child Welfare Information Gateway, https://www.childwelfare.gov/

National Center for Children in Poverty, http://nccp.org/ and http://www.nccp.org/publications /pub_1180.html

National Child Traumatic Stress Network, https://www.nctsn.org/ and https://www.nctsn.org/audi ences/families-and-caregivers

Robert Wood Johnson Foundation, https://www.rwjf.org/ and https:// www.rwjf.org/en/library/collections /aces.html

REFERENCES

AG Bell Academy for Listening and Spoken Language. (2019). Retrieved March 9,

2019 from https://agbellacademy.org/certification/

Bartlett, J. D., Smith, S., & Bringewatt, E. (2017). Helping young children who have experienced trauma: Policies and strategies for early care and education. (executive summary) Publication #2017-21. *ChildTrends.*

Bartlett, J., & Steber, K. (2019). How to implement trauma-informed care to build resilience to childhood trauma. *ChildTrends.*

Beardslee, W. R., Watson Avery, M., Ayoub, C. C., Watts, C. L., & Lester, P. (2010). Practical tips and tools: Building resilience: The power to cope with adversity. *Zero to Three, 31*(1), 50.

Bouvette-Turcot, A. A., Unternaehrer, E., Gaudreau, H., Lydon, J. E., Steiner, M., Meaney, M. J., & MAVAN Research Team. (2017). The joint contribution of maternal history of early adversity and adulthood depression to socioeconomic status and potential relevance for offspring development. *Journal of Affective Disorders, 207,* 26–31.

Brabeck, K., & Xu, Q. (2010). The impact of detention and deportation on Latino immigrant children and families: A quantitative exploration. *Hispanic Journal of Behavioral Sciences, 32*(3), 341–361.

Burke, N. J., Hellman, J. L., Scott, B. G., Weems, C. F., & Carrion, V. G. (2011). The impact of adverse childhood experiences on an urban pediatric population. *Child Abuse & Neglect, 35*(6), 408–413.

Center for Youth Wellness. (2013). An unhealthy dose of stress: The impact of adverse childhood experiences and toxic stress on childhood health and development. Retrieved from https://centerfor youthwellness.org/the-science/

Cohen, E., & Knitzer, J. (2004). *Young children living with domestic violence: The role of early childhood programs.*

Cohn-Vargas, B. (2015, March 25). Tackling implicit bias. Retrieved March 7, 2019 from https://www.tolerance.org/magazine/tackling-implicit-bias

Corr, C., & Danner, N. (2013). Court-appointed special advocate strong beginnings: Raising awareness across early childhood and child welfare systems. *Early Child Development and Care, 9–10,* 1–11. doi: 10.1080/03004430.2013.845564.

Council on Exceptional Children. (2018). CEC's policy on the prevention of and response to maltreatment. Retrieved March 10, 2019 from https://www.cec.sped.org/~/media/Files/Policy/CEC%20 Professional%20Policies%20and%20Posi tions/FINAL%20Policy%20on%20Mal treatment%2020180925.pdf

Division for Early Childhood. (2016). *Child maltreatment: A position statement of the DEC.* Washington, DC.

Dunst, C. J., & Trivette, C. M. (2009). Capacity-building family-systems intervention practices. *Journal of Family Social Work, 12*(2), 119–143.

Estabrooks, W., MacIver-Lux, K., & Rhoades, E. (2016). *Auditory-verbal therapy for young children with hearing loss and their families, and the practitioners who guide them* (pp. 507–543). San Diego, CA: Plural Publishing.

Forkey, H., & Szilagyi, M. (2014). Foster care and healing from complex childhood trauma. *Pediatric Clinics, 61*(5), 1059–1072.

Hands and Voices. (2019). Observe, understand & respond: O.U.R. children's safety project. Retrieved from http://www.hands andvoices.org/resources/OUR/index.htm

Harris, N. B. (2018). *The deepest well: Healing the long-term effects of childhood adversity.* Houghton Mifflin Harcourt.

Johnson, H. (2012). Protecting the most vulnerable from abuse. *The ASHA Leader, 17*(14), 16–19.

Johnson, S. B., Riis, J. L., & Noble, K. G. (2016). State of the art review: Poverty and the developing brain. *Pediatrics, 137*(4), e20153075.

Koball, H., & Jiang, Y. (2018). *Basic facts about low-income children: Children under 18 years, 2016.* New York, NY: National Center for Children in Poverty, Columbia

University Mailman School of Public Health.

Lipina, S. J., & Posner, M. I. (2012). The impact of poverty on the development of brain networks. *Frontiers in Human Neuroscience, 6*, 238.

Luterman, D. (2004). Counseling families of children with hearing loss and special needs. *Volta Review, 10*(4), 215–220.

Luterman, D. (2015). Being truly family-centered: An audiologist reflects on the value of including clients' family members in support groups and in planning and providing treatment. *The ASHA Leader, 20*(11), 96–96. https://doi.org/10.1044/leader.FPLP.20112015.96

McCormack, L., White, S., & Cuenca, J. (2017). A fractured journey of growth: Making meaning of a 'Broken' childhood and parental mental ill-health. *Community, Work & Family, 20*(3), 327–345.

McGill, T., Self-Brown, S. R., Lai, B. S., Cowart, M., Tiwari, A., LeBlanc, M., & Kelley, M. L. (2014). Effects of exposure to community violence and family violence on school functioning problems among urban youth: The potential mediating role of posttraumatic stress symptoms. *Frontiers in Public Health, 2*, 8.

McKinney-Vento Homeless Education Assistance Improvements Act of 2001 (42 USC §§11431–11435.) Retrieved from https://www2.ed.gov/policy/elsec/leg/esea02/pg116.html

McWilliam, R. A. (2010). *Routines-based early intervention: Supporting young children and their families*. Baltimore, MD: Brookes Publishing.

National Center for Children in Poverty (NCCP) at Columbia University. (2019). Retrieved March 9, 2019 from http://www.nccp.org/

National Research Council and Institute of Medicine. (2009). *Depression in parents, parenting, and children: Opportunities to improve identification, treatment, and prevention*. Washington, DC: The National Academies Press. Retrieved from https://doi.org/10.17226/12565

Noble, K. G., Houston, S. M., Brito, N. H., Bartsch, H., Kan, E., Kuperman, J. M., & Schork, N. J. (2015). Family income, parental education and brain structure in children and adolescents. *Nature Neuroscience, 18*(5), 773.

Robert Wood Johnson Foundation. (2017). Traumatic experiences widespread among US youth, new data show. Retrieved from https://www.rwjf.org/en/library/articles-and-news/2017/10/traumatic-experiences-widespread-among-u-s--youth--new-data-show.html

Rush, D., & Shelden, M. L. (2011). *The early childhood coaching handbook*. Baltimore, MD: Brookes Publishing.

Schenkel, L. S., Rothman-Marshall, G., Schlehofer, D. A., Towne, T. L., Burnash, D. L., & Priddy, B. M. (2014). Child maltreatment and trauma exposure among deaf and hard of hearing young adults. *Child Abuse & Neglect, 38*(10), 1581–1589.

Seibel, N., Britt, D., Gillespie, L. G., & Parlakian, R. (2006). *Preventing child abuse and neglect: Parent-provider partnerships in child care*. Washington, DC: Zero to Three.

Shonkoff, J. P., Garner, A. S., Siegel, B. S., Dobbins, M. I., Earls, M. F., McGuinn, L., . . . Committee on Early Childhood, Adoption, and Dependent Care. (2012). The lifelong effects of early childhood adversity and toxic stress. *Pediatrics, 129*(1), e232–e246.

Smith, V. C., & Wilson, C. R. (2016). Families affected by parental substance use. *Pediatrics, 138*(2), e20161575.

Substance Abuse and Mental Health Services Administration. (2012). *Supporting infants, toddlers, and families impacted by caregiver mental health problems, substance abuse, and trauma, a community action guide*. DHHS Publication No. SMA-12-4726. Rockville, MD.

Suskind, D. L., Graf, E., Leffel, K. R., Hernandez, M. W., Suskind, E., Webber, R., . . . Nevins, M. E. (2016). Project ASPIRE: Spoken language intervention curriculum for parents of low-socioeconomic status and their deaf and hard-of-hearing children. *Otology & Neurotology, 37*(2), e110–e117.

UNICEF. (2006). Behind closed doors: The impact of domestic violence on children. Retrieved from https://www.unicef.org /media/files/BehindClosedDoors.pdf

Van der Kolk, B. A. (2005). Developmental trauma disorder: Toward a rational diagnosis for children with complex trauma histories. *Psychiatric Annals, 35*(5), 401–408.

Voss, J. M., & Lenihan, S. (2016). Professional competence to promote resilience for children living in poverty. *Journal of Early Hearing Detection and Intervention, 1*(1), 34–56.

Wilson-Simmons, R., Jiang, Y., & Aratani, Y. (2017). *Strong at the broken places: The resiliency of low-income parents.*

Wing Sue, D. (2010, November 17). Microaggressions: More than just race. Retrieved March 9, 2019 from https:// www.psychologytoday.com/us/blog /microaggressions-in-everyday-life/2010 11/microaggressions-more-just-race

25

TELEPRACTICE AND AUDITORY-VERBAL THERAPY

Emma Rushbrooke, Monique Waite, and K. Todd Houston

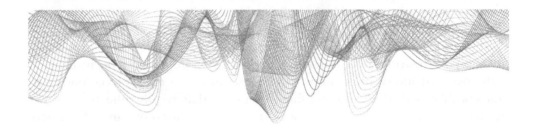

INTRODUCTION

Advances in telecommunications technology have greatly influenced the health care industry and can provide a bridge between clients and practitioners (Ribera, 2005; Rushbrooke & Houston, 2016; Swanepoel & Hall, 2010). This continuing evolution provides new and amazing opportunities and improves equity of access. This is especially important for highly specialized early intervention services like Auditory-Verbal Therapy (AVT).

Currently there are 466 million people with disabling hearing loss glob-ally, 34 million of whom are children who are unequally distributed across the world (World Health Organization [WHO], 2019) (see Chapter 1). Children who are deaf or hard of hearing and their families need access to appropriate early intervention services that are delivered by practitioners who are specialists in their chosen communication approach. In general, globally, there is a shortage of specialist hearing health care and early intervention practitioners and this is evident in relation to Auditory-Verbal practitioners (practitioners). As of September 2019, there are 894 certified practitioners worldwide, with 654 of them located in the United

States (AG Bell Association, 2019) (see Chapter 1).

Unfortunately, a lack of qualified practitioners, especially in remote and rural communities, combined with limited funding, can affect the quality of services that are provided to some children (Houston & Stredler-Brown, 2012). These facts highlight the urgent need for consideration of different models of service delivery, such as telepractice, to better meet this need. This chapter provides an overview of the telepractice delivery of AVT and discusses some of the factors that need to be considered to facilitate successful implementation. Additionally, it demonstrates that AVT is well suited to this model of service delivery and can deliver equivalent outcomes and high levels of client satisfaction.

The evidence shows that early identification of hearing loss combined with specialist intervention improves outcomes for both the child and family, and in general early intervention is likely to be more successful when it focuses as much on supporting parents as it does on working with the child (see Chapter 16). Specialist early intervention is essential to achieving the best communication outcomes for children who are deaf or hard of hearing. Most children born with hearing loss are born to typically hearing parents, many of whom will choose listening and spoken language as their desired outcomes for their child following AVT.

To achieve optimal listening and spoken language outcomes after the child is fitted with hearing technology, it is important that the child and family engage with an experienced, trusted, and qualified practitioner (Estabrooks, Houston, & McIver-Lux, 2014; Tye-Murray, 2009; von Muralt, Farwell, &

Houston, 2016). Evidence continues to show the shortage of practitioners who have the necessary knowledge and skills to deliver evidence-based and evidence-informed specialist early intervention services to children who are deaf or hard of hearing (Houston, Munoz, & Bradham, 2011; Houston & Perigoe, 2010; JCIH, 2007; Moeller, White, & Shisler, 2006; Shulman, Besculides, Saltzman, Ireys, & White, 2010; White, 2008).

Whilst specialist early intervention has traditionally involved direct person-to-person interaction, not every specialty can be represented in every community (Craig, 1999; Fried, 2001; Rushbrooke, 2012). Due to the small number of qualified practitioners worldwide, families of young children who are deaf or hard of hearing may struggle to find local programs. Specialist services are more likely to be available in larger towns or cities or via "outreach" services that require the practitioner to travel to different sites. These geographic barriers create many challenges for children and their families who live in rural and remote locations. Travel to services can impact significantly on education, family, and work life and may also result in financial strain (Darkins & Cary, 2000; Rushbrooke, 2012; Sevean, Dampier, Spadoni, Strickland, & Pilatzke, 2009). Alternatively, the provision of services via an outreach visit may not be time- or cost-efficient for the practitioner who is providing the service (Krumm, Ribera, & Schmiedge, 2005; Rushbrooke, 2012). In addition, some families, although not challenged by geographic location, may find regular attendance at a local service center, such as a private practice or a clinic, challenging due to issues such as mobility and transport. Telepractice may offer a solution to these barriers (Houston, 2014; Houston et al., 2011; Houston & Perigoe, 2010; JCIH, 2007; von Muralt et al., 2016).

Information and communication technologies are widely viewed as having great potential to transform the delivery of health care and support on a global scale. Advances in technology and telecommunication systems have extended the options for service delivery. Accessibility to specialist intervention is now better than ever before. This is because of improved real-time and video transmission, faster broadband Internet access, reduced costs, increased portability, and the rapid spread of wireless mobile devices (Armstrong, Giovinco, Joseph, Mills, & Rogers, 2011; Dzenowagis, 2009; Houston, 2014; Houston, Fleming, Brown, Weinberg, & Nafe, 2014; Rushbrooke & Houston, 2016; Xiaohui et al., 2013).

However, although these technological advances have provided many opportunities, it is important to emphasize that the technology is simply a tool (Brennan, 2013; Cohn, 2013; Rushbrooke & Houston, 2016). It will be the innovations of the practitioners using this technology that will enable the true integration of telepractice into their model of service delivery and provide equivalent support to children who are deaf or hard of hearing and their families, no matter what their location or circumstance.

RESEARCH EVIDENCE FOR THE USE OF TELEPRACTICE

Families and practitioners have reported overall satisfaction with telepractice ser-

vices (Blaiser, Behl, Callow-Heusser, & White, 2013; Constantinescu, 2012; Peters-Lalios, 2012). A small number of studies have also compared child outcomes in a telepractice service delivery model with those who received services in-person (Behl et al., 2017; Blaiser et al., 2013; Constantinescu et al., 2014). In each of these studies, young children with hearing loss and their families received a communication intervention program consisting of telepractice sessions supplemented by in-person sessions. Language outcomes were compared with those of matched children receiving in-person only services after 6 months of intervention (Behl et al., 2017; Blaiser et al., 2013) or two years post optimal amplification (Constantinescu et al., 2014). The studies found at least equivalent language outcomes for children in the telepractice and in-person groups at the end of the intervention period, as measured on standardized assessments. Further, Behl and colleagues also measured listening outcomes, with no significant differences between the two groups' achievements on the Auditory Skills Checklist (Caleffe-Schenck, 2006). There is also evidence of cost savings associated with telepractice services (Blaiser et al., 2013; Olsen, Fiechtl, & Rule, 2012), which increase as intensity of services increases (Blaiser et al., 2013).

APPROACHES TO SERVICE DELIVERY USING A TELEPRACTICE MODEL

Although there is no one correct telepractice model for the delivery of AVT, the implementation of the model requires careful planning, delivery, and evaluation to achieve optimal outcomes (see Chapter 17). In addition, connectivity and Internet capability will have an impact on this decision for both the practitioner and the family of the child with hearing loss. Consideration of these factors will allow the practitioner to decide the best options for service delivery that will ultimately meet the needs of the child, the family, and the Auditory-Verbal practitioner.

Types of telepractice:
A variety of methods and models can be described under the umbrella of telepractice. Telepractice may be used to provide individual sessions, group sessions, consultations, as well as supervision and training of professionals (Speech Pathology Australia, 2014). Services may be provided between discrete sites or across multiple sites (Speech Pathology Australia, 2014). In the context of early intervention for children who are deaf or hard of hearing, a variety of other terms are used for telepractice programs, including teleintervention, telehealth, teleschool, teletherapy, teleconsultation, teleaudiology, and telemedicine (Stredler-Brown, 2012). The models of service delivery are commonly described as either *asynchronous* (store-and-forward) or *synchronous* (real time). These different models relate to the timing of client-to-clinician or the clinician-to-clinician interactions (Craig & Patterson, 2006; Swanepoel, 2013; von Muralt et al., 2016).

The major models of telepractice are:

- synchronous: real-time communication between the practitioner and client through technologies such as videoconferencing and teleconferencing.
- asynchronous (store-and-forward): data are collected and then transmitted to the practitioner via the electronic communication system, e.g., email or videoconferencing software.
- hybrid: a combination of synchronous and asynchronous methods. The hybrid model is typically used to aid in assessment when there is unreliable infrastructure/connectivity (Keck & Doarn, 2014). A hybrid or blended approach may also refer to the use of both telepractice and in-person service delivery (ASHA, 2019).

Additionally, a telepractice model may incorporate mobile technologies and remote patient monitoring. The term *mHealth* refers to the use of mobile devices such as mobile phones, personal digital assistants, patient monitoring devices, and other wireless devices for health (World Health Organization, 2011).

In order to achieve the best possible outcomes with telepractice real-time services, the technology must enable the participants to communicate and relate in a way that is similar to an in-person consultation (Denton & Gladstone, 2005; Rushbrooke, 2012). This is particularly important when working with children and families, where it is essential to be able to observe behavioral responses and interact effectively with the parent, caregiver, or family member who is present with the child. AVT would be primarily delivered using the real-time (synchronous) model. However, the authors also believe that the service can be enhanced with the addition of some in-person contact (i.e., blended or hybrid) and by recording the AVT sessions (asynchronous), which enables parents to review the sessions as well as share them with extended family members and others involved in the child's care.

Research from the HEARing Cooperative Research Centre (CRC) in Australia, on the exploration of the use of telepractice in early intervention for children with hearing loss and their families, found that while there was variation across and within services, three broad telepractice models were used (Waite et al., 2019).

1. Telepractice only: Families received all parts of their service through telepractice and had infrequent or no in-person contact. This was a synchronous service utilizing real-time videoconferencing to connect the family with the early intervention professional.

2. Hybrid/blended with telepractice as primary service: Most families received services via this model, in which the majority or all AVT sessions were delivered via telepractice, supplemented by in-person services. The frequency of AVT sessions conducted via telepractice varied according to both the family's needs and child's progress, with most families receiving a therapy session weekly or fortnightly. Depending on the particular service, some assessment was administered via telepractice, including functional listening/speech perception tests and formal and informal communication assessments. However, some services conducted only informal communication assessment or assessed children via telepractice, only if the family could not attend an in-person assessment session. Under this

model, the frequency and nature of in-person contact also varied.

Most families had at least one and as many as four in-person sessions of service per year, but this may have been even more frequent—for example, if the family visited the city for other appointments (e.g., medical appointments, cochlear implant programming). In-person sessions typically took place in-center when the family had scheduled a visit to the town or city and/or at set times during the year when the service had scheduled an in-center intensive program (may also be called camps or residential programs). The in-center programs typically included individual AVT sessions, audiological and developmental assessments, group sessions for children, parent education including equipment demonstrations, and social activities for the child, parents, and siblings.

3. Hybrid/blended with telepractice as supplementary service: In contrast to the previous models, under this hybrid model most contact was in-person, with in-person AVT sessions being supplemented by telepractice sessions. This model was taken up by families who found it difficult or to travel regularly to the center for every therapy session or may have wished not to do so. Telepractice sessions occurred as frequently as every fortnight, alternating with the in-center session, or were infrequent/occasional, taking place when a family was not able to attend in-person due to poor weather or illness, etc.

Another option of this blended approach that could to be considered is the ability to include others in an in-center session via telepractice. That is, if one parent is attending in-person the other parent may videoconference in from work. In addition, grandparents who live in a different location or who have mobility issues can also participate. These telepractice participants can be included very easily by placing an iPad or tablet on the table where the AVT session is occurring. This research suggests that telehealth is most commonly used in conjunction with, or to complement, in-person services as opposed to a complete replacement.

In addition to individual AVT sessions, the services participating in the HEARing CRC study were increasingly using telepractice for group sessions and parent education. Services offering groups via telepractice reported both synchronous and asynchronous methods for delivering the groups. Families could attend a group via telephone or multi-point videoconference. Education sessions could be recorded for access by families via an online portal. Examples of groups offered via telepractice included parent advocacy, emotional coaching, parent education, as well as social skill development, music, and school readiness programs for children and families.

WHAT ARE THE BARRIERS?

Equitable access to specialized AVT sessions is a global issue. For example, families in low- and middle-income countries face poor access to devices and professional services (World Health Organization, 2013), a lack of hearing care practitioners (McPherson, 2011, 2014; McPherson & Amedofu, 2013), and prohibitive travel time and costs

(McPherson, 2011; McPherson & Amedofu, 2013). However, in higher-income countries, such as Australia and the United States, access to AVT may be difficult in regional and rural areas. A recent systematic review of Australian studies investigating the provision of services to children who are deaf or hard of hearing residing in regional, rural, and remote areas found families received services of both reduced frequency and quality (Barr, Duncan, & Dally, 2018). Specifically, the authors described issues in accessing specialized services associated with the following: a lack of qualified professionals, including experienced allied health professionals and educational support professionals; a high workforce turnover; lack of information and poor coordination and communication between services; access issues for Indigenous and other cultural minority groups; and reduced availability of support (Barr et al., 2018). However, as noted previously, families residing in metropolitan areas may also experience access barriers, including distances from specialist services, transport issues including difficulty accessing public transport, and family illness or disability making transport difficult. Families who work and who have many responsibilities may have difficulty attending sessions.

While telepractice offers a potential solution to equitable access, practitioners moving toward this type of service delivery must be aware of the potential challenges and learn how to advocate and promote this model of service delivery. Cuyler and Holland (2012) noted that even though telepractice has been used for some time, widespread adoption in the health care industry has not happened and it is often not well implemented (Rushbrooke, 2016). There are many factors noted in the literature that may be barriers to the successful implementation of telepractice delivery of AVT. Those include but are not limited to the following:

- Inadequate planning.
- Choosing the right equipment.
- Concerns about cost and funding.
- Practitioner confidence with technology.
- Poor quality picture and sound quality.
- Ability of the practitioner to establish rapport and have natural interactions.
- Concern about impact on outcomes and limited evaluation about the effectiveness of this modality.
- How standardized assessments are administered.
- Inadequate staff training.
- Concerns about privacy, confidentiality and consent.
- Practitioner licensing and reimbursement issues.
- Satisfaction with the service delivery, both family and practitioner.

(Constantinescu & Dornan, 2014; Craig, Russell, Paterson, & Wootton, 1999; Crutchley, Alvares, & Campbell, 2014; Cuyler & Holland, 2012; Rushbrooke, 2016; Singh, 2013; World Health Organization, 2010). It is beyond the limits of this chapter to explore all of these in great detail. However, both the benefits and challenges as perceived by parents and practitioners will be further discussed here later.

AUDITORY-VERBAL THERAPY IS WELL SUITED TO A TELEPRACTICE MODEL OF SERVICE DELIVERY

AVT promotes early diagnosis, access to hearing technology, and individual one-to-one therapy with a qualified practitioner. Parents and caregivers receive guidance, coaching, and support in their role as the child's most important teacher of language. They are encouraged to actively participate, so they will drive the majority of the child's therapy sessions and learning in everyday activities (see Chapters 1 and 17). AVT concentrates on developing the listening brain, and due to neural plasticity, there is a time locked period (the first 3 and half years of life) to get best outcomes (see Chapters 2 and 3). In view of this, telepractice can enable family access to qualified professionals, no matter where a family is located and in a timely fashion. In AVT telepractice, the very nature of the physical separation between child, family, and practitioner facilitates an immediate *handover* to the parent or caregiver from the practitioner.

EVIDENCE FOR AVT THROUGH TELEPRACTICE MODELS

There are many research studies that demonstrate the developmental, communicative, and social impacts of early intervention for young children who are deaf or hard of hearing (Apuzzo

& Yoshinaga-Itano, 1995; Calderón, 2000; Houston & Stredler-Brown, 2012; Mayne, Yoshinaga-Itano, & Sedey, 1998; Moeller, 2000; Pipp-Siegel, Sedey, Van-Leeuwen, & Yoshinaga-Itano, 2003; Yoshinaga-Itano, Sedey, Coulter, & Mehl, 1998). Telepractice is becoming more common in early childhood intervention for children with hearing loss and it has been validated in many areas of health care as an effective and equivalent model of service provision. Evidence to support its use in the delivery of family-centered early intervention, such as AVT, is still emerging, but while more research related to efficacy is needed, preliminary findings support the delivery of early intervention services, such as AVT, through various telepractice models (Houston & Stredler-Brown, 2012; McCarthy, Leigh, & Arthur-Kelly, 2019).

A scoping review was performed by McCarthy et al. (2018) and included 23 peer-reviewed publications that describe the current use of telepractice in the delivery of family-centered early intervention for children with hearing loss and their families. The authors noted that most of the publications (70%) showed anecdotal evidence relating to the challenges and benefits of telepractice. The remaining publications were studies that evaluated the effectiveness of early intervention delivered through telepractice. Of the 23 papers included, the majority (18) reported positively on the use of telepractice, while the remainder (5) showed mixed conclusions and the need for more data. It was suggested that many practitioners see telepractice as a supplement to traditional in-person services, and they concluded that, while there is evidence to indicate that telepractice can be an effective

model for delivering family-centered early intervention, more research is needed to verify telepractice as a viable alternative to in-person services (McCarthy et al., 2019).

Positive findings have emerged from a small number of studies looking specifically at telepractice and AVT. Constantinescu et al. (2014) conducted a retrospective study comparing the two-year outcomes of children who received AVT in-person with those who received AVT via telepractice. The participants were matched by chronological age, hearing age, degree of hearing loss, and type of hearing technology. In addition, inclusion criteria were very specific. The children had to have been identified at birth with hearing loss, received optimal auditory access with hearing aids and/or implants, and already been enrolled in AVT before 12 months of age. Language outcome scores in the telepractice group matched those of typically hearing peers. The telepractice group's mean scores for total language, auditory comprehension, and expressive communication were within the normal range of their hearing peers. The authors concluded that delivering AVT via telepractice is just as effective as in-person services and that telepractice allows more children to receive services than otherwise, due to geographic location. The authors acknowledged that a limitation of this research was the fact that the findings could not be generalized, due to the small sample size and single assessment results.

A similar pilot study by Chen and Liu (2017) looked at the effectiveness of telepractice for the delivery of AVT to Mandarin-speaking children with hearing loss. They compared language outcomes between matched groups of children receiving telepractice versus those receiving in-person AVT. While this study was also limited by a small sample size of five children in each group, equivalent outcomes were achieved. Parent and practitioner satisfaction were also assessed through a questionnaire. Satisfaction was generally rated high with regard to the telepractice delivery, and no significant differences were observed between parents and practitioners. However, it was noted that there were tendencies in their ratings that suggest differences between practitioner and parent perceptions of the program. Parents were generally more positive in their ratings in terms of the quality of the audio and the picture and technical issues. However, the authors did report that the practitioners became more comfortable as they gained more experience with this model of delivery. Both parents and practitioners felt positively about the convenience, and parents indicated significant cost savings and reduced travel time.

High levels of satisfaction were also reported in a study by Constantinescu (2012). Thirteen families who had been enrolled in the telepractice program for at least six months and five practitioners completed satisfaction questionnaires. Of note, parents' confidence and satisfaction with the equipment improved over time and with experience. Also, all parents reported being as comfortable in telepractice sessions and in-person sessions and 91% rated their child's level as comfortable also. All parents reported that they were as comfortable when discussing matters with the practitioner online and were satisfied with both their level and their child's level of interaction/rapport with the practitioner. All Auditory-Verbal practitioners were satisfied or very satisfied with the telepractice program.

The results of these studies, therefore, demonstrate the potential of telepractice service delivery for AVT for children with hearing loss, their families, and the practitioners who serve them.

AUDITORY-VERBAL THERAPY AND TELEPRACTICE: A PERFECT COMBINATION

AVT delivered through telepractice can be the answer when families struggle to find these services within their community. Families can have access to vital parent coaching, a central tenet of AVT, as they learn to be effective language facilitators and have direct interaction with a practitioner who is knowledgeable about listening and spoken language acquisition. With just a limited number of listening and spoken language specialists (LSLS) who provide AVT worldwide, finding an experienced therapist is one of the biggest challenges for many families. Thus, it appears that telepractice is a viable means of bridging the gap between supply and demand.

According to the Alexander Graham Bell (AG Bell) Academy for Listening and Spoken Language (AG Bell, 2012), 6 of the 10 core principles of listening and spoken language put the guidance and coaching of the parents front and center in their child's AVT, which is especially true through telepractice. Because AVT requires the active participation of the child's parents in each session, an effective practitioner needs to possess knowledge about many adult learning styles. This knowledge is critical to guiding the parents to become their child's primary facilitator of listening and spoken language (see Chapter 17).

Adults typically lean toward one of the general learning styles identified by most practitioners: auditory, verbal, or kinesthetic, but they often exhibit many variations and combinations therein. For adults to truly learn, they need to know: the why, the how, and the where of what they're learning.

- *Why*: Because of their life experience and problem-solving skills, the adult learner needs to understand the underlying principles and reasons of why they are doing something, and why they are doing it in a particular way or order.
- *How*: In spite of learning styles, most adults acquire skills through experience, critiqued (i.e., coached) performance, and affirmation.
- *Where*: It is essential for the adult learner to understand and remember where each task is going—the "big picture" goal.

Practitioners need to recognize the signs indicating when one or more of the above elements are missing. In conversations, a parent, for example, may exhibit a great deal of head nodding to coaching, guidance, or questions or too many responses such as: yes, uh huh, okay or sometimes no response but a glazed or quizzical look.

Sometimes adults may initially be high-maintenance learners, but once they have taken ownership of their role in their child's development and understand the why, how, and where, the practitioner is able to truly be an effective coach. The principles of adult learning and their importance in AVT are discussed in depth in Chapter 16. These are treated with the same respect, no matter where the AVT session (Chapter 17) takes place and of course, they fit perfectly with AVT telepractice.

HOW IS AUDITORY-VERBAL THERAPY DELIVERED VIA TELEPRACTICE?

This chapter outlines many considerations of developing a telepractice program for AVT. Successful programs need to align with a particular type of service delivery and will be influenced by connectivity, available technology, organizational or program needs, and funding. Ongoing monitoring and evaluation of both outcomes and satisfaction are needed to ensure the effectiveness of the program and that child and family outcomes are equivalent to those achieved in the in-person models. Auditory-Verbal practitioners need to have confidence in the suitability and sustainability of such programs (Jarvis-Selinger et al., 2008; von Muralt et al., 2016). Telepractice is an effective service delivery model if a practitioner and parents know that this mode of service delivery is yielding the desired outcomes. If not, then in-person sessions or consultations need to be arranged. This supports the benefit of considering a hybrid approach. Ultimately the needs of the child and family need to determine the service delivery model (von Muralt et al., 2016).

Auditory-Verbal practitioners, who are highly experienced at delivering in-person services, can be confident that they also have most of the foundational skills and expertise necessary for providing services via telepractice. However, some additional training and ongoing support may be required to ensure adaption to delivering telepractice (Houston, 2014a; Jarvis-Selinger, Chan, Payne, Plohman, & Ho, 2008; von Muralt et al., 2016). Some of the following skills need to be acquired:

- use of computer and other telecommunications technology and troubleshooting techniques;
- ability to modify service delivery and explain to the parent or caregiver how to carry out activities to achieve lesson goals rather than personally modeling this; and
- observation of performance and elicitation of feedback from parents and caregivers regarding the child's performance (Cason, 2009; von Muralt et al., 2016).

While there is no one correct telepractice model for the delivery of AVT, a growing number of practitioners is choosing to provide services by telepractice, with successful outcomes. Two programs that have developed innovative and successful telepractice programs for AVT service delivery are discussed here: the Hear and Say Centre in Brisbane, Australia, and the Telepractice and eLearning Laboratory (TeLL), the School of Speech-Language Pathology and Audiology at the University of Akron, Ohio.

Hear and Say Centre—Australia

Hear and Say has been delivering telepractice services since 1998. Over this time technology has changed, and much has been learned about this model of service delivery. For most families enrolled in the Hear and Say telepractice program, the service frequency is weekly. What may be unique to this service is the inclusion of regular planning sessions. In this model, the weekly telepractice sessions alternate between a session with the child and parent/s one week and a planning session with the parent/s on the alternate week. The planning sessions do not involve the child and include discussion of the child's goals and progress, review of the effectiveness of implementing the goals and activities into daily life, troubleshooting any concerns, and culminates in joint planning of the session that will occur in the alternate week.

These planning sessions are very important, as parents need to feel empowered to facilitate the sessions and prepare the resources/toys needed for the activities. The Auditory-Verbal practitioners write a plan during this session and the parent is encouraged to also take notes. Recording the session is also an option (with appropriate consent) and allows the parent to review what was discussed and/or share with other family members or persons in the child's circle of support. This approach fits well with the principles of adult learning, as parents are more likely to understand and retain the information they have learned if they are involved in the goal and activity setting and contribute their own ideas (see Chapter 16). An organized approach fosters confidence and supports the parents' ability to make connections and understand the effectiveness of the therapy. This also aligns well with the philosophy of AVT, where the practitioner is guiding and coaching the parents, and the parents are the natural language teachers of their child. Once completed, the lesson plan is emailed to the family prior to the next week's session with the child and parent/s, when the practitioner observes, guides, and coaches the parent in delivering and evaluating the AVT session (see Chapter 17). The practitioner documents the child's performance during a session, and the parent and therapist discuss the child's progress both during the therapy session and at the planning session.

Families enrolled in the Hear and Say Centre's telepractice program also receive age-appropriate "lesson boxes" that contain toys, puzzles, books, games, and other resources that can be used in lessons. These resources are loaned for a period of time, returned, and replaced with another lesson box. Auditory-Verbal practitioners are able to see the contents of the box on an electronic catalogue system, which helps with preparation and planning. Alternatively, inventories of home resources, crafts, and other items developed with the parent or caregiver may be used to plan sessions.

Families also receive in-person contact approximately four times each year in addition to weekly telepractice sessions. The practitioner travels to their home for a "home visit" as well as an inclusive educational setting visit for school-age children (providing consultation and advice on working with children who are deaf or hard of hearing). Families also attend the Hear and Say Centre to participate in in-person speech and language assessments, social skills groups, parent education sessions, and individual lessons. While service frequency may reduce, this cycle of support continues until the child enters school.

The Telepractice and eLearning Laboratory (TeLL)—University of Akron, Ohio

AVT requires full parent participation in each session, and as described above, the parent is the main "consumer" of the intervention. That is, the trained professional provides coaching and guidance to ensure that the parent becomes the primary facilitator of listening and spoken language in the child with hearing loss. As the parent's knowledge and skills increase, the child's auditory functioning and use of spoken language also improves. As indicated above, telepractice remains a valuable service delivery that can connect parents of who have chosen to follow AVT with qualified practitioners.

At the University of Akron, through the TeLL, families receive weekly Auditory-Verbal telepractice sessions. Because the University of Akron has two Listening and Spoken Language Specialists and Certified Auditory-Verbal Therapists (LSLS Cert. AVTs) on faculty, the commitment exists to provide comprehensive listening and spoken language services to children who are deaf or hard of hearing and their families through AVT. Furthermore, the School of Speech-

Language Pathology and Audiology remains one of only a few university training programs that incorporates Auditory-Verbal content in its courses and provides clinical practicum experiences in support of listening and spoken language outcomes for children with hearing loss. In fact, the School of Speech-Language Pathology and Audiology at the University of Akron is one of a limited number of university training programs that have received funding from the US Department of Education that support personnel preparation in the development of listening and spoken language for children with hearing loss. The Graduate Studies Consortium in Listening and Spoken Language was formed to provide coursework, practica, and field-based experiences to graduate students completing this training. Thus, through the TeLL, graduate students in speech-language pathology not only learn how to plan, deliver, and evaluate effective AVT in-person sessions (see Chapter 17), but also learn how to provide AVT sessions through a telepractice model.

Currently, the TeLL is housed in a converted treatment room in the Audiology and Speech Center. A Dell Optiplex 9010 desktop computer is connected to a 32-inch Toshiba flat screen television that is used as a monitor. The Phoenix USB Speakerphone serves as an integrated audio microphone and speaker. The webcam is a Logitech Orbit AF Quickcam. Because the University of Akron utilizes WebEx as its primary distance learning software, the same software is used for all telepractice sessions. Graduate students and faculty receive guided training on the use of the software and preferred practices for

delivering telepractice services prior to any treatment. Privacy, confidentiality, and appropriate software encryption are carefully monitored and maintained. Once treatment is initiated, graduate students continue to be closely supervised by experienced faculty.

Referrals of families with children who are deaf or hard of hearing are received primarily from pediatric audiologists, otolaryngology/otology practices, cochlear implant programs, speech-language pathologists, other parents of children who are deaf or hard of hearing, and through informal "word-of-mouth" connections. Typically, once a referral is received, the following process occurs:

1. a preliminary case history is gathered, usually over the telephone;

2. the child (and family) is scheduled for a comprehensive, in-person speech and language evaluation at the Audiology and Speech Center;

3. the diagnostic assessment is completed on functional hearing/speech perception with the child's hearing technology (e.g., digital hearing aids, cochlear implants, assistive listening device), speech production, receptive and expressive language, and oral-motor development (note: other assessment areas may be added—depending on the needs of the child);

4. once the assessment is completed, a determination is made regarding the use of service delivery models: telepractice or in-person, center-based AVT sessions; and

5. if telepractice is recommended, the parents complete a short questionnaire about the type of computer

equipment they have in their home or where they may have access to a computer with the necessary components (webcam, audio speakers, and microphone) as well as a broadband Internet connection;

a. if it is determined that the parents have the necessary computer equipment available to them, a session will be scheduled to "test" the connection and their comfort with the telepractice session; and

b. finally, if the connection is successful and the parents feel comfortable with the WebEx software, the first formal telepractice session is scheduled.

On occasion, a family who initially seemed to be excellent candidates for telepractice may have difficulty with the service delivery model. That is, there may be technological challenges that emerge or, after beginning services, the parents may find themselves struggling to incorporate the AVT strategies (see Chapter 15) through telepractice. Similarly, other behavioral or learning needs may be identified in the child that requires additional services that cannot be addressed entirely through telepractice. In these rare cases, a hybrid model of service delivery may be implemented whereby the family may come to the Audiology and Speech Center for in-person, center-based services on alternating weeks while they continue to gain confidence with telepractice. Subsequently, in-person sessions may be reduced as the family transitions to receiving all AVT services through telepractice. Ultimately, the top priority is to ensure that telepractice can provide an equivalent level of service delivery and that the child's (and family's) communication needs are being met. While some families may require a hybrid model of telepractice, most do not and usually adapt quickly.

After completing the initial speech and language assessment and the family's computer technology is tested (as outlined above), regular telepractice sessions are scheduled. Prior to each weekly 60-minute session, each family receives, via email, a session plan and materials to help meet the child's current goals in speech, language, and listening. Many of the materials, such as colorful scenes to foster language, can be printed at home and used during the AVT session in the form of PowerPoint files. In addition, the session plan may detail a list of toys of other household items that may be used in the session. The email also contains a web link that, once clicked, will launch WebEx. Parents then enter the "virtual classroom" and can see the beginning instructions or other materials as images on their computer screen.

Because WebEx provides teleconferencing with complete audio and video in real time, each AVT session begins with a discussion of the short-term objectives (STO) for speech, language, and listening objectives for that particular session (see Chapter 17). The discussion also includes how the parent has integrated previously demonstrated AVT strategies into daily living. The faculty member, graduate students, and parent discuss any new communication behaviors that might be relevant to the child's progress, such as new or emerging speech sounds, words, or listening behaviors that have been observed.

After discussing the materials and activities for the session, the faculty member and/or graduate students demonstrate the activity before asking the parent to engage the child. The parent repeats the activity while the faculty member and graduate students observe. This is when the practitioner's role shifts to that of a coach. The faculty member and/or graduate student provides positive reinforcement and constructive feedback to the parent based on how the activity was implemented and how the communication strategies that promote listening and spoken language were applied. This same scenario is repeated as one activity ends and a new activity is initiated. Throughout the session, the parent, the faculty member, and graduate students closely monitor the child's attention level and communication targets. Indeed, the model provided in Chapter 17 is perfectly applicable to AVT telepractice.

Following the session, the parent is able to discuss any concerns about the child's progress, to ask questions about short- or long-term goals, or to seek input about troubleshooting the child's hearing technology (e.g., digital hearing aids and/or cochlear implants, FM systems). Then, the faculty member and graduate students summarize the goals and facilitation strategies that were modeled and practiced during the AVT session and based on the child's performance and developmental stages in listening, talking, and thinking, new goals may be planned for the following week.

The AVT telepractice model offered in this facility continues to be a viable means by which to support children with hearing loss who are learning to listen and acquire spoken language.

WHAT ARE THE BENEFITS AND CHALLENGES OF AUDITORY-VERBAL THERAPY DELIVERED VIA TELEPRACTICE?

In order to further explore and confirm the benefits and challenges of AVT telepractice, the authors will discuss the findings from a study conducted by the HEARing CRC in Australia (Waite et al., 2019). This study explored the perceptions of parents, early-intervention practitioners, and managers involved in receiving or providing early intervention via telepractice and described many benefits and some challenges and considerations for the delivery of AVT via telepractice.

First, the benefits:

1. The telepractice model is responsive to the family's needs

Firstly, telepractice was a service-delivery model reported to be responsive to the family's needs. Models of service incorporating telepractice as well as different mHealth technologies (e.g., iPhones, iPads) could be implemented to meet the individual and sometimes changing needs of children and families. Telepractice provided families with more frequent and timely access to specialized services than was available in their local area and enabled them to choose a service that was best for their needs and priorities. In addition, families who lived far from the center were able to use telepractice alone or in a hybrid/blended format if they lived close to a center but found access difficult.

Overall, telepractice was described as a flexible and convenient service delivery model. It was able to be accessed anywhere, even when a family was on holiday. Similarly, other family members, such as grandparents, may be able to attend a session from another location. It was viewed to promote continuity of service; for example, if a family moved interstate or overseas, they could still attend AVT sessions. It may also facilitate flexibility in scheduling (frequency and timing of sessions).

2. *Telepractice makes use of naturalistic environments*

As telepractice typically took place in the family home, this service enabled AVT to be conducted within the family's natural communication and social environments. Families were reported to feel more comfortable in their own home because they did not have to travel far to access therapy. Some participants viewed the telepractice environment as less formal than a clinical environment, and some professionals reported they felt the environment was more intimate.

In addition to the inclusion of the child's important people in the AVT session, telepractice used the child's environment as stimuli. Sessions were built around family routines, including mealtimes. The practitioners and parents reported that by using the family's own materials and routines, they could more easily carry over listening, talking, and thinking strategies more easily in everyday life (see Chapter 15). Some practitioners were also able easily to observe and/or assess children's behavior and skills in this natural communication and social environment.

3. *Telepractice puts the family in the driver's seat*

In telepractice, the AV practitioner is not physically present with the child. This lack of physical proximity was reported to encourage the practitioner to take on the critical role of coaching family members and supporting them in all aspects of intervention. Families were viewed as being more engaged in sessions and having an increased role in the planning and delivery of sessions. Parents were engaged in suggesting goals and activities, preparing materials, delivering the session, managing behavior, observing, and reporting. As a result, families developed confidence and skills. Some professionals believed that telepractice families may learn these skills faster than families participating in the in-person model, and that the lack of physical proximity, and increased role of the family, had improved or consolidated the practitioner's skills in coaching families and encouraged therapists them to be more flexible.

4. *Supporting and training telepractice users*

A key learning from the research supported the need to support telepractice users (as previously discussed) as they adapted to this service delivery model. While the increased role facilitated the development of family skills and carryover, it also invited challenges. Challenges included behavior management, which could be impacted by being in the less formal home environment. Parents also reported added pressure of needing to suggest activities and prepare resources for the session to run according to the plan. Handover to another family member may also be difficult. It may be difficult for a parent to facilitate a session with an infant without a second pair of hands. Challenges for the practitioners included not being in control of the session, the materials and the child's behavior, difficulty with interrupting the parent to provide guidance and coaching, and difficulty modeling activities without being physically present.

The general telepractice hearing health care literature has called for a need for further training and support (e.g., guidelines) for professionals using telepractice (Behl & Kahn, 2015; Govender & Mars, 2017; McCarthy et al., 2019; Ravi, Gunjawate, Yerraguntla, & Driscoll, 2018). This study found that while there were few formal guidelines for professionals, there was varied training available, including mentoring and support, direct supervision, observation of other professionals (internal and external), professional development opportunities (group training and conferences), and knowledge sharing (Waite et al., 2019).

Overall, participants in the study perceived that practitioners utilized the same skills in telepractice as they did in-person management. However, the skills that were recognized as being particularly important include: rapport building, communication, flexibility and adaptability, and creativity and innovation. Clinical experience and skills were also seen as important for telepractice, and some organizations noted that they do not assign professionals with a telepractice caseload until they developed their in-person AVT skills. While some participants believed that specific skills in technology were important for professionals to have, others felt that these can be quickly acquired when using telepractice.

It is also important to consider the specific skills and any additional support or training that the family may need to successfully and confidently use telepractice. In this study participants identified a number of skills that they believed families needed. These included:

■ Specific technology skills including computer literacy and ability to troubleshoot technical issues. The development of a trouble shooting guide was suggested in addition to individual training and upskilling.

■ Behavior management training, if appropriate.

■ Organization, flexibility, creativity, and being natural in the role of agent of therapy with support from the Auditory-Verbal practitioner.

Also, having clear guidelines and setting expectations for how the telepractice service and individual sessions will run were considered important. This included the need for practitioners to take time to identify families' needs, negotiate roles, prepare families to take the lead, orient families to protocols and etiquette for using telepractice, and build trust. It was also reported that building a rapport with families and maintaining a positive therapeutic interaction may need to be more purposeful in telepractice, whereas in in-person intervention, it tends to be more informal and natural.

Another challenge that was observed was the overall lack of formal and practical policies and procedures for this type of service delivery. While most services in the study had a manual or guideline for professionals that contained information on equipment, technical troubleshooting, and best practices in service delivery, these were not always utilized or found to be useful. Finally, it is important to consider the need for technical support staff for the telepractice program. The study found that this level of support was more typically available for practitioners rather than families and that the practitioner often provided his or her own technical support and troubleshooting advice.

5. Comparisons to in-person AVT sessions

Another consideration for telepractice services is the potential need for and preference of in-person services. Although early intervention practitioners in the HEARing CRC study reported success with families who had not had any in-person contact, having some in-person contact was considered to be an important component of the telepractice model in order to conduct aspects of management not easily completed via telepractice. Building a relationship/rapport with families in-person was considered to be particularly important. It was also viewed as being useful to get a better observation/assessment of the child and to demonstrate AVT strategies to the parent. However, there is currently a lack of evidence for the amount of optimal in-person contact.

Although opinions varied, most families and practitioners in the study expressed a preference for in-person services. It is important to consider that those unfamiliar to telepractice may be uncertain that telepractice services are as effective as in-person services. Therefore, education to both staff and families on the current evidence for telepractice in AVT is important to help parents understand that it achieves the same level of service and outcomes as the in-person service.

6. Technology challenges

Technology issues continue to be among the top reported challenges for telepractice services. Although it was acknowledged that technology for telepractice was improving, an issue reported by some participants in this Australian study was poor Internet connectivity, leading to call dropouts, or other issues such as audio-visual lag, pixilation, and audio dropout. Other software and hardware issues may also cause interruptions to the AVT telepractice session. It is likely that in future higher bandwidths for videoconferencing will be more readily available (Behl et al., 2017). However, other means for overcoming these limitations, such as using the telephone as a back-up, or using store-and-forward methods for assessment, may need to be employed.

The HEARing CRC study highlighted the consideration needed in choosing technology that is usable and meets clinical needs. Services in the study often chose web-based videoconferencing systems that were easy to use. However, there may continue to be challenges associated with family confidence and ability to use the technology, highlighting an importance of providing adequate training and support. Some concerns have been reported about limitations in the quality and capability of the technology, including privacy and security concerns and audio-visual limitations. While further research is needed to determine the specific audio-visual conditions required for clinical tasks such as assessment, potential solutions to current limitations include using a parent or assistant to clarify what the child has said (Constantinescu, 2012), using asynchronous telepractice (Waite, Theodoros, Russell, & Cahill, 2010), or increasing bandwidth (Behl & Kahn, 2015).

7. *Access to telepractice*

Another current issue for telepractice service provision found in our study and in the broader literature is access to funding and telepractice technology. While research demonstrating that telepractice is a cost-effective service delivery model is emerging (Blaiser et al., 2013; Olsen et al., 2012), further research of particular models of telepractice is needed. Although telepractice was reported to reduce travel costs, it was acknowledged by participants in the HEARing CRC study that costs for telepractice may be a challenge for some families. Further, it was acknowledged that parts of the telepractice service may be costly for some service providers, including resources and equipment, and that cost is a factor in deciding what aspects of a service can be conducted by telepractice and whether a family accesses telepractice or in-person services.

8. *Child and family factors*

Child and family factors are important considerations when determining eligibility for telepractice services (Speech Pathology Australia, 2014) and for the planning, delivery, and evaluation of AVT sessions (see Chapter 17). Participants in the HEARing CRC study identified a number of child factors that were important considerations, including the child's age, familiarity with information and communication technology, en-

gagement, and behavior. These factors may impact timing and length of sessions, the choice of technology and the choice of activities. Further, age may impact how easily telepractice sessions are implemented. For example, some practitioners reported they found infants easier to manage in telepractice, because the interaction was more with the parent than the child. Some indicated that children with hearing loss may have difficulty with the auditory signal/non-live voice over videoconferencing. Finally, some children with multiple needs can be challenging to manage via telepractice, for both the practitioner and the parents.

Family factors were also considered important to the success of telepractice and included:

- the family structure
- family dynamics
- familiarity with the practitioner
- access to support systems, resources, and technology
- parent learning style and their preference for an intervention model (families who prefer a more *traditional model* of intervention may experience difficulty)
- the family's attitude, motivation, commitment, compliance, knowledge, and confidence in their ability to be the primary delivery agent

Family factors may influence their engagement, choice of technology parent and professional confidence, and the strategies that the early intervention professional uses in working with the family, and ultimately the outcomes of the program. However, some practitioners believe that all families have the ability to be successful in the telepractice environment.

9. *Preparation and follow-up*

It was generally noted by participants in the study that preparation and follow-up were necessary for intervention sessions via telepractice to be successful. Firstly, preparing the telepractice environment was important. This included selecting a suitable location for the family to access telepractice and that may not be the home, especially if connectivity is poor and setting up the room and furniture and information and communication technology are problematic. AV practitioners need to determine how to adapt activities to telepractice and to prepare the AVT session plan, timetable/schedule (considering time zones, when the child is alert), and resources (e.g., finding out what resources the family has, sending out resources to the family). In telepractice, preparation is seen as the responsibility of both the practitioner and the family. It was also seen as important to prepare families for each session by providing explicit communication about what will happen in the session and discussing telepractice etiquette. Finally, practitioners and parents need to be prepared to manage behavioral and technical interruptions (e.g., by having a back-up plan), and there must be follow-up (see Chapter 17).

CHAPTER SUMMARY

Children who are deaf or hard of hearing and their families need access to early intervention with an experienced and qualified Auditory-Verbal practitioner (Estabrooks et al., 2014; Tye-Murray, 2009; von Muralt et al., 2016). Unfortunately, there is a shortage of qualified practitioners who have the necessary knowledge and skills to deliver such evidence-based and evidence-informed intervention in clinics, private practices, and home and indeed by AVT telepractice, making access to this service model a challenge (Houston et al., 2011; Houston & Perigoe, 2010; Houston & Stredler-Brown, 2012; JCIH, 2007; Moeller et al., 2006; Shulman et al., 2010; White, 2008). Continued advances in telecommunication technology, a growing interest in the LSLS Cert. AVT credential, and a growing number of AV practitioners offering AVT by telepractice offer great opportunities for many families.

Although the current research is showing that equivalent outcomes and high levels of satisfaction can be achieved, there are challenges indeed, challenges for both the practitioner and families with this mode of AVT service delivery. However, research and practitioner feedback also suggest that there are great benefits that may not have been predicted that make AVT highly suited to telepractice as an effective mode of service delivery.

REFERENCES

AG Bell Association. (2019, July–August). By the numbers. *LSL Leading Edge.*

AG Bell Association. (2012). Principles of listening and spoken language. Retrieved from http://www.agbellacademy.org

American Speech-Language-Hearing Association. (2019). *Professional issues/teleprac-*

tice. Retrieved August, 2019 from http:// www.asha.org/Practice-Portal/Professional -Issues/Telepractice/

Apuzzo, M., & Yoshinaga-Itano, C. (1995). Early identification of infants with significant hearing loss and the Minnesota Child Development Inventory. *Seminars in Hearing, 16*, 124–139.

Armstrong, D. G., Giovinco, N., Joseph L. Mills, J. L., & Rogers, L. C. (2011). Face-Time for physicians: Using real time mobile phone-based videoconferencing to augment diagnosis and care in telemedicine. *EPlasty, 11*, 212–217.

Barr, M., Duncan, J., & Dally, K. (2018). A systematic review of services to DHH children in rural and remote regions. *Journal of Deaf Studies and Deaf Education, 23*, 118–130. doi: 10.1093/deafed /enx059

Behl, D. D., Blaiser, K., Cook, G., Barrett, T., Callow-Heusser, C., Brooks, B. M., . . . White, K. R. (2017). A multisite study evaluating the benefits of early intervention via telepractice. *Infants & Young Children, 30*(2), 147–161.

Behl, D. D., & Kahn, G. (2015). Provider perspectives on telepractice for serving families of children who are deaf or hard of hearing. *International Journal of Telerehabilitation, 7*(1), 3–12.

Blaiser, K. M., Behl, D., Callow-Heusser, C., & White, K. R. (2013). Measuring costs and outcomes of tele-intervention when serving families of children who are deaf/ hard-of-hearing. *International Journal of Telerehabilitation, 5*(2), 3–10.

Brennan, D. (2013). To move telepractice toward the future, we should look to the past. *SIG 18 Perspectives on Telepractice, 3*, 4–8.

Calderon, R. (2000). Parental involvement in deaf children's education programs as a predictor of child's language, early reading, and social-emotional development. *Journal of Deaf Studies and Deaf Education, 5*(2), 140–155.

Caleffe-Schenck N. (2006). *Auditory Skills Checklist*. Durham, NC: MED-EL Group.

Cason, J. (2009). A pilot telerehabilitation program: Delivering early intervention services to rural families. *International Journal of Telerehabilitation, 1*(1), 29–38.

Chen, P. H., & Liu, T. W. (2017). A pilot study of telepractice for teaching listening and spoken language to Mandarin-speaking children with congenital hearing loss. *Deafness and Education International, 19*(3–4), 134–143.

Cohn, E. (2013). SIG 18 Coordinator's column. *SIG 18 Perspectives on Telepractice, 3*, 3.

Constantinescu, G. (2012). Satisfaction with telemedicine for teaching listening and spoken language to children with hearing loss. *Journal of Telemedicine and Telecare, 18*, 267–272.

Constantinescu, G., Waite, M., Dornan, D., Rushbrooke, E., Brown, J., McGovern, J., . . . Hill, A. (2014). A pilot study of telepractice delivery for teaching listening and spoken language to children with hearing loss. *Journal of Telemedicine and Telecare, 20*(3), 135–140.

Craig, J. (1999). Introduction. In R. Wootton & J. Craig (Eds.), *Introduction to telemedicine* (pp. 3–17). London, UK: Royal Society of Medicine Press Ltd.

Craig, J., & Patterson, V. (2006). Introduction to the practice of telemedicine. In R. Wootton, J. Craig, & V. Patterson (Eds.), *Introduction to telemedicine* (2nd ed., pp. 3–14). London, UK: Royal Society of Medicine Press Ltd.

Craig, J., Russell, C., Patterson, V., & Wootton, R. (1999). User satisfaction with real-time teleneurology. *Journal of Telemedicine and Telecare, 5*, 237–241.

Crutchley, S., Alvares, R., & Campbell, M. (2014). Getting started: Building a successful telepractice program. In K. T. Houston (Ed.), *Telepractice in speech-language pathology* (pp. 51–81). San Diego, CA: Plural Publishing.

Cuyler, R., & Holland, D. (2012). *Implementing telemedicine*. Bloomington, IN: Xlibris Corporation.

Darkins, A. W., & Cary, M. A. (2000). *Telemedicine and telehealth: Principles, policies, performance, and pitfalls.* London, UK: Free Association Books.

Denton, D. R., & Gladstone, V. S. (2005). Ethical and legal issues related to telepractice. *Seminars in Hearing, 26*(1), 43–52.

Dzenowagis, J. (2009). Bridging the digital divide: Linking health and ICT policy. In R. Wootton, N. G. Patil, E. Richard, R. E. Scott, & K. Ho (Eds.), *Telehealth in the developing world* (pp. 9–26). London, UK: Royal Society of Medicine Press Ltd.

Estabrooks, W., Houston, K. T., & MacIver-Lux, K. (2014). Therapeutic approaches following cochlear implantation. In S. B. Waltzman & J. T. Roland (Eds.), *Cochlear implants* (3rd ed.). New York, NY: Thieme Medical Publishers.

Fried, M. P. (2001). The challenges and potential of otolaryngological telemedicine. *Archives of Otolaryngology–Head and Neck Surgery, 127*, 336.

Govender, S. M., & Mars, M. (2017). The use of telehealth services to facilitate audiological management for children: A scoping review and content analysis. *Journal of Telemedicine and Telecare, 23*(3), 392–401.

Houston, K. T., Fleming, A. M., Brown, K. J., Weinberg, T. R., & Nafe, J. M. (2014). History, definitions and overview of telepractice models. In K. T. Houston (Ed.), *Telepractice in speech-language pathology* (pp. 1–20). San Diego, CA: Plural Publishing.

Houston, K. T. (2014). *Telepractice in speech-language pathology.* San Diego: Plural Publishing.

Houston, K. T., & Bradham, T. S. (2011). Parent engagement in audiologic habilitation: Increasing positive outcomes for children with hearing loss. *The ASHA Leader, 16*(8), 5–6.

Houston, K. T., Munoz, K. F., & Bradham, T. S. (2011). Professional development: Are we meeting the needs of state EHDI programs? *The Volta Review, 111*(2), 209–223.

Houston, K. T., & Perigoe, C. B. (Eds.). (2010). Professional preparation for listening and spoken language practitioners. *The Volta Review, 110*(2), 86–354.

Houston, K. T., & Stredler-Brown, A. (2012). A model of early intervention for children with hearing loss provided through telepractice. *Volta Review, 112*(3), 283–296.

Hearing loss provided through telepractice. *The Volta Review, 112*(3), 283–296. Retrieved August 19, 2019 from https://www.learntechlib.org/p/113932/

Jarvis-Selinger, S., Chan, E., Payne R., Plohman, K., & Ho, K. (2008) Clinical telehealth across the disciplines: Lessons learned. *Telemedicine Journal and e-Health, 4*(7), 720–725.

Joint Committee on Infant Hearing. (2007). Year 2007 position statement: Principles and guidelines for early hearing detection and intervention programs. *Pediatrics, 120*(4), 898–921.

Keck, C. S., & Doarn, C. R. (2014). Telehealth technology applications in speech-language pathology. *Journal of Telemedicine and e-Health, 20*(7), 1–7.

Krumm, M., Ribera, J., & Schmiedge, J. (2005). Using a telehealth medium for objective hearing testing: Implications for supporting rural universal newborn hearing screening programs. *Seminars in Hearing, 26*, 3–12

Mayne, A. M., Yoshinaga-Itano, C., Sedey, A. L., & Carey, A. (2000). Expressive vocabulary development of infants and toddlers who are deaf or hard of hearing. *The Volta Review, 100*, 1–28.

McCarthy, M., Leigh, G., & Arthur-Kelly, M. (2019). Telepractice delivery of family-centred early intervention for children who are deaf or hard of hearing: A scoping review. *Journal of Telemedicine and Telecare, 25*(4), 249–260.

McPherson, B. (2011). Innovative technology in hearing instruments: Matching needs in the developing world. *Trends in Amplification, 15*(4), 209–214.

McPherson, B. (2014). Hearing assistive technologies in developing countries: Background, achievements and challenges. *Disability and Rehabilitation: Assistive Technology, 9*(5), 360–364.

McPherson, B., & Amedofu, G. (2013). Hearing aid candidacy and strategies in developing countries. *ENT and Audiology News, 22*, 88–90.

Moeller, M. P., White, K. R., & Shisler, L. (2006). Primary care physicians' knowledge, attitudes, and practices related to newborn hearing screening. *Pediatrics, 118*(4), 1357–1370.

Moeller, M. P. (2000). Early intervention and language development in children who are deaf and hard of hearing. *Pediatrics, 106*, E43

Olsen, S., Fiechtl, B., & Rule, S. (2012). An evaluation of virtual home visits in early intervention: Feasibility of "virtual intervention." *The Volta Review, 112*, 267–281.

Peters-Lalios, A. (2012). ConnectHear tele-intervention. *The Volta Review, 112*, 357–364.

Pipp-Siegel, S., Sedey, A. L., VanLeeuwen, A. M., & Yoshinaga-Itano, C. (2003). Mastery motivation and expressive language in young children with hearing loss. *Journal of Deaf Studies and Deaf Education 8*(2), 133–145.

Ravi, R., Gunjawate, D. R., Yerraguntla, K., & Driscoll, C. (2018). Knowledge and perceptions of teleaudiology among audiologists: A systematic review. *Journal of Audiology & Otology, 22*(3), 120.

Ribera, J. (2005). Interjudge reliability and validation of telehealth applications in a hearing in noise test. *Seminars in Hearing, 26*, 13–18.

Rushbrooke, E. (2012). *Remote MAPping for children with cochlear implants* (Unpublished master's thesis). Brisbane, Australia: The University of Queensland.

Rushbrooke, E. (2016). Models of service delivery: what should we consider? In E. Rushbrooke & K. Houston (Eds.), *Telepractice in audiology* (pp.23–45) San Diego, CA: Plural Publishing.

Rushbrooke, E., & Houston, K. T. (2016). History, terminology, and the advent of teleaudiology. In E. Rushbrooke &

K. Houston (Eds.), *Telepractice in audiology* (pp. 1–21) San Diego, CA: Plural Publishing.

Sevean, P., Dampier, S., Spadoni, M., Strickland, S., & Pilatzke, S. (2009). Patients and families' experiences with video telehealth in rural/remote communities in Northern Canada. *Journal of Clinical Nursing, 18*(18), 2573–2579.

Shulman, S., Besculides, M., Saltzman, A., Ireys, H., & White, K. R. (2010). Evaluation of the universal newborn hearing screening and intervention program. *Pediatrics, 126*, S19–S27.

Singh, G. (2013). Teleaudiology: Are patients and practitioners ready for it? Retrieved April 18, 2014 from http://www .phonakpro.com/content/dam/phonak/gc _hq/b2b/en/events/2013/chicago/Singh _SF_2013_Teleaudiology.pdf

Speech Pathology Australia. (2014). *Teleprac tice in speech pathology position state ment.* Melbourne, Australia: The Speech Pathology Association of Australia Ltd.

Stredler-Brown, A. (2012). The future of telepractice for children who are deaf and hard of hearing. *The Volta Review, 112*, 435.

Swanepoel, D. (2013). 20Q: Audiology to the people—combining technology and connectivity for services by telehealth. *AudiologyOnline*, Article 12183. Retrieved from http://www.audioloyonline.com

Tye-Murray, N. (2009). *Foundations of aural rehabilitation: Children, adults, and their family members* (3rd ed.). New York, NY: Delmar Cengage Learning.

von Muralt, M., Farwell, L., & Houston, K. T. (2016). Telerehabilitation in audiology. In E. Rushbrooke & K. Houston (Eds.), *Telepractice in audiology* (pp. 153–188). San Diego, CA: Plural Publishing.

Waite, M. C., Theodoros, D. G., Russell, T. G., & Cahill, L. M. (2010). Internet-based telehealth assessment of language using the CELF-4. *Language, Speech, and Hearing Services in Schools, 41*, 445–458.

Waite, M., Atkins, J., Scarinci, N., Meyer, C., Rushbrooke, E., Cowan, R., & Hickson,

(2019). Unpublished Project XR4.1.1 b. *Improving hearing healthcare access and outcomes: Paediatric stream*. Australia: HEARing CRC.

White, K. R. (2008). Newborn hearing screening. In J. R. Madell & C. Flexer (Eds.), *Pediatric audiology: Diagnosis, technology, and management* (pp. 31–41). New York, NY: Thieme.

World Health Organization. (2011). *mHealth New horizons for health through mobile technologies*. Geneva, Switzerland: Author. Retrieved August 21, 2019 from https://www.who.it/goe/publications/goe_mhealth_web.pdf

World Health Organization. (2013). *Multicountry assessment of national capacity to provide hearing care*. Geneva, Switzerland: Author. Retrieved August 21, 2019 from https://www.who.int/pbd/publications/WHOReportHearingCare_Englishweb.pdf

World Health Organization. (2019). Deafness and hearing loss. Retrieved August 29, 2019 from https://www.who.int/deafness/estimates/en/

Xiaohui, Y., Han, H., Jiadong, D., Liurong, W., Cheng, L., Xueli, Z., . . . Bleiberg, J. (2013). *mHealth in China and the United States: How mobile technology is transforming healthcare in the world's two largest economies* (Executive summary). Washington DC: Center for Technology Innovation at Brookings.

Yoshinaga-Itano, C., Sedey, A. L., Coulter, D. K., & Mehl, A. L. (1998). Language of early and later identified children with hearing loss. *Pediatrics, 102*(5).

Yoshinaga-Itano, C. (1995). Efficacy of early identification and intervention. *Seminars in Hearing, 16*, 115–120.

26

COACHING AND MENTORING PRACTITIONERS AND AUDITORY-VERBAL THERAPY

Helen McCaffrey Morrison
and Cheryl L. Dickson

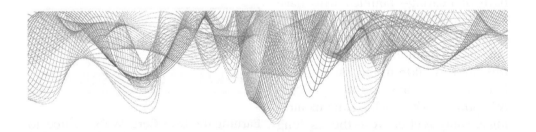

This chapter describes the process of coaching and mentoring to help practitioners master the knowledge and skills required for effective planning, delivery, and evaluation of Auditory-Verbal Therapy (AVT). Coaching and mentoring are long-standing traditions and hallmarks of Auditory-Verbal practice. As cited in Chapter 1, the history of AVT is, in fact, a story of coaching and mentoring, with each generation of practitioners passing on historic and accrued knowledge and skills to the next. Coaching and mentoring ensure fidelity of practice (Kretlow & Bartholomew, 2010), so that the 10 Principles of AVT remain in place to effectively support families who are helping their children who are deaf or hard of hearing to reach their maximum potential across the lifespan. This story is not yet fully told. The survey outcomes reported in Chapter 1 indicate that the future of AVT as envisioned by today's

LSLS Cert. AVT community is *growth*—growth that demands increased numbers of qualified AV practitioners on a global scale. Today, coaching/mentoring in AVT is more than a tradition. It is a necessity.

The journey to becoming an AV practitioner (practitioner) embodies two distinct areas of development: mastery of the theory and content encompassed by the knowledge domains that underlie competent practice patterns, and mastery of specific skills and strategies required to implement AVT. The aspiring practitioner is assisted by a coach/mentor who is able to support the learner as one masters both the required knowledge and skills over time. The coach/mentor model, however, is incomplete if one considers only the coach/mentor and the *aspiring* AV *practitioner.* AVT serves primary care givers and children who are deaf or hard of hearing—families who have chosen to work in partnership with a practitioner to chase the dreams of AVT that are a common theme throughout this book. Children and families are integral to coaching and mentoring in AVT, and as such, coaching and mentoring are only as effective as the resulting outcomes for the children and families served by the practitioner who receives coaching and mentoring support.

The authors begin here with a review of the protocols for earning certification as a LSLS Certified Auditory-Verbal Therapist. The certification process organizes the subsequent topics and suggestions. We recognize that not all practitioners will participate in a formal certification process. The topics offered here, therefore, are intended to be applicable regardless of whether coaching and mentoring take place within the LSLS certification framework

or on a more informal basis. Coaching and mentoring imply a relationship between two professionals—the coach/mentor and the aspiring AV practitioner, or mentee. The definitions, roles, and attributes of each are described in this chapter, along with principles of adult learning that shape the nature of coaching and mentoring practitioners in AVT.

Coaching and mentoring are active processes that follow logical steps, grounded in purpose, intended to help professionals become independent and competent practitioners who are highly effective in supporting families to help their children. Here we describe these steps, provide suggestions for how to implement the processes, and conclude with a discussion of the future of coaching and mentoring in AVT.

LISTENING AND SPOKEN LANGUAGE CERTIFIED AUDITORY-VERBAL THERAPIST (LSLS CERT. AVT)

Earning the LSLS Cert. AVT is a three- to five-year process culminating in passing the certification examination. The Academy for Listening and Spoken Language (the Academy) is the organization charged with administering the certification application process and examination. Table 26–1 displays the 10 requirements for LSLS Cert. AVT certification that are in place at the time this chapter is being written. For current and official information, the reader is encouraged to go directly to the website for the Academy (https://ag bellacademy.org) (see also Chapter 1 for certification history).

Table 26-1. Requirements for the LSLS Cert. AVT (AG Bell LSLS Academy, 2017a)

Requirement	Description
1. Academic	Bachelors/masters degree or international equivalent in audiology, speech-language pathology, or education of children who are deaf or hard of hearing
2. Credential	License, certificate, or credential required to practice independently in individual's location
3. Description of practice	Self-composed written description of applicant's Auditory-Verbal practice
4. Commitment to Principles of Auditory-Verbal Therapy	Signed commitments to AVT Principles, Principles of Professional Behavior and Rules of Conduct
5. Continuing education	80 hours, including 10 hours of observation of a LSLS Cert. AVT
6. Professional experience	900 clock hours of AVT: minimum of 750 hr in direct therapy, maximum 150 hr related activities (e.g., assessments, parent conferences, school consultations, audiological visits)
7. Mentored experience	20 1-hour therapy sessions observed by a LSLS certified coach/mentor distributed over the course of the 3- to 5-year certification period; a minimum of 3 mentored sessions per year
8. Parent recommendations	Letters of recommendation for certification from 2 families served
9. Professional recommendations	Two letters affirming competency, including one from a supervisor
10. Passing certification exam	AG Bell Academy gives permission to sit for the exam, dependent upon review of candidate's documentation of requirements 1–9.

The candidate for the LSLS Cert. AVT examination must have a university degree and certification/licensure to practice audiology, education of children who are deaf or hard of hearing, and/or speech-language pathology in their specific geographic location and must also acquire sufficient practice hours to have developed an in-depth understanding and competency for comprehensive planning, delivery, and evaluation of AVT. The Principles of Auditory-Verbal Therapy are a predominant theme throughout this process. The candidate for certification needs to demonstrate an understanding of the

Principles, the application of the Principles as observed by a mentor and in the applicant's own description of practice, and, most importantly, a signed commitment to the Principles. Certification is not an indicator of *readiness* to begin practice. It is an indicator of *mastery* of the knowledge and skills that are the foundation for competent and effective practice. The three- to five-year process for completing the journey to the eligibility for LSLS Cert. AVT certification exam is dependent upon the amount of time the candidate needs to accumulate the required professional experience.

When the candidate has met the first nine requirements, he or she may submit documentation for doing so to the Academy in an application to take the LSLS Certification Examination. The Certification Examination tests the application of knowledge in nine core content domains (AG Bell LSLS Academy, 2017b):

- hearing and hearing technology
- auditory function
- spoken language communication
- child development
- parent guidance and coaching
- strategies for listening and spoken language development
- history/philosophy/professional issues
- education
- emergent literacy

Coaching and mentoring are at the heart of the certification process. A LSLS Cert. AVT coach/mentor works closely with the candidate during the period leading up to eligibility for the Certification Examination. The AG Bell Academy refers to the certification candidate as the "mentee" and, for the purposes of this chapter, we will do the same. The LSLS Cert. AVT coach/mentor observes and provides feedback for 20 AVT sessions conducted by the mentee. Observation may be conducted live or via video. The 20 observations are distributed across the certification period at a rate of a minimum of 3 per year. The encounters and relationship between the coach/mentor and the mentee are far more robust and complex, however, than what might happen in a simple series of therapy observations and feedback sessions, as described below.

THE LSLS CERT. AVT COACH/MENTOR

Coaching and mentoring take place across a variety of professions. Descriptions of each can be found in published literature from business, healthcare, and education. Coaching and mentoring can each be defined in terms of the actors, the objectives, the activities, and the coach's or mentor's expertise. Mentoring has the longer history of the two. Mentoring is a helping relationship between a more experienced professional and one who has less experience (Rubinstein & Fox, 2018). The objective of mentoring is to help the recipient further his or her career objectives. Mentor support can include teaching, advising, counseling, and, of course, challenging the mentee who is working toward his or her professional objective (Johnson, 2016; Manza & Patrick, 2012). This might also include opening doors by making introductions to other professionals who can assist with employment, promotion, helping a new employee learn the protocols and culture in a work setting, or guiding a mentee through changing careers (Johnson & Ridley, 2018). Some definitions point to the mentor as a source of professional information or content knowledge, giving the mentor a role as a teacher (Hymans, 2018). The mentor's expertise is considered to be broad in comparison to that of the coach (Passmore, 2010).

Coaching is a helping relationship, although the coach may not necessarily be a more senior member of the profession. A coach holds expertise in a particular domain within the profession of the person who receives the coaching (van Nieuwerburgh, 2018). Coaching is less focused on furthering the recipient's career compared with mentoring (Hamlin, Ellinger, & Beattie, 2008). A coach typically assists in *skill development* as opposed to knowledge transfer. Coaching in education, for example, has been found to positively impact teacher strategies (Neuman & Cunningham, 2009) and student outcomes (Kraft, Blazar, & Hogan, 2018; Neuman & Cunningham, 2009).

The similarities between coaching and mentoring are more powerful than their differences. Both are valued means for helping professionals improve and expand practice in their respective fields. The principles that guide adult learning, change, and relationship building are fundamental to both. The overlapping characteristics and functions of coaching and mentoring have led some to describe these as falling on a continuum (Law, 2013). A hybrid model known as "coaching/mentoring" is used in the education profession as a more functional label that encompasses the range of services provided and the role flexibility

needed to help education professionals strengthen and improve their practice (Hymans, 2018; van Nieuwerburgh, 2018). The coach/mentor helps the educator in skill development, shares information as required, and points the recipient toward resources that will increase the professional's knowledge. The coach/mentor also functions as a sounding board and guide as the educator develops a perspective regarding the philosophy and ethics of the profession (Pask & Joy, 2007). The coach/mentor model is compatible with the process by which an experienced LSLS Cert. AVT supports a mentee as he or she works toward developing AVT practice. *This model is not unlike the service provided by the LSLS Cert. AVT to parents and caregivers, who are the primary agents of change in the lives of their children who are deaf or hard of hearing who choose to follow AVT.*

Sometimes, an organization asks a LSLS Cert. AVT who is a supervisor to also act as a coach/mentor to younger/newer employees who need to learn the knowledge and skills required for the planning, delivery, and evaluation of AVT. This is a difficult balancing act that can engender role conflict (Mellon & Murdoch-Eaton, 2015). A supervisor assesses performance and may have *influence* with regard to continued mentee employment, promotions, or increases in compensation. In contrast, the coach/mentor engages in non-judgmental interaction to encourage growth by providing vision, fostering reflection, and encouraging personal benchmarking against desired learning outcomes (Zachary 2000). When a supervisor is also a coach/mentor, aspects of the mentee's performance other than progress in AV skills and knowledge may potentially positively color or negatively cloud the coaching and/or mentoring. The imbalance of power between the supervisor and employee can prevent the creation of an effective mentoring relationship.

THE MENTEE

Aspiring AV practitioners seek a coach/mentor from a variety of starting points with regard to level of knowledge and skills. Mentees may be recent university graduates and fresh from training that may or may not have included AVT in the curriculum, may have experience in other approaches but are new to AVT, or may have experience in AVT and wish to enter the certification process. Mentees seek a coach/mentor with various motivations—to meet the interests and needs of families on their caseloads, to fulfill a mandated obligation to the family service plan or a child's independent educational plan, or to be competitive with AV practitioners in their community. Mentees also come from three related but different professions: audiology, education of children who are deaf or hard of hearing, and speech-language pathology.

What is common to all is that they enter into a relationship with a coach/mentor to learn new information and skills, and they do so as *adult learners*. Furthermore, regardless of their starting point as learners, mentees experience *positive change* while working with an AV coach/mentor. They change in *self-concept*, and they discover competencies they were not aware they possessed or were not aware that they needed to improve or acquire. They change their *knowledge structures* as they acquire new information that is important for AVT—information that is learned across the three professions that make up the work of AV practitioners. They change *attitudes and perspectives* as they take on new ways to think about serving families, coaching and guiding families, and they experience new expectations regarding what children who are deaf or hard of hearing are able to achieve. Change is more likely to be welcomed when it is generated from within the learner rather than imposed upon by the coach/mentor. Effective AV coach/mentors use strategies that maintain the locus of control with the mentee and help him or her to "meet change as a friend" (Lipscomb & An, 2010).

MENTEES AS ADULT LEARNERS

Coaching and mentoring in AVT are guided by principles of adult learning, or *andragogy* (Knowles, 1980; Knowles, Holton, & Swanson, 2005). Andragogy is different from pedagogy, the practice of teaching children, due to differences in brain development that enable adult learners to engage in higher order critical thinking and problem solving (Tokuhama-Espinosa, 2011), and life experience. Adults' varied life experiences necessitate that learning experiences be sufficiently flexible to allow for individualization. The process of coaching and mentoring in AVT is well suited to these aspects of adult learning, given the complexity of AVT and the individualized experience provided by the mentee's own caseload. Accordingly, coaching and mentoring shaped by adult learning principles is learner

Table 26-2. Principles of Adult Learning for AV Coach/Mentors (Knowles, Holton, & Swanson, 2005)

Adult learners	This means	AV Coach/mentors
Are self-directed	Adults are the agents (in charge) of their own learning	Stand back, providing models or examples, supportive feedback. Ultimately, adult learners choose what they will do.
Are experienced	Adults bring a lifetime of experience adapting to new circumstances, problem solving, and a knowledge base of their own.	Capitalize upon existing knowledge, skills, and experiences. Connect new skills to what adults already know and do.
Want to know "why"	When adults understand why new information and skills are important, they are more likely to take the time to add these to their repertoire.	Connect information and skills to goals that learners have selected for themselves and families they serve.
Are problem solvers	Knowledge and skills are more likely to be learned when they are needed to solve a problem to help children or families on the learner's caseload.	Listen and pay attention. Listen to discover what the learner perceives as a need. Pay attention and point out issues with children/families to invite a solution from the learner.

driven as opposed to coach/mentor directed. Table 26–2 gives examples of how adults approach learning and ways that AV coach/mentors can respond.

AV COACHING AND MENTORING IN ACTION

The following describes the work that takes place between the AV coach/mentor and mentee, laid out from the start of the relationship through the process of observing a mentee's work with children and families and the follow-up to the observation. This sequence is recycled until the relationship between the coach/mentor and mentee is finalized. Coaching and mentoring with a mentee may take place over several years; in the case of LSLS Cert. AVT certification, as stated earlier, the process may take three to five years. The sequence presented here is descriptive rather than prescriptive. AV coach/mentors and mentees move from one activity to another depending upon the needs and interests of the mentee.

Examining One's Own Motivation

An AV coach/mentor is advised to begin by examining why he or she wants to engage in coaching and mentoring: a monetary incentive, desire for professional development, desire to contribute to the future of the profession, et al. Coach/mentors who are self-aware bring insight to the coach/mentor–mentee relationship that is thoughtful and considered. Examining one's own motives helps the coach/mentor avoid the traps of an interest in power or a sense of superiority that can negatively impact the mentee (Johnson & Ridley, 2008; Manza & Patrick, 2012; Zachary, 2000).

The coach/mentor may also give some thought regarding his or her criteria for taking on a mentee. For example, in a global survey of LSLS Cert. AVTs who mentor, the top three criteria for accepting a mentee represented were: (1) possess academic and professionals credentials required to sit for LSLS exam, (2) commitment to AVT and motivation to learn, and (3) access to a sufficiently large Auditory-Verbal caseload for the mentee to obtain experience (Morrison, Perigoe, & Bernstein, 2010).

Starting Out with the Mentee

The relationship of coaches/mentors and mentees begins with a conversation, during which coaches/mentors invite mentees to tell their story of the journey that has led them to a desire to practice AVT (Tschannen-Moran & Tschannen-Moran, 2010). Having mentees tell their story helps clarify their own sense of urgency to take on the process, give voice to expectations, and identify possible roadblocks so that these can be addressed from the start. When mentees are mindful of their motivation for engaging an AV coach/mentor, they become more open to the changes in practice and knowledge that they will experience (Tschannen-Moran & Tschannen-Moran, 2010).

The coach/mentor and prospective mentee talk about the Principles of Auditory-Verbal Therapy in this very first conversation. This enables the coach/mentor to determine the mentee's level of understanding and commitment to the Principles. It is expected that a mentee will start out without a fully formed understanding and commitment. This is an opportunity to discover what the mentee may need from coaching and mentoring to fully embrace the practice of AVT. This opening conversation also provides an opportunity for both parties to discuss possible pitfalls and consider the best way forward.

Opening conversations, such as the above, help the coach/mentor and mentee determine whether they are compatible and ready to proceed. It is highly recommended that an agreement be composed in writing and signed by both parties to help ensure that both positively regard each person's roles and responsibilities and have a clear understanding of the activities and timelines that need to be anticipated. Possible items to address include, but are not limited to: method of communication (email, phone, text, internet communication platform), frequency of meetings, schedule of content to be addressed, coach/mentor expectations, mentee expectations, fees and other costs to the mentee, and strategies for miscommunication or failure to uphold the agreement. Including the Principles of Auditory-Verbal Therapy as an addendum to the agreement keeps all parties mindful of what they are working toward. It is imperative that mentees indicate on the agreement that they understand that working with an AV coach/mentor does not guarantee that they will be accepted by the Academy to sit for the certification examination, nor is there a guarantee that they will pass the examination if they are invited to take it. A sample mentoring Agreement can be found in the *AG Bell Academy LSLS Mentor Handbook* (AG Bell LSLS Academy, 2017c).

Mentee-Driven Goal Selection

Mentee-driven goal selection begins with self-assessment of current skills and knowledge. Self-assessment helps a mentee to recognize where to begin. Goal setting by the mentee puts that recognition into action (McLean, 2012). The mentee is more likely to be open to the changes that will be experienced in the learning process when there is recognition of the need for change and when the mentee is the person who selects the path toward achieving that change (Boyatzis, 2011).

At times the coach/mentor may believe that the mentee is not quite ready to take on a selected goal. The coach/mentor can guide the mentee toward a more appropriate selection by having a conversation about how he or she might work toward that goal. As the coach/mentor and mentee devise

a plan, they identify subskills that will help the mentee reach his or her desired outcome.

The Mentor's Guide to AV Competencies Years 1–3 (Dickson, Morrison, & Jones 2013) is a tool that can guide the mentee's goal selection. The guide was developed with an evidence-based practice model in mind, drawing from the clinical expertise of established LSLS Cert. AVTs (AVI, 2003; Caleffe-Schenck, 1992; Duncan, Kendrick, McGinnis, & Perigoe, 2010) and a survey of LSLS Cert. AVTs who mentor (Morrison et al., 2010).

The Mentor's Guide presents skills that a mentee develops in mastery of AVT, in nine practice areas:

- planning
- conduct of the therapy session
- audition
- spoken language and speech production
- literacy
- parent coaching
- assessment and reporting
- school inclusion
- professional qualities

These are distributed in a developmental sequence over a three-year period, the typical duration of work toward the LSLS Cert. AVT. Skills at year 3 are for the most part indicators that the mentee can not only demonstrate a particular skill, but also effectively coach a parent to do so. The assumption here is that it is more likely practitioners can effectively coach parents in skills they can perform well themselves. The guide does *not* assume, however, that parent coaching in a mentee's practice takes place only in year 3. Mentees guide and coach parents from the beginning of the process and are expected to improve over time. Examples of developmental mentee goals are found in Table 26–3.

The *Guide* is not intended to be prescriptive. It is simply a tool for self-assessment that can provide structure for conversations about skill development between the coach/mentor and mentee. If a mentee is able to demonstrate attainment of a year 1 level skill at the start of the process, the next level of skill development becomes a goal. If a mentee and coach/mentor observe that by the end of the first year of the process, skill development is not moving toward what is expected in the second year, a conversation about slower than expected progress is in order. Skill development and selection of subsequent skills are more effective in promoting mentee growth if they are revisited periodically.

A coach/mentor and mentee pair may also devise goals of their own making, using the practice aspects described above. It is possible for a mentee to become overwhelmed by all possible skills that an AV practitioner uses for effective planning, delivery, and evaluation of AVT (see Chapter 17). The coach/mentor can help the mentee to focus by suggesting only one or two practice areas at a time for mentee goal selection. A mentee may derive a long list of skills he or she wishes to attain. The coach/mentor can help the mentee prioritize skills and trim the number of selected skills so that the mentee is not overwhelmed.

Observation of the Mentee

Observation of a mentee's work is at the heart of AV coaching and mentoring. The observation illuminates a mentee's knowledge and skills. Each step in the observation process, from preparation to the final report, is an opportunity for the AV coach/mentor to learn about the mentee, and for the mentee to learn about AVT. The following describes a chronology of the session observation: (1) mentee collection and interpretation of child and family information, (2) mentee session review and reflection, (3) observation by the coach/mentor, (4) the feedback conversation, and (5) the written report.

Mentee Collection and Interpretation of Child and Family Information

The mentee gathers child and family information and prepares a description for the mentor about the child's and family's level of function at the time of the observation. Collecting and reading through child and family information serves several purposes:

- The mentee engages in diagnostic practice and learns more about one of the 10 Principles of AVT, "Administer ongoing formal and informal diagnostic assessments to develop individualized Auditory-Verbal treatment plans, to monitor progress and to evaluate the effectiveness of the plans for the child and family."
- Gathering information as a first step places the coach/mentor and mentee in a position to be mindful of the *child and family* in each mentoring session, a central ethical responsibility in the coaching and mentoring process.
- Understanding a child's level of function makes use of the knowledge domains in AVT and

Table 26–3. Examples of Developmental Mentee Goals from *The Mentor's Guide to Auditory-Verbal Competencies* (Dickson et al., 2013).

Year 1	Year 2	Year 3
Planning		
Writes lesson plans noting specific AV strategies and techniques to be used.	Writes lesson plans that include generalization of AV strategies for the family to use in daily routines in the home.	Aids parents to integrate auditory-based interactions in all environments (i.e., playground, library, sports)
Session		
Creates a favorable learning environment by achieving an appropriate ratio of experience based teaching *vs.* task specific testing.	Interweaves assessment of specific goals during play, decreasing formal testing.	Coaches parents to teach goals and assess the child's progress through play.
Audition		
Develops auditory targets based on a hierarchical model and typical auditory development.	Promotes a listening attitude to integrate listening into the child's personality through systematic development of auditory skills.	Assists parents to integrate audition into daily interactions to promote auditory neurological development.
Spoken Language and Speech Production		
Uses wait time and expectant looks to encourage the child to take turns listening and speaking.	Uses a variety of strategies to encourage the child's participation in dialogue, such as waiting, sabotage, following child's lead, recounting past events or retelling familiar stories, or responding to questions that cue language.	Coaches parents to use a variety of strategies to encourage their child's participation in dialogue.
Uses knowledge of speech acoustics and audiological information to select language and speech targets based on typical stages of development.	Adjusts child's targets in a timely manner based on prior performance and progress.	Coaches parents to recognize child's spoken language accomplishments and identify needs in order to adjust targets.

continues

Table 26–3. *continued*

Year 1		Year 2		Year 3
		Literacy		
Uses books, rhymes, and song to enhance vocabulary and language development.		Models and assists the parents in choosing books, rhymes, and songs to develop their child's vocabulary and language.		Coaches and guides the parents in using a variety of strategies to develop their child's vocabulary and language while engaged in books, rhymes, and songs.
		Parent Coaching		
Communicates Auditory-Verbal principles to parents in an effective manner.		Models Auditory-Verbal principles and assists parents to integrate these principles into their daily lives.		Assists parents to share Auditory-Verbal principles, theory, and practice with the child's wider community.
Guides parents to identify ideas for carryover of goals at home.		Coaches and guides parents to implement activities for carryover of goals at home.		Facilitates parent self-evaluation of carryover activities and provides feedback.

fosters critical thinking about the child by asking the guiding questions such as: "Is the diagnostic information consistent with the child's performance that I observe? If not, why not?"

A core set of documents helps the coach/mentor ascertain that the mentee is cognizant of a child's status and is able to collect information essential for providing service that moves a child and family forward: (1) the child's current level of function across the domains of audition, language, speech, and general development, (2) long-term goals, (3) AVT session plan, and (4) audiogram and current report of function with hearing technology. Each provides an opportunity for mentee learning.

1. *Child's current levels.* There are a number of documents/forms that can be used to summarize a child's level in the domains of audition, language, speech, and general development. "Level" can be interpreted as a child's equivalent language age or developmental age in each of the domains. The mentee also notes the child's performance on the Ling Six Sound Test and audiological information such as type and degree of hearing loss, technology used, and listening age. Information about a child's function may be obtained from informal or formal assessment (see Chapter 19) that needs to be conducted no earlier than three to six months prior to the observation session.

2. *Long-term goals.* Long-term goals in audition, language, speech, and cognition/general development need to have been set in the previous 3- to 6-month period. It is useful to encourage the mentee to include an expected rate of progress (e.g., one year or greater

increase in equivalent language age over a 12-month period).

3. *AVT session plan.* The AVT session plan includes (1) short-term objectives (STO) in audition, speech, language, communication, and cognition, (2) activities to reach each goal, (3) strategies, and (4) parent guidance (see Chapter 17).

4. *Audiogram and current report of function with hearing technology.* The AV coach/mentor encourages the mentee to ensure that scheduling for the audiological assessments and the information obtained adhere to the *Recommended Protocol for Audiological Assessment, Hearing Aid and Cochlear Implant Evaluation, and Follow-Up* (AG Bell, 2019). The AV coach/mentor encourages the mentee to think critically about the information on the audiogram and compare audiological information with the child's auditory functioning in therapy and at home (see Chapter 9). The mentee needs to think about the following question: Is functioning as expected based on audiological information or is there some discrepancy?

The mentee is likely to have versions of these documents that he or she uses regularly. It is recommended that the coach/mentor work with forms and documents that are required at the mentee's workplace and use those to help the mentee shape how to compose information to be consistent with what the practitioner needs to know in order to practice effectively.

Mentee Self-Observation and Reflection

The coach/mentor will either observe a mentee's session live or will view a recording. In either case, the mentee records the session to observe him/ herself. These questions guide the self-observation:

- What are highlights of the session?
- How was this session different than what I planned? What do I think accounted for those differences?
- What evidence from the session tells me whether the child and parent achieved the session objectives?
- How do I see myself demonstrating use of the skills I have selected to develop?
- How does this session demonstrate the application of the Principles of AVT?
- What aspects of the session do I especially want to discuss during my feedback conversation with my coach/mentor?

This purposeful self-observation is *reflection,* an evidence-based strategy that fosters change in adult learners (Mezirow, 1997). The self-observation and guiding questions assist the mentee to step away from the experience of doing AVT in real-time and become aware of the demonstrated skills and their effectiveness. This helps the mentee transform automatic, uncritical notions of what he or she is doing into a new perspective, leading to new ideas about how to practice (Taylor, 2007).

The mentee is advised to take notes in response to the questions above and share these with the coach/mentor. If the coach/mentor will be observing a recorded session, these notes can be given to the coach/mentor at the same time as the recording to guide the coach/

mentor's viewing. If the coach/mentor will be observing the session live, the mentee can bring the notes to the feedback session to help structure that conversation.

Observation by the Coach/Mentor

The observation needs to be conducted close in time to receiving the observation documents. Prior to the observation the coach/mentor reads the other supporting documents that describe the child and family and makes notes about what to look for during the observation and what might be points of discussion in the feedback conversation that follows. The coach/mentor also reads the mentee's summary and reflection of the session and uses this information to guide the observation. If the coach/mentor has questions, it is worthwhile to address these prior to watching the session so that there are no misconceptions during the observation.

The AG Bell Academy provides an official form, the F-1, that guides observation of mentees who are working toward the certification examination (AG Bell Academy, 2017a). Using the F-1, the coach/mentor records evidence of mentee skills in planning, audition, language, speech, literacy, parent guidance/coaching and participation, and professional qualities. Each area lists a number of skills considered critical for child and family development and as evidence that a mentee is mastering skills in AVT. The coach/mentor can indicate whether a skill was not applicable, not observed although an opportunity was present, seen at least once, or seen a multiple of times. Ultimately, the coach/mentor is looking for ways that the mentee is carrying out the Principles of Auditory-Verbal Therapy in practice.

It can be difficult to record directly onto a form like the F-1 during an observation, and often there is much to comment upon. A coach/mentor may simply make notes while watching, then go back and use the mentee's reflections and the Academy form as an organizational scheme. Careful observation may require more than one viewing of a recorded session. When coach/mentors are observing in real time they are mindful of what they are looking for, while at the same time noting serendipitous events that occur.

Real-time observation of an AVT session, either on site or through video conferencing, requires additional preparation with the mentee with regard to the level of participation by the coach/mentor. The session is under the control of the mentee, not the coach/mentor. It is important that the mentee remain the primary practitioner and that the coach/mentor refrain from jumping in and "rescuing" the session. A mentee might choose to invite the coach/mentor to take part if the mentee thinks that a demonstration might be helpful. In some cases, the child dictates participation. It is not uncommon for a young child to turn to this new adult in the room and hand over a toy—and who can resist that invitation?

The Feedback Conversation

The feedback conversation takes place after the observation and, like the observation, needs to be scheduled in a timely fashion. The word "conversation" is used with intention. Change and growth take place when the mentee par-ticipates in the exchange of information. The act of allowing another person to watch one's *performance* as an AV practitioner is an act of courage. When a coach/mentor is invited to observe an AVT session, the mentee is choosing to be vulnerable. When the coach/mentor is mindful of this courage and vulnerability, the feedback conversation is conducted with respect and sensitivity.

The feedback conversation is most effective when the mentee is able to maintain a sense of control. The mentee's own reflections and questions can set the agenda, or the coach/mentor can ask either prior to or at the start of the feedback conversation if there is anything in particular the mentee wants to start out with. Open-ended, nonjudgmental questions help the mentee to narrate the story of the AVT session in his or her own words, to consider new ways of thinking about a session, and discover insights into what worked and what might be done differently (Tschannen-Moran & Tschannen-Moran, 2010). The coach/mentor can listen for themes to discover any concerns that need to have priority in the conversation. The coach/mentor is advised to limit the number of issues that are raised in order to keep the mentee from being overwhelmed and to engender confidence that improvement is possible. *Asking rather than telling, inquiring rather than preaching, and suggesting rather than demanding are strategies that foster self-reflection and put the responsibility for growth on the mentee.*

Problem solving helps the mentee use new concepts and integrate old and new ideas for ways of doing things (Mezirow, 1997). Brainstorming is a form of problem solving. Rather than giving the mentee solutions, the coach/mentor can invite the mentee to join in to create a list of possible approaches that might be tried to help a child who is having difficulty or to help a mentee utilize a therapy strategy. The coach/mentor may then follow up by encouraging the mentee to devise some "experiments," create plans to try out a few of brainstorming ideas with specific children and their families (Tschannen-Moran & Tschannen-Moran, 2010). Those experiments can include hypothesizing with the coach/mentor about several possible outcomes to the plans and what the mentee might do when faced with the various outcomes.

The Principles of AVT ground the feedback conversation. Feedback and problem solving are referenced to the Principles: Is this a way to help the child learn through listening? Is the session parent-focused? Are the activities/goals/techniques developmentally appropriate? Are the expectations for child performance drawn from that expected from typical development?

Despite the admonition that the coach/mentor be sensitive and maintain mentee locus of control, honesty is critical. The mentee seeks out a coach/mentor because that individual has knowledge and skills and the mentee wants to learn. It is unethical for a coach/mentor to rely solely on strategies that require a mentee to come up with solutions. It's frustrating for a mentee when what is needed is information and a calibration regarding his or her performance. It is also unethical for a LSLS Cert. AVT coach/mentor to fail to address mentee performance in an AVT session when it hinders progress of the child and/or family.

The feedback conversation has a purposeful ending. The mentor/coach and mentee reflect and summarize the key elements of the conversation, with the mentee leading by suggesting the key information that he or she noted. The coach/mentor reviews any resources that can be shared with the mentee. Together, they plan how the ideas discussed in the conversation will be carried out.

They also look to the future and talk about what the next observation might entail. The mentee may suggest that the coach/mentor watch a session with the same or a similar child so that they can continue the conversation about the skills discussed following the current observation episode. The mentee may have concerns about a particular child and family and wishes input. The coach/mentor or mentee may wish to have an observation and conversation about a different age child and family or a child/family who require a different set of skills from the mentee. Subsequently, the coach/mentor can have a broader perspective about the mentee's skills. By planning for the next observation, the mentee moves forward.

The Written Report

The observation culminates in a written report that the coach/mentor delivers to the mentee, again in a timely fashion. We recommend the report not be written until after the feedback conference so that elements from the feedback conversation are included. Coach/mentors who have a mentee working toward the LSLS Cert. AVT will fill out the Academy F-1 form, which has space for narratives. The report might also include a list of pertinent resources and weblinks. It is the experience of many coach/mentors that mentees pay attention to, and refer frequently to, the written report. It merits careful, thoughtful, and informative writing.

Appraisal of Mentee Growth and Evaluation of the Coach/Mentor

The coach/mentor and mentee keep track of the mentee skill level by way of coach/mentor appraisal and through the mentee's own evaluation of progress using self-reflection and reference to the mentee's goals (Zachary, 2000). It can be helpful to schedule periodic, regular conversations that are not based on an observation session, but on mentee progress. Prior to the appraisal, the mentee and coach/mentor each review and reflect on the mentee's goals and documentation of performance, and consider next steps. Then, they do the same together in conversation. At times these conversations may be difficult (Johnson & Ridley, 2008) if the mentee has not kept up with obligations or has not demonstrated progress. It is observed that the more frequently the coach/mentor and mentee communicate and the more regularly appraisals are conducted, the more likely that mentees who are not viable candidates for AV practice will decide on their own to withdraw from the process.

The coach/mentor also needs to receive regular feedback and evaluation from the mentee. If the mentee points out difficulties, the coach/mentor has a responsibility to address these. If a coach/mentor is working with several mentees, anonymous evaluations can be collected using a platform such as *Survey Monkey* to avoid any fears that mentees might have about giving feedback.

Being "On Call"

The relationship between the mentee and coach/mentor extends beyond the session observation cycle. The mentee needs to feel comfortable getting in touch with the coach/mentor for guidance or to act as a sounding board throughout the relationship. Being "on call" is an integral part of the relationship between the coach/mentor and mentee, and this aspect of communication needs to be discussed when the mentoring agreement is first established. Some coach/mentors charge a fee for this time and the mentee needs to be aware of all costs related to the process.

THE FUTURE FOR COACHING AND MENTORING PRACTITIONERS IN AVT

At the beginning of this chapter, the authors referred to the growing interest in AVT from both families and practitioners and the need for mentoring to foster that growth. The survey reported in Chapter 1 also revealed that 50% of the responding LSLS Cert. AVTs engage in mentoring. This is promising and the profession is hopeful that it will increase. An increase in the number of LSLS Cert. AVTs who mentor, however, addresses only one aspect of this global need. Children and families don't just need more practitioners. They need highly qualified AV practitioners who provide high quality AVT.

The LSLS Cert. AVT coach/mentor has on average 8.8 years of experience as an AV practitioner (Morrison et al., 2010) and provides a strong experience and knowledge base for coaching and mentoring. The majority of LSLS Cert. AVTs who mentor (64.6%), however, report that they have received no specific training in coaching and mentoring (Morrison et al., 2010). This situation has been addressed by the AG Bell Academy in the creation of a Mentoring Committee charged with identifying and addressing mentor needs. The number of short courses and presentations at AG Bell meetings in coaching and mentoring has increased each year since the 2010 survey. It is anticipated that there will be even more systematic coaching and mentoring training, perhaps borrowing training strategies from other professions such as "mentoring the mentor" (Gandhi & Johnson 2016), training in coach/mentor and mentee communication, and strategies for fostering independence (Feldman et al., 2012; Pfund et al., 2016). The establishment of standards or at minimum guidelines for AV coach/mentors is in order, perhaps developed at the level of the Academy so that there can be more regularization of mentoring services.

CHAPTER SUMMARY

Families are seeking AVT in increasing numbers globally, creating a need for highly qualified AV practitioners. The development of the highest order of planning, delivery, and evaluation of AVT requires a focused effort on the part of the practitioner in partnership with an experienced coach/mentor who can *coach and guide* the practitioner toward knowledge and skill development. Coaching and mentoring in AVT requires an understanding of the learner as an adult who brings experience and specific interests to the coaching and mentoring process. Coaching and mentoring take place in an honest relationship with a mentee who maintains a locus of control throughout the process. The outcome of successful coaching and mentoring is measured not only in the development of highly qualified practitioners, but in outcomes to children and families.

REFERENCES

AG Bell Academy for Listening and Spoken Language. (2017a). *Listening and Spoken Language Specialist Certified Auditory-Verbal Therapist (LSLS Cert. AVT®) application packet*. Retrieved September 23, 2019 from https://agbellacademy.org/wp-content/uploads/2018/12/AVT-Application-2017.pdf

AG Bell Academy for Listening and Spoken Language. (2017b). *The AG Bell Academy for Listening and Spoken Language Certification Handbook*. Retrieved September 23, 2019 from https://agbellacademy.org/wp-content/uploads/2018/10/Certification-Handbook.pdf

AG Bell Academy for Listening and Spoken Language. (2017c). *The AG Bell Academy for Listening and Spoken Language Mentor Handbook*. Retrieved September 23, 2019 from https://agbellacademy.org/wp-content/uploads/2019/08/Mentor-Handbook.pdf

AG Bell Association for the Deaf. (2019). *Recommended protocol for audiological assessment, hearing aid and cochlear* implant evaluation, and follow-up. Retrieved July 6, 2019 from https://www .agbell.org/Advocacy/Alexander-Graham -Bell-Associations-Recommended-Proto col-for-Audiological-Assessment-Hearing -Aid-and-Cochlear-Implant-Evaluation -and-Follow-up

Auditory-Verbal International. (2003). *Auditory-Verbal International Standardized Curriculum*. Washington, DC: AVI.

Boyatzis, R. E. (2011). Managerial and leadership competencies: A behavioral approach to emotional, social and cognitive intelligence. *Vision, 15*(2), 91–100.

Caleffe-Schenck, N. (1992). The auditory-verbal method: Description of a training program for audiologists, speech language. pathologists, and teachers of children with hearing loss. *The Volta Review, 94*(1), 65–68.

Dickson, C. L., Morrison, H. M., & Jones, M. B. (2013). The mentor's guide to auditory-verbal competencies (years 1–3). Retrieved September 23, 2019 from https:// www.cochlear.com/intl/home/support /rehabilitation-resources/professional -resources

Duncan, J., Kendrick, A., McGinnis, M. D., & Perigoe, C. (2010). Auditory (re)habilitation teaching behavior rating scale. *Journal of the Academy of Rehabilitative Audiology, 43*, 65–86.

Feldman, M. D., Huang L., Guglielmo, B. J., Jordan, R., Kahn, J., Creasman, J. M., . . . Brown, J. S. (2009). Training the next generation of research mentors: The University of California San Francisco Clinical and Translational Science Institute Mentor Development Program. *Clinical and Translational Science, 2*, 216–221.

Gandhi, M., & Johnson, M. (2016). Creating more effective mentors: Mentoring the mentor. *AIDS and Behavior, 20*(2), 294–303.

Hamlin, R. G., Ellinger, A. D., & Beattie, R. S. (2008). The emergent "coaching industry": A wake-up call for HRD professionals. *Human Resource Development International, 11*(3), 287–305.

Hymans, M. (2018). *Coaching and mentoring staff in schools: A practical guide.* New York, NY: Routledge.

Johnson, W. (2016). *On being a mentor.* New York, NY: Routledge.

Johnson, W. B., & Ridley, C. R. (2008). *The elements of ethics for professionals.* New York, NY: St. Martin's Press.

Johnson, W. B., & Ridley, C. R. (2018). *The elements of mentoring: 75 practices of master mentors.* New York, NY: St. Martin's Press.

Knowles, M. S. (1980). *The modern practice of adult education: Andragogy versus pedagogy.* New York, NY: Association Press.

Knowles, M., Holton, E., & Swanson, R. (2005). *The adult learner: The definitive classics in adult education and human resource development.* New York, NY: Elsevier.

Kraft, M. A., Blazar, D., & Hogan, D. (2018). The effect of teacher coaching on instruction and achievement: A meta-analysis of the causal evidence. *Review of Educational Research, 88*(4), 547–588.

Kretlow, A. G., & Bartholomew, C. C. (2010). Using coaching to improve the fidelity of evidence-based practices: A review of studies. *Teacher Education and Special Education, 33*(4), 279–299.

Law, H. (2013). *The psychology of coaching, mentoring and learning.* Hoboken, NJ: John Wiley & Sons.

Lipscomb, R., & An, S. (2010). Mentoring 101: Building a mentoring relationship. *Journal of the American Dietetic Association, 1002–1008.*

Manza, G., & Patrick, S. K. (2012). *The mentor's field guide: Answers you need to help kids succeed.* Minneapolis, MN: Search Institute Press.

McLean, P. (2012). *The completely revised handbook of coaching: A developmental approach.* Hoboken, NJ: John Wiley & Sons.

Mellon, A., & Murdoch-Eaton, D. (2015). Supervisor or mentor: Is there a difference? Implications for pediatric practice. *Archives of Disease in Childhood, 100*, 873–878.

Mezirow, J. (1997). Transformative learning: Theory to practice. *New Directions for Adult and Continuing Education, 1997*(74), 5–12.

Morrison, H. M., Perigoe, C. B., & Bernstein, A. (2010). A survey of LSLS AVTs who mentor: Fostering independence to endow the future. *The Volta Review, 110*(2), 145–168.

Neuman, S. B., & Cunningham, L. (2009). The impact of professional development and coaching on early language and literacy instructional practices. *American Educational Research Journal, 46*(2), 532–566.

Pask, R., & Joy, B. (2007). *Mentoring-coaching: A guide for education professionals.* New York, NY: McGraw-Hill Education.

Passmore, J. (Ed.). (2010). *Excellence in coaching: The industry guide* (2nd ed.). London, UK: Kogan Page.

Pfund, C., Pribbenow, C. M., Branchaw, J., Lauffer, S. M., & Handelsman, J. (2006). The merits of training mentors. *Science, 311*(5760), 473–474.

Rubinstein, L., & Fox, E. (2018). BASHH/BHIVA mentoring scheme. *Sexually Transmitted Infections, 94*(4), 239–239.

Taylor, E. W. (2007). An update of transformative learning theory: A critical review of the empirical research (1999–2005). *International Journal of Lifelong Education, 26*(2), 173–191.

Tokuhama-Espinosa, T. (2011). Why mind, brain, and education science is the "new" brain-based education. *New Horizons for Learning, 9*(1), 1–15.

Tschannen-Moran, B., & Tschannen-Moran, M. (2010). *Evocative coaching: Transforming schools one conversation at a time.* Hoboken, NJ: John Wiley & Sons.

van Nieuwerburgh, C. (2018). *Coaching in education: Getting better results for students, educators, and parents.* New York, NY: Routledge.

Zachary, L. J. (2000). *The mentors guide: Facilitating effective learning relationships.* Indianapolis, IN: Wiley/Pfeiffer.

27

COST-BENEFIT OF AUDITORY-VERBAL THERAPY

Anita Grover, Ellie Goldblatt, and Sarah Hogan

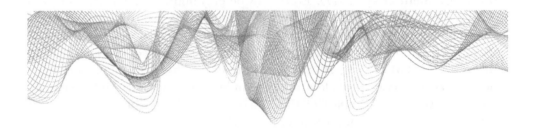

Effective program monitoring is essential to demonstrating the outcomes and impact of family-centered early intervention, and therefore it is essential to know the long-term costs and benefits of Auditory-Verbal Therapy (AVT) to the child, the family, and the economy.

A cost-benefit analysis is one way of quantifying the costs and benefits of AVT to help children with hearing loss develop listening and spoken language. This chapter explores the value of a cost-benefit analysis and how it helps practitioners, service providers, and families to understand the return on investment in early intervention. It sets out the key components of a cost-benefit analysis and practical steps to developing a model appropriate for any AVT program or service.

In the United Kingdom, the charity Auditory Verbal UK (AVUK) has drawn on robust evidence from around the world and developed a cost-benefit analysis of its Auditory-Verbal program using a model developed by the UK government and a 50-year project horizon. It demonstrates that the costs incurred in the child's early years can be seen as a sound investment in the child's future. The methodology, calculations, and outcomes used in this study are set out in this chapter.

UNDERSTANDING THE IMPACT OF AUDITORY-VERBAL PROGRAMS

There is a growing body of evidence from around the world that demonstrates the impact of Auditory-Verbal programs (Dornan, Hickson, Murdoch, & Houston, 2009; First Voice, 2017; Goldblat & Pinto, 2017; Hitchins & Hogan, 2018; Percy-Smith et al., 2017). Every year, new research highlights the impact of family-centered early intervention and the importance of getting it right from the start (AVUK, 2018). As practitioners, as service providers, and as parents, we see the impact of this as children progress through school, higher education, and future employment. We know the outcomes that are possible, but we need to be able to measure the long-term impact and economic case for investment in Auditory-Verbal Therapy.

Understanding the economic case for AVT is imperative for securing initial and sustained financial investment in AVT programs. It is vital for demonstrating the return on investment by the funding sources, such as a government agency, a charitable foundation, or a private investor or sponsor. It is vital for parents who may need to seek funds to enable their child to access a program. And it is important for speech-language pathologists, audiologists, or educators who may be considering professional training in AVT.

But how can we do this? We can look to other countries that have been running programs for longer and use the emerging evidence provided by longitudinal studies (First Voice, 2017; Lim, Goldberg, & Flexer, 2018). Recent studies have estimated the cost of late intervention on quality of life and the economy and have looked at the societal costs of permanent childhood hearing loss during the teenage years (Chorozoglou, Mahon, Pimperton, Worsfold, & Kennedy, 2018). But there are few studies that assess the full long-term impact of early intervention.

People responsible for making decisions often question studies produced by other countries as their circumstances and local costs are "different" to their own. So it is, therefore, critically important to use "recognized" measures to demonstrate the short-, medium-, and long-term impact of Auditory-Verbal Therapy in our respective countries or areas.

Drawing on a wide range of studies, the development of a comprehensive cost benefit analysis can demonstrate the local costs of programs and their benefits. The First Voice Network of listening and spoken language centers in Australia and New Zealand produced such a study in 2011 and updated it in 2017 in advance of the introduction of the National Insurance Disability Scheme and, indeed, provided the economic case and evidence base of outcomes in Auditory-Verbal Therapy (First Voice, 2011, 2017).

In this chapter, we will explore the issues around identifying an appropriate comprehensive cost-benefit model and look in-depth at the development of the Auditory Verbal UK cost-benefit analysis first developed in 2016 (AVUK, 2016).

DEVELOPING AN APPROPRIATE MODEL OF ANALYZING COSTS AND BENEFITS OF AN AUDITORY-VERBAL PROGRAM

Research continues to show that early identification of hearing loss, optimally fitted hearing amplification technology, and individualized intensive early intervention such as AVT result in better speech perception and language development outcomes (Goldblat & Pinto, 2017; Hitchins & Hogan, 2018; Percy-Smith et al., 2017). In addition to the primary service, there are gains in social values: wider economic, health, and social benefits, such as achievements in education, employment, and productivity. Historically, these "softer outcomes" have been harder to capture. In 2014, The Ear Foundation in the UK estimated the real financial cost of hearing loss and deafness to be over £30 billion ($39.4 billion) per annum on a conservative basis (Archbold, Lamb, O'Neill, & Atkins, 2014). These costs related to the direct costs of treating hearing loss, which were comparatively low, and the much larger costs of dealing with the health and social impacts of deafness. We wanted to find the best way to articulate the overall value of our service across a child's lifetime.

At the charity AVUK (2016), we first conducted a review of available studies to examine the cost-effectiveness of Auditory-Verbal Therapy programs. We found that no research had been published in the UK and only one study of this type existed globally at the time of development: "A Social Cost-Benefit Analysis: Early Intervention Programs

to Assist Children with Hearing Loss to Develop Spoken Language" (First Voice, 2011, 2017). This report provided a clear framework and methodology for how to measure the costs and benefits of Auditory-Verbal Therapy; the support of our Australian colleagues became invaluable during the design of AVUK's first cost-benefit analysis in 2016. We also examined models used by other charities in the UK to quantify the benefits of their services and specifically models used by other early intervention programs such as Place2Be (Pro Bono Economics, 2017). Rather than "reinvent the wheel," we were keen to adapt models that were known to be effective.

A cost-benefit analysis demonstrates the value of an intervention by calculating both the costs and the benefits. It may be used in the planning stages of a project or once the project has been delivered as an element of project evaluation. In our case, the cost-benefit analysis would examine the costs and the benefits that could be expected of the service, given the existing levels of expenditure in Auditory-Verbal Therapy by AVUK. If a positive cost-benefit ratio (CBR) were found, it would demonstrate the importance of investing in the training of professionals in the Auditory-Verbal approach and highlight the value of similar services being available more widely across the UK. It would also demonstrate the impact of an early intervention program of Auditory-Verbal Therapy at AVUK to potential funders.

We chose to use a cost-benefit analysis rather than a social return on investment model. Traditionally the latter uses stakeholders to identify proxies in order to value outcomes, which can result in different valuations of the same interventions. It was crucial that our analysis used accepted and published data, readily available in the public domain, to ensure the consistency and rigor of the results. Unlike in some other countries AVT receives no government funding in the UK. With the aim of changing this and making our analysis as verifiable as possible, we used the Office for National Statistics (ONS) and the Cabinet Office's Unit Cost Database (New Economy, 2015) to quantify outcomes, as well as three key documents to support the development of our cost-benefit analysis: HM Treasury and New Economy's cost-benefit analysis guidance (HM Treasury, 2014), HM Treasury's Green Book (HM Treasury, 2011), and Pro Bono Economics' Guide to cost-benefit analysis (Pro Bono Economics, 2015).

Our main challenge was to come to a reasonable assessment of the balance of the costs imposed on children, their families, and society at large, and the benefits that are generated by AVT. Access to AVT for children who are deaf or hard of hearing in the UK only became available from 2003 and as such, the first generation of beneficiaries of Auditory-Verbal Therapy are just reaching early adulthood. Evidence on the lifelong impacts of AVT is beginning to accumulate and as a result, highly accurate and scientifically robust estimates of long-term benefits of specific programs will become increasingly available over the coming years. Nonetheless, since investment decisions needed to be made, we were able to draw on considerable evidence from Australia and the United States where programs have been in place for 20 to 30 years (First Voice, 2015).

In line with other assessment reports on emerging health technologies, our cost-benefit analysis needed to make assumptions about future impacts. The approach taken throughout was to use conservative assumptions and to test any results using sensitivity analysis, as is standard practice. The following confidence grades for cost and benefit data were taken from HM Treasury and New Economy's cost-benefit analysis guidance, and an optimism bias correction was applied to all the data (see Figures 27–1 and 27–2).

A cost-benefit analysis requires a scenario with the investment to be compared with the situation without the investment. The latter is referred to as the "baseline" or "do nothing" scenario. We decided that the baseline would refer to what would happen in the absence of AVT (i.e., a child who has received hearing aids or cochlear implants but has not had the benefit of an Auditory-Verbal early intervention program). Amplification with hearing technology alone does not allow for optimal language development (Spencer & Marschark, 2010; Wilkins & Ertmer, 2002). Even if a child is diagnosed early and receives the optimal hearing technology, it is likely that he or she will experience some form of language delay and the wearing of hearing devices does not necessarily mean that sound will be perceived or interpreted. Through these listening devices, the child needs to learn to listen and understand that sounds have meaning (Chowdhry, 2010; Cole & Flexer, 2015). Auditory-Verbal Therapy, therefore, is complementary to the optimal hearing technology. This, of course, has implications for the attribution of value. In line with assumptions made in the 2011

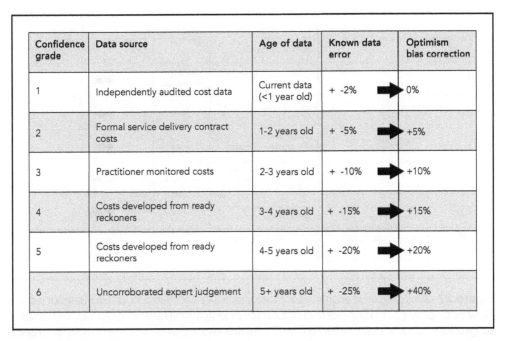

Confidence grade	Data source	Age of data	Known data error	Optimism bias correction
1	Independently audited cost data	Current data (<1 year old)	+ -2%	0%
2	Formal service delivery contract costs	1-2 years old	+ -5%	+5%
3	Practitioner monitored costs	2-3 years old	+ -10%	+10%
4	Costs developed from ready reckoners	3-4 years old	+ -15%	+15%
5	Costs developed from ready reckoners	4-5 years old	+ -20%	+20%
6	Uncorroborated expert judgement	5+ years old	+ -25%	+40%

Figure 27-1. Confidence grades for cost data. Modified from HM Treasury and New Economy. (2014) Supporting public service transformation: Cost benefit analysis guidance for local partnerships. Contains public sector information licensed under the Open Government License v3.0.

First Voice publication of "A Social Cost Benefit Analysis," a conservative assumption was made that for any improvement in health state that is achieved with technology and Auditory-Verbal Therapy, half was attributed to the technology and half to Auditory-Verbal Therapy (First Voice, 2015). We chose to use a 50-year project horizon to reflect the fact that the majority of the benefits flow later in life. HM Treasury recommends a 3.5% discount rate for projects between 0 and 30 years in length and a 3% discount rate for projects between 31 and 75 years (HM Treasury, 2011). We adopted this recommendation and used a 3.5% discount rate for the first 30 years, with a 3% discount rate for the final 20 years. The project horizon of 50 years is highly

conservative, given that the average life expectancy today is closer to 80 years in the UK.

Having decided on the model that we would use to analyze the costs and benefits of an Auditory-Verbal program, we undertook a literature review to establish whether AVT was effective at producing outcomes such as greater attainment at school and improved employment prospects. The literature review covered early intervention, the link between hearing loss and language delay, the role of early intervention in hearing loss and reviews of AVT. We included it within the publication of the cost-benefit analysis, but emphasized that it not be considered exhaustive. Rather, by providing relevant background information, the literature review

Confidence grade	Data source	Evidence base (engagement/Imapct)	Age of data	Known data error	Optimism bias correction
1	Figures taken from agency data systems	Randomised control trial in UK	Current data (<1 year old)	+ -2% ➡	0%
2	Figures derived from local stats	International randomised control trial	1-2 years old	+ -5% ➡	-5%
3	Figures based on national analysis in similar areas	Independent monitoring of outcomes with robust evaluation plan	2-3 years old	+ -10% ➡	-10%
4	Figures based on national analysis	Practitioner monitoring of outcomes with robust evaluation plan	3-4 years old	+ -15% ➡	-15%
5	Figures based on generic national analysis	Secondary evidence from a similar type of intervention	4-5 years old	+ -20% ➡	-25%
6	Uncorroborated expert judgement	Uncorroborated expert judgement	5+ years old	+ -25% ➡	-40%

Figure 27-2. Confidence grades for benefit data. Modified from HM Treasury and New Economy. (2014) Supporting public service transformation: Cost benefit analysis guidance for local partnerships. Contains public sector information licensed under the Open Government License v3.0.

helped to inform assumptions made in the cost-benefit analysis.

CASE STUDY: THE AUDITORY VERBAL UK COST-BENEFIT ANALYSIS

The AVUK cost-benefit analysis was developed in 2016 using data from 2015 to 2016. Costs included are in GBP (£) with a calculated equivalence in US dollars ($) with conversion according to exchange rates at the time of writing (March 2019).

What Are the Costs?

The cost-benefit analysis presented a comprehensive assessment of a range of costs involved in accessing AVT. The following estimated costs are incurred when a child is enrolled in the Auditory-Verbal program at AVUK.

Operational Costs

In 2015 to 2016 the total Early Intervention Program (EIP) costs for AVUK were £597,969 ($785,628). This included the direct cost of providing AVT, such as staff, travel, premises, training and courses, toys, books, and membership subscriptions. It also included the support costs, such as administrative and fundraising staff, information technology (IT), communications, and repairs and maintenance. With a caseload of 114, the cost per child was £6,557 ($8,622) per annum. Conservatively, it was assumed that the average amount of time a child stays on the program is

3.5 years. This takes some account of the greater program duration of a child with more complex needs: the average duration of a therapy program for a child without complex needs at AVUK is 2.5 years.

In-Kind Costs: Volunteer Staff Time and Free Use of Venues

In-kind costs are provided free of charge but need to be counted within a cost-benefit analysis because of the associated "opportunity cost"—if the resources were not used for this pro-

gram, they could be used elsewhere. In 2015, AVUK had four volunteers, two based in London and two based in Oxfordshire, who combined gave the equivalent time of a 1.1 full-time member of staff. The average yearly income for administrative staff, weighted both geographically and for different skills levels, was taken from a general market rate. A confidence grade of 4 was applied to this figure so an optimism bias correction of 15% was added, in line with HM Treasury and New Economy's recommendations in Figure 27–3. The average cost is outlined below:

Admin staff salary outside London	$19,740
Admin staff salary in London	$23,688
Highly skilled admin staff salary outside London	$32,900
Highly skilled admin staff salary in London	$36,848
Average Admin salary	$28,294
Average Admin salary for 1.1 member of staff	$31,123
Cost per child (114 caseload)	$272
Optimism Bias	15%
CBA Cost per child	$315

Figure 27-3. Volunteer staff time.

Four staff members were mentored by a human resources specialist. In total, this person gave 16 hours of support per year and charged £225 ($296) per hour. Normally there would be a charge for travel: a return trip of 204 miles, three times a year at £0.45 ($0.59) per mile. The total cost was £3,874.86 ($5,095.98), an in-kind cost of £34 ($45) per child. No optimism bias correction was required for this independently audited cost data.

An IT consultant also provided 10 days of consultancy work to optimize data collection methods. This was charged at £6,000 ($7,894), an in-kind cost of £53 ($70) per child. Again, no optimism bias correction was required for this independently audited cost data. The team also benefited from individual team profiles and a team awareness day from a consulting firm that specialized in organizational effectiveness. With consultancy fees of £5,000 ($6,578), seventeen profiles at £93.50 ($123) per person, £70 ($92) of printing costs, and £10 ($13) for travel, the total cost was £8,003 ($10,529) or an in-kind cost of £70 ($92) per child. Again, no optimism bias correction was required. Our organization also benefited from the free use of venues to hold an annual "team away" day. This alternated each year between London and Oxford. Weighted geographically, the cost of a conference room for 20 members of staff was estimated to be £147.50 ($194). With an optimism bias of 5%, this was an in-kind cost of £1.35 ($1.77) per child.

Travel

Detailed client surveys were not available to inform the discussion of this cost factor; however, it is clear that families travel to and from the AVUK centers in Bermondsey, London, and Bicester, Oxfordshire from throughout the UK. The cost-benefit analysis assumed that, on average, 20 trips to and from AVUK centers were made by each family each year. It was assumed that the average distance traveled was 200 miles in one return trip at £0.11 ($0.15) per mile. Parking was assumed to be free of cost. Using these assumptions and applying a 15% optimism bias, the average annual cost per child was estimated at £523 ($688).

Childcare for Siblings

Due to the nature of AVT and the focus on parent coaching, it may be necessary for siblings to be looked after by someone else while the parent(s) attends a therapy session, unless that session is offered in the home. According to the ONS, as of March 2013, 39% of the 7.7m families in the UK had 2 children and 14% had three or more children, giving a total of 53% of families with two or more children. For families like these, it is likely that some form of childcare would have to be organized for each session. Even if a child is in the care of a relative or friend, or being cared for by a volunteer, a value needed to be put on their time. Using a valuation of £7 ($9) per hour for either paid or unpaid childcare, with a five-hour requirement of childcare each time a sibling attends Auditory-Verbal Therapy, an economic cost of £35 ($46) per occasion was suggested. Assuming 20 trips per year on average, for 53% of the cohort to which this applies, this equated to a £427 ($561) cost per child per year, with a 15% optimism bias.

Caregiver's Loss of Income

There was no survey data available to determine whether a parent is more likely to give up work if their child were enrolled in AVT compared with parents of children who are deaf or hard of hearing who were not enrolled in AVT. However, we know anecdotally that at least one parent—if not both—may forgo income to bring their child to sessions. On average, including travel time and appointment time, parents can have to take at least five hours from work for each time their child attends AVT. It was conservatively assumed that this time equates to one parent taking a full day off work for each of the 20 sessions across the year.

In 2014, the labor participation rate in the UK was 76.5%: 74.6% for women and 83.1% for men (Office for National Statistics, 2014). The Office for National Statistics did not publish the participation rates of men dependent on child age. For women, their participation rate dropped to 65.0% when they had a child between the ages of 0 and 4 years and increased to 78.8% when a child was between the ages 5 and 10 years. Given that AVUK's caseload was split across ages 0 to 5 years, the average participation rate for mothers with children enrolled in AVT was estimated to be 67.9%. In addition, it was recognized that mothers of children with disabilities had a lower rate of workforce participation than other mothers; child disability was estimated to reduce maternal employment by 7.6% among women when they were secondary earners and by 10.8% when they were primary earners (Powers, 2001). As 31.0% of women were the primary household earners in 2014, we

estimated that there was, on average, an 8.6% reduction in employment among mothers of children with a disability (Ben-Galim & Thompson, 2013). This gap was acknowledged in the cost-benefit analysis by deducting 8.6% from the initial 67.9% participation rate identified previously. This means that 59.3% of the mothers of children in the Auditory-Verbal cohort could be expected to be in paid employment and 83.1% of men. Taken from the ONS, the average female salary in 2014 was £23,889 ($31,398) and the average male salary was £29,441 ($38,696) (Office for National Statistics, 2014). Conservatively assuming parents were working full time, this was a day rate of £113.23 ($148.82) and £91.88 ($121.74), respectively. It was recognized that each family will vary enormously but for the purpose of the cost-benefit analysis, it was assumed that the 59.3% of working mothers and 83.1% of working fathers would take off 10 days from work specifically for AVT appointments. The representative or average loss of income is, on this basis, estimated at £1,485.80 ($1,952.59) per year per child in an early intervention program of AVT at AVUK [(£113.22 × 10 × 0.831) + (£91.88 × 10 × 0.5931)]. With an optimism bias of 15% added, the average loss of parent income was £1,709 ($2,246).

Unquantifiable Costs

While the list of costs identified was highly conservative, there were a number of costs that were unquantifiable that we needed to acknowledge. One type of cost that was difficult to quantify was the greater effort that children who are deaf or hard of hearing have to put in to acquire language compared with hearing children (Hicks & Tharpe, 2002; McGarrigle et al., 2014). Another was related to cultural identity issues: children may identify less with the Deaf community and may feel rejected by it once they have completed their journey through their Auditory-Verbal program. Finally, as families adjust to the EIP, they may acquire literature and spend time researching different communication options. This clearly takes time and resources, but an estimation was not possible for our study.

Summary of Costs

The table below summarizes all of the costs described above for the 3.5 years that a child participates in the AVT program, using a 3.5% discount (Figure 27–4). After the child has left the program, approximately 5% of families request "ad hoc" support, but for the purposes of this analysis, it was assumed that no further follow-up takes place and costs consequently drop to zero for the rest of the project horizon.

The net present (discounted) value of all costs was £31,119 ($40,927). This can be seen as the investment that is made in the child's future. The total value of costs was much lower than the total value of costs in First Voice's 2011 Social Cost-Benefit analysis—£203,307 ($267,421) (£103,910 in 2014) ($136,717). The First Voice model is for 5 years from 0 to 5 years and includes an annual follow-up with children from the ages of 0 to 21 years. Additionally, the authors of the Australian study assumed that at least one member of the family stopped working for the 5 years that a child is in the

Cost	Value	Year 1	Year 2	Year 3	Year 3.5	Present Value
Operational	$8,629	$8,337	$8,055	$7,783	$3,760	$27,935
In Kind	$522	$504	$487	$471	$228	$1,690
Travel	$688	$666	$644	$621	$300	$2,231
Childcare for siblings	$562	$554	$524	$507	$245	$1,817
Carer's loss of income	$2,249	$2,173	$2,099	$2,028	$980	$7,280
Total Net Present Value						$40,953

Figure 27–4. Summary of costs over time, per child per year.

program. Our analysis did not make this assumption. Anecdotal evidence from parents of children in the AVUK program showed that if a parent did choose to stop working, pursuing AVT was not the reason for doing so.

What Are the Benefits?

Hearing loss, and the associated delays in language development, can have a number of well-documented negative impacts on a child's life (Miyamoto, Houston, Kirk, Perdew, & Svirsky, 2003; National Deaf Children's Society [NDCS], 2019; National Institute for Health and Care Excellence [NICE], 2009). AVUK's early intervention program aims to accelerate language development so that children achieve spoken language and communication skills that are on a par with their hearing peers and will enable them to flourish in a mainstream school. Where this is achieved, children are able to communicate better with their teachers and participate more actively alongside their typically hearing peers. In the short term, a key benefit is that the child will have better access to the language of the curriculum. Later on, this should translate into: stronger academic attainment and higher participation in further education; improved long-term earnings in the workplace; greater social integration, sense of achievement, and emotional well-being; and participation in a range of social and academic settings from childhood into adulthood.

Improved Quality of Life

There is a significant body of literature on the relationship between hearing loss, quality of life, and disability. The percentage of the Deaf community who say their health is poor is 10% compared with the national average of 6% and people with hearing loss are nearly five times more likely to have a visual impairment (9%) compared with 2% of the national average (Deaf Well-being Action Group in Nottinghamshire, 2001). A 2007 study into the health status of children with bilateral cochlear implants provided rigorous evidence of an association between bilateral permanent childhood hearing loss and diminished health-related quality of life preference-based outcomes during mid-childhood (Petrou et al., 2007). This literature clearly indicates that any intervention that improves hearing and enables more effective communication will improve quality of life.

Cost-effectiveness studies often report costs per quality adjusted life year (QALY) based on a variety of methodologies measuring health-related quality of life (HRQoL). QALY is a measure of the state of health of a person or group in which the benefits, in terms of length of life, are adjusted to reflect the quality of life (NICE, n.d.). The measurement of, and assumptions about, health states continues to be an active field of research. Our cost-benefit analysis used the method for valuing changes in QALY with the concept of the value of a life year (VOLY). The Interdepartmental Group on Costs and Benefits (IGCB, 2004) recommended the estimated VOLY to be valued at £27,000 ($35,530) (NERA Economic Consulting, 2007). This value was consistent with the value of a QALY used in recommendations by the UK National Institute for Clinical Excellence: about £30,000 ($39,502). This meant, for example, that

Site	Disability Weight	Notes
From Mathers (1999)		
Mild hearing loss	0.018 to 0.020	
Moderate hearing loss	0.104 to 0.120	
Severe hearing loss	0.324 to 0.370	
Global Burden of Disease study as shown in Mathers (2004)		
Deafness	0.224 (0.229)	At least moderate impairment resulting from meningitis
Hearing loss, adult onset (moderate or severe)	0.121	Cases of adult onset hearing loss due to ageing or noise exposure. Excludes hearing loss due to congenital causes, infectious diseases, other diseases or injury.

Figure 27-5. Disability weights.

a 10% reduction in disability (or improvement in quality of life) sustained over the course of a year would be valued at £2,700 ($3,555). Figure 27–5 lists disability weights from the World Health Organization's Global Burden of Disease study (Mathers, Vos, & Stevenson, 1999).

The figures presented indicate that if an intervention were to completely "remove" disability from hearing loss, it would be equivalent to a 2% reduction in disability for those with mild hearing loss, a 10% to 12% reduction for those with moderate hearing loss, and a 32% to 37% reduction for those with severe hearing loss. As mentioned, such a reduction could not be achieved without a hearing device, but it could also not be achieved without appropriate language development services. According to Anthony Hogan and colleagues:

The literature indicates that on average, the use of hearing aids and devices is associated with a 50% improvement in health related quality of life, but significant residual disability remains (Hogan, Shipley, Strazdins, Purcell, & Baker, 2011).

Our cost-benefit analysis conservatively assumed, with the use of modern technology and attendance at AVT, on average, a 50% change in the HRQoL. Half of this improvement was attributed to AVT and the other half to technology. Figure 27–6 shows that even before having optimal technology, the intervention was able to support children in increasing their rate of language development (Hogan, Stokes, White, Tyszkiewicz, & Woolgar, 2008). This increased further with a change in hearing technology.

The mid-point of the disability weights listed by Mathers et al. (1999) were used for mild, moderate, and severe hearing loss, and the improvement in HRQoL attributable to AVUK was weighted by the proportions of the AVUK cohort with corresponding levels

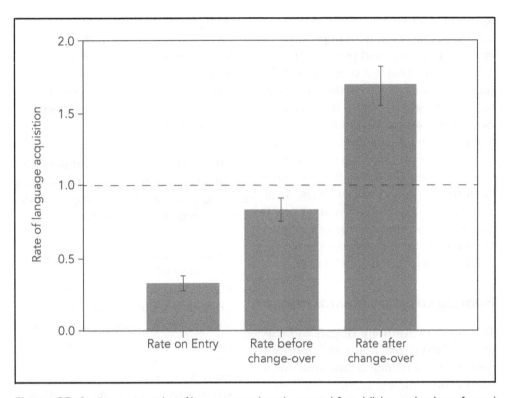

Figure 27-6. Average rate of language development for children who transferred from hearing aids to cochlear implant while on the program.

	Disability weight	50% change	Attribution to AVT	Proportion of cohort
Mild	0.02	1%	0.5%	5%
Moderate	0.11	6%	2.8%	20%
Severe and profound	0.35	17%	8.6%	75%
Change in health state (weighted average)	7%			
Annual value using VOLY of $35,573	$2,487			

Figure 27-7. Change in HRQoL attributable to AVT.

of hearing loss (Figure 27–7). The result was that, on average, a 7% improvement in HRQoL is attributed per child in the AVUK group. This is a conservative assumption—a figure two to three times as high would still be within the plausible range. It is assumed that this benefit flows from the date of enrollment in AVUK.

A 15% optimism bias correction was allocated as these figures have been based on national analysis. With a 3.5% discount rate for years 1 to 30 and a 3% discount rate for years 31 to 50, the total benefit over 50 years of a child's life was £39,669 ($52,215).

Hearing Loss and Mental Health

The paper by Anthony Hogan and colleagues (2011) also notes an important finding about mental health outcomes from other studies, namely that they appear to be independent of the degree of hearing loss:

> *"This insight is consistent with the hearing literature which observes that it is the degree of communicative difficulty experienced, rather than the measured degree of loss, which is most predictive of any restriction in social participation"* (p. 382).

According to the National Deaf Children's Society in the UK, over 40% of children with permanent hearing loss are estimated to have mental health difficulties at some point in childhood and early adulthood, compared with 10% of hearing children (NDCS, 2011). In a 2014 study, Harris reported that:

> Children and youth with hearing loss frequently experience difficulty

with peer relationships and are at a greater risk of social isolation and loneliness. Early social competence influences later peer and adult relationships, as well as academic success, school adjustment, and social-emotional development.

In a 2011 study of 27 children with cochlear implants, 56 children with hearing aids, and 117 hearing children, Theunissen et al. found that:

> Children with hearing loss reliably presented with more symptoms of depression than their typically hearing peers. Degree of hearing loss, socio-economic status, gender and age were unrelated to the level of depressive symptoms. But attending mainstream school or using exclusively speech for communication were related to fewer depressive symptoms.

The benefits of the overall improved quality of life include mental health outcomes within Mathers et al.'s disability weights. However, as evidence of improved self-confidence and reduced isolation for those who have followed AVT develops over time, it will be possible to quantify mental health outcomes separately.

Increased Educational Attainment, Employment, and Earnings

There is now a significant body of literature that indicates that children with untreated hearing loss do not achieve as well academically and may have a more negative long-term employment rate and income outlook than other children. In 2018, the Department for Education in the UK published data to show that only 48% achieved a grade 4/C or above in both English and Math, compared with 71% of children with no special educational needs (NDCS, 2019). This gap widens in post-16 year old education, with 34% of young people with hearing loss taking a level 3 qualification (A level, AS level, or equivalent) compared with more than 80% of 16- to 18-year-olds in the wider population. Of this 34%, fewer than 4% of children with hearing loss attain their qualification (Young, Oram, Squires, & Sutherland, 2015). Adults with hearing loss earn on average significantly less income than adults without hearing loss and are more likely to be unemployed (Jung & Bhattacharyya, 2012). Those that do graduate from postsecondary education, however, experience significant earning benefits (Schley et al., 2011). There is therefore a clear link between academic attainment and a child's long-term employment and earnings outlook in the future.

Employment

The potential benefit of early intervention on long-term employment opportunities will only accumulate over time as the number of children who have followed AVT reach employable ages and the data pool becomes large enough to be statistically robust. However, research strongly indicates that those who have attended early intervention programs will have significantly better prospects of being in paid work than those who were not enrolled in early intervention programs. The Office for National Statistics found that in 2015:

People with hearing loss are less likely to be employed (65% are in employment) when compared with people with no long-term health issue or disability (79%).

We considered how much of the 14% gap one can expect participation in AVT to close. Statistics available in 2014 (and subsequently in 2018) (Hitchins & Hogan, 2018) at AVUK indicated that at least 80% of children who spent 2+ years on the AVUK program had language and communication skills that were equivalent to those of their hearing peers. Data also showed that more than 30% of the AVUK children had additional needs. While a number of these children may not attain age-appropriate language, many of them do make accelerated progress through AVT. Assuming that the 65% of people with hearing loss had the advantage of hearing technology if appropriate, it was conservatively assumed that only half of the 14% gap identified by the ONS would be closed in the AVUK group. This meant that from the age of 18 years onward, a gain of £1,323 ($1,741) per year was applied to the child. This was based on the latest available ONS estimate of average wages for those in full-time paid employment (£27,000) ($35,541). A 15% optimism bias correction was allocated as these figures were based on national analysis. With a 3.5% discount rate for years 18 to 30 and a discount rate of 3% for years 31 to 50, the total benefit over 50 years of a child's life was £22,283 ($29,328).

Education and Earnings

The literature identified a link between hearing loss and earnings outlook. In

2014, the Ear Foundation calculated that, on average, people with hearing loss are paid £2,000 ($2,632) less per year than the general population (Archbold et al., 2014). This amounted to £4 billion ($5.3 billion) in lost income across the UK. A key benefit expected from early intervention is that educational outcomes improve and that consequently in the long term, enrollment in further education and acquisition of more advanced qualifications occur. Certainly, the early case studies of children who have followed the AV approach in the UK indicated that their hearing loss did not present a barrier to pursing higher education and managerial and professional positions. The economic literature on the returns of higher education is vast: a PricewaterhouseCoopers 2005 report into the economic benefits of higher education qualifications found that over a working life, the average graduate will earn about 23% more than his/her equivalent holding two or more A-Levels. Furthermore, the average monetary value in 2005 of completing a degree over and above two or more A-Levels was approximately £129,000 ($169,824). Similarly, an Australian report by Leigh and Ryan (2008) found that:

> At university level, Bachelor degrees and post-graduate qualifications are associated with significantly higher earnings, with each year of a Bachelor degree raising annual earnings by about 15%.

An important question for our cost-benefit analysis was how many years of additional education can one expect to result if a child participates in an early intervention program such as AVT. Dropout rates at all stages of education are currently higher for those with hearing loss than for others. The British Association of the Teachers of the Deaf (BATOD) reported in 2004 that 86% of their students leave school by age 16 years. In the UK, mandatory schooling is now from 5 to 18 years. In 2001, Goldberg and Flexer completed a survey of AVT graduates in the US and Canada et al. who were 18 years or older and had participated in AVT for at least 3 years. Their survey reported that more than 98% of the AVT graduates obtained a university education. The results were updated by Lim, Goldberg, and Flexer (2018) in a survey of more than 200 Auditory-Verbal graduates from around the world, and indicated that 63% of Auditory-Verbal graduates are awarded vocational, technical, or higher degrees. In the absence of long-term data at AVUK, it was assumed that participation in AVT, in addition to hearing technology, yields one additional year of education. This assumption was based on similar calculations made in First Voice's 2011 cost-benefit analysis, using long-term Australian data. Once again, this implies a highly conservative approach to valuation and we could expect this to increase in the future. Using the same ONS estimate of an average wage (£27,000) ($35,541), a 15% increase is the equivalent to £4,050 ($5,326). This was applied from years 21 to 50. A 15% optimism bias correction was allocated and with a 3.5% discount rate for years 21 to 30 and with a 3% discount rate for years 31 to 50, the total benefit over 50 years of a child's life was calculated at £64,938 ($85,477).

Lower Costs of Schooling

Improved language development and communication skills lead to more active participation in the classroom and an expectation that a child is more likely to attend a mainstream school and less likely to require extra assistance in the classroom. The benefits accrued by AVT in communication are considered here as an addition to the benefits of hearing technology. In the Australian "Listen Hear!" Report, the total "extra" cost of education for 20,918 children with hearing loss aged 5 to 16 years was estimated at AU$117.2 million (US$82.3 million) in 2005 (Access Economics, 2006). This equates to AU$5,603 ($3,936 USD) per child or £2,679 per child per annum. Again, the question for our analysis was to what extent can we expect these costs to be avoided as a result of a child enrolling in the AVT program at AVUK? It was assumed conservatively that children with additional needs in our group would continue to require additional support. For the remaining 70% of the children, the analysis assumed that a reduction in classroom support of 50% was possible. On this basis, a benefit saving of £938 ($1,235) per year was applied from the ages of 5 to 18. With a 15% optimism bias correction and a 3.5% discount rate, the total benefit from ages 5 to 18 years was £8,703.65 ($11,456.97)

Injuries Avoided

There has been comparatively little research into the link between hearing loss and an increased risk of injury. A Canadian cross-sectional study, conducted by Woodcock and Pole (2008), with a total of 131,535 respondents concluded that:

> Respondents classified as having a hearing problem were more likely to have achieved less education, less likely to be working and more likely to be experiencing higher rates of injury and work-related injury, compared with hearing respondents.

A 2007 US study by Mann, Zhou, McKee, and McDermott found that:

> Rates of injury treatment in children with hearing loss were more than twice that of the control group (17.72 vs 8.58 per 100). The relative rate (RR) remained significantly higher (RR = 1.51, 95% confidence interval, 1.30–1.75) after adjusting for age, race, sex and the number of hospital or emergency department encounters for treatment of non-injury-related conditions. Children with hearing loss had significantly higher treatment rates for every injury type, bodily location, and external cause, with a cell size sufficient for valid comparison.

There is no reason to believe that the situation would be different in the UK. In 2011, Public Health England reported that the annual number of hospital admissions in England was 46,771 for children between the ages of 0 and 5 years (approximately 423 in every 100,000 children). The short-term average cost per hospitalization for individual injury was £2,494 ($3,283) (Polinder, Toet, Mulder, & Van

Beeck, 2008). The cost was therefore estimated at £10.54 ($13.88) per year per child. Using the relative risk of 1.51 reported in the American study above, on average we expected 2,718 cases per 100,000 in the subgroup that were affected by hearing loss. For this subgroup, the estimated cost per child per year rose to £67.79 ($89.26), a difference of £57.25 ($75.34) compared with hearing children. It was assumed that AVT, coupled with appropriate hearing devices, would reduce this excess cost by 50% and half of this was attributed to the influence of AVT, making the expected benefit per child £14.31 ($18) per year. This benefit, though small, has been recognized in the cost-benefit analysis. We decided to apply the benefit for the 50-year project horizon. With a 15% optimism bias correction and a 3.5% discount rate for years 18 to 30 and a 3% discount rate for years 31 to 50, the total benefit over 50 years of a child's life was £300 ($395).

Unquantifiable Benefits

A number of additional benefits flowing from the AVUK early intervention program were identified but could not be quantified:

a. Benefits to caregivers over the long term

While the report emphasized the costs to parents who forgo income to attend appointments, it was also recognized that there is a long-term return to them. Parents undoubtedly value seeing their child benefit from intensive support and attaining better educational outcomes. Stress and anxiety levels may reduce over the long term as parents see their child integrate and succeed in mainstream school and beyond. No proxy could be readily identified to place a monetary value on this benefit of emotional well-being for parents. The ability to participate in fundraising and lobbying on behalf of AVUK was also seen by many parents as an empowering way to give something back to the wider community, but again, this benefit could not be quantified. Another benefit noted by families at AVUK was the strengthened bond between parent and child. This benefited not only the parent–child relationship, but also other siblings as the strategies used by parents could be used to support the language development of other children and improve family relationships. Interestingly, First Voice in Australia reported that the rate of marriage breakdown in families attending their programs was lower than might be expected in families with children with a disability (First Voice, 2011). Due to the absence of specific information on the differential in divorce rates between parents who chose AVT and other families with children who are deaf or hard of hearing, this benefit was not quantified.

b. Further social return

As highlighted, children who are deaf or hard of hearing frequently experience difficulties with peer relationships and are at greater risk of social isolation and loneliness, and over 40% of such children experience mental health difficulties during childhood or early adulthood (NDCS, 2010). While benefits to overall quality of life were included in the cost-benefit analysis, evidence of

Benefit	Value	Years	Net Present Value
Improved quality of life	$2,115	1-50	$52,204
Increased employment	$1,480	18-50	$29,324
Increased earnings	$4,532	21-50	$85,458
Lower cost of schooling	$1,049	5-18	$11,454
Injuries avoided	$16	1-50	$395
Total NPV			$178,835

Figure 27-8. Summary of benefits per child over 50 year project horizon.

improved self-confidence and reduced isolation for children in the AVUK cohort remains anecdotal and will develop further over time.

c. Demonstration and research value

The research by AVUK demonstrates the value of AVT to policymakers in the UK and worldwide who require information on approaches to rehabilitation. Building best practice and national standards are valuable in their own right. It was difficult to put a value on all the items summarized under the heading of demonstration, but we noted that the value could certainly be substantial.

Summary of Benefits

The table above summarizes the flow of benefits over time (Figure 27–8). The key finding of this analysis was that, even after discounting the future flow of benefits, the net present value (NPV) of benefits was £135,894 ($178.725).

THE BENEFIT-TO-COST RATIO (BCR)

When the quantified costs and benefits were compared, the costs were estimated at £31,119 ($40,927) in present value terms (2015) and the benefits were valued at £135,894 ($178,858). The BCR was therefore positive at 4:1. On average, it was estimated that for every £1 ($1.31) invested in AVT, £4 ($5.25) is returned. In this case the BCR was positive, despite a conservative approach to valuation (Figure 27–9).

Sensitivity Analysis

By adjusting the project horizons, we were able to calculate the BCR of AVT depending on a child's life span (Figure 27–10).

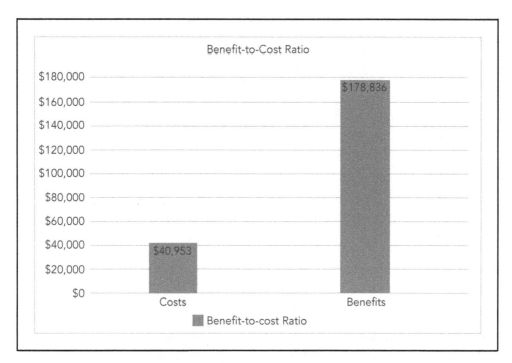

Figure 27-9. The costs and benefits of early intervention.

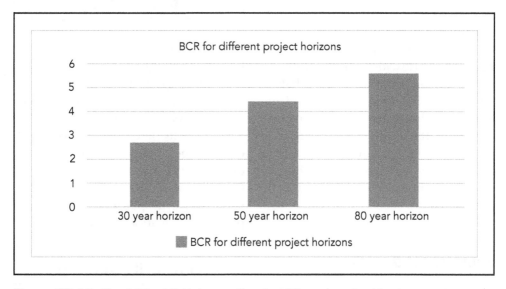

Figure 27-10. The BCR of AV intervention for different project horizons.

CONCLUSION

We want to see a world where all babies and young children who are deaf or hard of hearing have access to effective family-centered early intervention programs. Understanding the costs and benefits of such programs to the child, the family, and the economy is of critical importance.

Programs need to monitor the impact of their outcomes in the short, medium, and long term. This requires three key elements:

▪ Measures of a child's listening, talking, thinking, and social skills, using a defined set of assessments during and at the conclusion of a program.
▪ A mechanism for measuring progress of children in their school years.
▪ A measure of the costs and long-term benefits from an early intervention program.

A cost-benefit analysis is a useful way to demonstrate the long-term return on investment in an Auditory-Verbal early intervention program. It provides a mechanism for projecting the long-term benefits of a program. A cost-benefit analysis can provide "the final piece of the jigsaw" for practitioners and service providers seeking investment for their programs. A key lesson lies in the importance of using publicly recognized, validated data when calculating the costs and benefits and recognizing that they will vary from program to program and country to country. Local data always add weight to results.

The AVUK case study used a model and principles developed by the UK government and a 50-year project horizon to reflect the fact that the majority of benefits flow later in life. It drew on robust evidence from around the world. The accompanying literature review showed that the earlier the intervention begins, the better prognosis for language development and the greater the gains in areas such as quality of life, employment, and productivity, which are expected to be lifelong. The cost-benefit analysis concluded that the costs incurred in a child's early years can be seen as *a sound investment in the child's future.*

As more data become available through longitudinal studies on outcomes and new studies that will address benefits that are currently not quantified, the richness of cost-benefit analyses will improve over time. We are confident that society will continue to see the excellent returns provided by investment in Auditory-Verbal Therapy programs for babies and young children who are deaf or hard of hearing.

REFERENCES

Access Economics Pty Ltd. (2006). Listen Hear! The economic impact and cost of hearing loss in Australia [pdf file]. Retrieved from https://hearnet.org.au/wp-content/uploads/2015/10/ListenHear Final.pdf

Archbold, S., Lamb, B., O'Neill, C., & Atkins, J. (2014). The real cost of adult hearing loss: Reducing its impact by increasing access to the latest hearing technologies [pdf file]. Retrieved from https://www.earfoundation.org.uk/re

search/adult-strategy-reports/the-real
-cost-of-adult-hearing-loss-2014

AVUK (Auditory Verbal UK). (2016). Investing in a sound future for deaf children: A cost benefit analysis of auditory verbal therapy at Auditory Verbal UK [pdf file]. Retrieved from https://www.avuk.org/Handlers/Download.ashx?IDMF=12600eac-f5d5-4685-aed2-1ff2f5b26d38

AVUK. (2018). A sound future: Raising expectations for children with deafness [pdf file]. Retrieved from https://www.avuk.org/Handlers/Download.ashx?IDMF=401a8321-abaa-4a92-a654-a13e339c5a8a

Ben-Galim, D., & Thompson, S. (2013). Who's breadwinning? Working mothers and the new face of family support [pdf file]. Retrieved from https://www.ippr.org/publications/whos-breadwinning-working-mothers-and-the-new-face-of-family-support

Chorozoglou, M., Mahon, M., Pimperton, H., Worsfold, S., & Kennedy, C. R. (2018). Societal costs of permanent childhood hearing loss at teen age: A cross-sectional cohort follow-up study of universal newborn hearing screening. *BMJ Paediatrics Open, 2*(1) e000228.

Chowdhry, J. (2010). Auditory verbal therapy. *Otorhinolaryngology Clinics: An International Journal, 2*(2), 157–160.

Cole, E. B., & Flexer, C. (2015). *Children with hearing loss: Developing listening and talking, birth to six.* San Diego, CA: Plural Publishing.

Deaf Wellbeing Action Group in Nottinghamshire. (2001). A survey of deaf people's experiences of local health and social support [pdf file]. Retrieved from http://nottsdeafwellbeing.org.uk/onewebmedia/Deaf%20Wellbeing%20Survey%20report.pdf

Dornan, D., Hickson, L., Murdoch, B., & Houston, T. (2009). Longitudinal study of speech and language for children with hearing loss in auditory-verbal therapy programme. *The Volta Review, 109*, 61–85.

First Voice. (2011). A social cost-benefit analysis [pdf file]. Retrieved from https://www.firstvoice.org.au//wp-content/uploads/2016/09/02-Social-cost-benefit-analysis-summary-report-2.pdf

First Voice. (2015). Sound outcomes: First Voice speech and language data [pdf file]. Retrieved from https://www.firstvoice.org.au/reports-papers/

First Voice. (2017). Report on education, employment & social outcomes of first voice member centre graduates (18–28 years) [pdf file]. Retrieved from https://www.firstvoice.org.au/wp-content/uploads/2016/09/First-Voice-Graduate-Outcomes-Report.pdf

Goldberg, D. M., & Flexer, C. (2001). Auditory-verbal graduates: Outcome survey of clinical efficacy. *Journal of the American Academy of Audiology, 12*(8), 406–414.

Goldblat, E., & Pinto, O. Y. (2017). Academic outcomes of adolescents and young adults with hearing loss who received auditory-verbal therapy. *Deafness & Education International, 19*(3-4), 126-133. https://doi.org/10.1080/14643154.2017.1393604

Harris, L. G. (2014). Social-emotional development in children with hearing loss. *Master of Science dissertation, Department of Communication Sciences & Disorders, University of Kentucky*

Hicks, C. B., & Tharpe, A. M. (2002). Listening effort and fatigue in school-age children with and without hearing loss. *Journal of Speech, Language, and Hearing Research.* https://doi.org/10.1044/1092-4388(2002/046)

Hitchins, A. R., & Hogan, S. C. (2018). Outcomes of early intervention for deaf children with additional needs following an auditory verbal approach to communication. *International Journal of Pediatric Otorhinolaryngology, 115*, 125–132.

https://doi.org/10.1016/j.ijporl.2018 .09.025

HM Treasury. (2011). The green book: Appraisal and evaluation in central government [pdf file]. Retrieved from https:// www.gov.uk/government/publications /the-green-book-appraisal-and-evalua tion-in-central-governent

HM Treasury. (2014). Supporting public service transformation: Cost benefit analysis guidance for local partnerships [pdf file]. Retrieved from https://www.gov .uk/guidance/social-impact-bonds

Hogan, A., Shipley, M., Strazdins, L., Purcell, A., & Baker, E. (2011). Communication and behavioural disorders among children with hearing loss increases risk of mental health disorders. *Australian and New Zealand Journal of Public Health, 35*(4), 377–383. https://doi .org/10.1111/j.1753-6405.2011.00744.x

Hogan, S., Stokes, J., White, C., Tyszkiewicz, E., & Woolgar, A. (2008). An evaluation of auditory verbal therapy using the rate of early language development as an outcome measure. *Deafness & Education International, 10*(3), 143–167. https://doi .org/10.1179/146431508790559760

Jung, D., & Bhattacharyya, N. (2012). Association of hearing loss with decreased employment and income among adults in the United States. *Annals of Otology, Rhinology & Laryngology, 121*(12), 771– 775. https://doi.org/10.1177%2F000348 941212101201

Leigh, A., & Ryan, C. (2008). Estimating returns to education using different natural experiment techniques. *Economics of Education Review, 27*(2), 149–160. https://doi.org/10.1016/j.econedurev .2006.09.004

Lim, S. R., Goldberg, D. M., & Flexer, C. (2018). Auditory-verbal graduates— 25 years later: Outcome survey of the clinical effectiveness of the listening and spoken language approach for young children with hearing loss. *The Volta*

Review, 118(1-2), 5–40. https://doi.org /10.17955/tvr.118.1.2.790

Mann, J. R., Zhou, L., McKee, M., & McDermott, S. (2007). Children with hearing loss and increased risk of injury. *Annals of Family Medicine, 5*(6), 528–533.

Mathers, C., Vos, T., & Stevenson, C. (1999). The burden of disease and injury in Australia. Australian Institute of Health and Welfare [pdf file]. Retrieved from https:// www.aihw.gov.au/getmedia/6bd85f38 -dcb4-44fa-9569c48045634841/bdia.pdf .aspx?inline=true

McGarrigle, R., Munro, K. J., Dawes, P., Stewart, A. J., Moore, D. R., Barry, J. G., & Amitay, S. (2014). Listening effort and fatigue: What exactly are we measuring? A British Society of Audiology Cognition in Hearing Special Interest Group 'white paper.' *International Journal of Audiology, 53*(7), 433–445. https://doi .org/10.3109/14992027–2014.890296

Miyamoto, R. T., Houston, D. M., Kirk, K. I., Perdew, A. E., & Svirsky, M. A. (2003). Language development in deaf infants following cochlear implantation. *Acta Oto-Laryngologica, 123*(2), 241–244. https:// doi.org/10.1080/00016480310001079

National Deaf Children's Society. (2010). Deaf children at risk: NDCS briefing paper for the education select committee [pdf file]. Retrieved from https://www .ndcs.org.uk/

National Deaf Children's Society. (2011). A practitioner's guide social care for deaf children and young people: A guide to assessment and child protection investigations for social care practitioners [pdf file]. Retrieved from https://www .ndcs.org.uk/documents-and-resources /social-care-for-deaf-children-and-young -people-a-practitioners-guide/

National Deaf Children's Society. (2019). Note on department for education figures on attainment for deaf children in 2018 (England) [pdf file]. Retrieved from https://www.ndcs.org.uk/information

-and-support/information-for-professionals/research-and-data/

National Institute for Health and Care Excellence. (2009). Cochlear implants for children and adults with severe to profound deafness [pdf file]. Retrieved from https://www.nice.org.uk/guidance/ta166

National Institute for Health and Care Excellence. (n.d.). Glossary. Retrieved from https://www.nice.org.uk/glossary

NERA Economic Consulting. (2007). Human costs of a nuclear accident: Final report [pdf file]. Retrieved from http://www.hse.gov.uk/economics/research/humancost.pdf

New Economy. (2015). Unit cost database [Data file]. Retrieved from http://www.neweconomymanchester.com/our-work/research-evaluation-cost-benefit-analysis/cost-benefit-analysis/unit-cost-database.

Office for National Statistics. (2013). Trends in living arrangements including families (with and without dependent children), people living alone and people in shared accommodation, broken down by size and type of household [pdf file]. Retrieved from https://www.ons.gov.uk/peoplepopulationandcommunity/birthsdeathsandmarriages/families/bulletins/familiesandhouseholds/2013-10-31

Office for National Statistics. (2014). Annual survey of hours and earnings [pdf file]. Retrieved from https://www.ons.gov.uk/employmentandlabourmarket/peopleinwork/earningsandworkinghours/bulletins/annualsurveyofhoursandearnings/2014-11-19

Office for National Statistics. (2014). Participation rates in the UK labour market [pdf file]. Retrieved from https://www.ons.gov.uk/employmentandlabourmarket/peopleinwork/employmentandemployeetypes/compendium/participationratesintheuklabourmarket/2015-03-19

Percy-Smith, L., Tønning, T. L., Josvassen, J. L., Mikkelsen, J. H., Nissen, L., Dieleman, E., . . . Cayé-Thomasen, P. (2017). Auditory verbal habilitation is associ-ated with improved outcome for children with cochlear implant. *Cochlear Implants International, 19*(1), 38–45. https://doi.org/10.1080/14670100.2017.1389020

Petrou, S., McCann, D., Law, C. M., Watkin, P. M., Worsfold, S., & Kennedy, C. R. (2007). Health status and health-related quality of life preference-based outcomes of children who are aged 7 to 9 years and have bilateral permanent childhood hearing impairment. *Pediatrics, 120*(5), 1044–1052. https://doi.org/10.1542/peds.2007-0159

Polinder, S., Toet, H., Mulder, S., & Van Beeck, E. F. (2008). APOLLO: The economic consequences of injury. *Consumer and Safety Institute.*

Polinder, S. (2008). The economic consequences of injury in the European Union (report WP2.2 Apollo), Consumer Safety Institute, Amsterdam. Cited by Rogmans. W. (2009). *International Journal of Injury Control and Safety Promotion, 16*(2) 63–64.

Powers, E. T. (2001). New estimates of the impact of child disability on maternal employment. *American Economic Review, 91*(2), 135–139.

PricewaterhouseCoopers. (2005). The economic benefits of higher education qualifications. A report produced for the Royal Society of Chemistry and the Institute of Physics [pdf file]. Retrieved from https://www.iop.org/publications/iop/archive/file_52061.pdf

Pro Bono Economics. (2015). Our place guide to cost-benefit analysis [pdf file]. Retrieved from https://mycommunity.org.uk/resources/our-place-guide-to-cost-benefit-analysis/

Pro Bono Economics. (2017). Economic evaluation of Place2Be's counselling service in primary schools [pdf file]. Retrieved from https://www.place2be.org.uk/our-story/accounts-publications.aspx

Public Health England. (2011). Children (under 18, under 5, 5–17) hospital admissions due to injury cause, 2010/11 [Data file]. Retrieved from https://web archive.nationalarchives.gov.uk/2017 0106151057/http://www.apho.org.uk /resource/item.aspx?RID=115632

Schley, S., Walter, G. G., Weathers, R. R., Hemmeter, J., Hennessey, J. C., & Burkhauser, R. V. (2011). Effect of postsecondary education on the economic status of persons who are deaf or hard of hearing. *Journal of Deaf Studies and Deaf Education, 16*(4), 524–536. https:// doi.org/10.1093/deafed/enq060

Spencer, P. E., & Marschark, M. (2010). *Evidence-based practice in educating deaf and hard-of-hearing students* (pp. 44–45). New York, NY: Oxford University Press.

Theunissen, S. C., Rieffe, C., Kouwenberg, M., Soede, W., Briaire, J. J., & Frijns, J. H. (2011). Depression in hearing-impaired children. *International Journal of Pediatric Otorhinolaryngology, 75*(10), 1313–1317. https://doi.org/10.1016/j.ij porl.2011.07.023

Wilkins, M., & Ertmer, D. (2002). Introducing young children who are deaf or hard of hearing to spoken language: Child's Voice, an Oral School. *Language, Speech, and Hearing Services in Schools, 33*(3), 198–204. https://doi.org/10.1044/0161 -1461(2002/017)

Woodcock, K., & Pole, J. D. (2008). Educational attainment, labour force status and injury: A comparison of Canadians with and without deafness and hearing loss. *International Journal of Rehabilitation Research, 31*(4), 297–304. https://doi .org/10.1097/MRR.0b013e3282fb7d4d

Young, A., Oram, R., Squires, G., & Sutherland, H. (2015). Identifying effective practice in the provision of education and education support services for 16–19 year old deaf young people in further education in England. *National Deaf Children's Society.* http://www.ndcs.org.uk/docu ment.rm?id=9911 accessed 11/25/2019

AFTERWORD

The World Health Organization (WHO) estimates that by 2050 there will be more than 900 million people worldwide with hearing loss greater than 40 dB HL—double the number of 2018. One can surmise that today's number of 34 million children who are deaf or hard of hearing will surely also double—at least. We have much to do and a long way to go, therefore, to bring the gifts of listening and talking to children who are deaf or hard of hearing around the world. That mission is at the heart of this book.

Auditory-Verbal Therapy: Science, Research, and Practice is representative of the dedicated and collaborative work of practitioners who are inspired scientists, creative thinkers, motivated educators, committed coaches and mentors, ambitious researchers, lifelong learners, passionate advocates, critical innovators, and optimistic visionaries, who commit themselves to the entire AVT journey of children who are deaf or hard of hearing and their families.

Honored to be part of the plan, the delivery, and the outcomes of the journey, we are collectively in pursuit of hearing, listening, spoken language and spoken conversations, literacy competence, and academic and social interactions with others, in communities where children who are deaf or hard of hearing can thrive, as they grow up with resilience, self-actualization, and pride.

The foundational work of the pioneers of the Auditory-Verbal movement has led to the current abundant science, research, and excellence in practice that substantiate the proclivity of AVT.

As AV practitioners, we keep our hearts and minds focused on the desired outcomes of the families, and we work in tandem with teams of global allied professionals in the health and educational domains, as we coach and guide parents to *captain the ship* and lead the way forward, until their children who are deaf or hard of hearing are able to sail on their own.

We are committed to the evidence presented here and forward it with the intention to improve the functional, social, emotional, and economic impacts of hearing loss on the world's children, for today, tomorrow, and the years to come.

Warren Estabrooks
Helen McCaffrey Morrison
Karen MacIver-Lux
Summer, 2020

INDEX

Note: Page numbers in **bold** reference non-text material.

A